Congenital Heart Defects: Assessment and Management

Congenital Heart Defects: Assessment and Management

Editor: Hugo Winstead

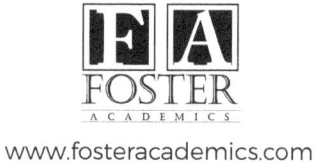

FOSTER
ACADEMICS

www.fosteracademics.com

www.fosteracademics.com

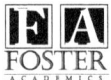

Cataloging-in-Publication Data

Congenital heart defects : assessment and management / edited by Hugo Winstead.
    p. cm.
Includes bibliographical references and index.
ISBN 978-1-63242-890-5
1. Congenital heart disease. 2. Congenital heart disease--Diagnosis. 3. Congenital heart disease--Treatment.
4. Heart--Abnormalities. I. Winstead, Hugo.
RC687 .C66 2020
616.120 43--dc23

Foster Academics,
118-35 Queens Blvd., Suite 400,
Forest Hills, NY 11375, USA

ISBN 978-1-63242-890-5 (Hardback)

Contents

Preface

The purpose of the book is to provide a glimpse into the dynamics and to present opinions and studies of some of the scientists engaged in the development of new ideas in the field from very different standpoints. This book will prove useful to students and researchers owing to its high content quality.

A congenital heart defect (CHD) refers to a congenital anomaly in the structure of the heart. It may manifest as abnormalities in the heart valves, the interior walls of the heart, and the large blood vessels that lead from and to the heart. The symptoms include poor weight gain, rapid breathing, feeling of exhaustion and bluish skin. It may be caused due to infections during pregnancy, use of certain drugs or medications, obesity or poor nutritional status in the mother and parents being closely related. CHDs can be classified into two main groups- cyanotic and non-cyanotic heart defects. Genetic conditions such as Down syndrome, Marfan syndrome and Turner syndrome are associated with such heart defects. Most CHDs can be diagnosed prenatally using fetal echocardiography. In other cases, the diagnosis can be made shortly after birth or sometimes several months and years after birth. A CHD is generally serious and requires surgery, medications or a combination of both. Most individuals with CHDs need specialized care throughout their lifetime. This book is compiled in such a manner, that it will provide in-depth knowledge about the assessment and management of congenital heart defects. It aims to present researches that have transformed the field of cardiology and aided its advancement. With state-of-the-art inputs by acclaimed experts of this field, this book targets students and professionals.

At the end, I would like to appreciate all the efforts made by the authors in completing their chapters professionally. I express my deepest gratitude to all of them for contributing to this book by sharing their valuable works. A special thanks to my family and friends for their constant support in this journey.

Editor

Variations of *CITED2* are Associated with Congenital Heart Disease (CHD) in Chinese Population

Yan Liu[1,2]⁹, Fengyu Wang[3]⁹, Yuan Wu[4]⁹, Sainan Tan[5], Qiaolian Wen[1,2], Jing Wang[6], Xiaomei Zhu[1,2], Xi Wang[1,2], Congmin Li[3]*, Xu Ma[1,2,7]*, Hong Pan[1,2]*

1 Graduate School, Peking Union Medical College, Beijing, China, 2 National Research Institute for Family Planning, Beijing, China, 3 Henan Research Institute of Population and Family Planning, Key Laboratory of Population Defects Intervention Technology of Henan Province, Zhengzhou, China, 4 Cardiac Surgery Department, Xiamen Heart Center, Organ Transplantation Institute of Xiamen University, Xiang'an District, Xiamen, China, 5 Key Laboratory of Genetics and Birth Health of Hunan Province, Family Planning Institute of Hunan Province, Chang sha, China, 6 Department of Medical Genetics, School of Basic Medical Sciences, Capital Medical University, Beijing, China, 7 World Health Organization Collaborating Centre for Research in Human Reproduction, Beijing, China

Abstract

CITED2 was identified as a cardiac transcription factor which is essential to the heart development. *Cited2*-deficient mice showed cardiac malformations, adrenal agenesis and neural crest defects. To explore the potential impact of mutations in *CITED2* on congenital heart disease (CHD) in humans, we screened the coding region of *CITED2* in a total of 700 Chinese people with congenital heart disease and 250 healthy individuals as controls. We found five potential disease-causing mutations, p.P140S, p.S183L, p.S196G, p.Ser161delAGC and p. Ser192_Gly193delAGCGGC. Two mammalian two-hybrid assays showed that the last four mutations significantly affected the interaction between *p300CH1* and *CITED2* or *HIF1A*. Further studies showed that four *CITED2* mutations recovered the promoter activity of *VEGF* by decreasing its competitiveness with *HIF1A* for binding to *p300CH1* and three mutations decreased the consociation of *TFAP2C* and *CITED2* in the transactivation of *PITX2C*. Both *VEGF* and *PITX2C* play very important roles in cardiac development. In conclusion, we demonstrated that *CITED2* has a potential causative impact on congenital heart disease.

Editor: Robert Dettman, Northwestern University, United States of America

Funding: This work was supported by the National Basic Research Program of China (2010CB529504), the National Natural Science Foundation of China (81300131) and the Applied Basic Research Program of Qinghai Province (QH2013-z-744). The funders had no role in study design, data collection and analysis, decision to publish, or preparation of the manuscript.

Competing Interests: The authors have declared that no competing interests exist.

* E-mail: 13838377996@163.com (CL); 13174483538@126.com (HP); nicgr@263.net (XM)

⁹ These authors contributed equally to this work.

Introduction

Congenital heart disease (CHD) is a most common defect caused by abnormal cardiac formation in fetuses and has become the leading reason of childhood mortality with an incidence around 1%[1–3]. In the past decades, a series of CHD-causing genes have been identified such as *NKX2-5*, *TBX5*, *GATA4* and *CITED2* [4–6]. It has been confirmed that their mutations can cause cardiac malformations through affecting the transcription activity of critical genes involved in heart development pathways.

CITED2 (Cbp/p300-interacting transactivator, with Glu/Asp-rich carboxy-terminal domain, 2) is one member of a new conserved family of transcriptional activators which includes four members: *CITED1* (*Msg1*), *CITED2* (*Mrg1/p35srj*), *CITED3* and *CITED4* (*Mrg2*) [7]. *CITED2* is a nuclear protein which binds closely to the CH1 region of *p300* and *CBP* by its CR2 region (including a conserved 32-amino acid sequence [8]). Meanwhile, many other transcription factors and transcription regulating factors such as *HIF1A*, *RXRα*, *NFk*, *Mdm2*, *Ets-1* and *Stat2* also bind to the CH1 region of *CBP/p300* [9,10]. Thus *CITED2* may act as a pivotal transcriptional modulator to regulate the expression of some specific genes. For example, *CITED2* decreased the expression of *HIF1A* (Hypoxia Inducible Factor 1) through its competitive binding to *CBP/p300CH1*[11,12], consequently interfering the transcription of genes induced by *HIF1A* such as *VEGF* (vascular endothelial growth factor) [13]. It has been confirmed that the overexpression of *vegf* is the main factor resulting in cardiac malformation in *cited2*⁻/⁻ mice [14].

Besides being a transcriptional repressor of *HIF1A*, *CITED2* acts as a transcriptional coactivator of *TFAP2* (transcription factor AP2, also called *Tcfap2*) [15]. Mutations of *TFAP2A* and *TFAP2B* result in neural tube, cranial ganglia defects and cardiac malformations [16,17]. This suggested that the coactivation of *TFAP2* with *p300*, *CITED2* and *CREBBP* is essential for the normal development of those structures. As a critical transcription factor, *TFAP2* can affect the transcription of many genes, including *PITX2C* (Paired-Like Homeodomain 2 C)which is critical in Nodal-*PITX2C* pathways [18]. In addition, it has been detected that *TFAP2* isoforms and *CITED2* work together on the *PITX2C* promoter1 which controls the expression of *PITX2C* in the heart of embryonic mice. The mice experiments already indicated that knocking out *pitx2c* gene can lead to valve defects, body wall dysraphism, gastroschisis, ectopia cordis and other multiple organs polymorphous defects [19].

CITED2 gene mutation in human congenital heart disease was first reported by Sperling *et al* [20] in 2005. They identified 3 mutations which alter the amino acid sequence and studied their association with *HIF1A* and *TFAP2C*. Their study confirms that *CITED2* is an important transcription factor in heart development and provides new insights into the molecular mechanism of congenital heart defects. Later, Yang *et al* found 3 new mutations in Chinese patients with congenital heart disease (2010) [21]and Chen *et al* [22]demonstrated another 3 new mutations in European CHD patients. Recently, Xu *et al* found 3 *CITED2* gene mutations, their research showed that *CITED2* gene mutations and methylation may play an important role in CHD. In their study, most of these mutations were in SRJ region. The mutations in our study were identified for the first time and located in SRJ region as well. Our work aimed to determine whether the new mutations also affect *HIF1A* or *TFAP2C* and finally lead to an abnormal expression of *VEGF* or *PITX2C* which play an important role in heart development.

Materials and Methods

Ethics statement

The study protocol conformed to the ethical guidelines of the 1975 Declaration of Helsinki and was approved by the Ethics Committee of the National Research Institute for Family Planning. Written informed consent was obtained from patients' parents or guardians.

Subjects

The study population comprised 700 patients who were diagnosed with CHD based on anthropometric measurement, physical examination for malformation and dysmorphism, and radiological evaluation. The patients with a phenotype of VSD, TOF and ASD accounted for 43.71%, 8.42% and 12% respectively. 250 unrelated healthy children were used as controls. Peripheral blood was collected from each affected individual and their parents and controls were from 6 months to 12 years old and most of them volunteered to participate in the study.

We sequenced the whole *CITED2* ORF in 700 CHD patients (Table 1) and 250 healthy controls recruited from Lanzhou University, Beijing Children's Hospital, Zhengzhou Children's Hospital, Henan provincial Chest Hospital and Children's Hospital of Fudan University.

Mutational analysis and bioinformatics

Genomic DNA was extracted from peripheral blood leukocytes using standard methods. The human *CITED2* gene is located on 6q24.1 and is encoded by two exons. One of the exons and splice sites of *CITED2* were amplified by polymerase chain reaction (PCR) using two pairs of *CITED2* gene-specific primers (Table 2). PCR products were sequenced using the appropriate PCR primers and the Big Dye Terminator Cycle Sequencing kit (Applied Biosystems, Foster City, CA, USA) and run on an automated sequencer, ABI 3730XL (Applied Biosystems), to perform mutational analysis.

Site-directed mutagenesis and plasmid construction

Human *CITED2* and *HIF1A* cDNA were obtained from OriGene True-Clone, and *TFAP2C* cDNA was purchased from GeneCopoeia. *CITED2* mutations were constructed by using the Quick Change Lightning Site-Directed Mutagenesis kit (Strata gene, La Jolla, CA, USA). Then the introduced mutations were confirmed by DNA sequence.

The WT and mutant *CITED2* were amplified by PCR from cDNA and inserted into the pEGFP-N1 vector (BD Biosciences, Palo Alto, CA, USA). The ORF of *HIF1A* and *TFAP2C* were also amplified by PCR from cDNA and inserted respectively into the pcDNA3.1(+) vector (Invitrogen, Carlsbad, CA, USA) to create the expression plasmid pcDNA3.1-*HIF1A* and pcDNA3.1-*TFAP2C*.

A 1300-bp fragment of the p300-CH1, *PITX2C* promoter and an 870-bp segment of *VEGF* promoter amplified by PCR from Human genomic DNA were cloned respectively into the GAL4-pCMX vector and the luciferase reporter PLG3-basic vector. GAL4-*HIF1A* was constructed by cloning DNA fragments into GAL4-pCMX vector at the Ecorv and Nhel sites. All primers of the PCRS were list in Table 2.

The VP16-pCMX vector with the potent transactivating domain of HSV, the promoter pGL3-basic vector with 4×GAL4 DNA-binding sites and the GAL4-pCMX vector containing GAL4-DBD were provided by Dr. Ronald M. Evans (Salk Institute for Biological Studies, USA).

Cell culture and transient transfection

293T and Hela cells were maintained in Iscove's modified Dulbecco's medium supplemented with 10% fetal bovine serum, 100 mg/ml penicillin, and 100 mg/ml streptomycin in a humidified atmosphere containing 5% CO_2 at 37°C. Transfection was carried out using a standard calcium phosphate method or Lipofectamine 2000 (Invitrogen Corporation, Carlsbad, CA, USA).

Table 1. Patients with congenital heart disease included in the study.

Phenotype	Total(n = 700)
Ventricular septal defect(VSD)	306
Tetralogy of Fallot(TOF)	59
Atrial septal defect(ASD)	84
Patent ductus arteriosus(PDA)	21
Pulmonal atresia or stenosis(PS)	21
double outlet right ventricle(DORV)	11
Aortic coarctation(COA)	4
Pulmonary hypertension(PH)	2
Other complex cardiac malformations	192

Table 2. Primers used for PCR.

Name	Primer pair
Primers for *CITED2*	F CCGGCTGTGTTATGAGTGGTAG
	R AGTTGGGGGTTTGATTTCTTTC
Middle Primer for *CITED2*	TCGGAAGTGCTGGTTTGTC
Primers for P140S	F TGCCGGATTTGCACTCTGCTGCA GGCCAC
	R GTGGCCTGCAGCAGAGTGCAAAT CCGGCA
Primers for S183L	F GCTCTGGCAGCAGCTTGGGCGGCG
	R CGCCGCCCAAGCTGCTGCCAGAGC
Primers for S196G	F AACAGCGGCGGCGGCGGCGGCAGCG GCAACA
	R TGTTGCCGCTGCCGCCGCCGCCGCC GCTGTT
Primers for Ser161delAGCAGC	F TGCAACCCCAAGCACGGCGGCAGCA GCACC TGCAACCCCAAGCACGGCGGCAGCAGCACC
	R GGTGCTGCTGCCGCCGTGCTTGGGG TTGCA
Primers for Ser192_Gly193delAGCGGC	F CGCGGGCAGCAGCAACGGCGGCAGC GGCAGCGGCAACAT
	R ATGTTGCCGCTGCCGCTGCCGCCGTT GCTGCTGCCCGCG
pEGFP-*CIITED2*	F GGGGTACCATGGCAGACCATATGATG
	R CGGGATCCCGACAGCTCACTCTGCTGG
pCDNA3.1(+)-*CITED2*	F CGGGGTACCTATGGCAGACCATATGA TGGC
	R TGCTCTAGAGTCAACAGCTCACTCTGCTG
pCMX-GAL4-*CITED2*	F CGGATATCAATGGCAGACCATATGA TGGC
	R CTAGCTAGCTCAACAGCTCACTCTGCT
pCMX-GAL4-*HIF1A*	F CGGATATCAATGGAGGGCGCCGGCG
	R CTAGCTAGCTCAGTTAACTTGATCCAA AGCT
pCMX-VP16-*P300CH1*	F CGCGGATCCTATGGCCGAGAATGTGG TGGAAC
	R CTAGCTAGCCCAACGGGTGCTCCAGT CAAA
pCDNA3.1(+)-*HIF1A*	F CGGGGTACCTATGGAGGGCGCCGGC
	R TGCTCTAGATCAGTTAACTTGATCCAAAGC
pCDNA3.1(+)-*TFAP2C*	F CGGGGTACCACGCCGGACGCCATGTTG
	R TGCTCTAGACTCTCCTAACCTTTCTTC GTTCC
PGL3basic-*VEGF* promoter	F GGGGTACCTTTGGGTTTTGCCAGACT
	R CCGCTCGAGAGGAGGGAGCAGGAATAG
PGL3basic-*PITX2C* promoter	F GGGGTACCGGGGACAAAAGGACTTTC
	R CCGCTCGAGCCCTGTTGGCCTAACATC

Subcellular localization

Hela cells were seeded in 12-well tissue culture plates 20 h prior to transfection at approximately 60% confluency. GFP-*CITED2* expression constructs containing wild-type and mutant *CITED2* were transfected using Lipofectamine 2000, according to the manufacturer's instructions. The empty vector pEGFP-N1 was transfected as a control. Forty hours after transfection, the cells were fixed and permeabilised in 4% paraformaldehyde for 15 min, 0.1% Triton X-100 for 20 min and the DNA was stained with 0.5 µg/ml DAPI for 3 min at room temperature. The cells were observed by fluorescence microscopy. All steps were operated in lucifugal conditions.

Mammalian two-hybrid assay and transcriptional assays

Mammalian two-hybrid assay plasmids including pCMX-VP16-*p300*, TK promoter reporter plasmid, the Renilla luciferase control plasmid pREP7-RLu and pCMX- GAL4-*CITED2* (wild-type or mutant) or pCMX-GAL4-*HIF1A* were contransfected into 293T cells. Thirty hours after transfection, cells were washed and

lysed in passive lysis buffer (Promega, Madison, WI, USA) and the transfection efficiency was normalised to paired Renilla luciferase activity by using the Dual Luciferase Reporter Assay System (Promega, Madison, WI, USA) according to the manufacturer's instructions.

In addition, the Dual LuciferaseReporter Assay System was used to study the effect of *CITED2* on the transcription of *VEGF* and *PITX2C*. Plasmids consisting of the Renilla luciferase control plasmid pREP7-RLu, pcDNA3.1-*CITED2* (wild-type or mutant), PGL3-*VEGF*-pro and pcDNA3.1-*HIF1A* or PGL3-*PITX2C*-pro and pcDNA3.1-*TFAP2C* were contransfected into 293T cells. Thirty hours after transfection, cells were treated the same way as above.

Statistical analysis

The results represent the means of three independent experiments performed in triplicate, and the bars denote the S.D. The independent-samples t test was adopted to determine statistical significance of unpaired samples. All data were analyzed by Prism Demo 5 software.

Table 3. Position of variations

Coding position	Amino acid position	Phenotype of mutation carrier
c.C418T	p. P140S,Pro-Ser	F4
c.C548T	p. S183L,Ser-Leu	VSD
c.A586G	p. S196G,Ser-Gly	VSD
c.481–483delAGC	p.Ser161delAGC	ASD
c.574–579delAGCGGC	p.Ser192_Gly193delAGCGGC	VSD

Results

Genetic and bioinformatics analysis

From a total of 700 non-syndromic CHD patients, we identified five novel *CITED2* nucleotide alterations (two amino acid deletions and three amino acid substitutions, table3). Three mutations (c.C548T, c.A586G and c.574-59delAGCGGC) were found in one, one and four patients with Ventricular septal defect (VSD) respectively. One mutation (c.C418T) was detected in one patient with Tetralogy of Fallot (TOF) and another mutation (c.481–483delAGC) was detected in one patient with Artrial septal defect (ASD).

All potential pathogenic mutations have not been reported in the NCBI dbSNP and are not included in the 1000 Genome Project database (http://browser.1000genomes.org/).

The result of sequence alignment of *CITED2* proteins among several species showed that three acid substitutions were located at highly conserved regions among different species (human,

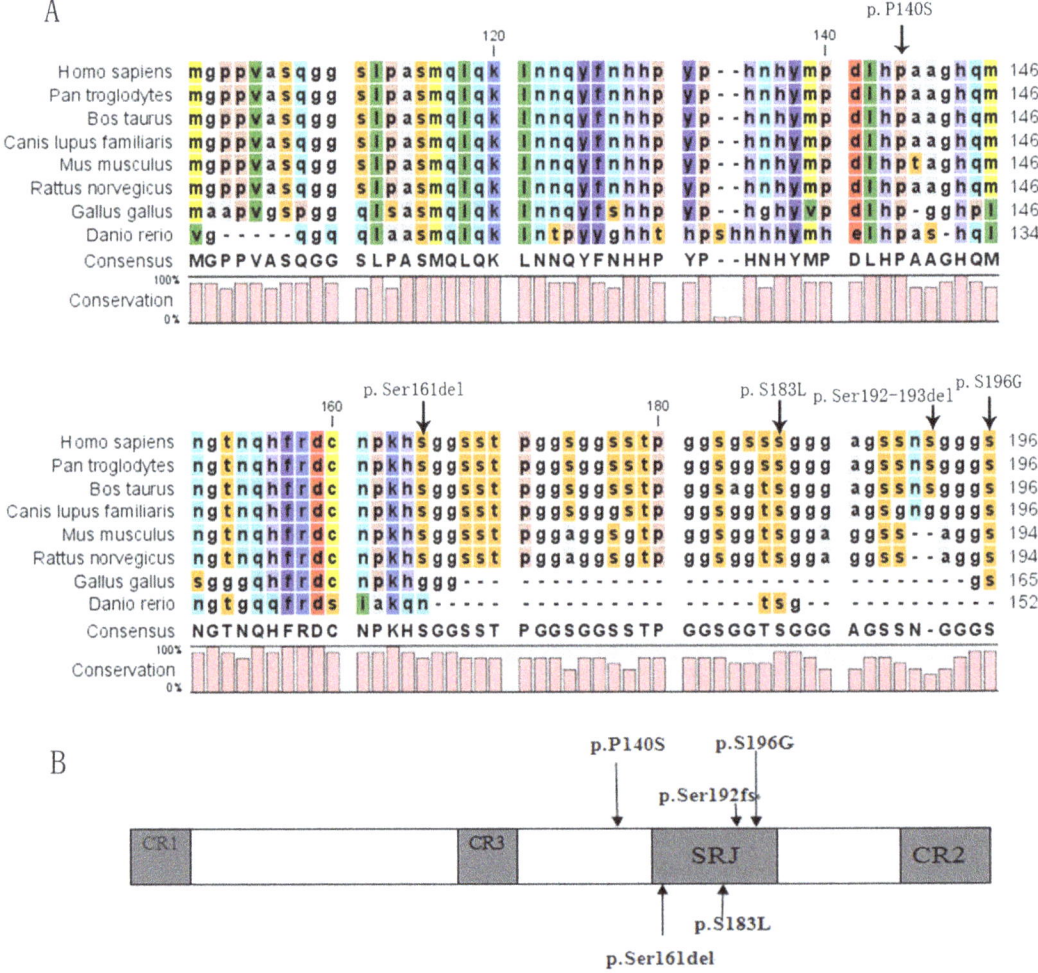

Figure 1. Structure of *CITED2*. A: Sequence alignment of *CITED2* proteins among several species. The figure showed that three acid substitutions were located at highly conserved regions among many species (human, chimpanzee, mice, dog, cattle, rat, chicken and zebrafish). **B**: Position of mutations in the *CITED2* protein identified in CHD patients. *CITED2* has three conserved regions CR1-3 and serine-glycine rich junction (SRJ). All other mutations were located in SRJ except p.P140S.

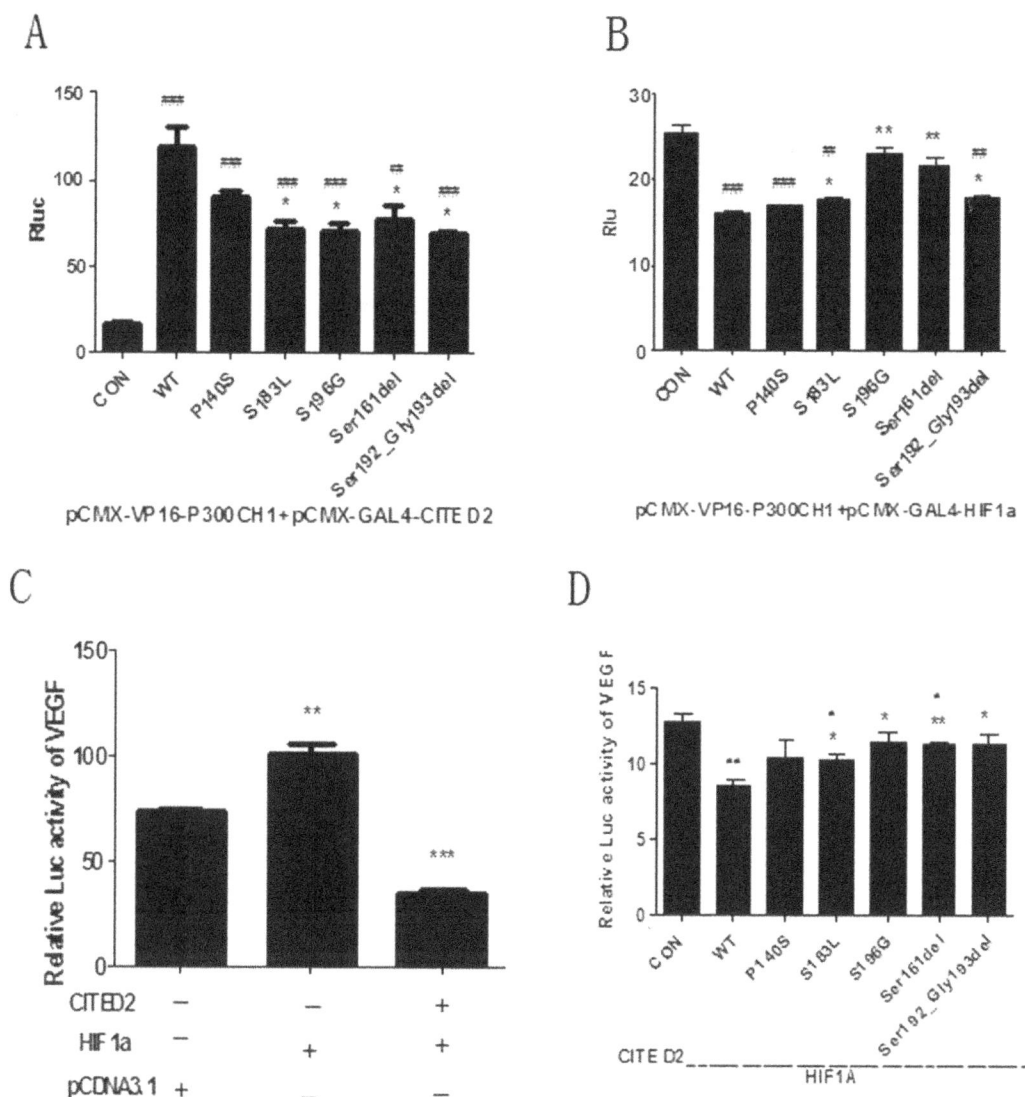

Figure 2. Effect of *CITED2* mutations on the transcriptional activation of *HIF1A* to its target gene *VEGF*. A: Effect of mutations on *CITED2-p300CH1* interactions. We cotransfected 293T cells with pCMX-VP16-*p300CH1*, TK promoter reporter plasmid, and the Renilla luciferase internal control plasmid, as well as empty vector pCMX-GAL4, GAL4-*CITED2* wild-type, and the mutants. The significance of differences was calculated using the independent-samples t test. (*p<0.05, **p<0.01 versus. wt-type, #p<0.05, ##p<0.01 versus.empty vector pCMX-GAL4.) **B**: Effect of mutations on *HIF1A-p300CH1* interactions. Cotransfection of pCMX-VP16-*p300CH1*, pCMX-GAL4-*HIF1A*, TK promoter reporter plasmid, and the Renilla luciferase internal control plasmid, as well as empty vector pcDNA3.1 (+), pcDNA3.1 (+)-*CITED2* wild-type, and the mutant. (* p<0.05, ** p<0.01 versus wt-type, # p<0.05, ## p<0.01 versus. empty vector pcDNA3.1 (+)) **C**: Effect of wt-type on the transcriptional activation of *VEGF*. Transfected the *VEGF* reporter plasmid and the expression vector for *HIF1A*, *CITED2* or pcDNA3.1 were transfected together in 293 T cells. The luciferase activity was normalized to Renilla activity.* p<0.05, **p<0.01 versus the untreated group (n = 3). **D**: Effect of *CITED2* mutants on transcription activation of *VEGF* compared with *CITED2*-wt. The rest report plasmids were same as above. (*p<0.05, **p<0.01 versus wt-type, #p<0.05, ##p<0.01 versus empty vector pcDNA3.1(+)). The results represent the means of 3 independent experiments performed in triplicate and the significance of differences was calculated using independent-samples t test.(*CITED2* = *Cbp/p300*-interacting transactivator, with Glu/Asp-rich carboxy-terminal domain, 2, *HIF1A* = Hypoxia Inducible Factor 1, *VEGF* = vascular endothelial growth factor)

chimpanzee, mice, dog, cattle, rat, chicken and zebrafish) and two amino acid deletions were not located at highly conserved regions among these species (Figure 1).

CITED2 mutations decrease *HIF1A* repression leading to up-regulation of *VEGF* expression

Two mammalian two-hybrid assays were used to evaluate whether the mutation affected the interaction between every two of *CITED2*, *p300CH1* and *HIF1A* (Figure 2). Cotransfection of both VP16- P300 and wild-type GAL4-*CITED2* with the TK

promoter reporter plasmid led to a nearly 10-fold increase in luciferase activity compared with VP16-P300 and empty vector of CMX-GAL4 (t test, p<0.01). The luciferase activity of p. P140S mutant was even the same as the wt-type, However, cotransfection of VP16-P300 and the four mutants (p.S183L, p.S196G, p.Ser161delAGC, p.Ser192_Gly193delAGCGGC) GAL4-*CITED2* showed weakened luciferase activity (t test, p<0.05) (Figure 2A) compared with wt-type. These findings indicated that the four mutations diminished protein-protein interactions be-

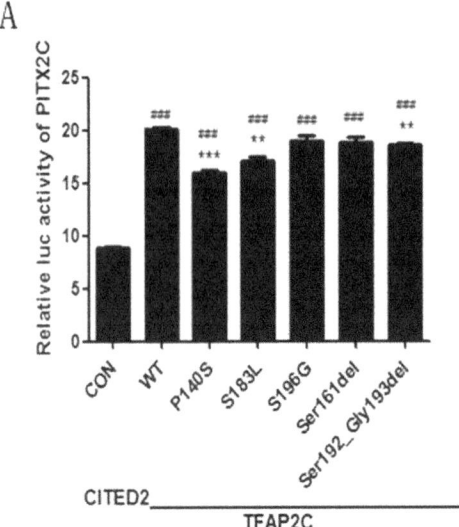

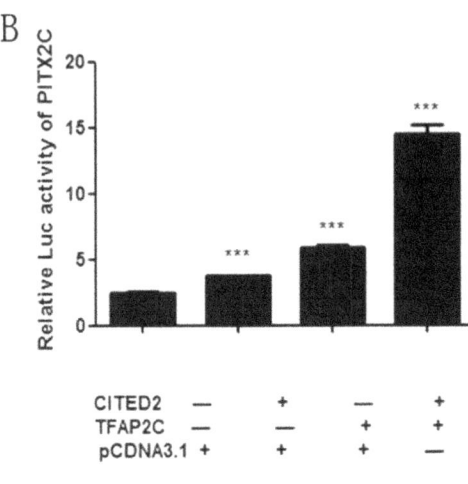

Figure 3. Effect of *CITED2* variants on the cooperation between *CITED2* and *TFAP2C* in the transactivation of the *PITX2C*. A: Effect of *CITED2* mutations on the transcription activation of *PITX2C*. (*p<0.05, **p<0.01 versus wt-type, #p<0.05, ##p<0.01 versus.empty vector pcDNA3.1(+)). **B:** *CITED2*-wt and *TFAP2C* working on the transcriptional activation of *PITX2C*. *PITX2C* reporter plasmid and the expression vector for *TFAP2C*, *CITED2*, or pcDNA3.1 alone were transfected respectively in 293 T cells. The luciferase activity was normalized to Renilla activity.(* p<0.05, **p<0.01 versus the untreated group (n = 3)).

tween p300 and *CITED2*, but the p.P140S mutant didn't alter the interactions.

Another mammalian two-hybrid assay was operated and analyzed to further evaluate whether the repression of *HIF1A* - p300 complex was influenced by *CITED2* mutation. The result showed that the luciferase activity of wt-type was only 60% of the control (t test, p<0.01) (Figure 2B). Compared with wild-type, the luciferase activity of mutants increased obviously except the p.P140S mutant. In conclusion, *CITED2* mutations weaken the *HIF1A* repression by diminishing the protein-protein interactions between *p300CH1* and *CITED2* on the one hand and by enhancing the interactions between *p300CH1* and *HIF1A* on the other hand.

As *HIF1A* can induce vascular endothelial growth factor (*VEGF*) potently, we supposed that *CITED2* mutations influenced the transcription of *VEGF* through their effect on *HIF1A*. This was confirmed by our dual luciferase assay (Figure 2C). Wild-type *CITED2* caused an approximately 32% decrease of activity compared with the control (t test, p<0.01). P140S showed no difference with wild-type in luciferase activity. As for the other four mutants, Ser161delAGCAGC showed an observable promotion of *VEGF*-promoter resulting in higher luciferase activity than wild-type (t test, p<0.01) and the rest mutants showed few differences compared with wt-type (t test, p<0.05) (Figure 2D).

CITED2 mutations impair *TFAP2C* coactivation resulting in abnormal transactivation of *PITX2C*

As a transcriptional coactivator of *TFAP2*, *CITED2* influenced cardiac left-right patterning by regulating the left-right patterning Nodal-*PITX2C* pathway. *PITX2C* is a critical gene of the Nodal-*PITX2C* pathway and controls the location of heart and intestines in embryo. Our study showed that *CITED2* mutations resulted in decreased luciferase activity of PITX2 by diminishing the coactivation of *CITED2* and *TFAP2C*. The luciferase activity of three mutants were decreased obviously compared with wt. (p.P140S vs. wt-type 80% (t test, p<0.01), p.S183L vs. wt-type 85% (t test, p<0.01), p.Ser192_Gly193delAGCGGC vs. wt-type

92% (t test, p<0.01)) (Figure 3A). The rest two mutants coactivated *TFAP2C* to the same level as wt-type.

In addition, we designed another test to prove the *TFAP2* coactivation with *CITED2*. The result showed that cotransfection of empty vector of pcDNA3.1 (+) with the luciferase reporter PGL3-*PITX2C*-pro was the lowest in all groups including pcDNA3.1-*TFAP2C* or wt–type pcDNA3.1-*CITED2* only and both of them (Figure 3B).

In conclusion, *CITED2* mutations contributed to the abnormal transactivation of *PITX2C*.

Impact of *CITED2* mutations on Subcellular Localization

To further study whether the functional changes are caused by changed subcellular localization of the protein, the transfections were performed using N-terminal GFP fusion constructs of wt and mutant *CITED2*, followed by fluorescence microscopy. The result indicated that the effects of *CITED2* mutations on *VEGF* and *PITX2C* were not caused by the incorrect localization of the protein. Whether in wt or mutant of *CITED2* the proteins were discovered mainly in nucleus and a lesser degree in the cytoplasm of Hela (Figure S1).

Discussion

Previous researches of *cited2*-/-mice confirmed that *cited2* plays a critical role in the development of heart and is essential for the normal creation of the left–right axis. *Cited2-/-* embryos showed a series of cardiac malformations such as VSD, ASD, outflow tract abnormalities and abnormal heart looping.

We screened the coding region and splice sites of the *CITED2* gene in 700 Chinese CHD patients. Two potential pathogenic amino acid deletions (p.Ser161delAGCAGC and p.Ser192_-Gly193delAGCGGC) and three potential pathogenic amino acid substitutions variants (p. P140S, p. S183L and p. S196G) were identified. These three regional highly conserved substitutions (conserved among Humans, chimpanzee, mice, dog, cattle, rat, chicken and zebrafish) were not identified in control group or the variant databases. Therefore, we supposed that these three mutations were possibly causative. Since, SRJ region is a research hot spot at present, the two potential pathogenic amino acid deletions in our study were found in SRJ region. As a result, the necessity of this study is highlight. Although the CHD phenotype was not seen in SRJ-deficient mice as observed in mutation carrying patients, we supposed that this could be due to species differences [23,24]in the function of *CITED2*, or some other unidentified factors[25] might interact with *CITED2* and modify its phenotype. Alternatively, it is also possible that CHD were present earlier in life but spontaneously closed at a later time in SRJ-deficient mice.

Mammalian two-hybrid analysis permits the semi-quantitative assessment of protein-protein interactions occurring within living cells. Cotransfection of wt or mutant *CITED2* and *p300CH1* in 293Tcells, the binding between *CITED2* and *p300CH1* activated the TK report gene expression in vivo. The functional study greatly supported the hypothesis that the mutations are causative and might affect the formation of heart. The last four mutated proteins (p. S183L, p. S196G, p.Ser161delAGCAGC and p.Ser192_Gly193delAGCGGC) showed significantly decreased reporter gene activation ability compared with wt-type. However, an opposite phenomenon occurred by transfecting *p300CH1*, *HIF1A* and wt or mutant *CITED2* together in cells. Taken together,the results indicated that the four mutated proteins decreased the interaction between *CITED2* and *p300CH1* compared with wt-type,causing a weakened competitive binding to p300 CH1 of *CITED2*. The increased interaction between *HIF1A* and *p300CH1* could up- regulate the promoter activity of *VEGF* according to our dual luciferase experiment.

Our study also showed that three mutations decreased the consociation of *TFAP2C* and *CITED2* in the transactivation of

pitx2c, an essential gene of the left–right axis establishment confirmed in mice and chick embryo. The mice experiments already indicated that knocking out *pitx2c* gene can lead to valve defects, body wall dysraphism, gastroschisis, ectopia cordis and other multiple organs polymorphous defects. In addition, there was no evidence that *CITED2* mutations were involved in the incorrect location of the protein in the subcellular localization experiment.

In conclusion, we identified five novel mutations among 700 CHD patients by screening the coding region and splice sites of the *CITED2* gene. To confirm our hypothesis that the mutations were pathogenic, we investigated the function and mechanism of them. Our study revealed that four mutations influenced the transcription regulatory properties of *VEGF* and three mutations reduced costimulation capacity to promote *PITX2C*. Further research showed that four *CITED2* mutations recovered the promoter activity of *VEGF* [26]caused by its decreased competitiveness with *HIF1A* to bind the *p300CH1*. Furthermore, three mutations also decreased the consociation of *TFAP2C* and *CITED2* in the transactivation of *PITX2C*. Our study confirmed that *CITED2* is a disease-causing gene of CHD and its mutations can result in the cardiac malformations.

Author Contributions

Conceived and designed the experiments: XM HP YL. Performed the experiments: YL. Analyzed the data: YL XZ XW. Contributed reagents/materials/analysis tools: FW YW ST QW JW XZ CL. Wrote the paper: YL.

References

1. Hoffman JI, Kaplan S (2002) The incidence of congenital heart disease. J Am Coll Cardiol 39: 1890–1900.
2. Crider KS, Bailey LB (2011) Defying birth defects through diet? Genome Med 3: 9.
3. Blue GM, Kirk EP, Sholler GF, Harvey RP, Winlaw DS (2012) Congenital heart disease: current knowledge about causes and inheritance. Med J Aust 197: 155–159.
4. Xiong F, Li Q, Zhang C, Chen Y, Li P, et al. (2013) Analyses of GATA4, NKX2.5, and TFAP2B genes in subjects from southern China with sporadic congenital heart disease. Cardiovasc Pathol 22: 141–145.
5. Ching YH, Ghosh TK, Cross SJ, Packham EA, Honeyman L, et al. (2005) Mutation in myosin heavy chain 6 causes atrial septal defect. Nat Genet 37: 423–428.
6. Garg V, Kathiriya IS, Barnes R, Schluterman MK, King IN, et al. (2003) GATA4 mutations cause human congenital heart defects and reveal an interaction with TBX5. Nature 424: 443–447.
7. Andrews JE, O'Neill MJ, Binder M, Shioda T, Sinclair AH (2000) Isolation and expression of a novel member of the CITED family. Mech Dev 95: 305–308.
8. Li Q, Pan H, Guan L, Su D, Ma X (2012) CITED2 mutation links congenital heart defects to dysregulation of the cardiac gene VEGF and PITX2C expression. Biochem Biophys Res Commun 423: 895–899.
9. Yin Z, Haynie J, Yang X, Han B, Kiatchoosakun S, et al. (2002) The essential role of Cited2, a negative regulator for HIF-1alpha, in heart development and neurulation. Proc Natl Acad Sci U S A 99: 10488–10493.
10. Xu M, Wu X, Li Y, Yang X, Hu J, et al. (2014) CITED2 mutation and methylation in children with congenital heart disease. J Biomed Sci 21: 7.
11. Freedman SJ, Sun ZY, Kung AL, France DS, Wagner G, et al. (2003) Structural basis for negative regulation of hypoxia-inducible factor-1alpha by CITED2. Nat Struct Biol 10: 504–512.
12. Amati F, Diano L, Campagnolo L, Vecchione L, Cipollone D, et al. (2010) Hif1alpha down-regulation is associated with transposition of great arteries in mice treated with a retinoic acid antagonist. BMC Genomics 11: 497.
13. Macdonald ST, Bamforth SD, Braganca J, Chen CM, Broadbent C, et al. (2013) A cell-autonomous role of Cited2 in controlling myocardial and coronary vascular development. Eur Heart J 34: 2557–2565.

14. Xu B, Doughman Y, Turakhia M, Jiang W, Landsettle CE, et al. (2007) Partial rescue of defects in Cited2-deficient embryos by HIF-1alpha heterozygosity. Dev Biol 301: 130–140.
15. Bamforth SD, Braganca J, Eloranta JJ, Murdoch JN, Marques FI, et al. (2001) Cardiac malformations, adrenal agenesis, neural crest defects and exencephaly in mice lacking Cited2, a new Tfap2 co-activator. Nat Genet 29: 469–474.
16. Satoda M, Zhao F, Diaz GA, Burn J, Goodship J, et al. (2000) Mutations in TFAP2B cause Char syndrome, a familial form of patent ductus arteriosus. Nat Genet 25: 42–46.
17. Bhattacherjee V, Horn KH, Singh S, Webb CL, Pisano MM, et al. (2009) CBP/p300 and associated transcriptional co-activators exhibit distinct expression patterns during murine craniofacial and neural tube development. Int J Dev Biol 53: 1097–1104.
18. Campione M, Ros MA, Icardo JM, Piedra E, Christoffels VM, et al. (2001) Pitx2 expression defines a left cardiac lineage of cells: evidence for atrial and ventricular molecular isomerism in the iv/iv mice. Dev Biol 231: 252–264.
19. Bamforth SD, Braganca J, Farthing CR, Schneider JE, Broadbent C, et al. (2004) Cited2 controls left-right patterning and heart development through a Nodal-Pitx2c pathway. Nat Genet 36: 1189–1196.
20. Sperling S, Grimm CH, Dunkel I, Mebus S, Sperling HP, et al. (2005) Identification and functional analysis of CITED2 mutations in patients with congenital heart defects. Hum Mutat 26: 575–582.
21. Yang XF, Wu XY, Li M, Li YG, Dai JT, et al. (2010) [Mutation analysis of Cited2 in patients with congenital heart disease]. Zhonghua Er Ke Za Zhi 48: 293–296.
22. Chen CM, Bentham J, Cosgrove C, Braganca J, Cuenda A, et al. (2012) Functional significance of SRJ domain mutations in CITED2. PLoS One 7: e46256.
23. Li DY, Whitehead KJ (2010) Evaluating strategies for the treatment of cerebral cavernous malformations. Stroke 41: S92–94.
24. Ruiz-Perez VL, Blair HJ, Rodriguez-Andres ME, Blanco MJ, Wilson A, et al. (2007) Evc is a positive mediator of Ihh-regulated bone growth that localises at the base of chondrocyte cilia. Development 134: 2903–2912.

25. Bentham J, Michell AC, Lockstone H, Andrew D, Schneider JE, et al. (2010) Maternal high-fat diet interacts with embryonic Cited2 genotype to reduce

24. Ruiz-Perez VL, Blair HJ, Rodriguez-Andres ME, Blanco MJ, Wilson A, et al. (2007) Evc is a positive mediator of Ihh-regulated bone growth that localises at the base of chondrocyte cilia. Development 134: 2903–2912.

Pitx2c expression and enhance penetrance of left-right patterning defects. Hum Mol Genet 19: 3394–3401.

26. Agrawal A, Gajghate S, Smith H, Anderson DG, Albert TJ, et al. (2008) Cited2 modulates hypoxia-inducible factor-dependent expression of vascular endothelial growth factor in nucleus pulposus cells of the rat intervertebral disc. Arthritis Rheum 58: 3798–3808.

2

Lifetime Costs and Outcomes of Repair of Tetralogy of Fallot Compared to Natural Progression of the Disease: Great Ormond Street Hospital Cohort

Rachael Maree Hunter[1]*, **Mark Isaac**[2], **Alessandra Frigiola**[2], **David Blundell**[3], **Kate Brown**[2], **Kate Bull**[2]

1 University College London, London, United Kingdom, 2 Great Ormond St Hospital NHS Foundation Trust, London, United Kingdom, 3 Leeds School of Medicine, Leeds, United Kingdom

Abstract

Background: Tetralogy of Fallot is a congenital heart disease that requires surgical repair without which survival through childhood is extremely rare. The aim of this paper is to use data from the mandatory follow-up of patients with Tetralogy of Fallot to model the health-related costs and outcomes over the first 55-years of life.

Method: A decision analytical model was developed to establish costs and outcomes for patients up to 55 years after diagnosis and first repair of Tetralogy of Fallot compared to natural progression. Data from Adult Congenital Heart Disease (ACHD) centres that follow up Tetralogy of Fallot patients and Great Ormond Street Hospital (GOSH), London, United Kingdom (UK) medical records was used to establish the cost and effectiveness of current interventions. Data from a Czech cohort was used for the natural, no intervention condition.

Results: The average cost per patient of a repair for Tetralogy of Fallot was £26,938 (SE = £4,140). The full life time cost per patient, with no discount rate, was £65,310 (95% CI £64,981–£65,729); £56,559 discounted (95% CI £56,159–£56,960). Patients with a repair had an average of 35 Quality Adjusted Life Years (QALYs) per patient over 55 years undiscounted and 20.16 QALYs discounted. If the disorder was left to take its natural course, patients on average had a total of 3 QALYs per patient with no discount rate and 2.30 QALYs discounted.

Conclusion: A model has been developed that provides an estimate of the value for money of an expensive repair of a congenital heart disease. The model could be used to test the cost-effectiveness of making amendments to the care pathway.

Editor: Giuseppe Biondi-Zoccai, Sapienza University of Rome, Italy

Funding: This project was funded by the Great Ormond Street Hospital Children's Charity. DB was supported by a bursary from Leeds University. The funders had no role in study design, data collection and analysis, decision to publish, or preparation of the manuscript.

Competing Interests: The authors have declared that no competing interests exist.

* E-mail: r.hunter@ucl.ac.uk

Introduction

Tetralogy of Fallot is the commonest cyanotic heart condition and was one of the first congenital heart diseases of any complexity to be repaired [1]. The condition affects about 0.31/1000 live births [2], with approximately 250 repairs of Tetralogy of Fallot being undertaken annually in the United Kingdom (UK) [3]. Survivors of the surgery in its ground-breaking era form a cohort of patients with a 'new disease' whose natural history they are themselves delineating.

Currently, the diagnosis of Tetralogy of Fallot may be achieved through pre-natal ultrasound screening or emerge at the time of an emergency presentation in infancy or during investigation of a murmur or an intercurrent illness. All patients require surgical repair without which survival through childhood is extremely rare. The repair is not fully 'corrective', primarily because obstruction in the area between right ventricle and pulmonary artery must be relieved, often sacrificing pulmonary valve function. Service

standards require lifetime follow up for all Fallot patients [4]. For some, surgical revision of the right ventricular outflow tract area is required later – most usually a pulmonary valve replacement (PVR). Though for an individual patient, the future need for PVR is hard to judge in early childhood, cohort studies are emerging that permit prediction of the proportions requiring later revision [5].

Achieving early surgical survival required a demanding learning curve – 30-day mortality rates were commonly around 25% in the 1960s and are currently around 10-times lower. Because early outcomes have been good for many years, the great majority of children currently treated leave 'childhood' services fit to face adult life [6]; they are looked after by a network of specialist Adult Congenital Heart Disease (ACHD) centres. With the benefit of a primary data source - a cohort of Fallot patients 1964–2009 - our aim was to estimate the first 55 years health-related costs and outcomes for patients with Tetralogy of Fallot born now and managed by current standards.

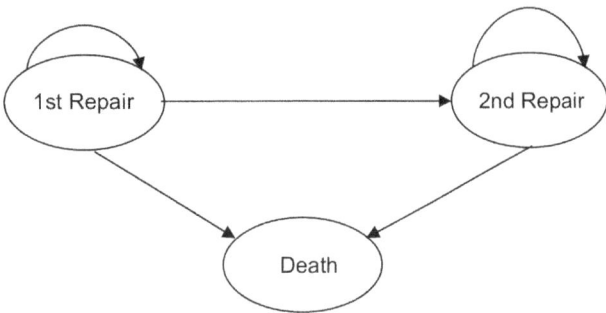

Figure 1. Markov model of health states for repair cohort.

Methods

Decision analytic models use the best available information from a range of sources to estimate the costs and consequences of a particular intervention or policy, providing they take into account the uncertainty associated with the variables contained in the model [7]. We developed a decision analytic model to calculate the health outcomes and costs of surgical repair of Tetralogy of Fallot over a 55 year time horizon. The primary data source is a complete consecutive list of all UK patients having repair of uncomplicated Tetralogy of Fallot at Great Ormond Street Hospital (GOSH), London, UK, from February 1964 to January 2009. Secondary data sources have been used where necessary.

Great Ormond Street Hospital Cohort

Data was available on all 1085 UK patients who had a repair of Tetralogy of Fallot at GOSH from February 1964 to January 2009. The GOSH medical records provided date and age at repair, dates of any PVRs and dates of death if these events occurred in childhood. Demographic data was also linked to NHS numbers, providing information about deaths since 1996 and collaborators from each ACHD centre used local databases to provide dates of any PVRs done for patients over the age of 16. The 46 patients lost to follow-up were censored on the last date of follow-up recorded.

Parents of current patients are asked to give written consent for patient details to be collected and stored for audit and research

purposes. The NHS Research Ethics Committee approved the collection and storage of resource use information from medical records from unconsented patients including the use of NHS numbers for later tracking.

Survival and Reoperation-free Survival

Natural survival for Tetralogy of Fallot patients with no repair was estimated from Samenek (1992) where data on incidence of congenital heart disease (CHD) was combined with date of death to determine the distribution of age at death for all children with CHD in Central Bohemia, Czechoslovakia, over a 27 year period [8]. No intervention for Tetralogy of Fallot was available at the time hence the observational study provides data on the attrition of the disease without intervention. This information was used to construct a parametric (Weibull) survival model.

The 1085 patients in the GOSH cohort data provided the inputs for the parametric models (Weibull) we used to summarise survival from birth, with and without PVR. This was done in line with methodology set out in Briggs et al [9].

All analyses were conducted in Stata v10.

Resource Usage: Frequencies

Age specific frequencies of routine health interventions were based on data from the cohort as follows:

Resource Usage: between Birth and Open Heart Repair

We used data from patients born since 2000 to populate the model for this phase. In clinical terms, this period includes the phase of presentation and diagnosis, preoperative investigations and surveillance. Of the 214 patients in the cohort born in this era, 30 were selected at random and the in-patient and outpatient events and investigations each received were aggregated from their clinical records. Presentation was coded as 'antenatal diagnosis', 'presentation with emergency hospital admission' or 'diagnosis achieved in an out-patient context'. Hospital lengths of stay, diagnostic and assessment investigations and numbers of out-patient visits were aggregated for these patients to represent the current pre-operative costs. There were no deaths in this interval.

Resource Usage: Admission for Open Heart Repair

Actual data from the same 30/214 patients were used to estimate multipliers for the current costs for the open heart

Table 1. Average resource use per patient: Mean (SE).

Resource	Birth to first repair	First decade following repair	Resource use per decade (2+)
	N = 30	N = 21	N = 14
Outpatient appointment	3.27 (0.42)		
ECHO	6.07 (0.4)	0.62 (0.02)	2 (0.62)
MRI	0.13 (0.1)	0.33 (0.14)	1.93 (0.41)
ECG	1.43 (0.2)	0.24 (0.15)	3.21 (0.75)
24 hr ECG	0.13 (0.06)	0.1 (0.07)	1.57 (0.37)
Ultrasound	0.73 (0.3)		
X-ray	8.77 (1.3)	0.14 (0.14)	2.5 (0.99)
ECMO	0.03 (0.03)		
Preliminary procedure	0.17 (0.03)		
Other Cardiac Surgery		0.05 (0.05)	0.07 (0.07)
Exercise lab		0.14 (0.08)	1.29 (0.41)

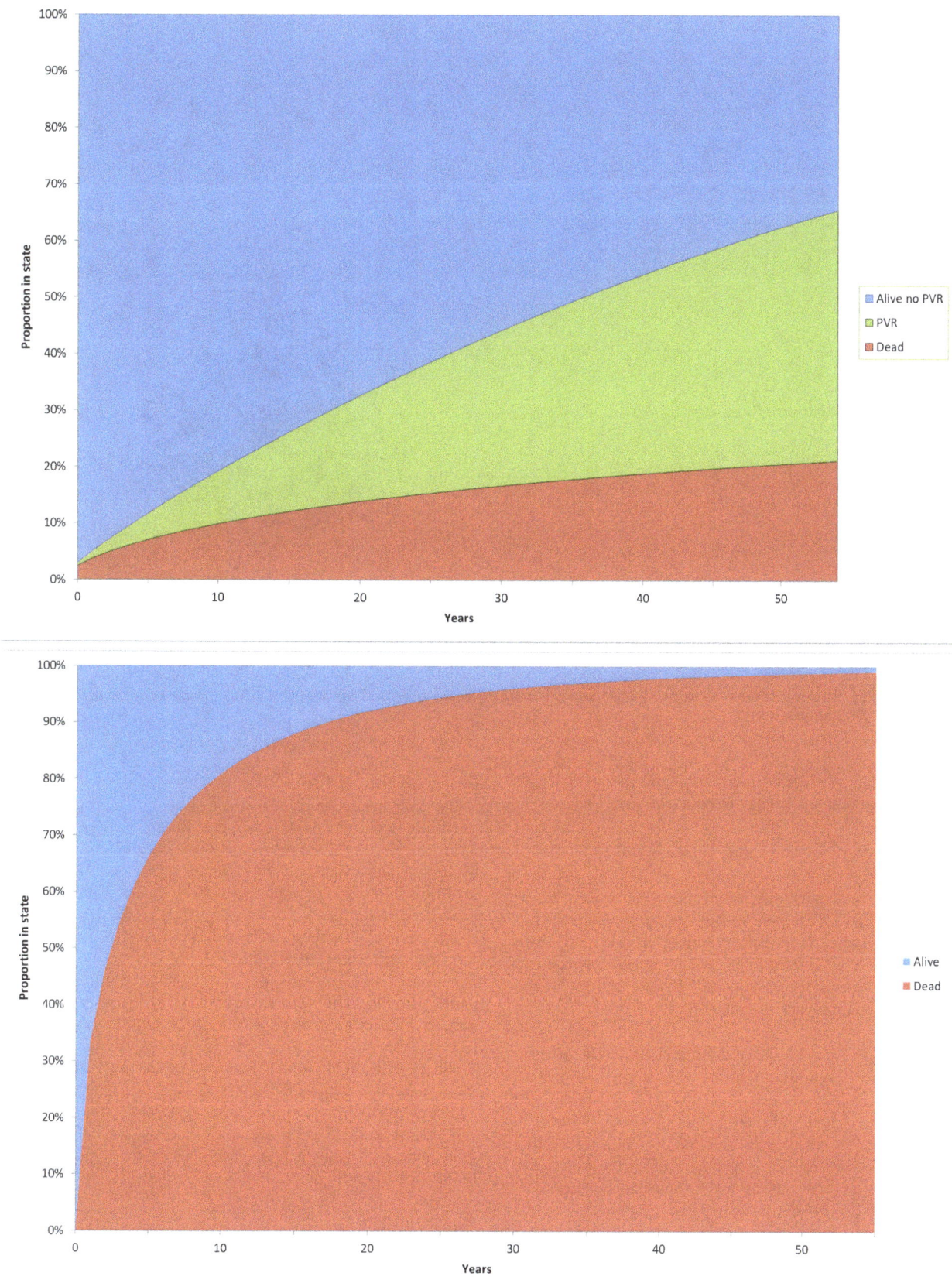

Figure 2. The changing proportion over time between 0 and 55 years in which patients are in 3 exhaustive and mutually exclusive states: 'dead', 'alive without PVR' and 'PVR'. A) With repair; B) Natural progression, no repair.

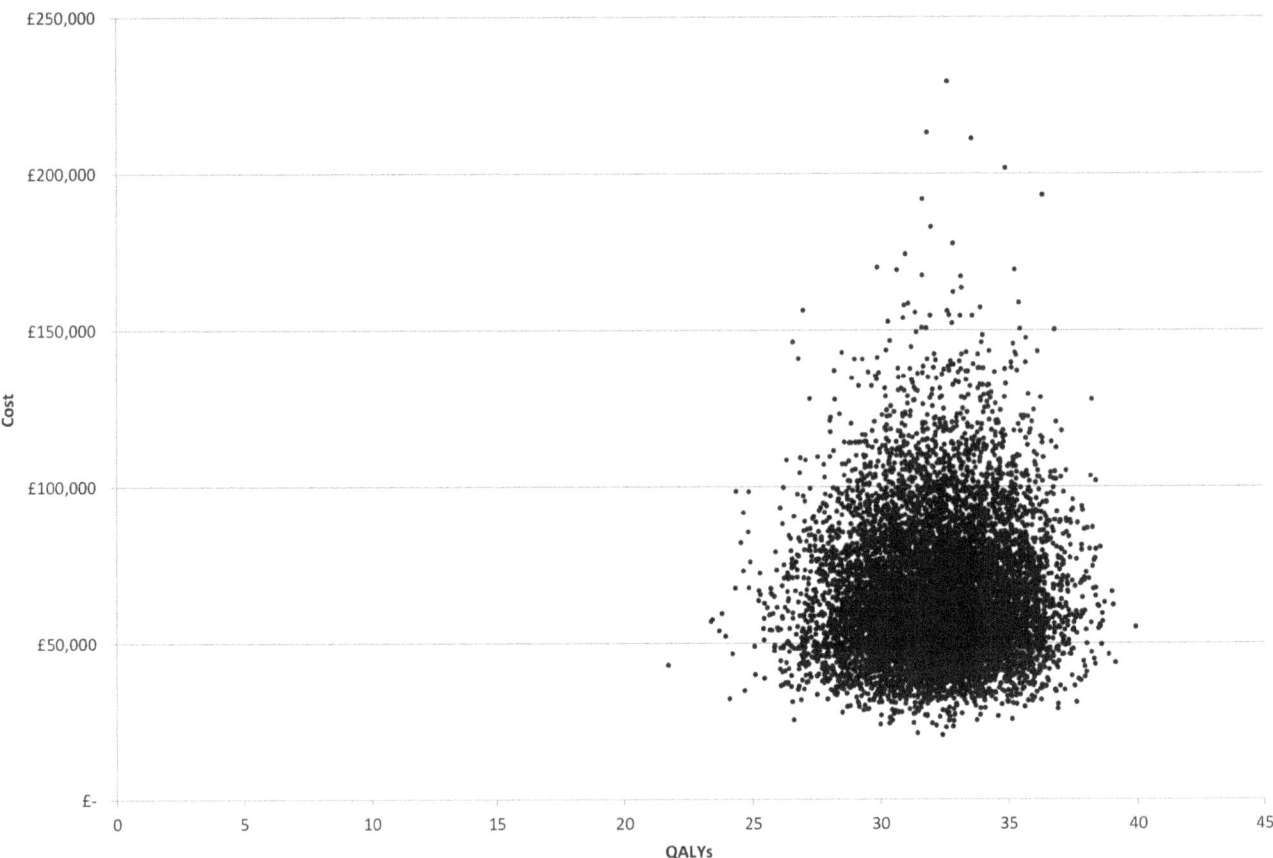

Figure 3. Cost-effectiveness plane – cost per Fallot patient over 55 years graphed against the QALY gained compared to natural progression –10,000 simulations.

operation. The data used included the cost of the operation, length of stay, ward type and any major postoperative complications.

Resource Usage: between Open Heart Repair and 10 Years of Age

Data from the same patients repaired since 2000 and who have not already required a PVR were used to estimate the current costs of postoperative surveillance, largely outpatient visits and investigations up to age 10. Interventions, whether catheter-based or surgical but which did not constitute a PVR were aggregated and the counts used as multipliers for these events.

Resource Usage: Age 10–20 and Subsequent Decades

Clinical events (primarily out-patient visits and investigations) from age 10–20 of all twenty-one surviving operated patients born in 1990 were aggregated and rendered as an annual estimate of the clinical event rate for patients aged 10–20. We assumed that the rate of clinic visits and investigations would remain at rates similar to those at ages 10–20 for subsequent decades. Re-interventions short of PVR were aggregated as before.

Cost of PVR

Data from the same 30/214 patients repaired since 2000 were used to estimate multipliers for the current costs for PVR. Data used related to length of stay and major postoperative interventions.

Resource Usage: Costs

Based on the above cohorts we calculated the average resource use from birth until first repair, per decade and per PVR for patients who have a second repair. Per decade costs were divided by 10 to obtain a weighted cost per patient per year. All costs were in British Pounds (£) and 2010/2011 values. Unit costs for interventions and investigations other than first repair, PVR and Extracorporeal Membrane Oxygenation (ECMO) were derived from reference costs 2010/2011 [10].

The cost of the open repair was obtained from the GOSH patient level costing system for 30/214 Tetralogy of Fallot patients. This was divided by the 2010 GOSH market forces factor to obtain a UK average cost of repair. It was assumed that a PVR operation itself would have the same cost as the primary repair operation, although additional costs for length of stay and additional procedures were handled separately.

The cost of ECMO was obtained from Brown et al, and was estimated at £10,539 per day over 6 days for a total cost per ECMO of £75,126, accounting for inflation [11].

Quality of Life

From the complete consecutive list, 50 survivors (10 from each surgical decade 1960's to 2000's) were chosen at random to receive a Quality of Life questionnaire; these patients (age 4–55) were assumed to be representative of survivors generally. In the absence of a generic quality of life instrument applicable across child and adult populations, the PEDSQL was administered to those age 1–18 and WHOQOL Bref to the adults.

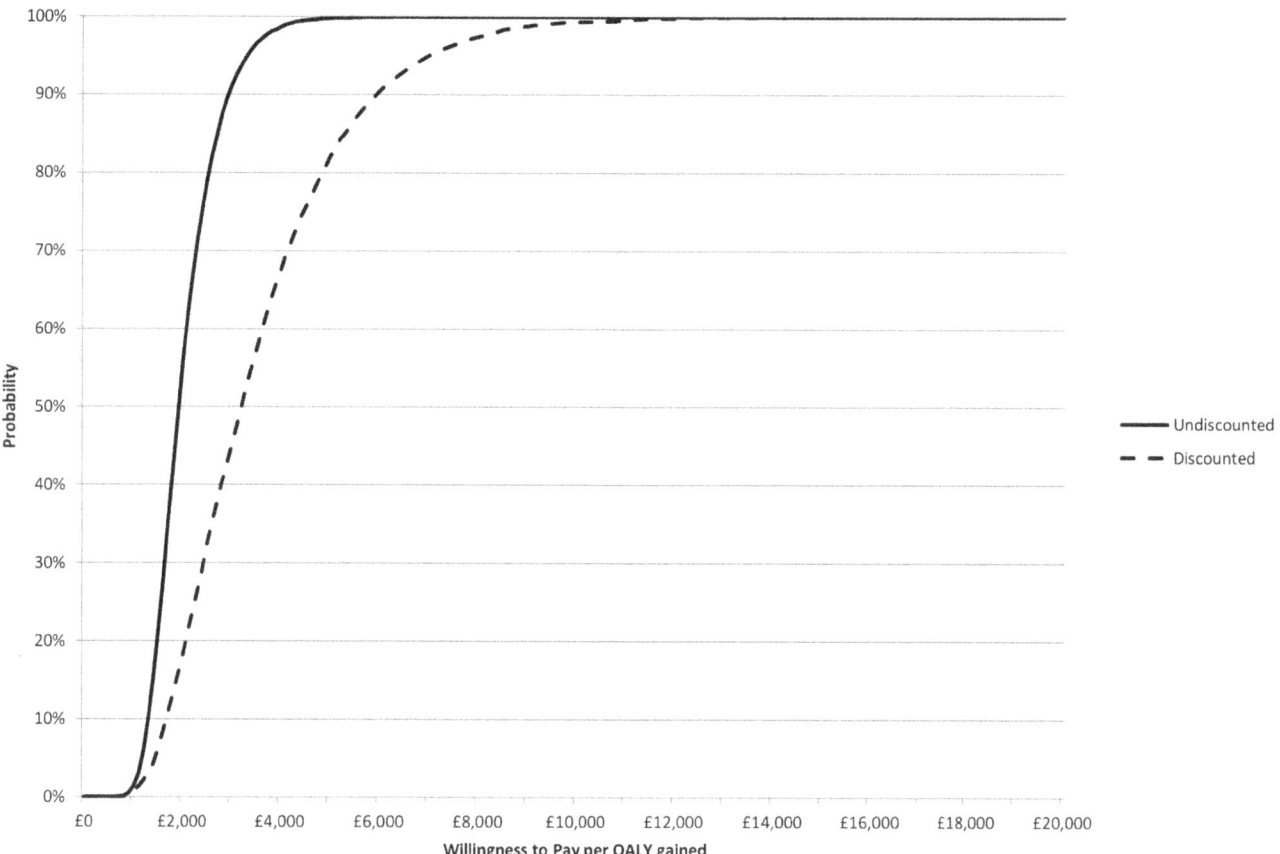

Figure 4. Cost effectiveness acceptability curve comparing repair of Tetralogy of Fallot with no repair: undiscounted (solid line) and discounted (dashed line).

The outcome measure used in the model was quality adjusted life years (QALYs). QALYs represent both the quality and quantity of health related quality of life, quality being measured by utility scores. A utility score of 1 represents perfect health and a utility of 0 death; negative values, representing states worse than death, are possible. QALYs are the recommended outcome for use in economic evaluations in the UK as they are a common unit that allow for comparable decisions about resource allocation across different diseases. In England, to ensure consistency of approach, the National Institute for Health and Clinical Excellence (NICE) recommends that utility scores used to calculate QALYs are calculated from the EuroQol 5D (EQ-5D), a 5 domain 3 level tool, and an algorithm developed by Dolan which is based on valuations of a selection of the 243 potential EQ-5D health states by 3,995 members of the general population [12].

There are no utility scores to calculate QALYs available for the WHOQOL. Instead we used a methodology similar to that used by Al Ruzzeh et al [13] to calculate utility scores from the WHOQOL; responses to WHOQOL questions which are similar to the EQ-5D dimensions were used to calculate utility scores. The utility values for the 5 level cross walk EQ-5D value set [14] were used so there was no need to covert the 5 levels of the WHOQOL to 3.

Similarly there are no utility scores available for PEDSQL, so the same methodology was used again but instead the questions are similar to those of the Child Health Utility 9D (CHU9D), for which utility scores are available [15]. We used the CHU9

algorithm applied to PEDSQL to calculate average utility for patients under 18.

As there is no quality of life (QoL) data available for the natural progression, for the 'no surgical repair' comparator cohort a random number between 0 and 1 was chosen to represent their utility scores.

Description of Model

The model used a time dependent Markov model, as described above, to simulate time to death from first repair, time to PVR and time to death from PVR over 55 years (see figure 1). The hypothetical population in the model is assumed to have the same characteristics as the cohort of patients described above.

The model was built in Microsoft Excel 2010 and is available as supporting material (Model S1).

Cost Effectiveness Analysis and Probabilistic Sensitivity Analysis

Cost effectiveness was calculated as the incremental cost, in British Pounds (£'s), per QALY gained from surgical repair of Tetralogy of Fallot compared to natural progression, no repair. This provides a summary of the incremental, or extra, costs of the surgical repair plus all heart related follow up appointments, divided by the incremental, or extra, benefits.

A probabilistic sensitivity analysis (PSA) was conducted to calculate the cost effectiveness of surgical repair using the net monetary benefit approach as set out in Briggs et al [9]. These values were used to generate a cost effectiveness acceptability

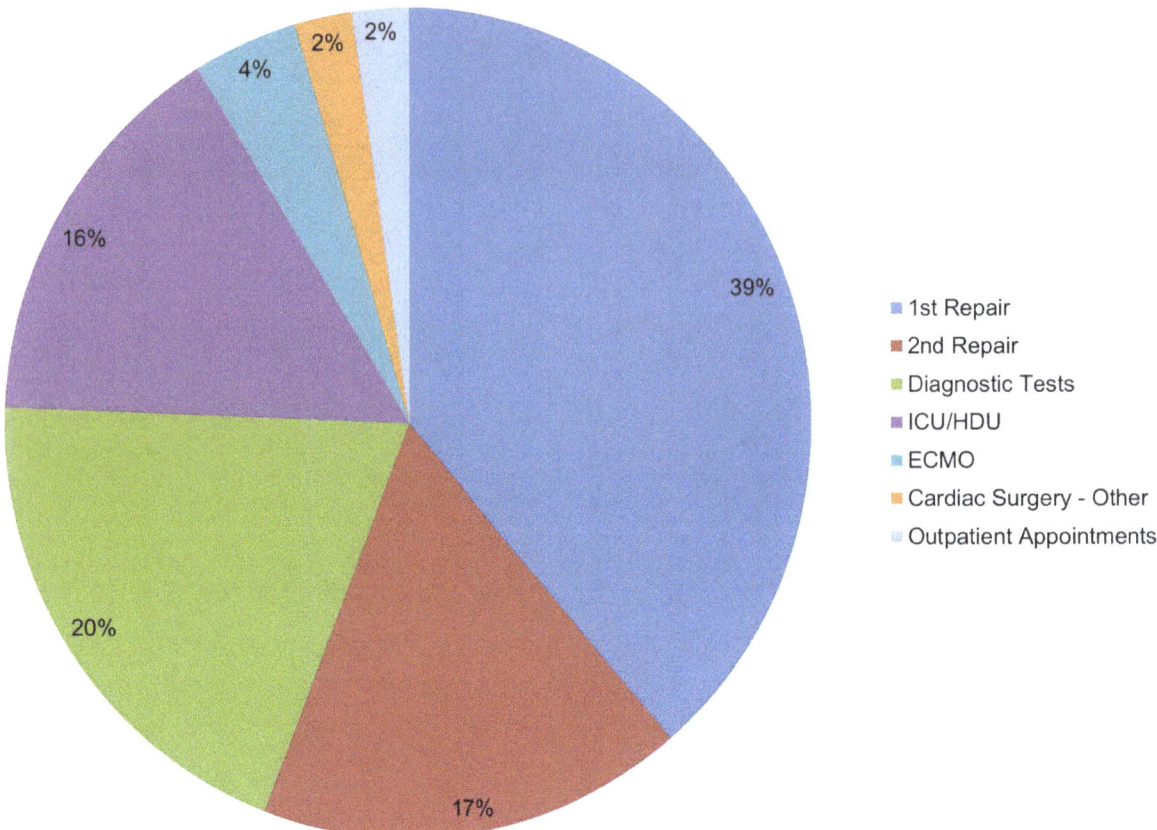

Figure 5. Breakdown of health care costs for Tetralogy of Fallot patients from birth to age 55: undiscounted.

curve to determine the probability that surgical repair of Tetralogy of Fallot is cost effective for a hypothetical willingness to pay for each additional QALY gained for values of between £0 and £20,000. Results are based on 10,000 simulations. We provided results for undiscounted and discounted models. The discount rate was randomly varied between 0% and 6% in line with NICE guidance [12].

Results

Costs

A summary of the average resource use per patient is reported in Table 1. The average cost per patient of the admission including repair of Tetralogy of Fallot was £26,938 (SE = £4,140). In 2010 GOSH had a market forces factor of 1.18 [16]. After applying the market forces factor, the average UK cost for a repair was calculated as £22,829. The mean full life time cost per patient, with no discount rate, is £65,310 (95% CI £64,981–£65,729) and £56,559 discounted (95% CI £56,159–£56,960).

Mortality and Quality of Life

Figure 2 provides a summary of the proportion of patients in each health state over time for the two models. The utility score for patients under 18 with a repair was 0.83 (SE = 0.031) and 0.72 (SE = 0.037) for adult patients. Patients with a repair had an average total of 35 QALYs with an average total of 3 QALYs for patients with no repair.

Incremental Cost per QALY Gained

The mean cost per QALY gained over 10,000 simulations was £2027 without discounting (£3168 discounted). All simulations fall into the north-east quadrant of the cost-effectiveness plane, in that all simulations result in more QALYs but also cost more (figure 3). Based on a willingness to pay of £20,000 per QALY gained there is a 100% chance that open repair of Tetralogy of Fallot is cost effective compared to doing nothing (figure 4).

Figure 5 shows the proportions of overall costs attributable to the surgery, inpatient stays in intensive care and high dependency units, outpatient appointments and investigations.

Discussion

This model provides information on the first 55 years costs of the common congenital heart problem Tetralogy of Fallot and compares it to the additional gain in QALYs. The first 55 years cost of a Fallot patient to the NHS is approximately £65,310. This cost is outweighed by the additional years of life gained in reasonably full health. Ungerleider et al [17] published estimates of hospital costs of repairing Tetralogy of Fallot, including an evaluation of the alternatives of primary repair versus repair after preliminary palliative procedures. However we believe this is the first time a full cost effectiveness evaluation has been attempted in the field of childhood heart disease.

Limitations

Surgery for Tetralogy of Fallot only emerged in the 1960's, hence the postoperative "natural history" beyond age 55 is unknown; Fallot patients' underlying biology makes it conceivable that heart related costs could escalate in later life. The natural progression, or no intervention, approach had only limited data from historical observational studies where no intervention was available, as it would be unethical to collect further information currently. None the less, this model presents confirmation of the benefit of expensive childhood interventions that significantly improve survival and quality of life of patients. Quality of life of surgical patients would need to decrease by 85% before the added life expectancy provided no additional benefit because of poor quality of life, even assuming perfect health for the 'do nothing' approach.

The results for both the discounted and undiscounted models have been presented; it is arguable which should be used in a context where surgery is offered to an infant as an 'investment' for their adult life. For patients living to the age of 55, using a discount rate of 3.5%, a year of life lived in perfect health is worth less than half a QALY. This seems to undermine the purpose of the intervention, which is to increase the chance that the patient reaches adult life in close to full health. This is supported by the evidence that people would like to give greater weight to younger people to represent the additional potential life they have to lose or gain. Trying to formalize the measurement of this though has proved difficult [18].

Conclusions

Repair of Tetralogy of Fallot is a worthwhile investment for the health care system given the QALYs gained. This model could be used as a baseline to test the cost-effectiveness of changes to the care pathway for Fallot babies. Such changes could include improving screening procedures, changes in conduct of the primary repair with a view to changing the long term incidence of PVR and trials of the impact of elective PVR in adult life – all substantive questions for the congenital heart disease community.

Author Contributions

Guidance and feedback: AF. Conceived and designed the experiments: RH Kate Bull Kate Brown. Analyzed the data: RH MI DB Kate Bull Kate Brown. Contributed reagents/materials/analysis tools: RH. Wrote the paper: RH Kate Bull Kate Brown.

References

1. Lillehei CW, Cohen M, Warden HE, Read RC, Aust JB, et al. (1955) Direct vision intracardiac surgical correction of the tetralogy of Fallot, pentalogy of Fallot, and pulmonary atresia defects; report of first ten cases. Ann Surg 142: 418–442.

2. Wren C, Richmond S, Donaldson L (2000) Temporal variability in birth prevalence of cardiovascular malformations. Heart 83: 414–419.

3. Central Cardiac Audit Database (2001) Procedures for congenital heart disease: Annual report. Available: http://www.ucl.ac.uk/nicor/audits/congenitalheartdisease/publicreports/pdfs/annualreport0001. Accessed 28 January 2013.

4. DH Vascular Programme Team (2006) A commissioning guide for services for young people and adults with congenital heart disease (also known as Grown Ups with Congenital Heart Disease or GUCH). London: Department of Health. 34 p.

5. Wray J, Frigiola A, Bull C (2012) Loss to specialist follow-up in congenital heart disease; out of sight, out of mind. Heart. heartjnl-2012-302831.

6. Bedard E, Shore DF, Gatzoulis MA (2008) Adult congenital heart disease: a 2008 overview. Br Med Bull 85: 151–180.

7. (2000) Decision analytic modelling in the economic evaluation of health technologies. A consensus statement. Consensus Conference on Guidelines on Economic Modelling in Health Technology Assessment. Pharmacoeconomics 17: 443–444.

8. Samanek M (1992) Children with congenital heart disease: probability of natural survival. Pediatr Cardiol 13: 152–158.

9. Briggs A, Claxton K, Schulper M (2006) Decision Modelling for Health Economic Evaluation. Oxford: Oxford University Press.

10. DH PbR Finance and Costing Team (2011) National Schedule of Reference Costs 2010–11 http://www.dh.gov.uk/health/2011/11/reference-costs/. Accessed 1 July 2012.

11. Brown KL, Wray J, Wood TL, Mc Mahon AM, Burch M, et al. (2009) Cost utility evaluation of extracorporeal membrane oxygenation as a bridge to transplant for children with end-stage heart failure due to dilated cardiomyopathy. J Heart Lung Transplant 28: 32–38.

12. NICE (2008) Guide to the methods of technology appraisal. London: National Institute of Health and Clinical Excellence. 76 p.

13. Al-Ruzzeh S, Epstein D, George S, Bustami M, Wray J, et al. (2008) Economic evaluation of coronary artery bypass grafting surgery with and without cardiopulmonary bypass: cost-effectiveness and quality-adjusted life years in a randomized controlled trial. Artif Organs 32: 891–897.

14. van HB, Janssen MF, Feng YS, Kohlmann T, Busschbach J, et al. (2012) Interim scoring for the EQ-5D-5L: mapping the EQ-5D-5L to EQ-5D-3L value sets. Value Health 15: 708–715.

15. Stevens K (2012) Valuation of the Child Health Utility 9D Index. Pharmacoeconomics 30: 729–747.

16. Department of Health (2008) Market Forces Factor Information. http://www.dh.gov.uk/en/Publicationsandstatistics/Publications/PublicationsPolicyAndGuidance/DH_091793. Accessed 21 July 2012.

17. Ungerleider RM, Kanter RJ, O'Laughlin M, Bengur AR, Anderson PA, et al. (1997) Effect of repair strategy on hospital cost for infants with tetralogy of Fallot. Ann Surg 225: 779–783.

18. Dolan P, Tsuchiya A, Armitage C, Brazier J, Bryan S, et al. (2012) What is the value to society of a QALY? http://www.hta.ac.uk/nihrmethodology/reports/1554.pdf. Accessed 14 November 2012.

3

Methodological Approaches to Evaluate Teratogenic Risk using Birth Defect Registries: Advantages and Disadvantages

Fernando A. Poletta[1,5], Jorge S. López Camelo[1,2,5]*, Juan A. Gili[1,5], Emmanuele Leoncini[3], Eduardo E. Castilla[1,4,5], Pierpaolo Mastroiacovo[3]

1 ECLAMC (Estudio Colaborativo Latinoamericano de Malformaciones Congénitas) at Centro de Educación Médica e Investigaciones Clínicas (CEMIC) (CONICET), Buenos Aires, Argentina, 2 ECLAMC at Instituto Multidisciplinario de Biología Celular (IMBICE) (CIC-CONICET), La Plata, Argentina, 3 Headquarters of the International Clearinghouse for Birth Defects Surveillance and Research, Rome, Italy, 4 ECLAMC at Instituto Oswaldo Cruz, Rio de Janeiro, Brazil, 5 INAGEMP (Instituto Nacional de Genética Médica Populacional), Rio de Janeiro, Brazil

Abstract

Background: Different approaches have been used in case-control studies to estimate maternal exposure to medications and the risk of birth defects. However, the performance of these approaches and how they affect the odds ratio (OR) estimates have not been evaluated using birth-defect surveillance programmes. The aim of this study was to evaluate the scope and limitations of three case-control approaches to assess the teratogenic risk of birth defects in mothers exposed to antiepileptic medications, insulin, or acetaminophen.

Methodology/Principal Findings: We studied 110,814 non-malformed newborns and 58,514 live newborns with birth defects registered by the Latin American Collaborative Study of Congenital Anomalies (ECLAMC) between 1967 and 2008. Four controls were randomly selected for each case in the same hospital and period, and three different control groups were used: non-malformed newborns (HEALTHY), malformed newborns (SICK), and a subgroup of SICK, only-exposed cases (OECA). Associations were evaluated using OR and Pearson's chi-square ($P<0.01$). There were no concordance correlations between the HEALTHY and OECA designs, and the average OR differences ranged from 3.0 to 11.5 for the three evaluated medicines. The overestimations observed for HEALTHY design were increased as higher OR values were given, with a high and statistically significant correlation between the difference and the mean. On the contrary, the concordance correlations obtained between the SICK and OECA designs were quite good, with no significant differences in the average risks.

Conclusions: The HEALTHY design estimates the true population OR, but shows a high rate of false-positive results presumably caused by differential misclassification bias. This bias decreases with the increase of the proportion of exposed controls. SICK and OECA odds ratios cannot be considered a direct estimate of the true population OR except under certain conditions. However, the SICK and OECA designs could provide practical information to generate hypotheses about potential teratogens.

Editor: Amit Singh, University of Dayton, United States of America

Funding: This study was supported by Agencia Nacional de Promoción Científica y Tecnológica (ANPCyT), grant number PICT 2008 0429, Argentina; Consejo Nacional de Investigaciones Científicas y Técnicas (CONICET), Argentina. The funders had no role in study design, data collection and analysis, decision to publish, or preparation of the manuscript.

Competing Interests: The authors have declared that no competing interests exist.

* E-mail: jslc@eclamc.org

Introduction

Different case-control study designs have been used to estimate the risk of birth defects after medication exposure. These approaches differ in their definition and selection of the control group. Case-control studies with healthy newborn controls are widely used, especially for studying rare events such as birth defects. In South America, the Latin American Collaborative Study of Congenital Anomalies (ECLAMC) has maintained a surveillance programme for birth defects since 1967 using a case-control design [1].

However, as has been laid out in previous works [2–7], these risk estimates from case-control studies are vulnerable to selection bias, confounding bias, and information bias (differential misclassification bias). In this sense, recall and interviewer bias (two types of information bias) are subjects of great concern in birth-defect epidemiology [8]. Recall bias may occur when mothers of babies with birth defects carefully report the use of medications or when they are thoroughly interviewed regarding medicine use as a possible cause of their infants' defects. In the latter case, mothers are more likely to recall medication exposure than are mothers of healthy controls with similar medication use [9]. Interviewer bias arises when the interviewers know who are the mothers of cases and who are the mothers of controls, and then the interviewers may have a higher tendency to determine the exposure histories of cases than the exposure histories for controls. Both biases may result in the over-estimation of the effect of medication (odds ratio) and a higher probability of false-positive results. Although previous studies have found little evidence of differential misclassification of exposures in case-control studies of birth defects (see refferences in Swan et al. [10]), potential reporting bias is a reasonable issue to be considered in studies to assess teratogenic effects of medications.

A useful system have been proposed to post-marketing surveillance of fetal effects of medications using available sources from existing birth defect surveillance programs and globally organized through the International Clearinghouse for Birth Defects Surveillance and Research (ICBDSR) [11]. Considering that methodology, coverage, and sources of ascertainment vary among these birth defects surveillance programs, approaches based on malformed controls and only-exposed controls has been suggested as practical designs to disclose potential teratogens [11–14].

The interpretation and usefulness of the epidemiological methods that include healthy and malformed controls have been discussed previously [11,15–18]; however, the performance of these approaches and how they affect the odds ratio estimates have not been evaluated using birth-defect surveillance programmes.

The aim of this study was to evaluate, using the ECLAMC's surveillance programme, the scope and limitations of three approaches to assess the teratogenic risk for birth defects in mothers exposed to specific medications during the first trimester of pregnancy: (a) antiepileptics, which are medications associated with a risk of birth defects; (b) insulin, which is a marker for pre-gestational diabetes, a chronic condition that is well known to be associated with birth defects; and (c) acetaminophen, which is a medication that is not associated with birth defects.

Materials and Methods

Sample and case definition

Live-birth cases were those that were registered by the ECLAMC network, involving 102 maternity hospitals from 11 South American countries from 1967 to 2008 and covering 3,939,474 births. A total of 58,514 live births with isolated or multiple birth defects were registered with ICD-X BPA codes [19]. Non-isolated (multiple malformed) cases were counted separately for each type of birth defect. Cases with aetiologic syndromes [20] and those with only a minor birth defect were excluded.

A total of 110,814 non-malformed newborns from the same database were used as healthy controls. Data regarding medication use and illnesses during pregnancy were obtained by qualified physicians using standard interviews of the mothers before their discharge from the hospital at which they had given birth. Data were collected, reviewed and coded by the ECLAMC following the same standardized procedure used since 1967 [1]. Medicines were coded with the standard ATC system [21]. The study protocol was approved by the ethics committee at CEMIC (*DHHS*-IRB #1745, IORG #1315).

Medicine exposure

The three medicines analyzed in this study were the following: antiepileptics (ATC code: N03A), including valproic acid (N03AG01); insulin (ATC code: A10A); and acetaminophen (ATC code: N02BE01). Exposures to vitamins and iron were excluded from the analysis in order to minimize bias, as exposure to these medications has not been proven to be teratogenic.

Epidemiological Designs

Figure 1a shows the four categories of association between the medications and types of birth defects in the sample. Risk 1

(M→BD) is the risk that the study medication ("M") causes the birth defect studied ("BD"); Risk 2 (M→OBD) is the risk that the study medication ("M") produces congenital anomalies other than the birth defect under study ("OBD"); Risk 3 (OM→BD) is the risk that other medicines ("OM") produce the birth defect studied ("BD"); and Risk 4 (OM→OBD) is the risk that other medications ("OM") cause other birth defects ("OBD"). In prospective studies, these associations could be estimated from the relative risks (*RR*). Similarly, in retrospective studies with non-malformed controls, the magnitude of each of these associations could be estimated by calculating the corresponding odds ratios (*OR*). As illustrated by the three-by-three table in Figure 1b, the ORs for these four associations are as follows:

$$OR_{(M \to BD)} = \frac{a \times i}{c \times g} \quad (1)$$

$$OR_{(M \to OBD)} = \frac{b \times i}{c \times h} \quad (2)$$

$$OR_{(OM \to BD)} = \frac{d \times i}{f \times g} \quad (3)$$

$$OR_{(OM \to OBD)} = \frac{e \times i}{f \times h} \quad (4)$$

These indicators are known to be sensitive to reporting bias, so different approaches including "malformed" and "only-exposed cases" controls were developed to try to reduce this bias.

Three different case-control designs were used in the present study:

a) HEALTHY design: This was the classical case-control design. Cases included those infants with any of the birth defects (alone or in combination with other birth defects). Four non-malformed controls were randomly selected for each case from all healthy newborns registered by ECLAMC in the same hospital and period. These controls showed no difference to total births with respect to maternal age, gravidity, and birth weight (Table S1; supplemental material).

Subjects were considered exposed if their mothers reported the use of the study medicine during the first trimester of pregnancy (with or without other medications) and were considered non-exposed when their mothers reported no medication use. The magnitude of this association (*OR-HEALTHY*) was calculated by the same method that was used for $OR_{(M \to BD)}$, (Figure 1b):

$$OR_{HEALTHY} = \frac{a \times i}{c \times g} \quad (5)$$

b) SICK design: This was a case-control design in which both the cases and controls were malformed. The cases were defined similarly to those in the HEALTHY design. Four newborns with birth defects other than the case were randomly selected from all malformed newborns registered by ECLAMC in the same hospital and period. The operative definition of exposed versus non-exposed was similar to that

a)

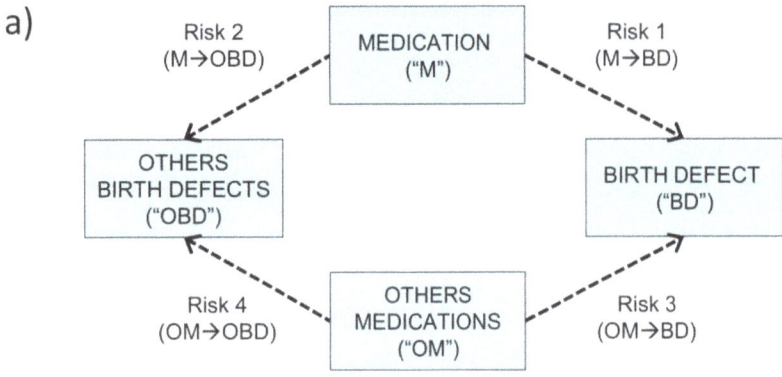

b)

	Cases with the study birth defect	Controls with malformations other than the study birth defect	Non-malformed Controls
Exposed to study medication	*a*	*b*	*c*
Exposed to other drug than the study medication	*d*	*e*	*f*
Non-exposed to any medication	*g*	*h*	*i*

Figure 1. Prenatal exposure to medications and birth defects occurrence. (a) Potential relationships between prenatal exposure to medications and birth defects occurrence in the population; **(b)** Three-by-three contingency table of malformed and non-malformed newborns with prenatal exposure to the study medication, exposure to other medications, and non-exposed; cell frequencies are represented by the letters *a, b, c, d, e, f, g, h,* and *i.*

for the HEALTHY design. The OR_{SICK} was calculated as follows (Figure 1b):

$$OR_{SICK} = \frac{a \times h}{b \times g} \qquad (6)$$

c) **OECA (Only-Exposed Cases) design:** This approach only included malformed newborns who were prenatally exposed to any type of medicine, so this is actually a subgroup of SICK. Cases and controls were defined similarly to those for the SICK design. Malformed newborns whose mothers reported the use of the study medication were considered exposed subjects, and those whose mothers reported the use of medicines other than the ones studied were included as non-exposed. The OR_{OECA} is represented as follows (Figure 1b):

$$OR_{OECA} = \frac{a \times e}{b \times d} \qquad (7)$$

Statistical methods and power

Associations between the medicines and birth defects were assessed using Odds ratios (ORs) and Pearson's chi-square test at a level of significance of 1% (P<0.01). Ninety-nine percent confidence intervals (99% CI) were calculated for all birth defects in HEALTHY design. Each birth defect was analysed separately for antiepileptics, insulin, and acetaminophen use during the first trimester of pregnancy.

For the available sample size and a medicine exposure around 1%, the minimum detectable OR is 2.0, with a power of 90% when the sample size is 2000 cases and 60% when sample size is 500 cases. Out of the 31 birth defects analysed in the present study, only two were found in less than 500 cases, and ten were found in more than 2000 cases.

Lin's concordance correlation coefficient (ρ_c) [22] was used as a measure of agreement between the three designs. This method combined measures of precision and accuracy to determine whether the $OR_{HELATHY}$ and OR_{SICK} estimates significantly deviated from the line of perfect concordance with the OR_{OECA} estimates (taken as the baseline). Lin's coefficient increases in value as a function of the nearness of the data's reduced major axis to the line of perfect concordance (a measure of accuracy of data) and of the tightness of the data about its reduced major axis (a measure of precision of data).

Bland-Altman analysis of the limits of agreement [23] was applied to compare the average difference between the designs, together with the variability of the differences and the overall trend. The correlation between the difference and mean (r_{d-m}) and the 95% limits of agreement (95% CI) were estimated and tested for significance using the Bradley-Blackwood test (F).

Potential reporting/selection biases (in percentages) were calculated according Swan et al. [10] as follows:

$$bias(\%) = \frac{(OR_i^B - OR_i^T)}{OR_i^T} \times 100$$

where OR^B ("biased" odds ratio) is the observed OR; OR^T ("true" odd ratio) is equals to 1, assuming there is not association among acetaminophen use and birth defects; and the letter i indicates SICK, OECA, or HEALTHY designs.

For each design, a linear regression model was applied to evaluate possible association between the bias and the proportion of exposed controls to acetaminophen:

$$bias(\%) = \beta_0 + \beta_1 \times Exp(\%) + e$$

where the β_0 coefficient is the bias-intercept and the β_1 coefficient evaluate the increment of bias as a function of the proportion of exposed controls (slope of the curve).

All statistical analyses were processed using Stata 12 SE (Stata Corporation, College Station, Texas).

Results

Medicine exposure during the first trimester of pregnancy

Out of the 3,939,474 total births that were registered by the ECLAMC, 58,514 newborns had a non-syndromic birth defect, of whom 48,971 had a single birth defect (83.7%), and 9,543 had two or more unrelated major birth defects (16.3%).

Table 1 summarises the frequencies of exposure to medicines during the first trimester of pregnancy among the malformed and non-malformed newborns. Twenty-six percent of the malformed newborns were prenatally exposed to some type of medication, while this percentage was around 19% among non-malformed newborns. Similar relative differences were observed between these groups for exposures to any other medication and for unknown exposures.

The frequencies of exposure to antiepileptics and insulin for malformed newborns were more than twice those observed for non-malformed babies. A minor difference between these groups was observed in the percentage of exposure to acetaminophen (Table 1). Considering only the total exposed subjects, 1.91% (294/15411), 1.48% (228/15411), and 11.60% (1788/15411) of these infants were prenatally exposed to antiepileptics, insulin, and acetaminophen, respectively.

Table 2 summarises the rate (per 10,000 births) of 30 birth defects and the frequency of medicine exposures during the first trimester of pregnancy registered by the ECLAMC in the study period.

Concordance among the three case-control approaches

When considering concordance, no significant correlation between the HEALTHY and OECA designs were observed for antiepileptics ($\rho_c = 0.07$; 95%CI: 0.02–0.11), insulin ($\rho_c = 0.06$; 95%CI: 0.02–0.10), and acetaminophen ($\rho_c = 0.02$; 95%CI: 0.01–0.04). The average difference between these designs ($OR_{HEALTHY} - OR_{OECA}$) was 6.1 (95%CI: −1.9–14.0) for antiepileptics, 11.5 (95%CI: −11.8–34.7) for insulin, and 3.0 (95%CI: 0.98–5.06) for acetaminophen. The overestimations observed for HEALTHY design were increased as higher odds ratio values were given, with high and statistically significant correlations between the difference and mean (r_{d-m}) for antiepileptics ($r_{d-m} = 0.98$; F = 863.3; P<0.001), insulin ($r_{d-m} = 0.99$; F = 976.9; P<0.001), and acetaminophen ($r_{d-m} = 0.95$; F = 1474.9; P<0.001).

In contrast, significant concordance correlations were obtained between the SICK and OECA methods for antiepileptics ($\rho_c = 0.95$; 95%CI: 0.92–0.98), insulin ($\rho_c = 0.98$; 95%CI: 0.97–0.99), and acetaminophen ($\rho_c = 0.68$; 95%CI: 0.51–0.85). There were no significant differences in the average values between OR_{SICK} and OR_{OECA} for antiepileptics (0.13; 95%CI: −0.21–0.47), insulin (0.15; 95%CI: −0.25–0.56), and acetaminophen (0.11; 95%CI: −0.17–0.39).

Significant associations identified by SICK, OECA, and HEALTHY designs

The associations between each birth defect and exposure to antiepileptics, insulin, and acetaminophen estimated by the three case-control designs are presented as smile plots in Figure 2. In each smile plot, P values are plotted on the y-axis on a reverse log

Table 1. Frequency of exposed to medicines during the first trimester of pregnancy in 58,514 subjects with single or multiple birth defects (excluding minor anomalies and syndromes) and 110,814 non-malformed newborns.

	Malformed newborns (N = 58,514)		Non-malformed newborns (N = 110,814)	
	N	% (95% CI)	N	% (95% CI)
Total newborns exposed to medicine[1]	15,411	26.3 (26.0–26.7)	20,783	18.8 (18.5–19.0)
Exposed to antiepileptics[2] (ATC code: N03A)	294	0.50 (0.45–0.56)	254	0.23 (0.20–0.26)
Exposed to insulin[2] (ATC code: A10A)	228	0.39 (0.34–0.44)	161	0.15 (0.12–0.17)
Exposed to acetaminophen[2] (ATC code: N02BE01)	1,788	3.06 (2.92–3.20)	2,730	2.46 (2.37–2.56)
Exposed to any other medicine	11,286	19.3 (19.0–19.6)	14,897	13.4 (13.2–13.6)
Unknown exposure	4,215	7.20 (7.00–7.42)	5,285	4.77 (4.64–4.89)
Total Non-exposed newborns[1]	43,103	73.7 (73.3–74.0)	90,031	81.3 (81.0–81.5)

References: (1): Prenatal medication exposure during the first trimester of pregnancy according to maternal report; (2): Exposed to the study medication, alone or in combination with other medications; (ATC code) Anatomical Therapeutic Chemical classification system.

Table 2. Number of cases; rate per 10,000 births; and frequencies of exposed to antiepileptics, insulin, and acetaminophen registered by the ECLAMC during 1967–2008.

| | Cases | | Prenatal Medication Exposure[1] | | | | | | | |
| | | | Antiepileptics | | Insulin | | Acetaminophen | | Others | |
Birth Defects	N	Rate[2]	N	%	N	%	N	%	N	%
Ambiguous genitalia/Intersexual organs, ambiguous	592	1.5	6	1.0	4	0.7	18	3.0	146	24.7
Anencephaly	1,262	3.2	6	0.5	4	0.3	27	2.1	291	23.1
Anophthalmia	527	1.3	2	0.4	3	0.6	17	3.2	126	23.9
Anorectal atresia/stenosis	1,509	3.8	6	0.4	3	0.2	47	3.1	307	20.3
Atrial septal defect	560	1.4	6	1.1	7	1.3	34	6.1	107	19.1
Axial skeleton malformation	615	1.6	4	0.7	14	2.3	12	2.0	150	24.4
Cardiac left ventricle obstructive defect	548	1.4	1	0.2	9	1.6	20	3.7	115	21.0
Cardiac outflow tract defect	496	1.3	3	0.6	7	1.4	14	2.8	96	19.4
Cardiac right ventricle obstructive defects	615	1.6	3	0.5	2	0.3	27	4.4	119	19.4
Cleft lip with or without palate	4,267	10.8	32	0.8	11	0.3	115	2.7	838	19.6
Cleft palate (included Pierre Robin)	1,439	3.7	13	0.9	6	0.4	49	3.4	295	20.5
Cystic kidney	918	2.3	8	0.9	6	0.7	49	5.3	193	21.0
Encephalocele	720	1.8	4	0.6	4	0.6	27	3.8	172	23.9
Gastroschisis	935	9.5	1	0.1	1	0.1	31	3.3	160	17.1
Hip dislocation	5,432	13.8	15	0.3	9	0.2	116	2.1	1061	19.5
Hydrocephaly	3,072	7.8	13	0.4	8	0.3	125	4.1	649	21.1
Hydronephrosis - Ureter stenosis/atresia	2,025	5.1	15	0.7	6	0.3	107	5.3	424	20.9
Hypospadias	3,390	8.6	22	0.7	11	0.3	122	3.6	701	20.7
Intestinal atresia/stenosis	928	2.4	7	0.8	6	0.7	37	4.0	191	20.6
Levo transposition of great arteries	318	0.8	0	0.0	6	1.9	11	3.5	58	18.2
Limb reduction defect	2362	6.0	8	0.3	7	0.3	65	2.8	583	24.7
Microcephaly	1,096	2.8	10	0.9	10	0.9	23	2.1	207	18.9
Multiple malposition/contractures	894	2.3	5	0.6	1	0.1	20	2.2	207	23.2
Oesophageal atresia/stenosis	1,021	2.6	1	0.1	3	0.3	28	2.7	216	21.2
Omphalocele	800	8.1	5	0.6	4	0.5	26	3.3	194	24.3
Patent Ductus Arteriosus	375	1.0	2	0.5	5	1.3	15	4.0	72	19.2
Severe ear malformation	1,838	4.7	3	0.2	13	0.7	46	2.5	362	19.7
Spina bifida	3,058	7.8	29	1.0	5	0.2	94	3.1	625	20.4
Unilateral/Bilateral kidney a/dysgenesis	524	1.3	2	0.4	8	1.5	20	3.8	118	22.5
Ventricular septal defect	2,216	5.6	9	0.4	22	1.0	116	5.2	372	16.8

References: (1): Prenatal medication exposure during the first trimester of pregnancy according to maternal report; (2) Rate per 10,000 live births.

scale against the estimated odds ratios on the x-axis. Therefore, statistically significant positive associations are plotted in the upper right quadrant of each smile plot.

A significant association between antiepileptics exposure and Spina bifida (Q05) was identified by SICK and OECA approaches. While eighteen significant associations (including Spina bifida) with ORs ranging between 2.8 and 18.3 were observed using HEALTHY design (see Figure 2, row 1). Full details of odds ratios, P values and 99% CI estimates for the association between the antiepileptic medications and each birth defect by the three approaches are shown in Table S2 (supplemental material).

Atrial septal defect (Q21.1), axial skeletal malformations (Q67.5; Q76.0–Q76.8), severe ear malformation (Q16.0 and Q17.2), and ventricular septal defect (Q21.0) showed a strong association with insulin exposure using SICK and OECA approaches. Fifteen significant associations (including the four birth defect groups

described above) with ORs ranging between 4.2 and 74.6 were identified by HEALTHY design (Figure 2, row 2). All odds ratios, P values, and 99% CI for insulin and each birth defect are presented in Table S3 (supplemental material).

There were no significant associations between the birth defects and acetaminophen (paracetamol) using the SICK and OECA designs, with the unique exception of a negative association (OR<1) with multiple joint contractures (Q74.3) using OECA approach. On the other hand, twenty-nine significant associations with ORs ranging between 2.3 and 6.3 were observed using HEALTHY design (Figure 2, row 3). Details of all odds ratios, P values, and 99% CI for acetaminophen exposure are shown in Table S4 (supplemental material).

Table 3 summarizes the statistically significant results obtained using SICK or OECA approaches. The estimated OR and P values are shown for SICK and OECA designs, while OR and

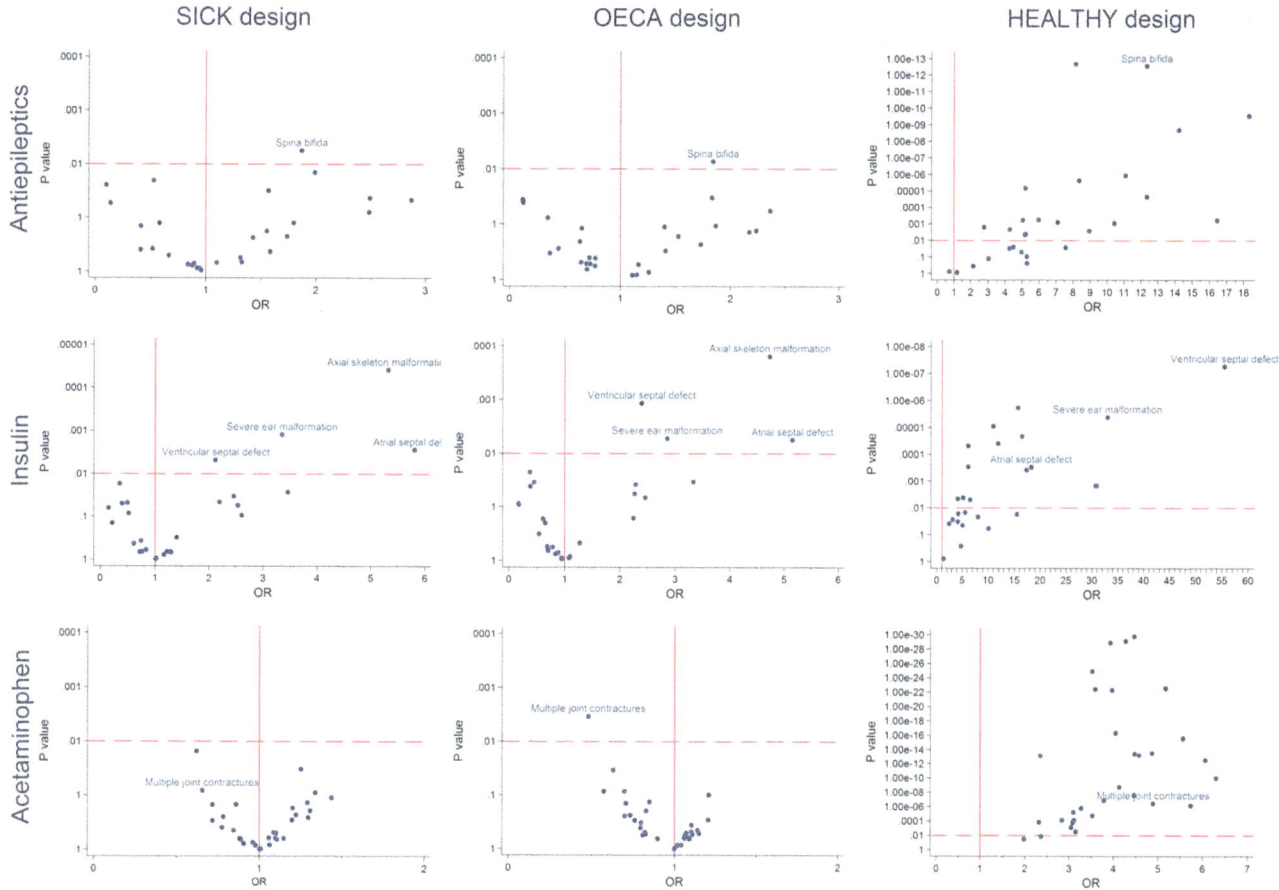

Figure 2. Associations between medications and birth defects for SICK, OECA and HEALTHY designs. The smile plots summarize the associations between each birth defect and exposure to antiepileptics, insulin, and acetaminophen for the three case-control designs. In each smile plot, P-values are plotted on the y-axis on a reverse log scale against the estimated odds ratios on the x-axis. So, the higher the P-values up the y-axis the more significant they are. The vertical full red line represents no association between medication exposure and birth defect (OR equals to 1), and the horizontal dashed red line represents the cut-off P value (0.01).

99%CI are shown for the four measures of association calculated from non-malformed controls.

Potential bias in each approach

Figure 3 shows bias as a function of the proportion of exposed controls to acetaminophen for 31 birth defect groups in the SICK, OECA, and HEALTHY designs.

The average proportions of exposure to acetaminophen in the 31 control groups (± SD) were 4.6% (±1.2); 12.9% (±2.9); and 1.3% (±0.4) for SICK, OECA, and HEALTHY design, respectively. While the mean biases (± SD) were 2.6% (±21.7) for SICK; −8.4% (±20.0) for OECA; and 293.4% (±112.1) for HEALTHY design.

No significant associations between the proportion of exposed controls and bias were detected for SICK (β_1 coeff. = −4.93; P = 0.127), and OECA (β_1 coeff. = −0.81; P = 0.526) approaches, with overall R-squared of 0.08 (F = 2.46; P = 0.127) and 0.01 (F = 0.41; P = 0.525), respectively. On the other hand, a significant decrease in bias with the increasing proportion of exposed controls was observed for HEALTHY design (β_1 coeff. = −141.0; P = 0.002), with an overall R-squared of 0.28 (F = 11.3; P = 0.002),

In addition we have calculated the associations between acetaminophen and each of 31 birth defects by the four odds ratios that use non-malformed controls (see Figure 1 and formulas

1 to 4). The average odds ratio (± SD) between acetaminophen and the birth defects studied (M→BD) was 3.9 (±1.1). Between acetaminophen and congential anomalies other than the birth defect under study (M→OBD) was 3.9 (±0.9). Furthermore, the average odds ratio observed for other medications and the birth defect studied (OM→BD) was 4.9 (±0.8), and for other medications and other birth defects (OM→OBD) was 4.4 (±0.3).

Discussion

This study evaluates the scope and limitations of three different approaches used to assess the teratogenic risk of prenatal exposure to medications, applying these methods to the data from ECLAMC's birth-defect surveillance programme. For this purpose, the association between the use of three well-known medicines during the first three months of pregnancy and the risk for 31 types of birth defects were assessed by means of case-control methodology using three types of controls: non-malformed newborns ("HEALTHY" design), malformed newborns ("SICK" design), and malformed newborns exposed to certain medications ("OECA" design).

Table 3. Statistically significant results obtained using SICK or OECA approaches.

Birth Defect	Exposure[5]	Malformed Controls				Non-malformed Controls				
		SICK		OECA		HEALTHY (M→BD)[1]		(M→OBD)[2]	(OM→BD)[3]	(OM→OBD)[4]
		OR	P value	OR	P value	OR (99% CI)	P value	OR (99% CI)	OR (99% CI)	OR (99% CI)
Spina bifida	ANTI	1.8	0.006	1.9	0.003	12.3 (5.1–30.0)	<0.00001	6.6 (2.9–14.9)	4.6 (4.0–5.2)	4.5 (4.0–5.0)
Severe ear malformation	INSU	3.4	0.001	2.9	0.005	33.0 (4.6–234.6)	<0.00001	9.9 (1.4–68.2)	5.0 (4.2–6.0)	4.3 (3.7–4.9)
Ventricular septal defect	INSU	2.1	0.005	2.4	0.001	55.5 (8.2–373.3)	<0.00001	26.2 (4.0–169.7)	3.9 (3.3–4.6)	4.4 (3.9–5.0)
Atrial septal defect	INSU	5.8	0.003	5.2	0.006	18.3 (2.3–145.3)	<0.001	3.2 (0.4–27.3)	4.4 (3.2–6.0)	3.9 (3.0–4.9)
Axial skeletal malformations	INSU	5.3	<0.0001	4.7	0.002	74.6 (5.1–689.8)	<0.00001	14 (3.2–96.7)	4.8 (3.6–6.5)	4.3 (3.4–5.4)
Multiple joint contractures	ACET	0.7	0.082	0.5	0.003	4.9 (2.2–10.9)	<0.00001	7.5 (4.1–13.6)	5.9 (4.5–7.6)	4.3 (3.5–5.3)

References: (1): (M→BD) is the risk that the study medication ("M") causes the birth defect studied ("BD"); (2): (M→OBD) is the risk that the study medication ("M") produces congenital anomalies other than the birth defect under study ("OBD"); (3): (OM→BD) is the risk that other medicines ("OM") produce the birth defect studied ("BD"); (4): (OM→OBD) is the risk that other medications ("OM") cause other birth defects ("OBD"); (5): Exposure: (ANTI) antiepileptic medications, (INSU) insulin, (ACET) acetaminophen.

Methodological considerations: measures of the association for the HEALTHY, SICK, and OECA designs

The interpretation of the measures of association obtained with the different methodological approaches using non-malformed, malformed, or exposed malformed newborns as the control groups in the research on medication teratogenicity has been extensively discussed [11–13,15,16,24]. Although some of the formulas displayed in this work (from No. 1 to No. 14) are certainly basic, we summarised this discussion and applied these basic concepts to real data from a birth defects surveillance programme in order to better understand the relationships among these measures.

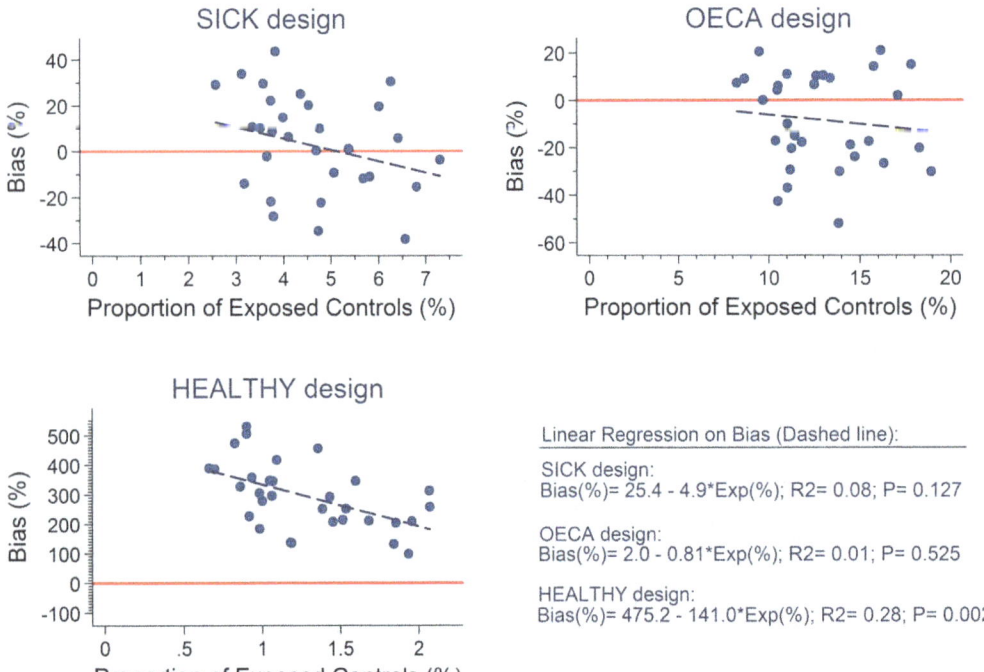

Linear Regression on Bias (Dashed line):

SICK design:
Bias(%)= 25.4 - 4.9*Exp(%); R2= 0.08; P= 0.127

OECA design:
Bias(%)= 2.0 - 0.81*Exp(%); R2= 0.01; P= 0.525

HEALTHY design:
Bias(%)= 475.2 - 141.0*Exp(%); R2= 0.28; P= 0.002

Figure 3. Bias in SICK, OECA and HEALTHY designs. The potential bias (%) is shown as a function of the proportion of exposed controls to acetaminophen (%) in the 31 birth defect groups and for the three evaluated designs. The linear function is defined as follows: Bias(%) = $\beta_0 + \beta_1$*Exp(%); R-squared (R2) and the overall P value for the regression model are shown for each design.

Beyond the control group used, these risk estimates from case-control studies of birth defects are vulnerable to both reporting bias and selection bias ([10,18,25]. Although effects of selection and reporting bias on the odds ratio are expected to act in opposite directions and it could be difficult to predict in each particular design which are of greater magnitude, both are shown to be algebraically equivalent [10]. Thus, both sources of bias could be combined through a unique term and any of the types of association (Figure 1) estimated by each OR calculated from the formulas *(1)* to *(7)* could be expressed as follows:

$$OR_i^B = OR_i^T \times k_i \qquad (8)$$

where the observed ("biased") odds ratio (OR^B) depends on the true value (OR^T) and k that indicates the effect of bias on the estimated measures of association for each particular approach (i).

If cases and non-malformed controls have differential mis-sclasification bias (reporting bias), then $k_i > 1$ and the OR^B will over-estimate the true OR^T. If, however, malformed controls are used and at least some of the malformations in the control group were positively associated with the study medication, this introduces a selection bias so-called teratogenicity non-specific bias [18], then $k_i < 1$ and the OR^T will be under-estimated. Another possibility is that cases and non-malformed controls have poor recall but with non-differential misclassification bias of exposure; or that the use of malformed controls could be to balance out the selective recall by parents of cases, then $k_i \approx 1$ and the effect of bias could be considered negligible.

It is important to note that the k_i term is a function of the ratio of the observed odds of exposure to the true odds of exposure in cases to that in controls. Therefore, it is equivalent to the "selection odds ratio" describe by Kleinbaum [26] and to the inverse of "gamma" (γ) defined by Swan et al. [10].

HEALTHY design. This is the classic retrospective case-control design (Figure 1). Considering the formulas *(1)*, *(5)*, and *(8)*, $OR_{HEALTHY}$ can be expressed as follows:

$$OR_{HEALTHY} = OR_{(M \to BD)}^B = OR_{(M \to BD)}^T \times k_{(M \to BD)} \qquad (9)$$

Therefore, this design is unable to reduce the bias ($k_{(M \to BD)}$) or quantify the magnitude of bias on the estimated $OR_{HEALTHY}$, unless the measurement of prenatal exposure has been collected before the birth-defect diagnosis (a prospective cohort design as a "gold standard").

Our results showed high-sensibility and low-specificity to detect significant associations between each of the three medications and each birth defect using HEALTHY approach. Furthermore, the overestimations that were observed using this design were increased with higher odds ratios. Thus, we might assume that most of these associations are false positive results caused by differential misclassification bias (maternal recall bias or ascertainment bias by the interviewer).

We have shown also that, at least in the case of acetaminophen, this bias effect inflates in average near to 300 percent the odds ratio and that the bias decrease with the increase of proportion of exposed controls. Therefore, if this bias acts in a similar way for different exposures, we expect a higher bias effect for rare medications. This interpretation is in agreement with our observations for antiepileptics and insulin, which have showed very low proportion of exposed and high odds ratios estimated by HEALTHY design for the majority of evaluated birth defects.

The main advantage of using non-malformed controls in retrospective studies of potential teratogens is the possibility of

estimating the "true" population odds ratio, but as it is shown in this and previous papers [10,15], the effects of bias on the observed odds ratio could be considerable and difficult to quantify. One possible approach to quantify this bias when non-malformed controls are used, is to calculate the four associations that has been proposed in this work (formulas 1 to 4), under the hypothesis that reporting bias should affect in a similar way the four odds ratios. In this paper, acetaminophen exposure showed average odds ratios around 4 for these associations, showing the lack of specificity of the association between acetaminophen and the study birth defect (M→BD), acetaminophen and other birth defects (M→OBD), of other medications and the birth defect studied (OM→BD), and other medications with other birth defects (OM→OBD). We may regard this value as a rough measure of the magnitude of the overestimation due to reporting bias in this particular study and to use it to adjust the observed measure of association between the study medication and the birth defect studied (M→BD).

Our results are in agreement with the estimate of reporting bias for the retrospective ascertainment of exposure reported by Bar-Oz et al. [15]. These authors investigated the recall bias for itraconazole exposure at least during the first trimester of pregnancy using pharmaceutical-industry data by comparing two cohorts, retrospective and prospective. The authors showed that the chances of the occurrence of a major birth defect after first-trimester exposure to itraconazole were four times higher when the woman or her physician filed the report during the postpartum period than when women were followed up prospectively. As expected, the authors showed that women whose children have major birth defects, or their physicians, are more likely to report the "exposure" than those with healthy newborns.

SICK design. This approach uses malformed newborns as the control group. Based on equations *(1)*, *(2)*, *(6)*, and *(8)*, OR_{SICK} can be expressed as follows:

$$OR_{SICK} = \frac{OR_{(M \to BD)}^B}{OR_{(M \to OBD)}^B} = \frac{OR_{(M \to BD)}^T \times k_{(M \to BD)}}{OR_{(M \to OBD)}^T \times k_{(M \to OBD)}} \qquad (10)$$

If minor birth defects and well-known associations were excluded from the analysis, and the biases were therefore dependent on the type of medication but to a lesser extent on the birth defect studied, then $k_{(M \to BD)} \approx k_{(M \to OBD)}$, and consequently:

$$OR_{SICK} = \frac{OR_{(M \to BD)}^T \times k_{(M \to BD)}}{OR_{(M \to OBD)}^T \times k_{(M \to OBD)}} \approx \frac{OR_{(M \to BD)}^T}{OR_{(M \to OBD)}^T} \qquad (11)$$

Therefore, the OR_{SICK} is a measure of the relationship between the risk of the study medication causing the birth defect studied (M→BD) and the risk of the study medication producing congenital anomalies other than the birth defect under study (M→OBD). This OR_{SICK} is then a measure of the teratogenic specificity of the medication, as previously reported [16]. If the medicine under study is associated with other birth defects, this introduces a type of selection bias known as teratogenicity non-specific bias [18], and then the SICK approach under-reports the true odds ratio. However, if the medications under study has a specific teratogenic effect, then $OR_{(M \to OBD)}^T \approx 1$ and OR_{SICK} will be a good approximation of the true odds ratio of interest ($OR_{(M \to BD)}^T$).

In the present work, acetaminophen exposure showed no significant associations using SICK approach with average odds ratios around 1.0. Moreover, the observed average bias could be considered negligible (2.6%) with no relationship with the frequency of exposure. Thus, unlike $OR_{HEALTHY}$, this approach affords the opportunity, under certain assumptions, to reduce the effect of reporting bias on the measure of association. Although it is important to reiterate that OR_{SICK} is not a direct estimate of the true population odds ratio unless there is no association between the medications and other birth defects.

OECA design. This methodology uses malformed newborns exposed to certain medications as the control group. We can develop the previous formulas *(1)*, *(2)*, *(3)*, *(4)*, *(7)*, and *(8)*, and OR_{OECA} can be expressed as follows:

$$OR_{OECA} = \frac{OR^B_{(M\to BD)} \times OR^B_{(OM\to OBD)}}{OR^B_{(M\to OBD)} \times OR^B_{(OM\to BD)}} \qquad (12)$$

$$= \frac{OR^T_{(M\to BD)} \times k_{(M\to BD)} \times OR^T_{(OM\to OBD)} \times k_{(OM\to OBD)}}{OR^T_{(M\to OBD)} \times k_{(M\to OBD)} \times OR^T_{(OM\to BD)} \times k_{(OM\to BD)}}$$

Similar to the SICK design, if the bias is mainly dependent on the kind of medication, then $k_{(M\to BD)} \approx k_{(M\to OBD)}$ and $k_{(OM\to BD)} \approx k_{(OM\to OBD)}$. On the other hand, if the bias is mainly dependent on the type of birth defect, then $k_{(M\to BD)} \approx k_{(OM\to BD)}$ and $k_{(M\to OBD)} \approx k_{(OM\to OBD)}$. Under either of these two scenarios, the measure of association can be expressed as follows:

$$OR_{OECA} = \frac{OR^T_{(M\to BD)} \times k_{(M\to BD)} \times OR^T_{(OM\to OBD)} \times k_{(OM\to OBD)}}{OR^T_{(M\to OBD)} \times k_{(M\to OBD)} \times OR^T_{(OM\to BD)} \times k_{(OM\to BD)}}$$

$$\approx \frac{OR^T_{(M\to BD)} \times OR^T_{(OM\to OBD)}}{OR^T_{(M\to OBD)} \times OR^T_{(OM\to BD)}} \qquad (13)$$

Thus, as previously reported [24], the magnitude of this association depends on a complex relationship between the risk of the study medication to cause the birth defect studied (M→BD), the risk of other medications to cause other birth defects (OM→OBD), the risk of the study medication to produce congenital anomalies other than the birth defect under study (M→OBD), and the risk of other medicines to produce the birth defect studied (OM→BD).

Despite this complex relationship, if the study medication has a specific teratogenic effect ($OR^T_{(M\to BD)} > 1$ and $OR^T_{(M\to OBD)} \approx 1$), and well-known associations are excluded from the analysis ($OR^T_{(OM\to OBD)} \approx 1$), then OR_{OECA} will be almost equal to the quotient between $OR^T_{(M\to BD)}$ and $OR^T_{(OM\to BD)}$. Therefore, the OR_{OECA} could be a measure of the degree of aetiological specificity of the defect under study. Then, if the study birth defect were related to other medications, the OECA approach would under-estimate the odds ratio of interest ($OR^T_{(M\to BD)}$). However, when the study medication is a major cause of the birth defect under study ($OR^T_{(M\to BD)} > 1$ and $OR^T_{(OM\to BD)} \approx 1$), then OR_{OECA} will be a good approximation of the true population odds ratio.

In the present study, acetaminophen exposure showed no significant associations using OECA approach and the observed average odds ratio slightly under-estimated the expected value of 1.0. Thus, as for the SICK approach and under certain assumptions, the OECA design could reduce the effect of bias on the measurement of association. Nevertheless, it cannot be considered a direct estimate of the true population odds ratio except under certain conditions as described above.

SICK vs. OECA designs

Under certain assumptions described in the formulas *(11)* and *(13)*, the relation between OR_{SICK} and OR_{OECA} can be expressed as follows:

$$OR_{OECA} \approx OR_{SICK} \times \frac{OR^T_{(OM\to OBD)}}{OR^T_{(OM\to BD)}} \qquad (14)$$

From this relation, and taking into account our results, some general considerations can be outlined:

If the observed odds ratios for the SICK and OECA designs are similar, then it can be inferred that the odds ratio between other medications and other birth defects is equivalent to the odds ratio between other medications and the birth defect under consideration ($OR^T_{(OM\to OBD)} \approx OR^T_{(OM\to BD)}$). This was observed in our results, where good concordance correlations were found between SICK and OECA designs for atiepileptics, insulin and acetaminophen. Among the significant associations found, this was mainly evident in the case of antiepileptic and spina bifida.

If $OR_{OECA} > OR_{SICK}$, then it can be concluded that other medication are associated with other birth defects to a greater extent than with the birth defect under study ($OR^T_{(OM\to OBD)} > OR^T_{(OM\to BD)}$). This was observed, for example, for insulin and ventricular septal defects although with small differences in absolute values.

On the other hand, if $OR_{OECA} < OR_{SICK}$ we would expect the opposite relationship ($OR^T_{(OM\to OBD)} < OR^T_{(OM\to BD)}$). While only minor differences were observed among the significant associations found, this was the case for, e.g. insulin and severe ear malformation, atrial septal defect, and axial skeletal malformations; and for acetaminophen and multiple joint contractures.

If other medication are associated with other birth defects in a different extent than with the birth defect under study ($OR^T_{(OM\to OBD)} \neq OR^T_{(OM\to BD)}$), then only OECA is affected while the SICK is not.

If the study medication is associated with other birth defects apart from the one studied ($OR^T_{(M\to OBD)} > 1$), then both SICK and OECA will under-estimate the true population odds ratios of interest ($OR^T_{(M\to BD)}$).

In view of these considerations and the results discussed in the present work, it is important to exclude all known associations between medications and birth defects from the control groups before obtaining odds ratios values using SICK and OECA designs.

Findings and comparison of results

Antiepileptics. The three approaches identified the recognised association between anti-epileptic exposure during pregnancy and spina bifida. When we used HEALTHY design the odds ratio for spina bifida was twelve times higher than for non-exposed mothers. A cohort study in Finland [27] found a relative risk for spina bifida of 11.3 (95%CI: 2.3–108), which is similar to that from our findings, despite the low accuracy of the estimator. Other recent studies using malformed controls found significant associations between spina bifida and monotherapy with valproic acid [14,28] and with carbamazepine [29]. Furthermore, using "exposed case-only" (like our OECA approach) and data from twelve registries of congenital birth defects (including ECLAMC), Lisi et al. [11] found significant associations between spina bifida and fatty acid (mainly valproic acid); carboxamide, and other antiepileptic medications.

In the present paper, spina bifida was the only birth defect significantly associated with antiepileptic medications using both SICK and OECA approaches. In addition to spina bifida, previous studies found significant associations between antiepileptics exposure and cardiac defects, cleft lip with or without cleft palate, hypospadias, anomalies of brain, anomalies of circulatory system, limb reduction defects, and hypertelorism [14]; and between antiepileptics exposure and hypospadias, cleft lip with or without cleft palate, polydactyly, cardiac outflow tract defects, cleft palate, limb deficiency, atrial septal defect, and craniosynostosis using OECA design [11].

Insulin. Insulin was used as an indicator of clinically significant diabetes, a well-known teratogen that can produce different types of birth defects (see review by Stothard et al. [30]). Severe ear malformation, ventricular septal defect, atrial septal defect, and axial skeletal malformations were significantly associated with insulin by SICK, OECA and HEALTHY designs in our work. With the exception of the first one, all of these associations were in agreement with Lisi et al. [11], who only used the OECA design. Unlike previous reports [11,30,31], no relevant associations were detected in our study for cardiac defects, kidney a/dysgenesis, patent ductus arteriosous, holoprosencephaly, choanal atresia, and levo transposition of great arteries.

Acetaminophen. For acetaminophen exposure, no significant associations were detected using the SICK design, while an unexpected negative association was found with multiple joint contractures using the OECA approach. The higher odds ratios observed for acetaminophen and other birth defects $(OR_{(M \to OBD)})$, and for other medications and multiple joint contractures $(OR_{(OM \to BD)})$ in relation to the two odds ratios in the denominator, could explain this last finding.

Moreover, using HEALTHY design, twenty-nine birth defects were significantly associated with acetaminophen exposure. These results disagree with a recent study conducted by the NBDPS (National Births Defects Prevention Study, USA) that showed that single-ingredient acetaminophen use during the first trimester of pregnancy does not appear to increase the risk for major birth defects [32]. Whereas acetaminophen has no proven teratogenic effect [33], the HEALTHY design in our study increased the number of false-positive associations compared to SICK and OECA designs. Interestingly, we also observed that this bias increases with decreasing proportion of exposed controls. Therefore the differences between the NBDPS study [32] and our study using the HEALTHY design could be related to the ascertainment of exposure and a different selection of controls. While NBDPS reported an average frequency of exposure of 46.9% in cases and 45.8% in controls, we observed frequencies of 3.06% and 2.46%, respectively. The NBDPS study assigned the exposure as "single-ingredient acetaminophen" consumption according to maternal medication use and the information of the Slone Epidemiology Center Drug Dictionary, which identifies product-specific ingredients. While we used a seven-digit ATC code (N02BE01) that could be a more specific exposure classification than that used in the NBDPS study, the use of other drugs together with acetaminophen cannot be ruled out in our study. In addition, the NBDPS study selected the controls from population-based registries, while our work used non-malformed controls from a hospital-based registry.

Finally, the partial discrepancies between our results for the three medications evaluated and previous reports could be due to differences in the sample size, differences in reporting the exposure, differences in the definition of the exposure, differences in the use of a specific medication in different countries, and chance or true differences in exposure risks.

Strengths and pitfalls

An important issue discussed here is the selection of control group as a potential source of bias. In this regard, it is interesting to consider the strengths and pitfalls of the present work under the framework of the three principles of comparability described by Wacholder et al. in their classical series of papers [2–4]: (1) the study base principle, (2) the deconfounding principle, and (3) the comparable accuracy principle.

Because the ECLAMC is a hospital-based program the trade-off between principles No. 1 and No. 3 is a reasonable concern, thus selection bias and information bias cannot be completely discarded. But while the selection bias could affect especially the malformed cases due to referral of prenatally diagnosed cases to hospitals serving high-risk pregnancies; we expect that the referral it be independent of the exposure assessment. Furthermore, the non-malformed controls registered by ECLAMC are not the typical "hospital controls", that is to say, that were hospitalized for some different disease than cases, but they are selected from the total newborns from each hospital that participates in the ECLAMC program. Thus, the controls are also independently selected of the exposure assessment. In the present work, the non-malformed controls were randomly selected from all healthy newborns registered by ECLAMC in the same hospital and period of time (year) as the cases, and they showed no difference to total births with respect to maternal age, gravidity, and birth weight. In this sense, given that more than 95 per cent of births in South America occur in hospitals, it could be expected that these cases and non-malformed controls are representative samples from the same study population ("the study base"). With regards to principle No. 2, it is plausible that confounding structure may be specific for the study base of each hospital and period of time. Because the confounding by a factor is theoretically eliminated by eliminating variability in that factor, we have selected a random sample of controls born in the same hospital and same year as cases (case-control ratio of 1:4) to try to control most of the underlying confounding structure.

Another potential pitfall could be that the medications were grouped as acetaminophen, antiepileptics (irrespective of the type of medication), and insulin as a proxy for diabetes. However, we believe there is no major limitation because this study attempts to analyse the performance of case-control studies using three types of controls and does not evaluate the biological significance of the medication exposures and birth defects.

The main strengths in this study are the standardised method in the diagnostic procedures for all malformed and healthy newborns included in the study, and the standardised procedure for medications reported using ATC codes. In addition, medicines and birth defects were reviewed and coded centrally.

Conclusion

Case-control designs using three control types were compared. The approach using non-malformed controls (HEALTHY) showed a high rate of false-positive results presumably caused by differential misclassification bias. We have shown also that, at least in the case of acetaminophen, this bias decreases with the increase of the proportion of exposed controls. The methods using malformed (SICK) or only-exposed cases (OECA) showed a good concordance for antiepileptics, insulin and acetaminophen. Both approaches could yield similar results, depending on the relationship of the other medications with other birth defects (OM→OBD), and the relationship of other medications with the birth defect under study (OM→BD).

SICK and OECA odds ratios cannot be considered a direct estimate of the true population odds ratio except under certain conditions. However, the SICK design could be effective to determine the teratogenic specificity of the medication, whereas the OECA approach could be useful to estimate the aetiological specificity of the defect under study.

In birth defect surveillance programs that have not access to recruit non-malformed controls, the comparison between SICK and OECA designs could provide practical information to generate hypotheses about potential teratogens.

Supporting Information

Table S1 Maternal age, gravidity and birth weight differences between the study sample of non-malformed controls and the total births in the period 1967–2008.

Table S2 Odds ratios, 99% confidence intervals, and P values of Antiepileptics exposure for birth defects, according to three case-control approaches: HEALTHY, OECA and SICK designs.

Table S3 Odds ratios, 99% confidence intervals, and P values of Insulin exposure (as a proxy of maternal diabetes) for birth defects, according to three case-control approaches: HEALTHY, OECA and SICK designs.

Table S4 Odds ratios, 99% confidence intervals, and P values of Acetaminophen exposure for birth defects, according to three case-control approaches: HEALTHY, OECA and SICK designs.

Acknowledgments

The authors want to thank all physicians collaborating on ECLAMC network.

Author Contributions

Conceived and designed the experiments: FAP JLC JAG EL EEC PM. Performed the experiments: FAP JLC JAG EL EEC PM. Analyzed the data: FAP JLC JAG EL EEC PM. Contributed reagents/materials/analysis tools: FAP JLC JAG EL EEC PM. Wrote the paper: FAP JLC JAG EL EEC PM.

References

1. Castilla EE, Orioli IM (2004) ECLAMC: the Latin-American collaborative study of congenital malformations. Community Genet 7: 76–94.
2. Wacholder S, McLaughlin JK, Silverman DT, Mandel JS (1992) Selection of controls in case-control studies. I. Principles. Am J Epidemiol 135: 1019–1028.
3. Wacholder S, Silverman DT, McLaughlin JK, Mandel JS (1992) Selection of controls in case-control studies. III. Design options. Am J Epidemiol 135: 1042–1050.
4. Wacholder S, Silverman DT, McLaughlin JK, Mandel JS (1992) Selection of controls in case-control studies. II. Types of controls. Am J Epidemiol 135: 1029–1041.
5. Elwood J, Little J (1992) Epidemiology and Control of NTDs: Oxford, Oxford University Press.
6. Elwood JM (1992) Causal relationships in medicine: a practical system for critical appraisal: Oxford University Press.
7. Infante-Rivard C, Jacques L (2000) Empirical study of parental recall bias. Am J Epidemiol 152: 480–486.
8. Coughlin SS (1990) Recall bias in epidemiologic studies. J Clin Epidemiol 43: 87–91.
9. Mackenzie SG, Lippman A (1989) An investigation of report bias in a case-control study of pregnancy outcome. Am J Epidemiol 129: 65–75.
10. Swan SH, Shaw GM, Schulman J (1992) Reporting and selection bias in case-control studies of congenital malformations. Epidemiology 3: 356–363.
11. Lisi A, Botto LD, Robert-Gnansia E, Castilla EE, Bakker MK, et al. (2010) Surveillance of adverse fetal effects of medications (SAFE-Med): findings from the international Clearinghouse of birth defects surveillance and research. Reprod Toxicol 29: 433–442.
12. Kallen B, Castilla EE, Robert E, Lancaster PA, Kringelbach M, et al. (1992) An international case-control study on hypospadias. The problem with variability and the beauty of diversity. Eur J Epidemiol 8: 256–263.
13. Kallen B, Robert E, Mastroiacovo P, Martinez-Frias ML, Castilla EE, et al. (1989) Anticonvulsant drugs and malformations is there a drug specificity? Eur J Epidemiol 5: 31–36.
14. Arpino C, Brescianini S, Robert E, Castilla EE, Cocchi G, et al. (2000) Teratogenic effects of antiepileptic drugs: use of an International Database on Malformations and Drug Exposure (MADRE). Epilepsia 41: 1436–1443.
15. Bar-Oz B, Moretti ME, Mareels G, Van Tittelboom T, Koren G (1999) Reporting bias in retrospective ascertainment of drug-induced embryopathy. Lancet 354: 1700–1701.
16. Prieto L, Martinez-Frias ML (1999) Case-control studies using only malformed infants: are we interpreting the results correctly? Teratology 60: 1–2.
17. Prieto L, Martinez-Frias ML (2000) Response to "What kind of controls to use in case control studies of malformed infants: recall bias versus 'teratogen nonspecificity' bias". Teratology 62: 372–373.
18. Hook EB (2000) What kind of controls to use in case control studies of malformed infants: recall bias versus "teratogen nonspecificity" bias. Teratology 61: 325–326.
19. WHO (2007) World Health Organization. International Statistical Classification of Diseases and Related Health Problems 10th Revision Version for 2007. Available: http://apps.who.int/classifications/apps/icd/icd10online/. Accessed May 1, 2011.
20. Castilla EE, Orioli IM, Lopez-Camelo JS (1985) On monitoring the multiply malformed infant. I: Case-finding, case-recording, and data handling in a Latin American program. Am J Med Genet 22: 717–725.
21. WHO (2010) Collaborating Centre for Drug Statistics Methodology - WHOCC. Available: http://www.whocc.no/. Accessed May 10, 2011.
22. Lin LI (1989) A concordance correlation coefficient to evaluate reproducibility. Biometrics 45: 255–268.
23. Bland JM, Altman DG (1986) Statistical methods for assessing agreement between two methods of clinical measurement. Lancet 1: 307–310.
24. Prieto L, Martinez-Frias ML (2000) Case-control studies using only malformed infants who were prenatally exposed to drugs. What do the results mean? Teratology 62: 5–9.
25. Hook EB (1993) Normal or affected controls in case-control studies of congenital malformations and other birth defects: reporting bias issues. Epidemiology 4: 182–184.
26. Kleinbaum DG, Morgenstern H, Kupper LL (1981) Selection bias in epidemiologic studies. Am J Epidemiol 113: 452–463.
27. Artama M, Ritvanen A, Gissler M, Isojarvi J, Auvinen A (2006) Congenital structural anomalies in offspring of women with epilepsy–a population-based cohort study in Finland. Int J Epidemiol 35: 280–287.
28. Jentink J, Loane MA, Dolk H, Barisic I, Garne E, et al. (2010) Valproic acid monotherapy in pregnancy and major congenital malformations. N Engl J Med 362: 2185–2193.
29. Jentink J, Dolk H, Loane MA, Morris JK, Wellesley D, et al. (2010) Intrauterine exposure to carbamazepine and specific congenital malformations: systematic review and case-control study. BMJ 341: c6581.
30. Stothard KJ, Tennant PW, Bell R, Rankin J (2009) Maternal overweight and obesity and the risk of congenital anomalies: a systematic review and meta-analysis. JAMA 301: 636–650.
31. Becerra JE, Khoury MJ, Cordero JF, Erickson JD (1990) Diabetes mellitus during pregnancy and the risks for specific birth defects: a population-based case-control study. Pediatrics 85: 1–9.
32. Feldkamp ML, Meyer RE, Krikov S, Botto LD (2010) Acetaminophen use in pregnancy and risk of birth defects: findings from the National Birth Defects Prevention Study. Obstet Gynecol 115: 109–115.
33. Scialli AR, Ang R, Breitmeyer J, Royal MA (2010) A review of the literature on the effects of acetaminophen on pregnancy outcome. Reprod Toxicol 30: 495–507.

4

Characteristic Face: A Key Indicator for Direct Diagnosis of 22q11.2 Deletions in Chinese Velocardiofacial Syndrome Patients

Dandan Wu[1,9], Yang Chen[1,9], Chen Xu[1], Ke Wang[2], Huijun Wang[3], Fengyun Zheng[4], Duan Ma[3,4]*, Guomin Wang[1]*

1 Department of Oral & Cranio-maxillofacial Science, Shanghai 9th People's Hospital, College of Stomatology, School of Medicine, Shanghai Jiao Tong University, Shanghai Key Laboratory of Stomatology, Shanghai, P. R. China, 2 Department of Oral and Maxillofacial Surgery, The Affiliated Hospital, Medical School, Qingdao University, Qingdao, P. R. China, 3 Children's Hospital, Fudan University, Shanghai, P. R. China, 4 Key Laboratory of Molecular Medicine, Ministry of Education, Department of Biochemistry and Molecular Biology, Institute of Medical Sciences, Shanghai Medical College, Fudan University, Shanghai, P. R. China

Abstract

Velocardiofacial syndrome (VCFS) is a disease in human with an expansive phenotypic spectrum and diverse genetic mechanisms mainly associated with copy number variations (CNVs) on 22q11.2 or other chromosomes. However, the correlations between CNVs and phenotypes remain ambiguous. This study aims to analyze the types and sizes of CNVs in VCFS patients, to define whether correlations exist between CNVs and clinical manifestations in Chinese VCFS patients. In total, 55 clinically suspected Chinese VCFS patients and 100 normal controls were detected by multiplex ligation-dependent probe amplification (MLPA). The data from MLPA and all the detailed clinical features of the objects were documented and analyzed. A total of 44 patients (80.0%) were diagnosed with CNVs on 22q11.2. Among them, 43 (78.2%) presented with 22q11.2 heterozygous deletions, of whom 40 (93.0%) had typical 3-Mb deletion, and 3 (7.0%) exhibited proximal 1.5-Mb deletion; no patient was found with atypical deletion on 22q11.2. One patient (1.8%) presented with a 3-Mb duplication mapping to the typical 3-Mb region on 22q11.2, while none of the chromosomal abnormalities in the MLPA kit were found in the other 11 patients and 100 normal controls. All the 43 patients with 22q11.2 deletions displayed characteristic face and palatal anomalies; 37 of them (86.0%) had cognitive or behavioral disorders, and 23 (53.5%) suffered from immune deficiencies; 10 patients (23.3%) manifested congenital heart diseases. Interestingly, all patients with the characteristic face had 22q11.2 heterozygous deletions, but no difference in phenotypic spectrum was observed between 3-Mb and 1.5-Mb deletions. Our data suggest that the characteristic face can be used as a key indicator for direct diagnosis of 22q11.2 deletions in Chinese VCFS patients.

Editor: Bart Dermaut, Pasteur Institute of Lille, France

Funding: This study was supported by the funds from National Natural Science Foundation of China (No. 81070813), Nation Science Supporting Plan (No. 2006BAI5A09), and Hospital Foundation of Shanghai Ninth People's Hospital (No. 201212). The funders had no role in study design, data collection and analysis, decision to publish, or preparation of the manuscript.

Competing Interests: The authors have declared that no competing interests exist.

* E-mail: guomin@sh163.net (GW); duanma@yahoo.cn (DM)

9 These authors contributed equally to this work.

Introduction

VCFS, also known as DiGeorge syndrome, conotruncal anomalies face syndrome, and CATCH 22, is firstly termed by *Shprintzen et al.* in 1978 and exhibits an expansive phenotype with more than 180 clinical features involving almost every organ and system [1,2]. The major symptoms include congenital heart disease, particular conotruncal malformation, characteristic face, palatal abnormality, immune deficiency, and cognitive or behavioral disorder. Its minor features involve growth retardation, neonatal hypocalcemia, feeding difficulty, hearing loss, limb deformity, and so on. The penetrance of each clinical feature is different; no single phenotype occurs in all patients, and none is obligatory [3].

VCFS is also one of the most common human genomic disorders with a population prevalence ranging from approximately 1:2000 to 1:7000 [4]. Only about 5–15% patients inherit the disease from parents, while most of them are sporadic (*de novo*) due to a heterozygous deletion caused by nonallelic homologous recombination (NAHR), mainly mediated by the low copy repeats (LCRs) on 22q11.2. Three types of deletion on 22q11.2 have been reported so far. While most the cases have typical 3-Mb deletion with breakpoints flanked by LCR A and D, some cases carry proximal 1.5-Mb deletion flanked by LCR A and B within the typically deleted region (TDR); only a few cases show atypical deletions overlapping or nonoverlapping with the TDR [5]. Researchers also found that certain cases with 22q11.2 duplication or CNVs on other chromosomes, such as 4q, 8p, 10p, and 17p, presented with clinical phenotypes similar to those of VCFS; these cases were also defined as VCFS by some geneticists and clinicians, who believed that such cases increased the diversity of genetic mechanism of VCFS [6–10].

Although recent studies have improved our understanding of the pathogenesis of VCFS, the correlations between the phenotypes and genotypes of CNVs remain ambiguous [11]. While discordant types of CNVs can occur in the cases with identical phenotypes, concordant chromosomal aberrations may result in variable expressions, even within families or between homozygotic twins [12,13]. Thus, exactly determining the specified clinical features for each type of CNVs will facilitate genetic counseling and health care.

This study has detected 55 clinically-suspected Chinese VCFS patients by MLPA, with 100 healthy subjects as control, aiming to reveal the types and sizes of CNVs in VCFS patients with different phenotypes and explore the correlations between CNVs and clinical findings in Chinese VCFS patients.

Methods

Patients

All 55 patients enrolled in this study were from the Center for Cleft Lip and Palate, Shanghai Ninth People's Hospital, Shanghai Jiao Tong University School of Medicine, and all the clinical findings in these patients were confirmed with physical or auxiliary examinations by specialists. Patients from No. 1–43 commonly presented with characteristic face and palatal abnormality, and most of them displayed other features such as congenital heart diseases, immune deficiency, and cognitive or behavioral disorders. Patients No. 44 presented with palatal abnormality, immune deficiency, mild mental retardation, low set ears, and conductive hearing disturbance. Patients No. 45–54 commonly presented with congenital heart diseases and palatal abnormality, and some of them showed other features too. Patients No. 55 presented with palatal abnormality, mild mental retardation, and conductive hearing disturbance (Table 1). The identified congenital heart diseases included tetralogy of Fallot, interrupted aortic arch, ventricular septal defect, atrial septal defect, and patent ductus arteriosus. The characteristic face consisted of vertically long face, narrow palpebral fissures, fleshy nose with a broad nasal root, flattened malar region, and retrognathia (Figure 1). The palatal abnormalities involved congenital velopharyngeal insufficiency, submucosal cleft palate, occult submucous cleft palate, and overt cleft palate. Patients who had thymic hypoplasia, T-cell deficiency, or history of recurrent infections, were diagnosed with immune deficiency. All the cognitive or behavioral disorders in VCFS patients were mild.

The present study was carried out according to the principles of the Declaration of Helsinki and approved by the Shanghai Ninth People's Hospital Ethics Committee. Written informed consents were obtained from all participants, and written permission to use the images in this study was also obtained from the participated patients or their parents.

DNA Extraction

Genomic DNA was extracted from the whole peripheral blood using QIAGEN kit (QIAGEN, Hilden, Germany) according to the manufacturer's instructions, and a concentration of 10–50 ng/uL DNA was suitable for MLPA detecting.

MLPA Analysis

The MLPA detection was performed using SALSA MLPA KIT P250-B1 DiGeorge (MRC-Holland, Amsterdam, Netherlands) according to the provider's protocol. Amplification products were detected and quantified by capillary electrophoresis on an ABI 3130XL Genetic Analyser (Applied Biosystems, Foster City, CA). Finally, the files of electropherograms were imported into and analyzed in GeneMarker software V1.8 (Softgenetics, State College, PA).

The MLPA kit used in this study contained 48 probes for 48 different genes. There were 29 probes targeting 22q11 region, among which 9 probes were between LCR A and B; 3 probes between LCR B and C; 2 probes between LCR C and D; 3 probes between LCR D and E; 4 probes between LCR E and F; 2 probes between LCR F and G; 1 probe between LCR C and D; and 5 probes in Cat Eye syndrome region proximal to LCR A. The other 19 probes located in other locus outside 22q11. Among them, 2 probes were on 4q34-qter; 3 probes on 8p23; 2 probes on 9q34.3; 6 probes on 10p14; 4 probes on17p13.3; and 2 probes on 22q13.

Each sample was detected in triplicate by MLPA, and the replicates were detected on different days.

Results

Of the 55 patients, 44 (80.0%) were confirmed with CNVs on 22q11.2 by MLPA analysis. Among them, 43 cases (78.2%) showed 22q11.2 heterozygous deletion, of whom 40 (93.0%) exhibited typical 3-Mb deletion with breakpoints between LCR A and D, while 3 (7.0%) displayed proximal 1.5-Mb deletion between LCR A and B; no case was found with atypical deletion on 22q11.2. Additionally, 1 case (1.8%) had 3-Mb duplication mapping to the typical 3-Mb region on 22q11.2 (Figure 2 and 3). None of the chromosomal abnormalities in the MLPA kit were detected in the rest 11 patients and 100 normal controls.

According to the clinical features, all 55 VCFS patients (100%) had palatal anomalies; 43 patients (78.2%) exhibited characteristic face; 40 patients (72.7%) displayed cognitive or behavioral disorders; 24 patients (43.6%) had immune deficiency; and 20 patients (36.4%) suffered from congenital heart diseases. Other features with lower frequencies were ear deformities, conductive hearing disturbance, exotropia, cleft lip, tooth hypocalcification, congenital odontosteresis, brachydactyly, syndactyly, preaxial polydactyly, digital hyperextensibility, epilepsy, hypocalcemia, growth retardation, small stature, partial sternal absence, bifid rib, cryptorchidism, hypospadias, oblique inguinal hernia, anal fistula, and hypomyotonia (Table 1). Of the 43 patients with 22q11.2del (No. 1–43), all (100%) exhibited characteristic face and palatal anomalies; 37 patients (86.0%) showed cognitive or behavioral disorders; 23 patients (53.5%) had immune deficiency; and 10 patients (23.3%) suffered from congenital heart diseases (Figure 4). The patient with 22q11dup (No. 44) displayed palatal abnormality, immune deficiency, mild mental retardation, low set ears, and conductive hearing disturbance.

Comparing the clinical findings and molecular diagnosis, we found that all the cases with characteristic faces harbored 22q11.2 heterozygous deletions, but there was no difference in phenotypic spectrum between the 3-Mb and 1.5-Mb deletions.

Discussion

As a multiple anomaly syndrome, VCFS's phenotypes are complex and diverse with expression variable in each patient. There are no definitive or minimal diagnostic criteria for this disorder, and most of the clinical findings are easy to overlap with other genetic disorders such as, Noonan syndrome, Alagille syndrome, Goldenhar syndrome, and Smith-Lemli-Opitz syndrome, as well as CHARGE and VATER associations [3]. Therefore, the clinical diagnosis of VCFS largely depends on clinicians' experience and hence is often biased or wrong. However, accurate diagnosis of this disorder is crucial for treatment [14]. Some features not presenting at birth may have

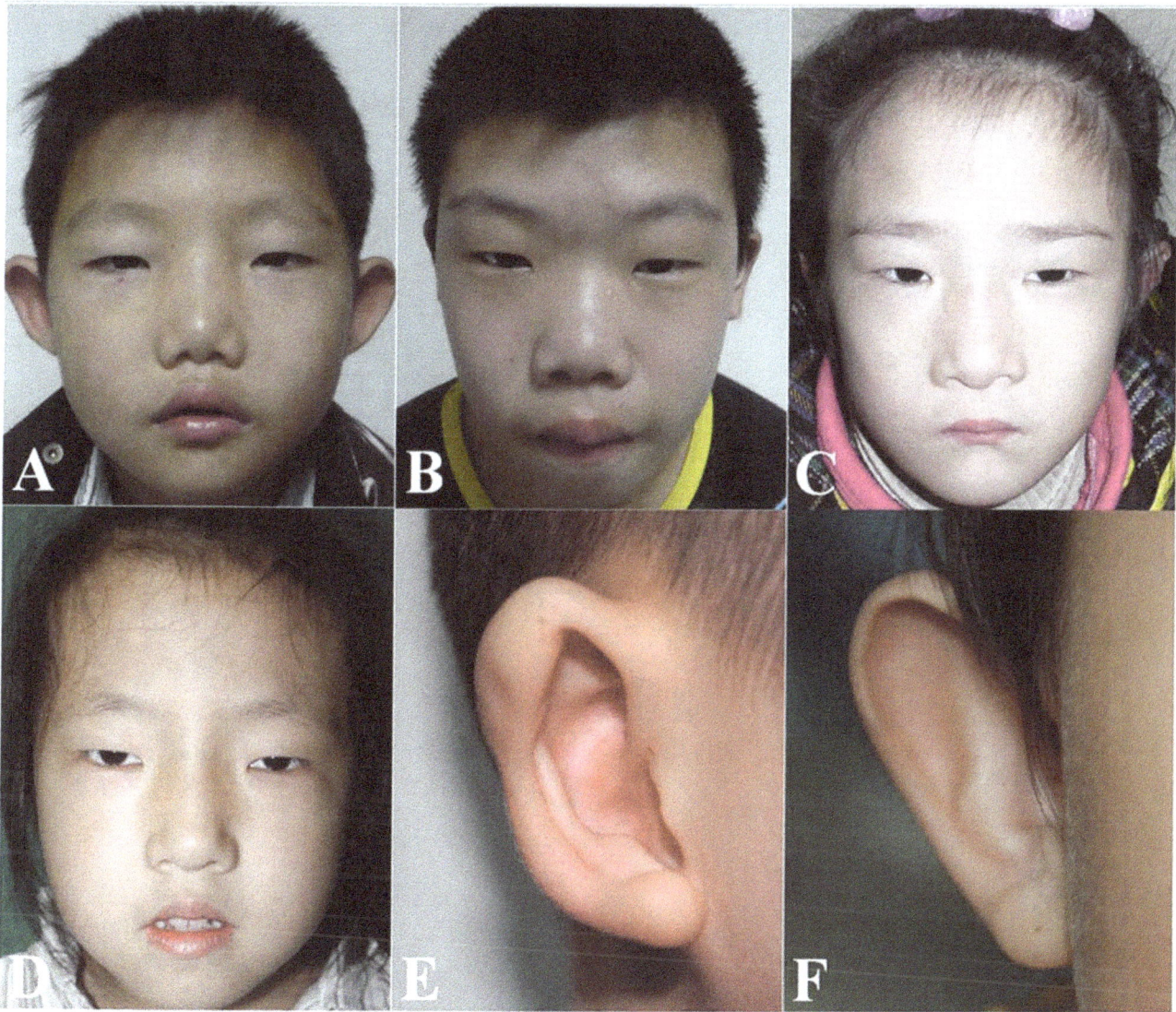

Figure 1. Characteristic face of VCFS. These Chinese VCFS patients all presented with a characteristic face, consisting of vertically long face, narrow palpebral fissures, fleshy nose with a broad nasal root, flattened malar region, retrognathia, and sometimes overfolded helix (E) or cup-shaped ear (F).

a late onset; thus, an early identification can lead to more effective therapeutic regimen with better prognosis [15].

Molecular diagnosis is considered as a more advanced and accurate method for defining VCFS [16]. Studies showed that more than 90% VCFS cases have microdeletion on 22q11.2, among which 85–90% were typical 3-Mb deletion; 10–12% proximal 1.5-Mb deletion, and only a few were atypical deletions [5]. Moreover, a small number of VCFS-like cases harboring a microduplication on 22q11.2 or CNVs on other chromosomes (4q, 8p, 10p, and 17p), such as partial monosomies and trisomies, have also been reported as etiologic heterogeneity that causes clinical variability [17]. Identification of these variant cases is of particular interest, because it may provide insight into the genes or genomic regions, which are crucial for specific phenotypic manifestations, and may help to elucidate the mechanisms of deletion and duplication [18]. Oh *et al.* analyzed phenotypes of 16 patients with 22q11.2 deletions and revealed the correlation of characteristic face and small stature with 22q11.2 deletions [19]. Rauch *et al.* stated that atypical clinical findings related to atypical 22q11.2

deletions, and that the distally nested interval of TDR containing the gene of *CRKL* contributed to major mental impairment [20]. Yatsenko *et al.* found that atrial septal defect might be the most common cardiac anomaly associated with haploinsufficiency of genes on 10p, a commonly accepted second critical region for DiGeorge syndrome [21]. However, most of the investigators failed to define any correlations between molecular diagnosis and clinical findings.

This study mainly has analyzed the major compositions of phenotypes and types of associated chromosomal aberrations and identified the correlations between CNVs and clinical features in Chinese VCFS patients. Our data indicated that 43 cases (78.2%) among all patients suspected for VCFS presented with 22q11.2 heterozygous deletions; of them, 40 (93.0%) exhibited typical 3-Mb deletion, and 3 (7.0%) displayed proximal 1.5-Mb deletion. In theory, both deletion and duplication events should occur in equal proportions, as a result of NAHR due to unequal crossovers of LCRs [22]. However, the reported frequency of 22q11.2 duplications was much lower than that of 22q11.2 deletions [23–

Table 1. Summary of patient data.

Case no.	Sex	Age (years)	Phenotypes						Molecular diagnosis
			CHD	Characteristic face	Palatal anomaly	Immune deficiency	Cognitive/ behavioral disorder	Other features	
1	M	5	+	+	+	+	+	Epilepsy	3Mb 22q11del
2	F	5	−	+	+	−	+	−	3Mb 22q11del
3	F	10	−	+	+	+	+	−	3Mb 22q11del
4	M	6	−	+	+	+	−	Hypocalcemia	3Mb 22q11del
5	F	8	−	+	+	+	+	Epilepsy	3Mb 22q11del
6	F	12	−	+	+	−	+	Low set ears	3Mb 22q11del
7	F	21	−	+	+	+	+	−	3Mb 22q11del
8	F	6	−	+	+	+	+	−	3Mb 22q11del
9	M	5	−	+	+	−	+	Cup-shaped ears, anal fistula	3Mb 22q11del
10	F	4	−	+	+	+	+	Cup-shaped ears, hypospadias	3Mb 22q11del
11	M	6	−	+	+	+	−	−	3Mb 22q11del
12	M	13	−	+	+	+	+	Cup-shaped ears	3Mb 22q11del
13	M	12	+	+	+	−	+	Hypocalcification of teeth	3Mb 22q11del
14	F	13	−	+	+	−	+	−	3Mb 22q11del
15	F	11	−	+	+	−	+	−	3Mb 22q11del
16	F	10	−	+	+	+	+	Brachydactyly	3Mb 22q11del
17	M	8	+	+	+	+	+	−	3Mb 22q11del
18	M	6	+	+	+	+	+	−	3Mb 22q11del
19	F	3	−	+	+	−	+	Growth retardation, overfolded helix, oblique inguinal hernia	3Mb 22q11del
20	M	13	+	+	+	−	+	−	3Mb 22q11del
21	M	2	+	+	+	+	+	Overfolded helix, oblique inguinal hernia	3Mb 22q11del
22	M	7	−	+	+	−	+	Cup-shaped ears	3Mb 22q11del
23	F	11	+	+	+	−	+	Cup-shaped ears	3Mb 22q11del
24	F	6	−	+	+	+	+	Overfolded helix	3Mb 22q11del
25	M	20	−	+	+	+	+	Epilepsy	3Mb 22q11del
26	M	2	+	+	+	−	−	Epilepsy, hypomyotonia	3Mb 22q11del
27	M	8	−	+	+	+	+	Growth retardation	3Mb 22q11del
28	F	4	−	+	+	+	+	Growth retardation, cup-shaped ears	3Mb 22q11del
29	M	18	−	+	+	−	+	Overfolded helix	3Mb 22q11del
30	F	5	−	+	+	+	−	Cup-shaped ears	3Mb 22q11del
31	M	3	−	+	+	+	−	Cup-shaped ears	3Mb 22q11del
32	M	14	−	+	+	−	+	Low set and cup-shaped ears	3Mb 22q11del

Table 1. Cont.

Case no.	Sex	Age (years)	Phenotypes						Molecular diagnosis
			CHD	Characteristic face	Palatal anomaly	Immune deficiency	Cognitive/behavioral disorder	Other features	
33	M	13	−	+	+	−	+	Overfolded helix	3Mb 22q11del
34	F	10	−	+	+	−	+	Overfolded helix	3Mb 22q11del
35	M	15	−	+	+	−	+	−	3Mb 22q11del
36	F	5	−	+	+	−	−	Cup-shaped ears	3Mb 22q11del
37	F	12	−	+	+	+	+	Epilepsy	3Mb 22q11del
38	M	11	−	+	+	+	+	Small stature, low set ears, congenital odontosteresis, digital hyperextensibility, cryptorchidism	3Mb 22q11del
39	F	13	+	+	+	+	+	−	3Mb 22q11del
40	M	4	+	+	+	+	+	Overfolded helix	3Mb 22q11del
41	M	17	−	+	+	−	+	Small stature, cup-shaped ears, oblique inguinal hernia	1.5Mb 22q11del
42	F	18	−	+	+	−	+	−	1.5Mb 22q11del
43	F	12	−	+	+	−	+	Cup-shaped ears	1.5Mb 22q11del
44	M	4	−	−	+	+	+	Low set ears, conductive hearing disturbance	3Mb 22q11dup
45	F	2	+	−	+	−	−	Low set ears	−
46	F	2	+	−	+	−	−	Exotropia, cup-shaped ears, syndactyly	−
47	M	7	+	−	+	−	+	Exotropia, cleft lip, preaxial polydactyly, oblique inguinal hernia, bifurcation of the left third rib, growth retardation	−
48	F	2	+	−	+	−	−	−	−
49	M	2	+	−	+	−	−	−	−
50	F	2	+	−	+	−	−	Growth retardation	−
51	M	24	+	−	+	−	−	Cleft lip	−
52	F	21	+	−	+	−	−	Growth retardation, partial sternal absence, bifurcation of the right fourth rib	−
53	F	3	+	−	+	−	−	Cleft lip	−
54	F	2	+	−	+	−	−	−	−
55	M	5	−	−	+	−	+	Conductive hearing disturbance	−

M, male; F, female; CHD, congenital heart disease; +, presence of symptoms; −, absence of symptoms or no CVNs in MLPA detection; del, deletion; dup, duplication.

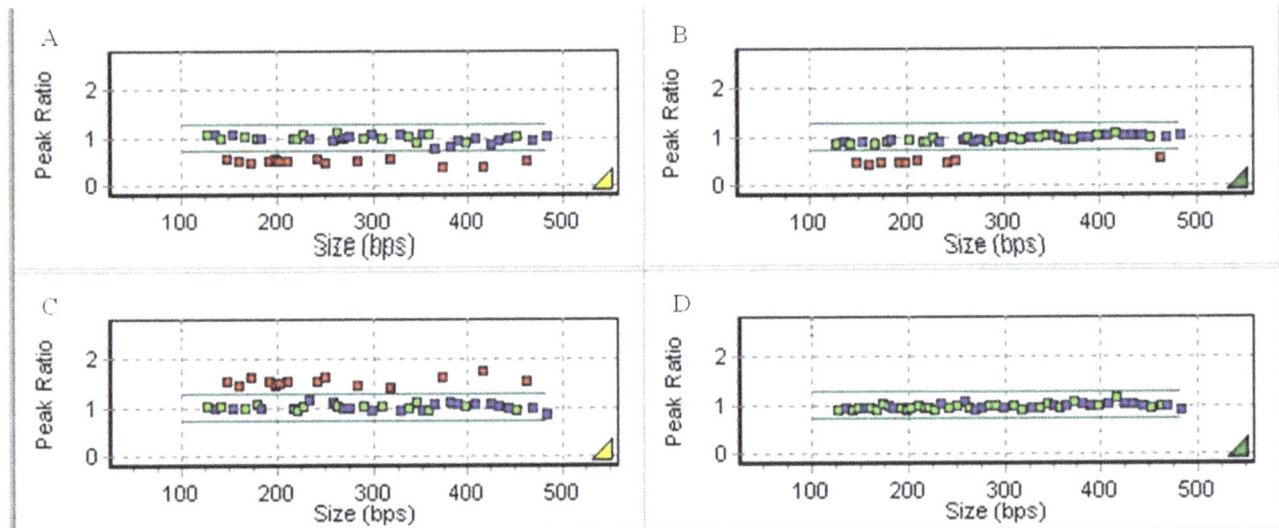

Figure 2. Data of MLPA analysis with P250-B1 DiGeorge kit. The four graphs represent four patients' data analyzed by MLPA. In each graph, the spots represent MLPA probes, the upper green line indicates a peak ratio of 1.3 and any probes above this line represent a duplication, the lower green line indicates a peak ratio of 0.75 and any probes below this line represents a deletion, and the probes between the two lines are considered as normal two copies. (**A**): A patient with 22q11.2 deletion spanning 3Mb TDR (red spots). (**B**) A patient with 22q11.2 deletion spanning proximal 1.5Mb (red spots) within TDR. (**C**): A patient with 22q11.2 duplication (red spots) mapping to 3Mb TDR. (**D**) A patient with normal copy probes.

25]. In consistence, only 1 case (1.8%) in this study showed 3-Mb duplication mapping to the TDR on 22q11.2.

In terms of phenotype, all the 43 patients (100%) with 22q11.2del displayed the characteristic face and palatal abnormalities, indicating that both features, the characteristic face and palatal abnormalities, may strongly associate with the 22q11.2 deletions in Chinese patients. The frequencies of cognitive/behavioral disorders and immune deficiency were 86.0% and 53.5% respectively, similar to those of recent reports [26,27],

suggesting that these are also common features demand more attentions during the patients' growth and development. Surprisingly, congenital heart diseases, the major symptoms of 22q11.2del according to some scholars [4,5], were observed in only 23.3% cases in this study. Variable penetrance in different races or bias in patient selection may be responsible for this phenomenon. Some investigators suggested that the absence of cardiac anomalies should not impede the clinical diagnosis for a patient with VCFS [28,29]. In addition, the clinical manifestations of thepatient with

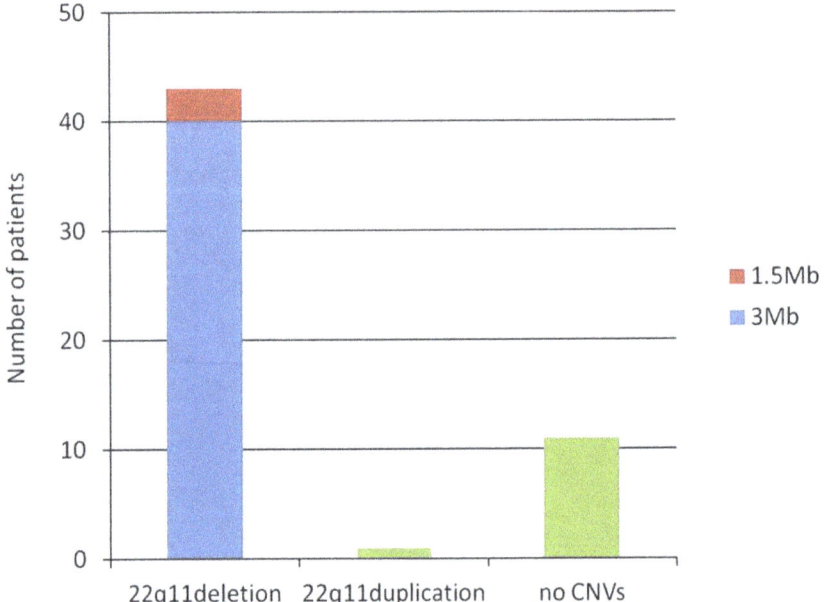

Figure 3. The results of 55 patients detected by MLPA. A total of 43 cases (78.2%) showed 22q11.2 heterozygous deletion, of whom 40 (93.0%) exhibited typical 3-Mb deletion, while 3 (7.0%) showed proximal 1.5-Mb deletion; no case was found having atypical deletion on 22q11.2. Only 1 case (1.8%) had 3-Mb duplication. None of the chromosomal abnormalities in the MLPA kit were found in the other 11 patients.

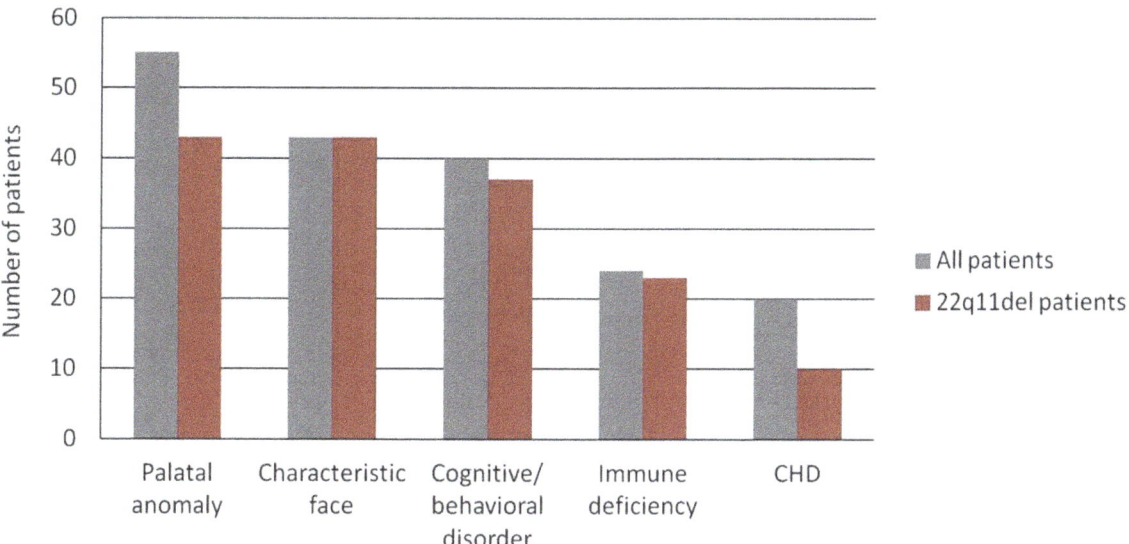

Figure 4. Number of patients presenting with major clinical features of VCFS. All cases with characteristic faces exhibited 22q11.2 heterozygous deletions.

22q11dup seem milder than those of patients with 22q11del herein. Most importantly, our data indicate that all cases with the characteristic face exhibited 22q11.2 heterozygous 3-Mb or 1.5-Mb deletion, suggesting that characteristic face that commonly presents in the majority of Caucasian individuals [30] forms an indicative factor for direct diagnosis of 22q11.2 deletions in Chinese VCFS patients. There seems to be a discrepancy between the present study and the study of Xu et al. [31], in which some of the 13 Chinese 22q11del patients did not show a characteristic face. This may be explained by that the patients in their study were mostly infants, whose facial characteristics might not have been yet recognizable, i.e., the phenotypes were not manifested yet. The phenotypic spectrums between 3-Mb and 1.5-Mb deletions show no difference in this study, which is consistent with previous reports [4,32]. The proximal 1.5-Mb region, nested in 3-Mb TDR, is considered as the critical region for the syndrome; many genes in this region have been tested for causative effects, especially *TBX1*, which has been defined as a major candidate gene for this disorder [16]. However, whether *TBX1* mutations in human cause VCFS remains controversial. Only 9 patients with VCFS have been identified to have *TBX1* mutations [33–35], while a large number of patients were determined to be negative for *TBX1* mutations [36,37], and it seems that this disease was not caused by a single gene mutation or dosage alteration, but resulted from a combined effect of many genes [38].

In comparison to the standard fluorescence *in situ* hybridization (FISH), MLPA used in this study has been recognized as a more rapid, highly cost-effective, and sensitive method for detecting various types of CNVs, especially in the 22q11.2 region [39]. It not only can identify certain atypical aberrations on 22q11.2 that the commercially available FISH probe of TUPLE1 or N25 is unable to detect, but also can provide the sizes of these aberrations simultaneously [40]. The MLPA of P250-B1 DiGeorge kit containing probes targeting 22q11 and other above described VCFS-associated chromosomes may serve as a more reliable tool for the molecular diagnosis of VCFS.

Nonetheless, the present study has limitations. Firstly, our results were obtained by analyzing 55 suspected VCFS cases;

further studies with a larger sample size may provide more detailed and accurate data. Secondly, since all the cases were from one center that mainly engages in craniofacial researches, selection bias may exist; future multicenter researches by multidisciplinary teams may avoid the possible inclusion bias. Thirdly, the 11 cases without CNVs may relate to other chromosomal aberrations out of MLPA locus, suggesting that more genetic approaches should be used in future to grasp larger sets of data. Overcoming these limitations will improve our ability to determine the types of CNVs contributing to specified abnormal phenotypes, and to eventually facilitate a more consistent application of these techniques in genetic counseling.

Conclusions

VCFS presents with variable phenotypes and diverse chromosomal aberrations. Accurate diagnosis of VCFS not only benefits the genetic counseling and patient care, but also helps patients to obtain effective therapeutic regimen and good prognosis. This study has analyzed the clinical phenotypes and molecular diagnosis of 55 Chinese VCFS patients and revealed that all the cases with characteristic face exhibited 22q11.2 heterozygous 3-Mb or 1.5-Mb deletion, indicating that the characteristic face can be used as a key indicator for direct diagnosis of VCFS with 22q11.2 deletions in Chinese patients.

Acknowledgments

We are grateful to the patients and their families for participating in our study, and being gracious with their time and effort. We also thank the research teams of Birth Defect Research Center & Pathology Research Center, Fudan University, Shanghai, China, who helped with this research.

Author Contributions

Conceived and designed the experiments: DM GW. Performed the experiments: DW YC. Analyzed the data: DW YC CX. Contributed reagents/materials/analysis tools: KW HW FZ. Wrote the paper: DW YC.

References

1. Shprintzen RJ, Goldberg RB, Lewin ML, Sidoti EJ, Berkman MD, et al. (1978) A new syndrome involving cleft palate, cardiac anomalies, typical facies, and learning disabilities: velo-cardio-facial syndrome. Cleft Palate J 15: 56–62.

2. Shprintzen RJ (2000) Velo-cardio-facial syndrome: a distinctive behavioral phenotype. Ment Retard Dev Disabil Res Rev 6: 142–147.

3. Robin NH, Shprintzen RJ (2005) Defining the clinical spectrum of deletion 22q11.2. J Pediatr 147: 90–96.

4. Shprintzen RJ (2008) Velo-cardio-facial syndrome: 30 Years of study. Dev Disabil Res Rev 14: 3–10.

5. Gothelf D, Frisch A, Michaelovsky E, Weizman A, Shprintzen RJ (2009) Velo-Cardio-Facial Syndrome. J Ment Health Res Intellect Disabil 2: 149–167.

6. Portnoï MF (2009) Microduplication 22q11.2: a new chromosomal syndrome. Eur J Med Genet 52: 88–93.

7. Tsai CH, Van Dyke DL, Feldman GL (1999) Child with velocardiofacial syndrome and del (4)(q34.2): another critical region associated with a velocardiofacial syndrome-like phenotype. Am J Med Genet 82: 336–339.

8. Devriendt K, De Mars K, De Cock P, Gewillig M, Fryns JP (1995) Terminal deletion in chromosome region 8p23.1–8pter in a child with features of velo-cardio-facial syndrome. Ann Genet 38: 228–230.

9. Van Esch H, Groenen P, Fryns JP, Van de Ven W, Devriendt K (1999) The phenotypic spectrum of the 10p deletion syndrome versus the classical DiGeorge syndrome. Genet Couns 10: 59–65.

10. Greenberg F, Courtney KB, Wessels RA, Huhta J, Carpenter RJ, et al. (1988) Prenatal diagnosis of deletion 17p13 associated with DiGeorge anomaly. Am J Med Genet 31: 1–4.

11. Friedman MA, Miletta N, Roe C, Wang D, Morrow BE, et al. (2011) Cleft palate, retrognathia and congenital heart disease in velo-cardio-facial syndrome: a phenotype correlation study. Int J Pediatr Otorhinolaryngol 75: 1167–1172.

12. Bassett AS, Chow EW, Husted J, Weksberg R, Caluseriu O, et al. (2005) Clinical features of 78 adults with 22q11 deletion syndrome. Am J Med Genet A 138: 307–313.

13. Driscoll DA, Boland T, Emanuel BS, Kirschner RE, LaRossa D, et al. (2006) Evaluation of Potential Modifiers of the Palatal Phenotype in the 22q11.2 Deletion Syndrome. Cleft Palate Craniofac J 43: 435–441.

14. McDonald-McGinn DM, Sullivan KE (2011) Chromosome 22q11.2 deletion syndrome (DiGeorge syndrome/velocardiofacial syndrome). Medicine (Baltimore) 90: 1–18.

15. Looman WS, Thurmes AK, O'Conner-Von SK (2010) Quality of life among children with velocardiofacial syndrome. Cleft Palate Craniofac J 47: 273–283.

16. Kobrynski IJ, Sullivan KE (2007) Velocardiofacial syndrome, DiGeorge syndrome: the chromosome 22q11.2 deletion syndromes. Lancet 370: 1443–1452.

17. Fernández L, Lapunzina P, Pajares IL, Palomares M, Martínez I, et al. (2008) Unrelated chromosomal anomalies found in patients with suspected 22q11.2 deletion. Am J Med Genet A 146A: 1134–1141.

18. Emanuel BS (2008) Molecular mechanisms and diagnosis of chromosome 22q11.2 rearrangements. Dev Disabil Res Rev 14: 11–18.

19. Oh AK, Workman LA, Wong GB (2007) Clinical correlation of chromosome 22q11.2 fluorescent in situ hybridization analysis and velocardiofacial syndrome. Cleft Palate Craniofac J 44: 62–66.

20. Rauch A, Zink S, Zweier C, Thiel CT, Koch A, et al. (2005) Systematic assessment of atypical deletions reveals genotype-phenotype correlation in 22q11.2. J Med Genet 42: 871–876.

21. Yatsenko SA, Yatsenko AN, Szigeti K, Craigen WJ, Stankiewicz P, et al. (2004) Interstitial deletion of 10p and atrial septal defect in DiGeorge 2 syndrome. Clin Genet 66: 128–136.

22. Ensenauer RE, Adeyinka A, Flynn HC, Michels VV, Lindor NM, et al. (2003) Microduplication 22q11.2, an emerging syndrome: clinical, cytogenetic, and molecular analysis of thirteen patients. Am J Hum Genet 73: 1027–1040.

23. Wentzel C, Fernström M, Ohrner Y, Annerén G, Thuresson AC (2008) Clinical variability of the 22q11.2 duplication syndrome. Eur J Med Genet 51: 501–510.

24. Ou Z, Berg JS, Yonath H, Enciso VB, Miller DT, et al. (2008) Microduplications of 22q11.2 are frequently inherited and are associated with variable phenotypes. Genet Med 10: 267–277.

25. Lundin J, Söderhäll C, Lundén L, Hammarsjö A, White I, et al. (2010) 22q11.2 microduplication in two patients with bladder exstrophy and hearing impairment. Eur J Med Genet 53: 61–65.

26. Kitsiou-Tzeli S, Kolialexi A, Fryssira H, Galla-Voumvouraki A, Salavoura K, et al. (2004) Detection of 22q11.2 deletion among 139 patients with Di George/Velocardiofacial syndrome features. In Vivo 18: 603–608.

27. Sandrin-Garcia P, Abramides DV, Martelli LR, Ramos ES, Richieri-Costa A, et al. (2007) Typical phenotypic spectrum of velocardiofacial syndrome occurs independently of deletion size in chromosome 22q11.2. Mol Cell Biochem 303: 9–17.

28. Lipson AH, Yuille D, Angel M, Thompson PG, Vandervoord JG, et al. (1991) Velocardiofacial (Shprintzen) syndrome: an important syndrome for the dysmorphologist to recognise. Med Genet 28: 596–604.

29. Sandrin-Garcia P, Richieri-Costa A, Tajara EH, Carvalho-Salles AB, Fett-Conte AC (2007) Fluorescence in situ hybridization (FISH) screening for the 22q11.2 deletion in patients with clinical features of velocardiofacial syndrome but without cardiac anomalies. Genet Mol Biol 30: 21–24.

30. McDonald-McGinn DM, Minugh-Purvis N, Kirschner RE, Jawad A, Tonnesen MK, et al. (2005) The 22q11.2 deletion in African-American patients: an underdiagnosed population? Am J Med Genet A 134: 242–246.

31. Xu YJ, Wang J, Xu R, Zhao PJ, Wang XK, et al. (2011) Detecting 22q11.2 deletion in Chinese children with conotruncal heart defects and single nucleotide polymorphisms in the haploid TBX1 locus. BMC Med Genet 12: 169–177.

32. Paylor R, Lindsay E (2006) Mouse models of 22q11 deletion syndrome. Biol Psychiatry 59: 1172–1179.

33. Yagi H, Furutani Y, Hamada H, Sasaki T, Asakawa S, et al. (2003) Role of TBX1 in human del22q11.2 syndrome. Lancet 362: 1366–1373.

34. Paylor R, Glaser B, Mupo A, Ataliotis P, Spencer C, et al. (2006) Tbx1 haploinsufficiency is linked to behavioral disorders in mice and humans: implications for 22q11 deletion syndrome. Proc Natl Acad Sci USA 103: 7729–7734.

35. Zweier C, Sticht H, Aydin-Yaylagül I, Campbell CE, Rauch A (2007) Human TBX1 missense mutations cause gain of function resulting in the same phenotype as 22q11.2 deletions. Am J Hum Genet 80: 510–517.

36. Gong W, Gottlieb S, Collins J, Blescia A, Dietz H, et al. (2001) Mutation analysis of TBX1 in non-deleted patients with features of DGS/VCFS or isolated cardiovascular defects. J Med Genet 38: E45.

37. Conti E, Grifone N, Sarkozy A, Tandoi C, Marino B, et al. (2003) DiGeorge subtypes of nonsyndromic conotruncal defects: evidence against a major role of TBX1 gene. Eur J Hum Genet 11: 349–351.

38. Scambler PJ (2000) The 22q11 deletion syndromes. Hum Mol Genet 9: 2421–2426.

39. Vorstman JA, Jalali GR, Rappaport EF, Hacker AM, Scott C, et al. (2006) MLPA: a rapid, reliable, and sensitive method for detection and analysis of abnormalities of 22q. Hum Mutat 27: 814–821.

40. Jalali GR, Vorstman JA, Errami A, Vijzelaar R, Biegel J, et al. (2008) Detailed analysis of 22q11.2 with a high density MLPA probe set. Hum Mutat 29: 433–440.

5

The Ciliary Protein Ftm is Required for Ventricular Wall and Septal Development

Christoph Gerhardt, Johanna M. Lier, Stefanie Kuschel, Ulrich Rüther*

Institute for Animal Developmental and Molecular Biology, Heinrich Heine University, Düsseldorf, Germany

Abstract

Ventricular septal defects (VSDs) are the most common congenital heart defects in humans. Despite several studies of the molecular mechanisms involved in ventricular septum (VS) development, very little is known about VS-forming signaling. We observed perimembranous and muscular VSDs in *Fantom* (*Ftm*)-negative mice. Since Ftm is a ciliary protein, we investigated presence and function of cilia in murine hearts. Primary cilia could be detected at distinct positions in atria and ventricles at embryonic days (E) 10.5–12.5. The loss of Ftm leads to shortened cilia and a reduced proliferation in distinct atrial and ventricular ciliary regions at E11.5. Consequently, wall thickness is diminished in these areas. We suggest that ventricular proliferation is regulated by cilia-mediated Sonic hedgehog (Shh) and platelet-derived growth factor receptor α (Pdgfrα) signaling. Accordingly, we propose that primary cilia govern the cardiac proliferation which is essential for proper atrial and ventricular wall development and hence for the fully outgrowth of the VS. Thus, our study suggests ciliopathy as a cause of VSDs.

Editor: Robert Dettman, Northwestern University, United States of America

Funding: This work was supported by the Deutsche Forschungsgemeinschaft (Sonderforschungsbereiche 590 and 612) to U.R. The funders had no role in study design, data collection and analysis, decision to publish, or preparation of the manuscript.

Competing Interests: The authors have declared that no competing interests exist.

* E-mail: ruether@hhu.de

Introduction

One of 100 newborns suffers from a congenital heart defect [1]. Among these human congenital cardiac diseases ventricular septal defects (VSDs) are the most common [2,3] and occur in approximately 1 of 1000 births [4]. The most prevalent VSD subtype is the perimembranous VSD [5,6] which is characterized by the loss of the membranous part of the ventricular septum (VS) and a defect in the development of a second part of the VS - the muscular septum. Interestingly, the membranous VS does not start to grow before the muscular VS generation has been finished [7] indicating that membranous VS development is probably initiated by an interaction of the inlet muscular VS and the atrioventricular endocardial cushion cells (ECCs) [8,9] The membranous VS arises solely from the ECCs and not from the muscular VS [4]. Although the molecular background of muscular VS development is only poorly understood [10,11], two different hypothesis have been debated for its formation and outgrowth. The first theory describes VS generation as an active process of cell growth in the apical region of the muscular septum [12,13], while the second ascribes muscular septal length gain to a passive process based on the increase of the ventricular cavities. According to this hypothesis, the formation of the muscular septum is carried out by proliferation of cells at distinct regions in the left and right ventricle [14–17], so that it consists of cardiomyocytes with both left-ventricular and right-ventricular identities [11,18,19].

Ftm (alias Rpgrip1l)-negative mice display abnormal heart development particularly a VSD and suffer from a dysfunction of primary cilia [20] indicating a potential relation between heart formation and ciliary action. The Ftm protein is localised at the base of cilia [20] and appears to be present at every cilium. The

fact that mutations of *FTM* in humans were already found in ciliopathies like Meckel-Gruber syndrome, Joubert syndrome and nephronophthisis [21,22] accentuates the importance of this gene in human development.

Primary cilia are hairlike, 1–15 μm long protrusions on most vertebrate cells. They function as the cells "antenna" receiving and mediating signals from the environment. These signals, in turn, control important cellular processes like proliferation, apoptosis, migration, differentiation and cell cycle regulation [23]. Consequently, defective primary cilia provoke severe human diseases [24]. Several signaling pathways are thought to be associated with cilia, including Sonic hedgehog (Shh), platelet-derived growth factor receptor α (Pdgfrα) as well as canonical and non-canonical Wnt signaling [25–35]. While the connection between cilia and Wnt signaling has been frequently discussed and remains the subject of fierce debate [34–36], it is well-known that Shh and Pdgfrα signaling can be mediated by cilia [25–27,29,30,35].

Shh is a member of the Hedgehog (Hh) family of evolutionary conserved signaling molecules and binds to its receptor Patched (Ptc) which in vertebrates is localized in the ciliary membrane and regulates the activity of Smoothened (Smo), a seven-transmembrane receptor. Recruited to the cilium active Smo invokes Glioblastoma (Gli) transcription factors. In vertebrates three Gli isoforms exist – Gli1, 2 and 3. They regulate the expression of Shh target genes like for example *Ptc1* and thereby cell differentiation, proliferation, survival and growth [37,38]. Gli1 functions as a constitutive activator [39,40], whereas Gli2 and Gli3 have a C-terminal transcriptional activator domain and a N-terminal transcriptional repressor domain [41]. Full-length Gli3 (Gli3-

190) protein can be transformed into a transcriptional activator (Gli3-A) most likely by modifications [42,43]. Importantly, the full-length protein can be proteolytically processed into a transcriptional repressor (Gli3-R, also known as Gli3-83) [44]. The ratio of activator and repressor forms controls cellular processes dependend on Shh signaling.

Signaling by Pdgfrα relates also to cilia [29]. Pdgfrα is localized to cilia and becomes dimerized and phosphorylated after being bound by its ligand Pdgf-AA which also functions as a dimer. Activated Pdgf receptors regulate essential cell processes like proliferation, anti-apoptosis, migration, differentiation, actin reorganization and cell growth [45–47]. Stimulation of Pdgfrα drives the activation of signal transduction through the Mek1/2-Erk1/2 and Akt/PKB pathways mediated by primary cilia, whereas Pdgfrα signaling gets blocked in the absence of cilia [29].

We used *Ftm*-deficient mice to investigate whether cardiac cilia are functionally involved in heart development, especially in VS formation. Furthermore, we analysed which signals are mediated by these cilia. We were able to identify components of Shh and Pdgfrα signaling pathways in or at ventricular cilia giving evidence that these signals are cilia-mediated in embryonic murine hearts. According to ciliary dysfunction caused by Ftm deficiency [21,48,49], Shh and Pdgfrα signaling are downregulated in *Ftm*-negative ventricles. We propose these signaling defects as the cause of reduced ventricular cell proliferation that in turn results in diminished ventricular wall thickness and VSDs.

Materials and Methods

Ethics Statement and Animal Husbandry

All mice (Mus musculus) used in this study were on the C3H background and kept under standard housing conditions with a 12/12 hours dark-light cycle and with food and water ad libitum. All experiments were performed in accordance with the relevant national guidelines for the Care and Use of Laboratory Animals, with approval from the authority for animal work at the Heinrich Heine University (Permit Number: O18/99). Generation of *Ftm* mutant mice was designed and carried out as described [20].

Antibodies

We used primary antibodies to actin (Sigma #A2066), Arl13b (Proteintech #17711-1-AP), Gapdh (Sigma #G8795), acetylated α-tubulin (Sigma #T6793), γ-tubulin (Sigma #T6557), detyrosinated tubulin (Millipore #AB3201), BrdU (Developmental Studies Hybridoma Bank #G3G4), Pdgfrα (Santa Cruz #sc-338), pericentrin (Covance #PRB-432C), pMek1/2 (Cell Signaling Technology #9121), Gli3 (kindly gift of B. Wang), Gli3 (R&D systems #AF3690), ErbB3 (Santa Cruz #sc-285), DDR2 (kindly gift of E.C. Goldsmith) and Tropomyosin (AbD Serotec #9200-0504). The creation of polyclonal antibodies against Ftm was delineated formerly [20]. Polyclonal antibodies to Gli3-190 were generated by immunizing rabbits with a His-Gli3 fusion protein encompassing the Gli3-C-terminal region (3473–4806 bp) by Pineda antibody services. Antibodies were affinity-purified with the antigen coupled to Ni-NTA agarose (Qiagen #30230).

Apoptosis Studies

Apoptotic nuclei were labeled *in situ* by the TdT-mediated dUTP-biotin nick end labeling (TUNEL) method [50] using Apop Taq Plus Peroxidase *in situ* Apoptosis Kit (Millipore #S7101) and following manufacturer's instructions.

Genotyping

Genotyping of the mice was performed as previously described [20].

Histochemistry

Histochemical stainings were performed as described [20].

Histology and Paraffin Embedding

Embryos were dissected and fixed in 4% paraformaldehyde (PFA) overnight at 4°C. Then they were serially dehydrated using ethanol, embedded in paraffin and sectioned (12 μm). Afterwards, sections were stained with hematoxylin and eosin or used for *in situ* hybridisation.

Immunofluorescence

Embryos were fixed in 4% PFA and incubated in 30% sucrose (in PBS) overnight at 4°C. Next day they were embedded in Tissue-Tek O.C.T. compound (Sakura Finetechnical #4583) and then stored at −80°C. Transverse cryostat sections (7 μm in thickness) were prepared, washed with PBS and permeabilized with PBS/0.5% Triton-X-100. Blocking was performed with 10% FCS in PBS/0.1% Triton-X-100. The sections then were incubated with the primary antibodies diluted in blocking solution overnight at 4°C. After three washing steps, they underwent an incubation in the secondary antibody (diluted in blocking solution) for 2 hours and then were washed again. Finally, they were embedded in Mowiol containing DAPI (Merck #1.24653).

In situ Hybridisation

In situ hybridisation on paraffin sections were performed as previously described [51].

Proliferation Studies

Mice received an intraperitoneal injection of 10 μl BrdU (Sigma #B5002-1G) per g body weight 2 hours before they were killed. After killing embryos were dissected and embedded in Tissue-Tek O.C.T. compound (Sakura Finetechnical #4583) as described before. Cryosections were undergone BrdU immunohistochemical stainings like described before with the exception of two additionally steps after the first washings: These steps include incubation in 2 N HCl for 10 minutes at 37°C and then in 50% formamide/2×SSC for 45 minutes at 65°C. Anti-BrdU (Developmental Studies Hybridoma Bank #G3G4) antibody was used as primary antibody.

Real-time PCR Analysis

Atrial and ventricular RNA was isolated by using RNeasy Kit (Qiagen #74104) and RNase-Free DNase Set (Qiagen #79254). Isolated RNA was converted into cDNA by utilising Expand Reverse Transcriptase (Roche #11785826001). Quantitative Real-time PCR was carried out by employing a Step One Real-Time PCR System Thermal Cycling Block (Applied Biosystems #4376357) and the TaqMan Universal PCR Master Mix, No AmpErase UNG (Applied Biosystems #4324020). The following primer/TaqMan probe sets were used: *Gapdh* (Assay ID: Mm99999915_g1), *Ptc1* (Assay ID: Mm00970977_m1) and *Hif1α* (Assay ID: Mm00468878_m1). Real-time PCR was carried out with 50 ng of cardiac cDNA of each sample in triplicate reactions in a 20 μl volume containing 100 nM primers and 50 nM probe. Cycling conditions were 50°C for 2 minutes and 95°C for 10 minutes, followed by a 40-cycle amplification of 95°C for 15 seconds and 60°C for 1 minute. The analysis of real-time data was performed by using included StepOne Software version 2.0.

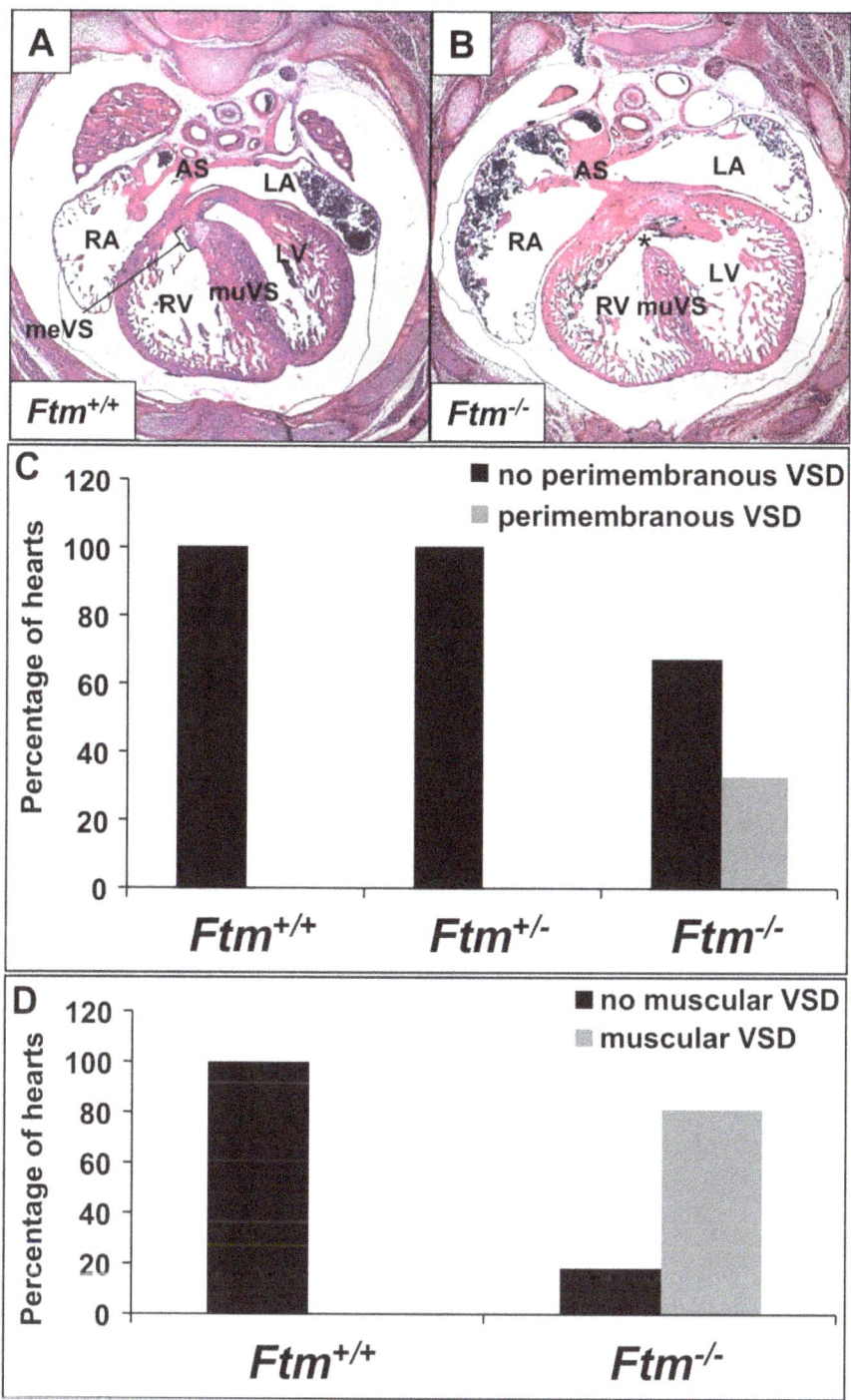

Figure 1. *Ftm*-deficient murine embryos show perimembranous and muscular ventricular septal defects. (A, B) Hematoxylin and Eosin stainings at E14.5 on transverse heart sections. (A) In wild-type mouse embryos, the ventricular septum consists of a muscular part (muVS) and a membranous part (meVS). (B) In *Ftm*$^{-/-}$ embryos, the muscular VS displays a shorter and thinner shape and the membranous VS is missing (indicated by the asterisk) representing a perimembranous ventricular septal defect. (C) While in *Ftm*$^{+/+}$ (n = 23) and *Ftm*$^{+/-}$ mice (n = 21) the heart develops normally, 33% of *Ftm*$^{-/-}$ mice (n = 27) show perimembranous ventricular septal defects. This statistics is based on investigations of mice at E13.5, E14.5, E15.5, E16.5 and E17.5. (D) *Ftm*$^{+/+}$ mouse embryos (n = 23) do not suffer from muscular ventricular septal defects. 81.5% of all analyzed *Ftm*$^{-/-}$ embryos (n = 27) display muscular ventricular septal defects. Embryos at E13.5, E14.5, E15.5, E16.5 and E17.5 were examined in this context. LA, left atrium; RA, right atrium; LV, left ventricle; RV, right ventricle; meVS, membranous ventricular septum; muVS, muscular ventricular septum; AS, atrial septum.

Semiquantitative PCR Analysis

RNeasy Kit (Qiagen #74104) was used to isolate mRNA from pooled embryonic hearts (E11.5). Reverse transcription was carried out by utilising High Capacity RNA-to-cDNA Master Mix (Applied Biosystems #4390777). The sets of primers were as following: *Hprt*: 5′-CAC AGG ACT AGA ACA CCT GC

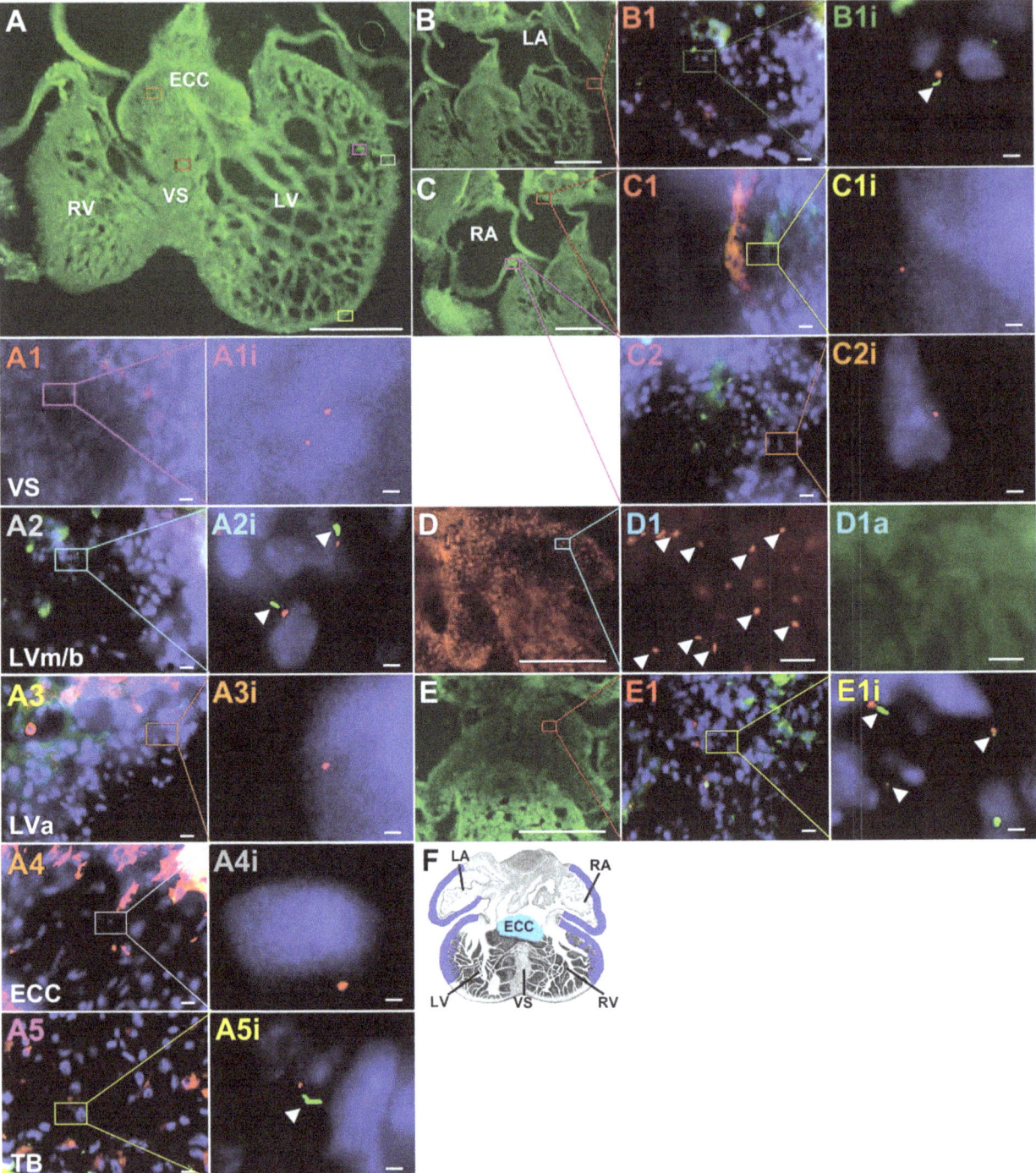

Figure 2. Distribution of primary cilia in murine embryonic hearts. (A, B, C, D, E, A1–5, B1, C1+2, D1, E1, A1i–A5i, B1i, C1i, C2i, D1a, E1i) Immunofluorescence on transverse heart sections at E12.5. (A, B, C) Tubulin cytoskeleton of cardiac cells is stained in green by acetylated α-tubulin resulting in a total view of ventricles (A) and atria (B, C). Cilia are stained in green by acetylated α-tubulin, basal bodies in red by pericentrin and cell nuclei in blue by DAPI (A1–5, B1, C1+2, A1i–A5i, B1i, C1i, C2i). Scale bars (in white) represent a length of 0.5 mm (A, B, C, D, E), 10 μm (A1–5, B1, C1+2, D1, D1a, E1) or 2 μm (A1i–A5i, B1i, C1i, C2i, E1i). (A, B, C, D, E) Coloured squares mark cardiac regions which are presented magnified in A1–5, B1, C1+2, D1+1a and E1. (A1–A5, B1, C1+2, E1) Coloured squares mark cardiac regions which are shown magnified in A1i-A5i, B1i, C1i, C2i and E1i. (A, B, C, D, E, A1–A5, B1, C1, C2, D1, D1a, E1, A1i–A5i, B1i, C1i+2i, E1i) The colour of the square correlates with the colour of the number of the magnified figures. (D) Arl13b is stained in red resulting in a total view of ECCs. (D1) Arl13b staining reveals ciliary presence on ECCs, while these cilia cannot be detected by staining acetylated α-tubulin in green (D1a). (E) Tubulin cytoskeleton of cardiac cells is stained in green by detyrosinated tubulin resulting in a total view of the ECCs. (E1, E1i) Cilia are stained in green by detyrosinated tubulin, basal bodies in red by γ-tubulin and cell nuclei in blue by DAPI. (F) Schematic illustration of ciliary distribution in embryonic mouse hearts. We found cilia exclusively at E10.5–12.5 and solely in distinct ventricular and atrial regions (blue lines) and on ECCs (turquoise staining). ECC, endocardial cushion cells; LA, left atrium; RA, right atrium; LV, left ventricle; LVa, left ventricle apical; LVm/b left ventricle medial/basal; RV, right ventricle; TB, trabecular formations; VS, ventricular septum.

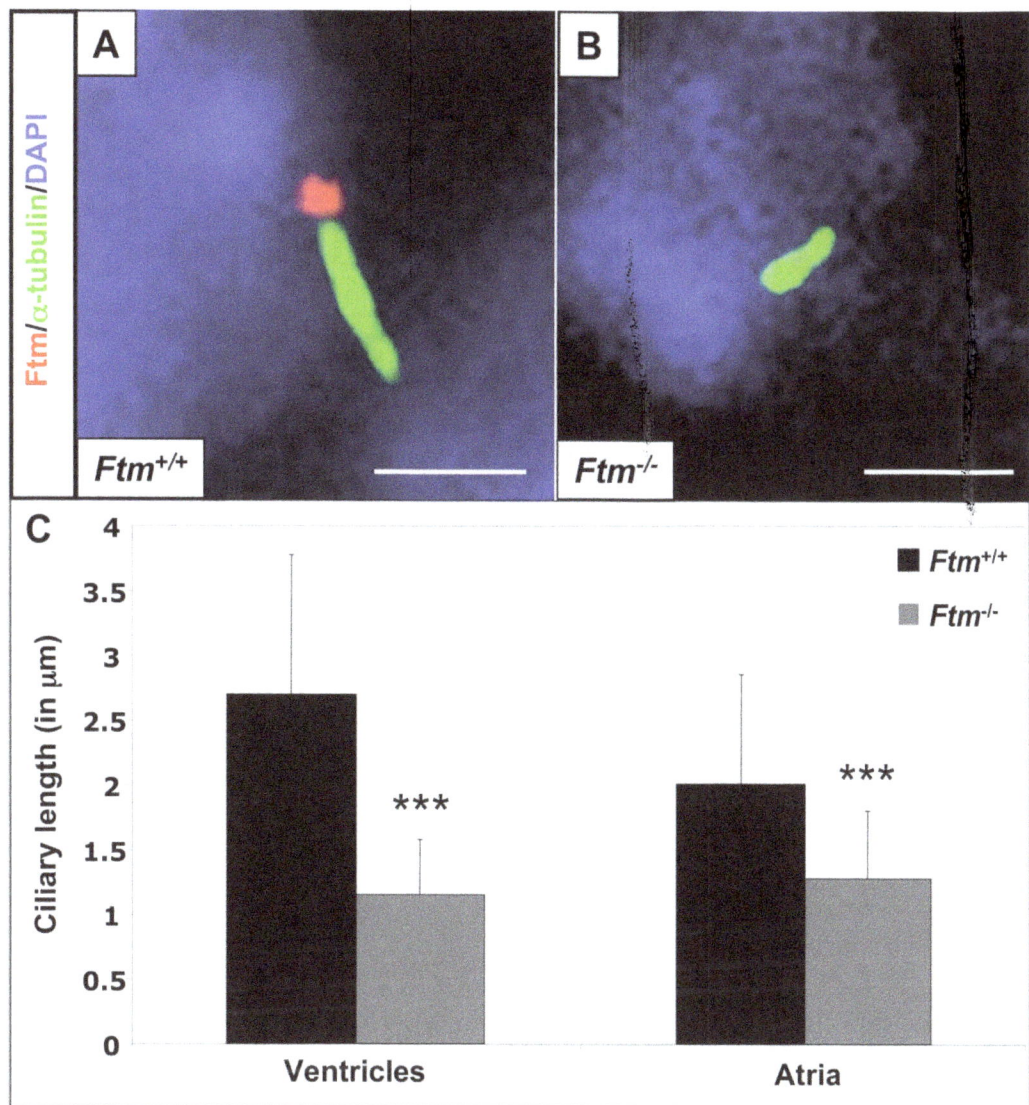

Figure 3. Loss of Ftm leads to shorter cardiac cilia. (A, B) Immunofluorescence on transverse heart sections at E11.5. Cilia are stained in green by acetylated α-tubulin and cell nuclei in blue by DAPI. Scale bars (in white) represent a length of 2 μm. Ftm is localised at cardiac cilia (A), but is absent from *Ftm*-negative cilia (B). (C) Comparison of wild-type and *Ftm*-deficient ciliary length in ventricles and atria (n = 50 cilia, respectively). *Ftm*-negative cilia are significantly shorter in both ventricles (p = 3.41E−12) and atria (p = 2.79E−06).

(forward), 3′-GCT GGT GAA AAG GAC CTC T (reverse); *Cyclin E*: 5′ CTG GCT GAA TGT TTA TGT CC (forward), 3′-TCT TTG CTT GGG CTT TGT CC (reverse); *p27*:5′-AAC CTC TTC GGC CCG GTG GAC CAC (forward), 3′-GTC TGC TCC ACA GAA CCG GCA TTT (reverse).

Statistical Data

To compare percentage of proliferating cells and percentage of apoptotic cells in wild-type and *Ftm*-mutant hearts, we counted BrdU or TUNEL marked cells and total number of cells (DAPI-marked) in distinct regions on ten different, transverse sections per heart, averaged over them and related them to each other. All heart chambers could be analysed on every section. Thereby, we differentiated between ciliary, former ciliary and non-ciliary regions.

To contrast wild-type with *Ftm*-negative cardiac wall thickness, the measurements of wall thickness were performed at distinct regions on ten different, transverse sections per heart. All four heart chambers were uncovered on every section. The measured values per heart were averaged.

Data are presented as mean ± standard deviation. Student's *t* test was performed to compare percentage of proliferating cells, cardiac wall thickness, RNA-expression levels and percentage of apoptotic cells in wild-type and *Ftm*-mutant hearts by using Graphpad and Microsoft Excel. A *p* value <0.05 was considered to be statistically significant (one asterisk), a *p* value <0.01 was regarded as statistically very significant (two asterisks) and a *p* value <0.001 was accounted statistically high significant (three asterisks).

Western Blotting

Western blot studies were done essentially as described using anti-Gli3 antibody or anti-pMek1/2 antibody [44]. Anti-actin antibody and anti-Gapdh antibody were used as control for loading. Visualising of Gli3, pMek1/2, actin and Gapdh bands

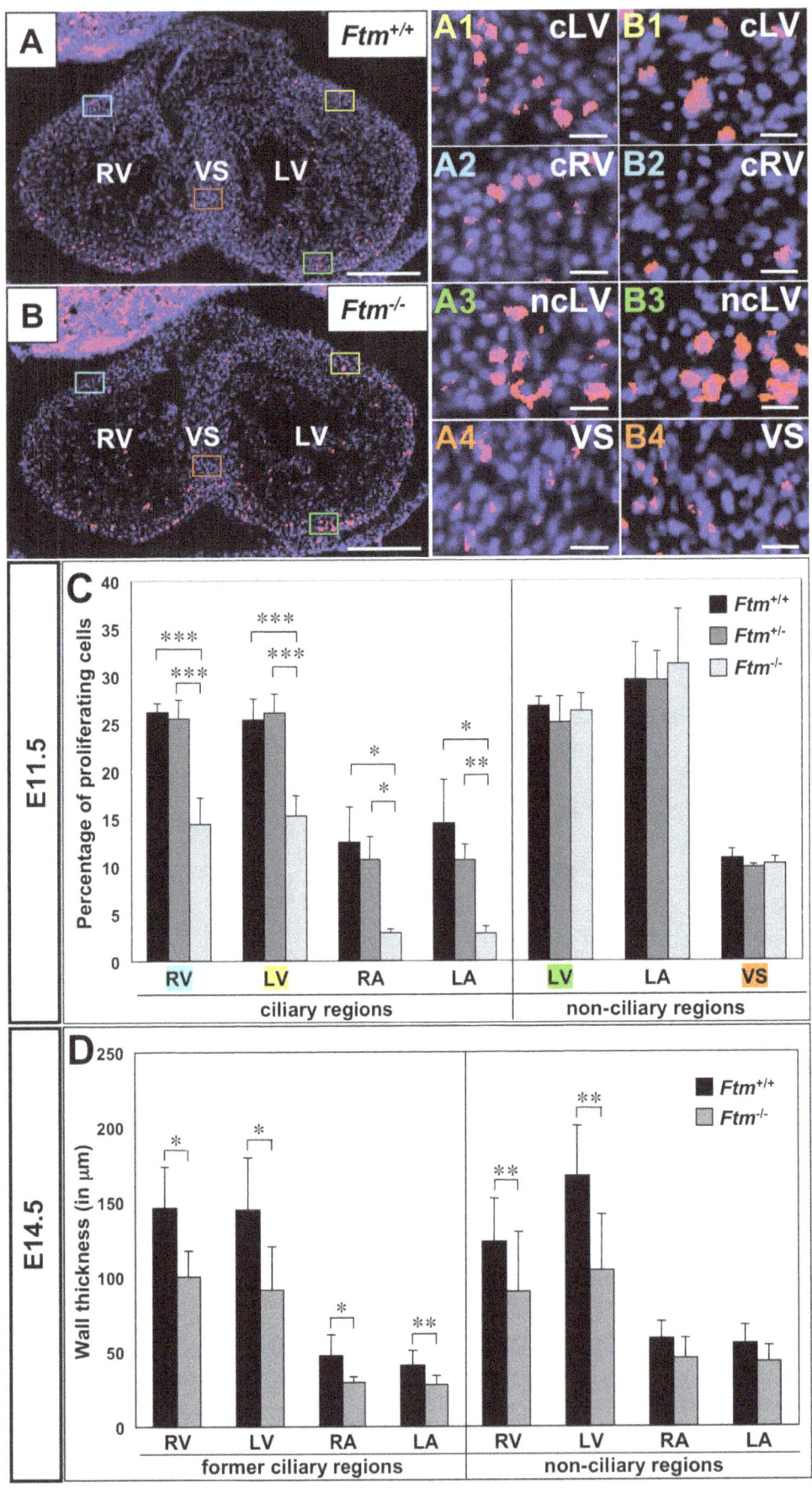

Figure 4. Reduced proliferation in ciliary regions of *Ftm*-deficient murine hearts and thickness decrease of *Ftm*-negative walls. (A, B, A1–4, B1–4) Immunofluorescence on transverse ventricular sections at E11.5. Dividing cells (red staining) are marked by BrdU and cell nuclei (blue staining) by DAPI. Scale bars (in white) represent a length of 0.5 mm (A, B) or 20 μm (A1–4, B1–4). (A, B) Coloured squares mark cardiac regions which are presented magnified in A1–4 and B1–4, respectively. The colour of the square correlates with the colour of the number of the magnified figures. (C) Proliferation rate is determined by the relation of dividing (BrdU-marked) cells to the number of all cells in this heart region at E11.5 (*Ftm*$^{+/+}$: n = 6; *Ftm*$^{+/-}$: n = 11; *Ftm*$^{-/-}$: n = 5). There is significantly less proliferation in the ciliary regions of ventricles and atria compared to non-ciliary regions. (D) Cardiac wall thickness measurements of wild-type (n = 6) and *Ftm*-deficient (n = 6) atria and ventricles in former ciliary and non-ciliary regions at E14.5. Walls are significantly thinner in all former ciliary regions. Additionally, ventricular, non-ciliary regions show a reduction in wall thickness, while atrial, non-ciliary regions do not differ significantly. LA, left atrium; RA, right atrium; LV, left ventricle; cLV, ciliary region of the left ventricle; ncLV, non-ciliary region of the left ventricle; RV, right ventricle; ciliary region of the right ventricle; VS, ventricular septum.

was realised by LAS-4000 mini (Fujifilm #8692184). Bands were measured in intensity using Adobe Photoshop 7.0.

Results

Ftm-negative, Murine Embryos Display Muscular and Perimembranous Ventricular Septal Defects

33% of all analysed *Ftm*-homozygous mutant embryos (9 of 27 embryos) show perimembranous VSDs marked by the combination of a significantly thinner muscular part of the VS and the absence of the membranous part of the VS (Figure 1B, C), while none of the *Ftm*-heterozygous mutants exhibits an abnormal heart phenotype (Figure 1C). We measured the length and thickness of ventricular and atrial septa in *Ftm*$^{+/+}$ and *Ftm*$^{-/-}$ hearts, respectively, and found out that the atrial septum (AS) displays no differences between the wild-type and *Ftm*-negative state (data

not shown). Furthermore, we did not observe any morphological AS abnormalities. In contrast to the atria, *Ftm*-deficient ventricles display defects, but the length measurements do not reflect a significant alteration at different embryonic days (Figure S1A, D, G, J, M). This is due to the fact that the frequency of perimembranous VSDs in the absence of Ftm is too low during embryonic development (Figure S1B, E, H, K, N). At E13.5 40% of all analyzed *Ftm*$^{-/-}$ mouse embryos (2 of 5) suffer from perimembranous VSDs, at E14.5 50% (3 of 6), at E15.5 67% (2 of 3), at E16.5 0% (none of 4) and at E17.5 22% (2 of 9). Compared to the length measurements, the width of *Ftm*-negative VS is significantly reduced (Figure S1A, D, G, J, M) characterizing a muscular VSD. 81, 5% of all analyzed *Ftm*$^{-/-}$ embryos (22 of 27 embryos) suffer from muscular VSDs (Figure 1D). The reduction of muscular VS width is significant at all analyzed embryonic days from E13.5 to E17.5 (Figure S1A, D, G, J, M), since the frequency

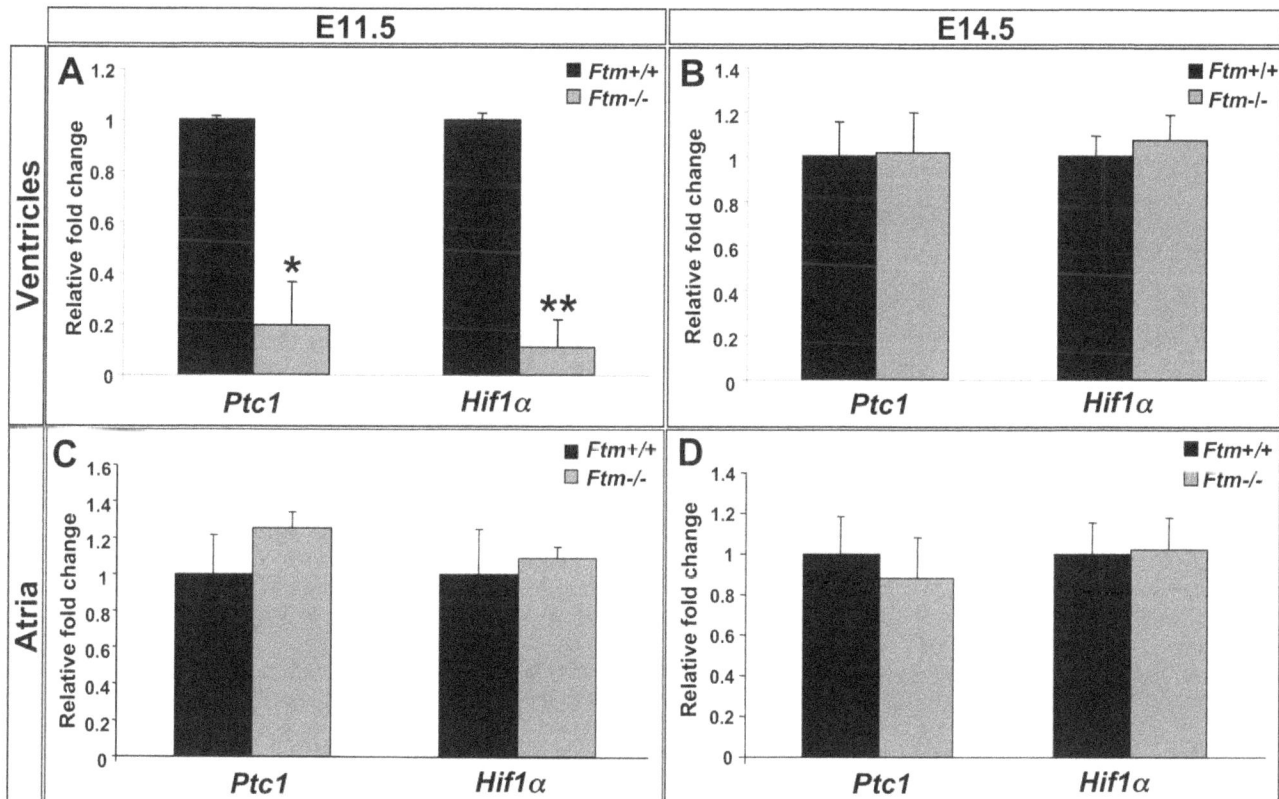

Figure 5. Shh and Pdgfrα signals are downregulated in *Ftm*-negative murine hearts. (A–D) Real-time PCR analysis of wild-type and *Ftm*-deficient ventricular (A, B) and atrial tissue (C, D) at E11.5 (A, C) and E14.5 (B, D). (A) Shh target gene expression of *Ptc1* and Pdgfrα target gene expression of *Hif1α* are significantly downregulated in E11.5 *Ftm*$^{-/-}$ ventricles (n = 3, respectively; *Ptc1*: p = 0.013; *Hif1α*: p = 0.005). (B) At E14.5, both signaling pathways are unaffected in *Ftm*-negative ventricles (n = 6, respectively). (C, D) In *Ftm*$^{-/-}$ atria, Shh and Pdgfrα signaling are not significantly altered at E11.5 (n = 6 atria, respectively; C) and at E14.5 (n = 6 atria, respectively; D).

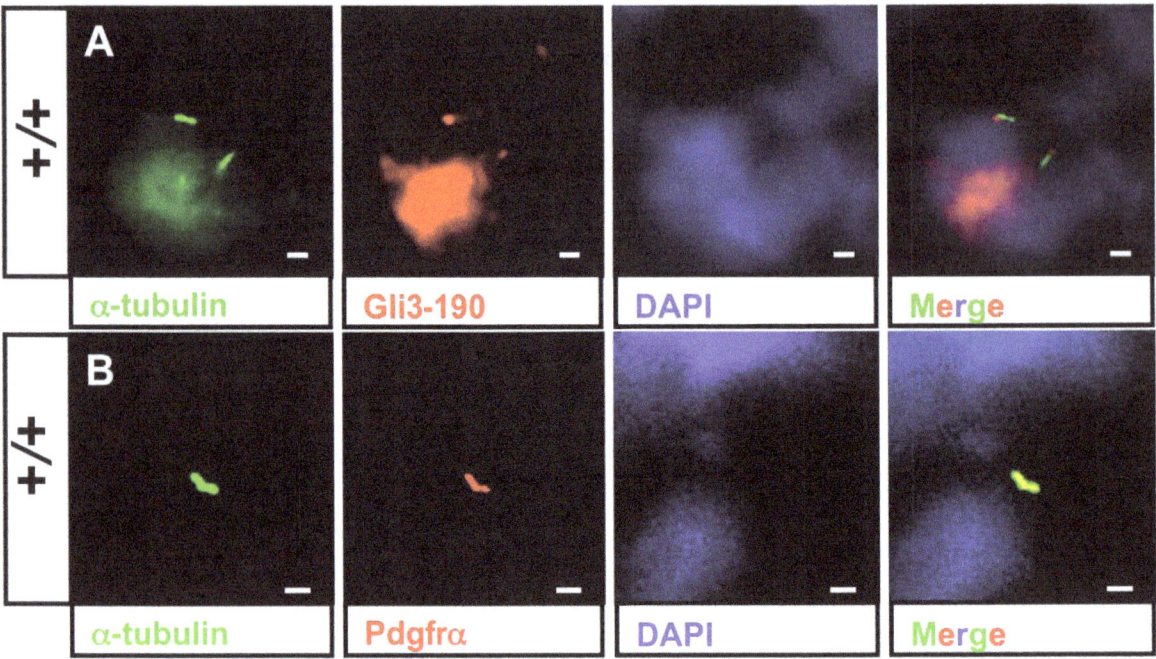

Figure 6. Shh and Pdgfrα signaling components localize at cardiac cilia. (A+B) Immunofluorescence on transverse heart sections at E11.5. Cilia are stained in green by acetylated α-tubulin and cell nuclei in blue by DAPI. Scale bars (in white) represent a length of 2 μm. (A) Ciliary Gli3-190 localisation (red staining) in wild-type ventricles demonstrates that Shh signaling is transduced by ventricular cilia. (B) Pdgfrα (red staining) is distributed along cardiac cilia in wild-type ventricles.

of muscular VSDs is high in all embryonic stages (Figure S1C, F, I, L, O). At E13.5 muscular VSDs can be observed in 80% of all analysed *Ftm*-negative embryos (4 of 5), at E14.5 in 83% (5 of 6), at E15.5 in 100% (3 of 3), at E16.5 in 50% (2 of 4) and at E17.5 in 89% (8 of 9). These data indicate that the muscular VS defect takes place in a high frequency even if the loss of the membranous VS occurs only in a minority of all *Ftm*$^{-/-}$ embryos leading to the conclusion that muscular VS development is severely disturbed in most *Ftm*-deficient embryos.

To test if the appearance of perimembranous VSDs correlates with other defects of *Ftm*-deficient mice, we looked for the entire phenotype of all analyzed mice. Comparing the different phenotypes, there seems to be no correlation between the occurrence of perimembranous VSDs and other abnormalities (Table S1).

Cilia are absent from the VS in E10.5 to E12.5 murine hearts. Since Ftm is a cilia-associated protein [20], we assumed that the cause of heart phenotype in *Ftm*-negative mice could be a ciliary dysfunction, although never before a ciliopathy was regarded as the elicitor of VSDs. The pre-condition for this assumption is the presence of cilia in murine hearts. In previous studies, cardiac cilia were detected in mice [52,53], but it was not mentioned if the VS is ciliated. We observed monocilia in a very distinct spatial distribution from E10.5 to E12.5 (Figure 2), but could never detect any cilia on VS cells (Figure 2A1, A1i). Furthermore, we could not demonstrate the presence of cilia on those ventricular cells which are close to the base of the muscular VS (Figure 2A3, A3i). Interestingly, cilia on ECCs were hardly detectable by visualizing acetylated α-tubulin (Figure 2D1a). Instead, the detection of Arl13b reveals ciliary presence also on the surface of these cells (Figure 2D1). Since acetylated α-tubulin serves as a marker for the ciliary axoneme, we tested if ECC cilia lack axonemes. Therefore, we used an antibody to detyrosinated tubulin which is another tubulin modification indicative for the

ciliary axoneme [54]. Detyrosinated tubulin was detected on ECCs (Figure 2E, E1, E1i) demonstrating that ECC cilia exhibit an axoneme. To proof if cilia can be observed on VS cells by using other ciliary marker instead of labelling acetylated α-tubulin, we performed antibody stainings with an anti-Arl13b antibody. But even by marking Arl13b, we could not detect cilia on VS cells (Figure S2) or in other non-ciliary regions. Marking different cardiac cell types, we found cardiac cilia poking out of myocardial and endocardial cells (Figure S3A, B), but not from cardiac fibroblasts (Figure S3C).

Cardiac cilia are shortened in Ftm-homozygous mutant mice. We previously showed that Ftm is present at the base of cilia in cell culture [20] and others observed Ftm at cilia of murine eyes and brains [48], but nothing is known about the localisation of Ftm at cardiac cilia. Consequently, we looked for Ftm in wild-type hearts. The staining of Ftm and acetylated α-tubulin (indicative for the ciliary axoneme) in combination with the partly overlapping staining of Ftm and γ-tubulin (basal body marker) reveals that Ftm is located at the base of atrial and ventricular cilia (Figure 3A; Figure S4A). Meanwhile, Ftm is completely missing in *Ftm*-negative embryos (Figure 3B; Figure S4B). Since the loss of Ftm in some cilia leads to a change in ciliary morphology (e.g. nodal cilia; [20]) and since the alteration of ciliary length leads to ciliary dysfunction [27,55–57], we analysed the length of *Ftm*-homozygous mutant, cardiac cilia at E11.5. Cilia of *Ftm*-deficient ventricles and atria are clearly shorter than in the wild-type (Figure 3C) arguing for a possible ciliary dysfunction in those hearts. Thus, Ftm is necessary for regulating the length of cardiac cilia.

Less proliferation at ciliary regions in Ftm-deficient hearts. The VS does not fully grow out in *Ftm*-negative mice (Figure 1B). From other tissue and cell culture experiments, it is known that monocilia mediate proliferative and apoptotic signals [23]. Since ventricular cilia appear at the time, when the muscular

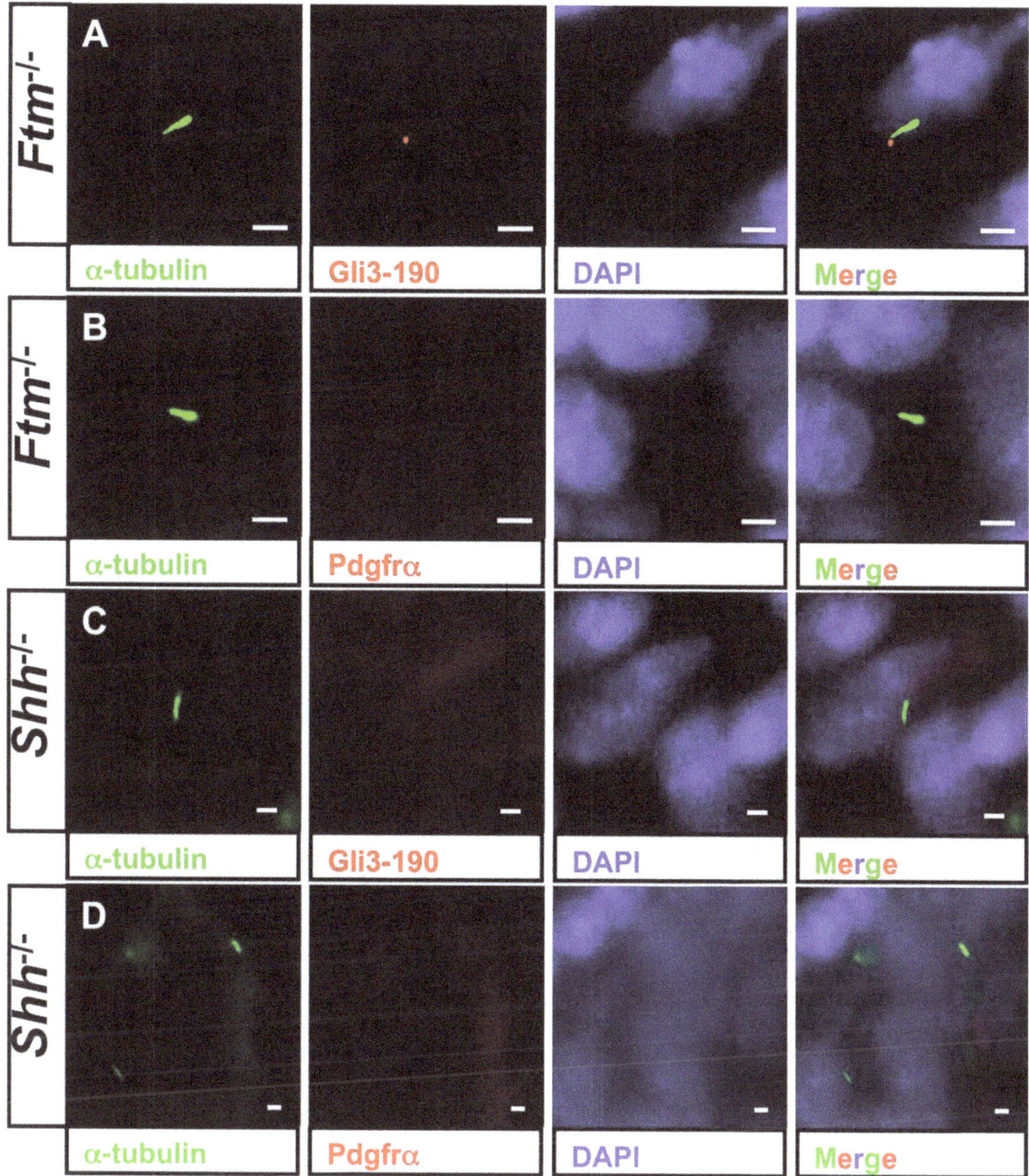

Figure 7. Shh signaling acts upstream of Pdgfrα signals in cardiac cilia. (A–D) Immunofluorescence on transverse heart sections at E11.5. Cilia are stained in green by acetylated α-tubulin and cell nuclei in blue by DAPI. Scale bars (in white) represent a length of 2 μm. (A) Gli3-190 (red staining) still shows a ciliary localisation in ventricular $Ftm^{-/-}$ cilia. (B) Pdgfrα (red staining) is absent in cilia of Ftm-deficient ventricles. (C) Gli3-190 protein is not observed at cilia of $Shh^{-/-}$ ventricles. (D) Pdgfrα cannot be detected in cilia of Shh-negative ventricles.

VS is growing out [58], and at those regions, where the proliferation of cells effects the outgrowth of the VS [11], we investigated proliferation and apoptosis via bromodeoxyuridine (BrdU) staining to determine the rate of proliferation and by means of TdT-mediated dUTP-biotin nick end labeling (TUNEL) staining to look for cell death at E11.5. Whereas the apoptosis study was inconspicuous (Figure S5A), there were differences in the proliferation rate between wild-type, Ftm-heterozygous and Ftm-homozygous mutant hearts. The proliferation in all Ftm-negative, ciliary areas in ventricles and atria was significantly diminished, while no proliferation differences could be observed in non-ciliary regions (Figure 4B1–B4, C). So in embryonic hearts, cilia seem to be necessary to mediate proliferative signals which in

turn are responsible for a part of cardiac cell proliferation. Consequently, when cilia are absent at a later point of time, the rate of proliferation of wild-type, Ftm-heterozygous and Ftm-homozygous mutant embryos should not differ significantly. Performing the same proliferation assays in E14.5 hearts, we found that, indeed, the proliferation in all areas, which were investigated, was similar in wild-type and Ftm-deficient hearts (Figure S5B). The diminished proliferation in Ftm-homozygous mutant hearts is in agreement with the results of semiquantitative Reverse transcription-PCRs. These experiments uncovered a change of expression levels of *cyclin E* and *p27* that are involved in cell cycle regulation and proliferation (Figure S6) substantiating suspicion of a proliferation defect in Ftm-deficient hearts.

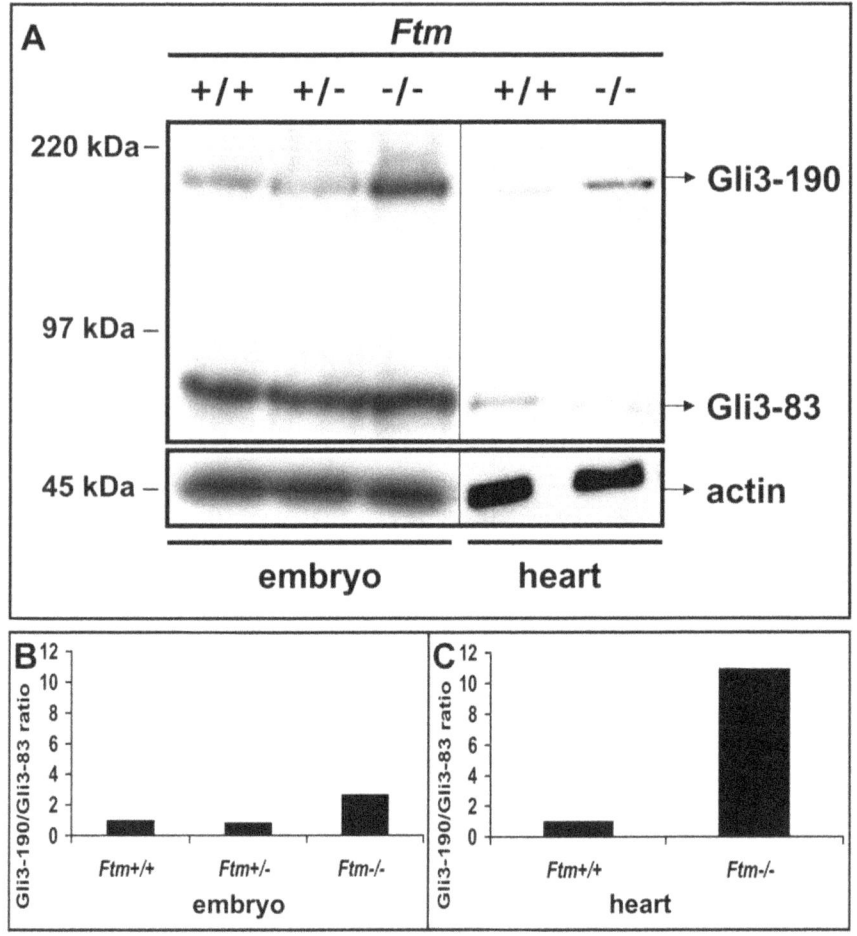

Figure 8. *Ftm*-negative hearts display a disturbance in Gli3 processing. (A) Western blot analysis of E11.5 embryo and heart protein lysates. Actin serves as loading control. In *Ftm*-negative embryos (n = 3), there is more Gli3-190 protein than in wild-type littermates, but an equal amount of Gli3-83. The amount of Gli3-190 protein is higher in *Ftm*-deficient than in wild-type hearts (n = 12, respectively), while conversely, there is less Gli3-83 in *Ftm*$^{-/-}$ hearts indicating a processing defect in *Ftm*-negative hearts. (B, C) Graphical evaluation of the Gli3-190/Gli3-83 ratio in wild-type and *Ftm*-deficient embryos and hearts, respectively. (B) The ratio of Gli3-190/Gli3-83 is 2.64 fold elevated in *Ftm*-homozygous mutant embryos. (C) Gli3-190/Gli3-83 ratio is 10.94 fold increased in *Ftm*-negative hearts.

Reduction of wall thickness in Ftm-negative hearts. Suggesting ciliary dysfunction is responsible for the decline of cell number in *Ftm*-deficient ventricular walls, we supposed that ventricular walls could be thinner in *Ftm*-negative than in wild-type mice. Analysis of ventricular wall sizes reveals a decrease of wall thickness in all regions of *Ftm*-negative hearts at E14.5, where cilia were present at E11.5 (Figure 4D). Furthermore, ventricular walls of *Ftm*-deficient mice without ciliary presence at any time are significantly thinner than those of wild-type mice at E14.5 (Figure 4D). These walls reside close to the base of the muscular VS. We also detected a reduction of wall thickness in all ciliary atrial areas, but not in non-ciliary regions of the atria (Figure 4D). Remarkably, 100% of all analyzed *Ftm*-negative embryos (6 of 6) display a decreased wall thickness in atria and ventricles (data not shown).

Shh and Pdgfrα signals are downregulated in Ftm-deficient hearts. Primary cilia are mediators of signaling pathways, which activate certain cellular processes. To elucidate, which signals are indispensable for cilia-controlled, cardiac proliferation, we looked for target gene expression of signaling pathways from which is known that they are mediated by cilia [25,35]. Thereby, *Patched1* (*Ptc1*) is used as target gene of Shh

signaling [59] and *Hypoxia-inducible factor 1, α subunit* (*Hif1α*) of Pdgfrα signaling [60]. Gene expression studies were performed at a ciliary as well as at a non-ciliary period (E11.5 and E14.5, respectively) and the hearts got subdivided into the ventricular and the atrial part to differ between ventricular and atrial ciliary signal mediation. At E11.5, *Ftm*-deficient ventricles show a significant downregulation of Shh and Pdgfrα signaling (Figure 5A), but these signaling pathways are unaltered in *Ftm*-negative atria (Figure 5C). At the non-ciliary stage E14.5, we do not see expression alterations of the analysed target genes in the *Ftm*$^{-/-}$ state (Figure 5B,D). Taken together, these results show a downregulation of signaling pathways in *Ftm*-homozygous mutant hearts at E11.5, but no differences at the non-ciliary stage E14.5.

Most likely Shh signaling acts upstream of Pdgfrα signaling in ventricular cilia and is disturbed in Ftm-deficient hearts owing to a Gli3 processing defect. To elucidate if these signaling pathways are mediated by cardiac cilia, we performed immunofluorescence stainings of proteins which are essential for Shh and Pdgfrα signaling, respectively. The Shh signaling mediator Gli3-190 [41] can be clearly observed at the base of ventricular cilia (Figure 6A, Figure S7A, B) and Pdgfrα is present all along ventricular cilia (Figure 6B). We could neither

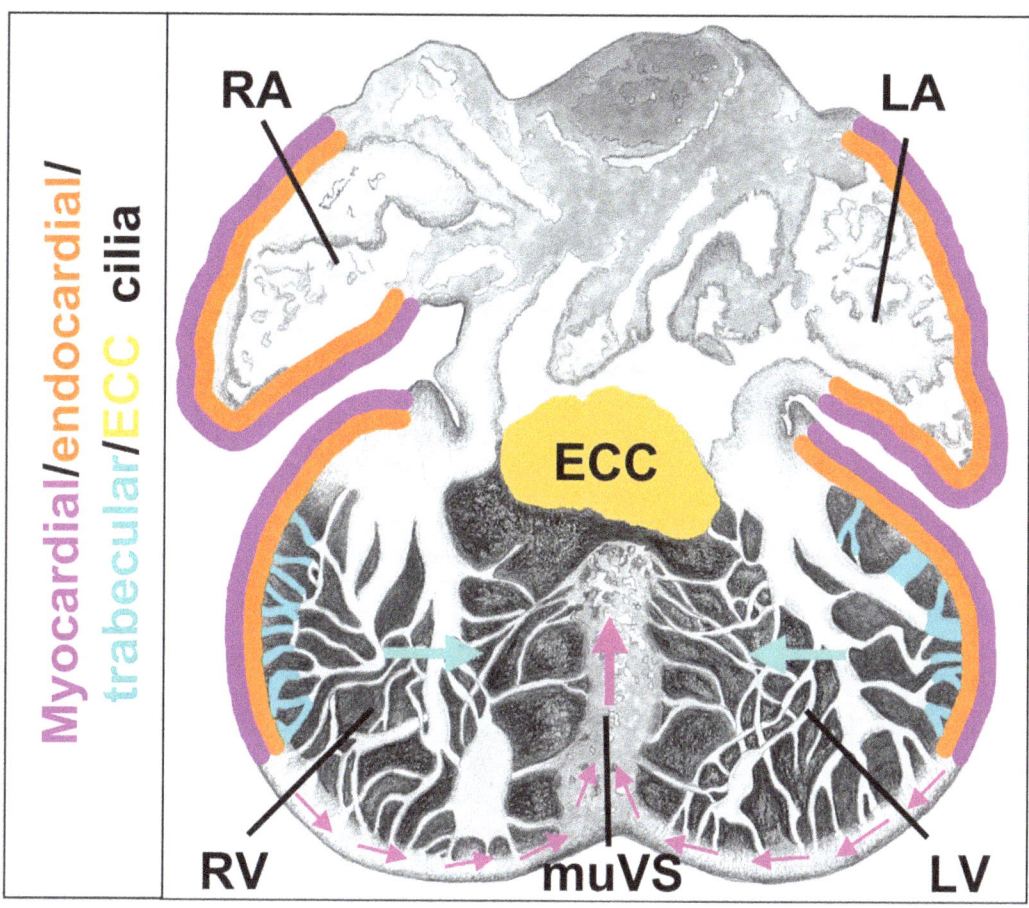

Figure 9. Model of VS development. Myocardial (violett), endocardial (orange) and most likely trabecular cilia (turquoise) regulate proliferation at distinct cardiac regions. In the ventricles, the cell proliferation in these regions results in wall thickness control, trabecular formation and a push of cells toward the base of the muscular ventricular septum (indicated by pink arrows). ECC cilia (yellow) seem to be different from the other cardiac cilia, since they do not regulate ECC proliferation. LA, left atrium; RA, right atrium; LV, left ventricle; RV, right ventricle; muVS, muscular ventricular septum.

detect Gli3-190 nor Pdgfrα at E11.5 atrial cilia (data not shown). This indicates that both signaling pathways are mediated by cilia in ventricles but not in atria at E11.5. Since we already detected a downregulation of Shh and Pdgfrα signaling in *Ftm*-deficient hearts via qRT-PCR, we looked for Gli3-190 and Pdgfrα localisation in *Ftm*-negative cardiac cilia. In these cilia, Gli3-190 is still present (Figure 7A), while Pdgfrα gets lost in ventricular cilia (Figure 7B). These results let assume that Pdgfrα signaling acts downstream of Shh signaling. To confirm this hypothesis, we investigated Gli3-190 and Pdgfrα localisation at *Shh*-deficient cilia in the heart. Gli3-190 and Pdgfrα are absent in ventricular cilia (Figure 7C, D) resulting in the conclusion that Pdgfrα signaling functions downstream of Shh signaling in ventricular cilia. The dependency of ventricular Pdgfrα signaling on Shh signaling is confirmed by a smaller amount of the Pdgfrα signaling component pMek1/2 in $Shh^{-/-}$ ventricles (Figure S8). This is indicative of a downregulation of Pdgfrα signaling in *Shh*-negative ventricles.

Since the phenotype of *Shh*-deficient hearts, which display atrioventricular septal defects, appears to be much stronger than in *Ftm*-negative embryos [61], Ftm functions most likely downstream of Shh ligand in this pathway. The phenotypes of mice, which are negative for Ptc1 and Smo, two components of the Shh pathway downstream of its ligand, are also more severe than the *Ftm*-deficient phenotype [57,62], so that we focused on the next players

within this signaling cascade – the Gli proteins. We examined Gli3 processing by western blot analysis, using an antibody against the N-terminus of Gli3 that detects both the full-length (Gli3-190) and processed short, repressor (Gli3-83) forms. Previously, we were able to show that the ratio of Gli3-190/Gli3-83 is higher in *Ftm*$^{-/-}$ whole embryo protein lysates than in wild-type or *Ftm*-heterozygous ones (Figure 8A, B) [20]. In *Ftm*-deficient hearts, we also detected an increase of the Gli3-190/Gli-83 ratio at E11.5 (Figure 8A,C) confirming our assumption of a Gli3 processing defect. The ratio of Gli3-190/Gli3-83 in *Ftm*-negative embryos is 2.64 fold higher than in the wild-type (Figure 8B), while in *Ftm*-deficient hearts, the Gli3-190/Gli3-83 ratio is 10.94 fold higher than in their wild-type counterparts (Figure 8C).

Membranous ventricular septal defects in *Ftm*-negative mice are most likely not due to endocardial cushion defects. An interaction of inlet muscular VS and atrioventricular ECCs seems to be required for the beginning of membranous VS formation [8,9]. Previously, it was suggested that defective ciliary function leads to a decreased cellularity of the ECCs [52]. So we looked for endocardial cushion morphology, the expression of marker genes and ECC proliferation (Figure S9). Morphologically, ECCs show a normal shape in *Ftm*$^{-/-}$ mice (Figure S9B) and also the marker gene expression of *Msh homeobox 1-like protein* (*Msx1*; Figure S9B) gives no hints indicating an abnormality in endocardial cushion development. Moreover, the number of proliferating ECCs is not altered in *Ftm*-deficient hearts at E11.5 (Figure S9C) and the atrioventricular valves exhibit a normal shape (data not shown). Since cilia are present on the surface of ECCs, it is interesting that the loss of Ftm does not seem to affect ECC proliferation. The proliferation in murine ventricles seems to be controlled mainly by Shh signals and so we examined ECC cilia-mediated signaling by analysing the ciliary localisation of Gli3. Interestingly, we did not detect Gli3 in or at wild-type ECC cilia (Figure S9D) indicating that these cilia do not transduce Shh signaling at all. Thus, although Ftm is present at the base of ECC cilia (Figure S9E), these cilia seem to be different from ventricular cilia as already suggested by the absence of acetylated α-tubulin (Figure 2D1). These data let suppose that the origin of perimembranous VSDs in *Ftm*-homozygous mutant hearts is not due to ECC dysfunction, but might be a defective outgrowth of the muscular VS.

Discussion

VSDs of *Ftm*-negative Mice are not only a Consequence of Impaired Left-right (LR) Asymmetry

Until now, the molecular mechanisms underlying VS development are largely unknown, but some factors have been elucidated which lead to the appearance of VSDs. One favoured reason for the occurrence of these congenital heart defects is the disturbancy of LR asymmetry. There is a high association between VSDs and LR asymmetry defects [63,64]. Previously, we published that *Ftm*-deficient mice suffer from an impairment of LR asymmetry due to a dysfunction of nodal cilia [20]. This fact raises the possibility that the VSDs observed in the absence of Ftm are caused by randomized heart looping. 19% of *Ftm*$^{-/-}$ murine embryos display an abnormal heart looping [20], while 33% of these mice exhibit perimembranous VSDs. Thus, this laterality defect cannot be the exclusive reason for VSDs in *Ftm*-negative mice. Furthermore, other studies about hearts from embryos with abnormal LR development due to paralyzed node cilia show proper cardiac wall thickness [52], but 100% of all analyzed *Ftm*$^{-/-}$ embryos suffer from reduced wall thickness supporting evidence for other VSD-causing reasons.

Preliminarily, it was suggested that primary cilia in murine hearts contribute to proper cardiac development [52]. Since Ftm deficiency has been shown to result in ciliary dysfunction [20,49], we examined in this study if *Ftm*-negative cardiac cilia cause perimembranous and muscular VSDs. The impact of Ftm absence on cardiac cilia is obvious, because *Ftm*-deficient cilia are shorter in atria and ventricles (Figure 3C). As an alteration of ciliary length gives a hint on a ciliary dysfunction, we investigated which molecular signals are mediated by cardiac cilia and if signaling is defective in the *Ftm*-negative state.

Do cardiac cilia mediate proliferative and hence muscular VS-generating signals?. We identified two signaling pathways which might be mediated by murine, ventricular cilia from E10.5 to E12.5, namely Shh and Pdgfrα signaling. The fact that atrial cilia do not transduce both pathways seems to be due to a difference in signal transduction of ventricular and atrial cells. Nevertheless, the correlation between ciliary presence and proliferation reduction as well as diminished wall thickness within the atria indicates that atrial cilia are associated with the proliferation of atrial cells at distinct regions. The control of this cilia-regulated atrial proliferation might be realized by mediating other signals than Shh or Pdgfrα signaling.

Our data let assume that there is a hierarchy between Shh and Pdgfrα signaling. In wild-type ventricles, Pdgfrα is located at cilia

(Figure 6B). Since Pdgfrα is missing at *Shh*-negative, ventricular cilia (Figure 7D), Shh signaling seems to have an effect on Pdgfrα signaling in cardiac cilia of embryonic ventricles. In some cases, the loss of Pdgfrα alone already leads to VSDs in mice [65]. These findings provide the indication that the defect in *Ftm*-negative mice firstly seems to perturb Shh signaling and then secondly Pdgfrα signaling. Considering the heart phenotypes of *Shh*- [61], *Ptc1*- [62] and *Smo*-deficient mouse embryos [57], we suggest that the interruption in Shh signaling appears downstream of Smo, because the heart defects of these mutants are more severe than the cardiac phenotype of *Ftm*$^{-/-}$ embryos. Since the ratio of Gli3-190 to Gli3-83 is changed in *Ftm*-deficient embryonic hearts at E11.5 (Figure 8A, C), this could be the step in Shh signaling where the disturbance firstly takes place. The fact that not as much full-length Gli3 is cleaved to its shorter repressor form as in the wild-type implicates a defect in proteolytic processing of Gli3. Hence, *Ftm*-negative hearts display a higher amount of Gli3-190. Nevertheless, Shh signaling is downregulated in *Ftm*-deficient ventricles at E11.5 (Figure 5A). An explanation for this discrepancy could be a defect in the transformation of full-length Gli3 to its transcriptional activator form leading to a reduced activation of Shh target genes.

Since we measured a reduced expression of Shh and Pdgfrα target genes in E11.5 *Ftm*-deficient ventricles (Figure 5A) indicating a downregulation of both pathways and detected a reduction of proliferation at those regions of *Ftm*$^{-/-}$ ventricles where cilia are present, it is possible that cilia control ventricular proliferation by mediating Shh and Pdgfrα signals. We could not detect cardiac cilia on muscular VS cells (Figure 2A1i) and the proliferation rate of these cells is not significantly altered (Figure 4B1–B4, C). Hence, we suggest that VS formation is not based on cell proliferation in the apical region of the muscular VS.

Remarkably, ECC cilia which are clearly visible by detecting Arl13b (Figure 2D1) or detyrosinated tubulin (Figure 2E1i), but not by using an antibody against acetylated α-tubulin (Figure 2D1a), do not display the presence of Gli3 (Figure S9D) leading to the assumption that cilia of the ECCs do not mediate Shh or Pdgfrα signaling. Consequently, ECC proliferation is not significantly affected by Ftm deficiency. Since we did not find any morphological or molecular ECC alterations in *Ftm*-negative hearts (Figure S9), it is unlikely that defective ECCs are the reason for VSD appearance in *Ftm*$^{-/-}$ mice.

Reduced proliferation influences the thickness of cardiac walls and VS development. We detected a decrease in the thickness of atrial and ventricular walls at those positions where cilia previously acted (Figure 4D) in 100% of all *Ftm*-negative hearts. Since wall thickness is diminished in all cases, but the attenuation of muscular VS thickness occurs in 81.5% of all analysed *Ftm*-negative hearts and perimembranous VSDs only appear in 33% of *Ftm*-deficient hearts, the decline of the wall thickness seems to be the primary defect of cardiac ciliary dysfunction, while the VSD is a consequence of it. The entire phenotype of *Ftm*-negative mouse embryos is subject to a variation reaching from embryos with extrinsically mild defects to severly deformed embryos. Nevertheless, all *Ftm*$^{-/-}$ embryos die at latest around birth. The reason for the phenotype variation is unknown, but maybe, it is the same, which causes differences in VS development of *Ftm*-deficient hearts. Potentially, the number of functional cilia plays a decisive role in the phenotype variation. If there is a threshold of cilia-mediated signals determing the severity of the mutant phenotype, it could be possible that the fewer cilia are present the stronger shapes the phenotype.

Interestingly, the percentage of perimembranous VSDs is higher in *Ftm*$^{-/-}$ hearts at E13.5 (40%) (Figure S1B) than at E17.5 (22%) (Figure S1N) suggesting that the defective VS development in the absence of Ftm occurs due to a developmental delay. Another explanation is that mice displaying a stronger phenotype and therefore a perimembranous VSD die earlier within the embryonic development than those with a milder phenotype. The second possibility is supported by the following facts: It is obvious that lethality at early embryonic stages (e.g. E13.5) takes place when Ftm is missing. *Ftm*-deficient embryos which suffer from multiple defects die earlier than those displaying a milder phenotype. Consequently, we observe exclusively milder mutant phenotypes at late embryonic stages (Table S1). Remarkably, some *Ftm*-negative embryos at late embryonic days which show mild mutant phenotypes suffer from perimembranous VSDs meaning that most organs of these embryos develop properly and indicating that a possible developmental delay only affects heart development. This argues clearly against a developmental delay. Moreover, muscular VSDs are detected in a high frequency at late embryonic days like E17.5 (89%) (Figure S1O) demonstrating that the observed VSDs are hardly based on a developmental delay.

The analysis of wall thickness in *Ftm*-negative hearts results in a clear subdivision appearing in the atria. We observed thinner walls where cilia had been present and normal wall thickness at those sites which never showed any cilia. However, ventricular walls display reduced wall thickness at both ciliary and non-ciliary regions (Figure 4D). It is known that the muscular VS consists of cardiomyocytes with both left-ventricular and right-ventricular identities [11] indicating that the ciliary dysfunction leads to a decrease of ventricular proliferation and hence to the appearance of VSDs. In contrary to ventricular development, atrial septal formation seems to be independent of ciliary function, because the atrial septum appears to be unaffected in *Ftm*-negative embryos.

Model of VS formation. Assuming that cardiac cilia regulate proliferation, our data allow us to propose a model for how the VS is generated. Ventricular cells at distinct positions assemble monocilia on their surface. These cardiac cilia contain components of Shh and Pdgfrα signaling most likely permitting them to mediate those signals. Thus, target genes of those signaling pathways are activated in cilia-possessing, ventricular cells. Interestingly, in ventricular cilia Pdgfrα signaling acts downstream of Shh signaling. In the end, the mediation of these different signals by cardiac cilia stimulates the cells to proliferate and this proliferation leads to a push of cells to the base of the muscular VS (Figure 9). Thus, in *Ftm*-negative ventricles the wall thickness of non-ciliary regions near the base of the muscular VS is significantly thinner (Figure 4D) due to the numeral reduction of cells which are pushed towards the base of the muscular VS. Both, the pushed cells and the trabecular formations shape the muscular VS which on its part grows to a certain point and then interacts molecularly with the ECCs. In turn, the ECCs start to shape the membranous VS which then grows towards the muscular VS. When they meet, they fuse and the development of the VS is finished. So finally, the muscular VS consists of cells which descend from the left and right ventricular walls and from the trabecular formations. Thus, our model supports the idea of muscular septal formation as a product of a passive process based on proliferation of cells at distinct regions in the left and right ventricles.

Supporting Information

Figure S1 Defects of VS development in *Ftm*-negative mice are most likely not due to a developmental delay. Septum length and width was measured as well as the percentage of murine hearts suffering from perimembranous and muscular VSDs was determined at E13.5 (A, B, C), at E14.5 (D, E, F), at E15.5 (G, H, I), at E16.5 (J, K, L) and at E17.5 (M, N, O). (A, D, G, J, M) Septum measurements of wild-type and *Ftm*-deficient ventricles at E13.5 (A), E14.5 (D), E15.5 (G), E16.5 (J) and E17.5 (M). Septum width was measured at different levels of the VS – apical, medial and basal. The results of all levels together were used to compile statistics. (A) At E13.5, *Ftm*-negative VS (n = 5) are significantly thinner (p = 0.017) than their wild-type counterparts (n = 5), while the length of $Ftm^{-/-}$ VS (n = 5) is not significantly altered in comparison to the wild-type ones (n = 5). (D) At E14.5, *Ftm*-negative VS (n = 6) are significantly thinner (p = 0.003) than their wild-type counterparts (n = 6), while the length of $Ftm^{-/-}$ VS (n = 6) is not significantly altered in comparison to the wild-type ones (n = 6). (G) At E15.5, *Ftm*-negative VS (n = 3) are significantly thinner (p = 0.046) than their wild-type counterparts (n = 3), while the length of $Ftm^{-/-}$ VS (n = 3) is not significantly altered in comparison to the wild-type ones (n = 3). (J) At E16.5, *Ftm*-negative VS (n = 4) are significantly thinner (p = 0.007) than their wild-type counterparts (n = 4), while the length of $Ftm^{-/-}$ VS (n = 4) is not significantly altered in comparison to the wild-type ones (n = 4). (M) At E17.5, *Ftm*-negative VS (n = 9) are significantly thinner (p = 0.003) than their wild-type counterparts (n = 5), while the length of $Ftm^{-/-}$ VS (n = 9) is not significantly altered in comparison to the wild-type ones (n = 5). Percentages of hearts affected by perimembranous or muscular VSDs were calculated from the very same number of embryos used in A, D, G, J and M. None of the wild-type embryos displays a VSD. (B) At E13.5, 40% of all analyzed *Ftm*-deficient embryos exhibit a perimembranous VSD, (E) at E14.5 50%, (H) at E15.5 67%, (K) at E16.5 0% and at E17.5 22%. (C) At E13.5, 80% of all analyzed *Ftm*-deficient embryos show a muscular VSD, (E) at E14.5 83%, (H) at E15.5 100%, (K) at E16.5 50% and at E17.5 89%. VS, ventricular septum; VSD, ventricular septal defect.

Figure S2 Cilia are not present on VS cells. Immunofluorescence on transverse heart sections at E12.5. Cilia are stained in red by marking Arl13b and cell nuclei in blue by the use of DAPI. Scale bar (in white) represents a length of 100 µm. ECCs are encircled by a yellow line, VS cells by a green line. White arrowheads point to cilia which are present on trabecular cells, but not on VS cells.

Figure S3 Primary cilia are present on myocardial and endocardial cells. (A–C) Immunohistochemistry on transverse heart sections at E11.5. Cilia are stained in green by acetylated α-tubulin and cell nuclei in blue by DAPI. Scale bars (in white) represent a length of 2 µm. (A–C) White arrows point to cilia. (A, B) Myocardial cells (A; red staining; marked by tropomyosin) and endocardial cells (B; red staining; marked by ErbB3) possess cilia. (C) Cardiac fibroblasts (red staining; marked by DDR2) do not show any cilia. (D) Schematic illustration of ciliary distribution in embryonic mouse hearts. We found cilia at E10.5–12.5 on myocardial cells (violett), endocardial cells (orange), ECCs (yellow) and trabecles (turquoise). LA, left atrium; RA, right atrium; LV, left ventricle; RV, right ventricle; muVS, muscular ventricular septum.

Figure S4 Co-localisation of Ftm with the basal body and centrosome marker γ-tubulin. (A, B) Immunohistochemistry on transverse heart sections at E11.5. Centrosomes/basal bodies are marked in green by γ-tubulin and cell nuclei in blue by DAPI. Scale bars (in white) represent a length of 2 µm. (A) Ftm staining (red) partially overlaps with the staining of the centrosome/basal body (green). (B) In *Ftm*-negative hearts, Ftm is missing at the centrosome/basal body of cilia.

Figure S5 Apoptosis at E11.5 and proliferation rate at E14.5 is unaltered in *Ftm*-deficient hearts. (A) Apoptosis studies by TUNEL stainings in E11.5 hearts. No significant differences can be detected in wild-type (n = 3), *Ftm*-heterozygous mutant (n = 3) and *Ftm*-homozygous mutant (n = 3) heart compartments. (B) Proliferation rate is determined by the relation of dividing (BrdU-marked) cells to the number of all cells in distinct heart regions at E14.5 (*Ftm*$^{+/+}$: n = 3 hearts; *Ftm*$^{-/-}$: n = 3 hearts). In none of the investigated *Ftm*-negative heart compartments, cell proliferation is significantly altered.

Figure S6 Expression alterations of genes involved in cell cycle progression and proliferation in atria and ventricles. Semi-quantitative PCR analysis of wild-type and *Ftm*$^{-/-}$ atrial and ventricular tissue at E11.5. *Hprt* serves as loading control. Expression of *cyclin E* is downregulated and expression of *p27* is upregulated in *Ftm*-negative atria and ventricles suggesting a disturbance in cell cycle progression and proliferation.

Figure S7 Gli3-190 localizes at the base of ventricular cilia. Immunohistochemistry on transverse heart sections at E11.5. (A) Centrosomes/basal bodies are marked in green by γ-tubulin and cell nuclei in blue by DAPI. Scale bar (in white) represents a length of 2 µm. Gli3-190 staining (red) partially overlaps with the staining of the centrosome/basal body (green). (B) Pericentriolar material at the base of cilia is stained in blue by pericentrin and the ciliary axoneme in green by acetylated α-tubulin. Gli3-190 (red staining) co-localizes with pericentrin and hence is present at the base of ventricular cilia.

Figure S8 pMek1/2, a Pdgfα signaling pathway component, is downregulated in *Shh*-negative ventricles. Western blot analysis of E11.5 ventricular protein lysates. Gapdh serves as loading control. In *Shh*-negative ventricles (n = 3), there is less phosphorylated Mek1/2 protein than in wild-type littermates.

Figure S9 Endocardial cushion development is not altered in *Ftm*-negative embryos. (A, B) In situ hybridizations on heart sections at E11.5. Endocardial cushion marker expression of *Msx1* is unchanged in *Ftm*-deficient, murine hearts (compare inlets in A and B). (C) Proliferation rate is determined by the relation of dividing (BrdU-marked) ECCs to the number of all ECCs in this region at E11.5 (*Ftm*$^{+/+}$: n = 3 hearts; *Ftm*$^{-/-}$: n = 3 hearts). The number of proliferating ECCs is not significantly altered in *Ftm*-negative hearts. (D, E) Immunofluorescence on transverse heart sections at E11.5. ECC cilia are marked in red by Arl13b. Scale bars (in white) represent a length of 2 µm. (D) Gli3 (green) is missing at ECC cilia. (E) Ftm (green) is present at ECC cilia.

Table S1 Phenotypes of all analyzed *Ftm*-negative embryos. The phenotypes of all analyzed *Ftm*-negative embryos in the developmental stages E13.5 to E17.5 is depicted in this table. The "x" symbolizes the appearance of the defect. pVSD, perimembranous ventricular septal defect; mVSD, muscular ventricular septal defect.

Acknowledgments

The authors thank Drs. Renate Dildrop and Jürgen Schrader for critical reading of the manuscript; Wioletta Hörschken and Peter Sikorski for technical assistance; Kerstin Rose for generating the Gli3-190 antibody; and Edie C. Goldsmith and Baolin Wang for providing antibodies. The antibody against BrdU developed by Dr. Stephen J. Kaufman was obtained from the Developmental Studies Hybridoma Bank developed under the auspices of the NICHD and maintained by The University of Iowa, Department of Biological Sciences, Iowa City, IA 52242.

Author Contributions

Conceived and designed the experiments: CG UR. Performed the experiments: CG JL SK. Analyzed the data: CG JL. Wrote the paper: CG JL UR.

References

1. Kovacs AH, Sears SF, Saidi AS (2005) Biopsychosocial experiences of adults with congenital heart disease: review of the literature. Am Heart J 150: 193–201.
2. Lloyd-Jones D, Adams R, Carnethon M, De Simone G, Ferguson T, et al. (2009) Heart disease and stroke statistics–2009 update: a report from the American Heart Association Statistics Committee and Stroke Statistics Subcommittee. Circulation 119: 480–486.
3. Scully B, Morales D, Zafar F, McKenzie E, Fraser CJ, et al. (2010) Current expectations for surgical repair of isolated ventricular septal defects. Ann Thorac Surg 89: 550–551.
4. Komatsu K, Wakatsuki S, Yamada S, Yamamura K, Miyazaki J, et al. (2007) Meltrin beta expressed in cardiac neural crest cells is required for ventricular septum formation of the heart. Dev Biol 303: 82–92.
5. Soufflet V, Van de Bruaene A, Troost E, Gewillig M, Moons P, et al. (2010) Behavior of unrepaired perimembranous ventricular septal defect in young adults. Am J Cardiol 105: 404–407.
6. Reller MD, Strickland MJ, Riehle-Colarusso T, Mahle WT, Correa A (2008) Prevalence of congenital heart defects in metropolitan Atlanta, 1998–2005. J Pediatr 153: 807–813.
7. İçten N, Tetik S (1996) The membranous portion of the interventricular septum in neonates. An anatomic study in neonatal cadavers. Surg Radiol Anat 18: 97–101.
8. Meredith M, Hutchins G, Moore G (1979) Role of the left interventricular sulcus in formation of interventricular septum and crista supraventricularis in normal human cardiogenesis. Anat Rec 194: 417–428.
9. Lamers W, Moorman A (2002) Cardiac septation: a late contribution of the embryonic primary myocardium to heart morphogenesis. Circ Res 91: 93–103.
10. Sakata Y, Kamei C, Nakagami H, Bronson R, Liao J, et al. (2002) Ventricular septal defect and cardiomyopathy in mice lacking the transcription factor CHF1/Hey2. Proc Natl Acad Sci U S A 99: 16197–16202.
11. Franco D, Meilhac S, Christoffels V, Kispert A, Buckingham M, et al. (2006) Left and right ventricular contributions to the formation of the interventricular septum in the mouse heart. Dev Biol 294: 366–375.
12. Patten BM (1964) The heart. Foundation of Embryology, McGraw Hill, New York (1964): 545–569.
13. Harh JY, Paul MH (1975) Experimental cardiac morphogenesis. I. Development of the ventricular septum in the chick. J Embryol Exp Morphol 33: 13–28.
14. Goor D, Edwards J, Lillehei C (1970) The development of the interventricular septum of the human heart; correlative morphogenetic study. Chest 58: 453–467.
15. Rychter Z, Rychterová V, Lemez L (1979) Formation of the heart loop and proliferation structure of its wall as a base for ventricular septation. Herz 4: 86–90.
16. Steding G, Seidl W (1980) Contribution to the development of the heart. Part 1: normal development. Thorac Cardiovasc Surg 28: 386–409.
17. Van Mierop L, Kutsche L (1985) Development of the ventricular septum of the heart. Heart Vessels 1: 114–119.
18. Bruneau BG, Logan M, Davis N, Levi T, Tabin CJ, et al. (1999) Chamber-Specific Cardiac Expression of Tbx5 and Heart Defects in Holt-Oram Syndrome. Dev Biol 211: 100–108.
19. Takeuchi JK, Ohgi M, Koshiba-Takeuchi K, Shiratori H, Sakaki I, et al. (2003) Tbx5 specifies the left/right ventricles and ventricular septum position during cardiogenesis. Development 130: 5953–5964.
20. Vierkotten J, Dildrop R, Peters T, Wang B, Rüther U (2007) Ftm is a novel basal body protein of cilia involved in Shh signalling. Development 134: 2569–2577.
21. Delous M, Baala L, Salomon R, Laclef C, Vierkotten J, et al. (2007) The ciliary gene RPGRIP1L is mutated in cerebello-oculo-renal syndrome (Joubert syndrome type B) and Meckel syndrome. Nat Genet 39: 875–881.

22. Wolf M, Saunier S, O'Toole J, Wanner N, Groshong T, et al. (2007) Mutational analysis of the RPGRIP1L gene in patients with Joubert syndrome and nephronophthisis. Kidney Int 72: 1520–1526.

23. Satir P, Christensen S (2008) Structure and function of mammalian cilia. Histochem Cell Biol 129: 687–693.

24. D'Angelo A, Franco B (2009) The dynamic cilium in human diseases. PathoGenetics 2: 3.

25. Eggenschwiler J, Anderson K (2007) Cilia and developmental signaling. Annu Rev Cell Dev Biol 23: 345–373.

26. Corbit K, Aanstad P, Singla V, Norman A, Stainier D, et al. (2005) Vertebrate Smoothened functions at the primary cilium. Nature 437: 1018–1021.

27. Haycraft C, Banizs B, Aydin-Son Y, Zhang Q, Michaud E, et al. (2005) Gli2 and Gli3 localize to cilia and require the intraflagellar transport protein polaris for processing and function. PLoS Genet 1: e53.

28. Ross A, May-Simera H, Eichers E, Kai M, Hill J, et al. (2005) Disruption of Bardet-Biedl syndrome ciliary proteins perturbs planar cell polarity in vertebrates. Nat Genet 37: 1135–1140.

29. Schneider L, Clement C, Teilmann S, Pazour G, Hoffmann E, et al. (2005) PDGFRalphaalpha signaling is regulated through the primary cilium in fibroblasts. Curr Biol 15: 1861–1866.

30. Rohatgi R, Milenkovic L, Scott M (2007) Patched1 regulates hedgehog signaling at the primary cilium. Science 317: 372–376.

31. Gerdes J, Liu Y, Zaghloul N, Leitch C, Lawson S, et al. (2007) Disruption of the basal body compromises proteasomal function and perturbs intracellular Wnt response. Nat Genet 39: 1350–1360.

32. Corbit K, Shyer A, Dowdle W, Gaulden J, Singla V, et al. (2008) Kif3a constrains beta-catenin-dependent Wnt signalling through dual ciliary and non-ciliary mechanisms. Nat Cell Biol 10: 70–76.

33. Germino G (2005) Linking cilia to Wnts. Nat Genet 37: 455–457.

34. Wallingford J, Mitchell B (2011) Strange as it may seem: the many links between Wnt signaling, planar cell polarity, and cilia. Genes Dev 25: 201–213.

35. Berbari N, O'Connor A, Haycraft C, Yoder B (2009) The primary cilium as a complex signaling center. Curr Biol 19: R526–535.

36. Lancaster M, Gleeson J (2010) Cystic Kidney Disease: the Role of Wnt Signaling. Trends Mol Med 16: 349–360.

37. Satir P, Pedersen L, Christensen S (2010) The primary cilium at a glance. J Cell Sci 123: 499–503.

38. Ruiz i Altaba A, Sánchez P, Dahmane N (2002) Gli and hedgehog in cancer: tumours, embryos and stem cells. Nat Rev Cancer 2: 361–372.

39. Hynes M, Stone D, Dowd M, Pitts-Meek S, Goddard A, et al. (1997) Control of cell pattern in the neural tube by the zinc finger transcription factor and oncogene Gli-1. Neuron 19: 15–26.

40. Ruiz i Altaba A (1999) The works of GLI and the power of hedgehog. Nat Cell Biol 1: E147–148.

41. Sasaki H, Nishizaki Y, Hui C, Nakafuku M, Kondoh H (1999) Regulation of Gli2 and Gli3 activities by an amino-terminal repression domain: implication of Gli2 and Gli3 as primary mediators of Shh signaling. Development 126: 3915–3924.

42. Chen M, Wilson C, Li Y, Law K, Lu C, et al. (2009) Cilium-independent regulation of Gli protein function by Sufu in Hedgehog signaling is evolutionarily conserved. Genes Dev 23: 1910–1928.

43. Humke E, Dorn K, Milenkovic L, Scott M, Rohatgi R (2010) The output of Hedgehog signaling is controlled by the dynamic association between Suppressor of Fused and the Gli proteins. Genes Dev 24: 670–682.

44. Wang B, Fallon J, Beachy P (2000) Hedgehog-regulated processing of Gli3 produces an anterior/posterior repressor gradient in the developing vertebrate limb. Cell 100: 423–434.

45. Christensen S, Pedersen S, Satir P, Veland I, Schneider L (2008) The primary cilium coordinates signaling pathways in cell cycle control and migration during development and tissue repair. Curr Top Dev Biol 85: 261–301.

46. Yun S, Lee M, Ryu J, Song C, Han H (2009) Role of HIF-1alpha and VEGF in human mesenchymal stem cell proliferation by 17beta-estradiol: involvement of PKC, PI3K/Akt, and MAPKs. Am J Physiol Cell Physiol 296: 317–326.

47. Schild C, Wirth M, Reichert M, Schmid R, Saur D, et al. (2009) PI3K signaling maintains c-myc expression to regulate transcription of E2F1 in pancreatic cancer cells. Mol Carcinog 48: 1149–1158.

48. Arts H, Doherty D, van Beersum S, Parisi M, Letteboer S, et al. (2007) Mutations in the gene encoding the basal body protein RPGRIP1L, a nephrocystin-4 interactor, cause Joubert syndrome. Nat Genet 39: 882–888.

49. Besse L, Neti M, Anselme I, Gerhardt C, Rüther U, et al. (2011) Primary cilia control telencephalic patterning and morphogenesis via Gli3 proteolytic processing. Development 138: 2079–2088.

50. Gavrieli Y, Sherman Y, Ben-Sasson S (1992) Identification of programmed cell death in situ via specific labeling of nuclear DNA fragmentation. J Cell Biol 119: 493–501.

51. Moorman A, Houweling A, de Boer P, Christoffels V (2001) Sensitive nonradioactive detection of mRNA in tissue sections: novel application of the whole-mount in situ hybridization protocol. J Histochem Cytochem 49: 1–8.

52. Slough J, Cooney L, Brueckner M (2008) Monocilia in the embryonic mouse heart suggest a direct role for cilia in cardiac morphogenesis. Dev Dyn 237: 2304–2314.

53. Clement C, Kristensen S, Møllgård K, Pazour G, Yoder B, et al. (2009) The primary cilium coordinates early cardiogenesis and hedgehog signaling in cardiomyocyte differentiation. J Cell Sci 122: 3070–3082.

54. Van der Heiden K, Groenendijk B, Hierck B, Hogers B, Koerten H, et al. (2006) Monocilia on chicken embryonic endocardium in low shear stress areas. Dev Dyn 235: 19–28.

55. May S, Ashique A, Karlen M, Wang B, Shen Y, et al. (2005) Loss of the retrograde motor for IFT disrupts localization of Smo to cilia and prevents the expression of both activator and repressor functions of Gli. Dev Biol 287: 378–389.

56. Haycraft C, Zhang Q, Song B, Jackson W, Detloff P, et al. (2007) Intraflagellar transport is essential for endochondral bone formation. Development 134: 307–316.

57. Tran P, Haycraft C, Besschetnova T, Turbe-Doan A, Stottmann R, et al. (2008) THM1 negatively modulates mouse sonic hedgehog signal transduction and affects retrograde intraflagellar transport in cilia. Nat Genet 40: 403–410.

58. Henderson D, Copp A (1998) Versican expression is associated with chamber specification, septation, and valvulogenesis in the developing mouse heart. Circ Res 83: 523–532.

59. Marigo V, Tabin C (1996) Regulation of patched by sonic hedgehog in the developing neural tube. Proc Natl Acad Sci U S A 93: 9346–9351.

60. Nilsson M, Zage P, Zeng L, Xu L, Cascone T, et al. (2010) Multiple receptor tyrosine kinases regulate HIF-1alpha and HIF-2alpha in normoxia and hypoxia in neuroblastoma: implications for antiangiogenic mechanisms of multikinase inhibitors. Oncogene 29: 2938–2949.

61. Goddeeris M, Rho S, Petiet A, Davenport C, Johnson G, et al. (2008) Intracardiac septation requires hedgehog-dependent cellular contributions from outside the heart. Development 135: 1887–1895.

62. Goodrich L, Milenkovic L, Higgins K, Scott M (1997) Altered neural cell fates and medulloblastoma in mouse patched mutants. Science 277: 1109–1113.

63. Tan S, Rosenthal J, Zhao X, Francis R, Chatterjee B, et al. (2007) Heterotaxy and complex structural heart defects in a mutant mouse model of primary ciliary dyskinesia. J Clin Invest 117: 3742–3752.

64. Franco D, Icardo J (2001) Molecular characterization of the ventricular conduction system in the developing mouse heart: topographical correlation in normal and congenitally malformed hearts. Cardiovasc Res 49: 417–429.

65. Richarte A, Mead H, Tallquist M (2007) Cooperation between the PDGF receptors in cardiac neural crest cell migration. Dev Biol 306: 785–796.

6

Serotonin Potentiates Transforming Growth Factor-beta3 Induced Biomechanical Remodeling in Avian Embryonic Atrioventricular Valves

Philip R. Buskohl[1], Michelle L. Sun[2], Robert P. Thompson[3], Jonathan T. Butcher[2]*

1 Department of Mechanical and Aerospace Engineering, Cornell University, Ithaca, New York, United States of America, **2** Department of Biomedical Engineering, Cornell University, Ithaca, New York, United States of America, **3** Department of Cell Biology and Regenerative Medicine, Medical University of South Carolina, Charleston, South Carolina, United States of America

Abstract

Embryonic heart valve primordia (cushions) maintain unidirectional blood flow during development despite an increasingly demanding mechanical environment. Recent studies demonstrate that atrioventricular (AV) cushions stiffen over gestation, but the molecular mechanisms of this process are unknown. Transforming growth factor-beta (TGFβ) and serotonin (5-HT) signaling modulate tissue biomechanics of postnatal valves, but less is known of their role in the biomechanical remodeling of embryonic valves. In this study, we demonstrate that exogenous TGFβ3 increases AV cushion biomechanical stiffness and residual stress, but paradoxically reduces matrix compaction. We then show that TGFβ3 induces contractile gene expression (RhoA, aSMA) and extracellular matrix expression (col1α2) in cushion mesenchyme, while simultaneously stimulating a two-fold increase in proliferation. Local compaction increased due to an elevated contractile phenotype, but global compaction appeared reduced due to proliferation and ECM synthesis. Blockade of TGFβ type I receptors via SB431542 inhibited the TGFβ3 effects. We next showed that exogenous 5-HT does not influence cushion stiffness by itself, but synergistically increases cushion stiffness with TGFβ3 co-treatment. 5-HT increased TGFβ3 gene expression and also potentiated TGFβ3 induced gene expression in a dose-dependent manner. Blockade of the 5HT2b receptor, but not 5-HT2a receptor or serotonin transporter (SERT), resulted in complete cessation of TGFβ3 induced mechanical strengthening. Finally, systemic 5-HT administration *in ovo* induced cushion remodeling related defects, including thinned/atretic AV valves, ventricular septal defects, and outflow rotation defects. Elevated 5-HT *in ovo* resulted in elevated remodeling gene expression and increased TGFβ signaling activity, supporting our *ex-vivo* findings. Collectively, these results highlight TGFβ/5-HT signaling as a potent mechanism for control of biomechanical remodeling of AV cushions during development.

Editor: Michael Schubert, Ecole Normale Supérieure de Lyon, France

Funding: This project was funded by the American Heart Association (0830384N, JTB; www.heart.org), National Institutes of Health (HL110328, JTB; HL91452, RPT; www.NIH.gov), The Hartwell Foundation (JTB; www.thehartwellfoundation.org) and the National Science Foundation (CBET-0955172, JTB; DGE0841291, PRB; www.nsf.gov). The funders had no role in study design, data collection and analysis, decision to publish, or preparation of the manuscript.

Competing Interests: The authors have declared that no competing interests exist.

* E-mail: jtb47@cornell.edu

Introduction

Biomechanical remodeling is the process by which living tissues reorganize, reshape, and refit their microstructure in adaptation to changing internal and external forces. This process defines much of embryogenesis, during which initially indistinct cellular masses acquire shape and functional specificity through production and manipulation of the extracellular matrix (ECM). This is particularly important for the morphogenesis of the heart, which is critically responsible for distributing nutrients as the embryo grows. The heart transitions rapidly from a tubular structure into a multi-chambered pumping organ, simultaneously growing over 100-fold in volume [1]. The hemodynamic environment inside the heart increases dramatically in severity during this process [2–4], which means the biomechanical properties of the forming valves must be precisely tuned to maintain efficient unidirectional blood flow. Atrioventricular (AV) valve morphogenesis is characterized by rapid ECM accretion and turnover [5,6], which is hypothesized to be stimulated by a dynamic interaction of molecular and mechanical signaling. While numerous molecular agents important for valve morphogenesis have been identified [7–10], less is known about how these signals affect valve mechanics, which is a key readout of valve function.

The transforming growth factor-beta (TGFβ) superfamily is critically important for a wide range of cellular processes [11–13], and is heavily involved in directing morphogenesis of AV cushions [14–18]. In the chick, TGFβ2 and TGFβ3 isoforms are necessary for the endothelial to mesenchymal transition (EMT) which initiates AV cushion development [19]. TGFβ2 induces initial cell-cell separation of valve endothelial cells, while TGFβ3 stimulates their invasion and subsequent mesenchymal phenotype shift [15,16]. During post-EMT, these mesenchymal cells facilitate a transition in the cushion microstructure from glycosaminoglycans (GAGs) (hyaluronan, versican) toward fibrous structural proteins (collagen I, IV, V, fibronectin, periostin) [5,20,21]. This shift in ECM content translates into increased valve stiffness [22], and coincides with elevated expression of TGFβ3 in the cushions and AV canal [23]. Furthermore, TGFβ3 upregulates collagen I and periostin in post-EMT AV cushion explants [24], suggesting that TGFβ3 is a key modulator of cushion ECM content, and consequent mechanical properties. An aim of this study is to better understand this remodeling potential of TGFβ3 through a combined analysis of cushion stiffness, matrix compaction, cell proliferation, and ECM synthesis.

The capacity of TGFβ3 to stimulate valvular remodeling events underscores the importance of identifying molecular signals which modulate TGFβ activity. Recent studies indicate that serotonin (5-HT) interacts with TGFβ signaling in adult heart valves [25,26], and can also alter valve mechanical properties [27,28]. 5-HT, which is a monoamine neurotransmitter derived from the essential amino acid tryptophan [29], increased the stiffness of porcine aortic valve cusps with the endothelial layer denuded [27], and under cyclic stretch [30]. Serotonin also increased collagen synthesis in human and sheep valve interstitial cells (VICs) [25,31]. Reports in adult VICs indicate that 5-HT can upregulate TGFβ, resulting in cell differentiation and aberrant connective tissue accumulation [25,26,32]. In development, serotonin is active in key events such as cardiac progenitor patterning, left-right laterality, and migration of the neural crest [33–37]. Murine AV cushions express the serotonin receptors 5-HT2a and 5-HT2b, and the serotonin transporter (SERT) by the completion of EMT [38,39], which is when TGFβ3 expression increases in the cushions [18,40]. Latent TGFβ binding protein and serotonin binding protein are also expressed in murine post-EMT endocardial cushions [41,42], highlighting each pathway's capacity to regulate expression of their ligands. The proximity of these TGFβ and 5-HT signaling components suggests that they may be interacting partners in post-EMT cushion development. Furthermore, a recent study reported TGFβ1 upregulation in murine SERT KO hearts at near fetal stages, which was hypothesized to be a consequence of excess 5-HT signaling due to SERT inhibition [43]. In light of these signaling interactions in both adult and development models, we hypothesize that this mechanically relevant crosstalk of TGFβ and 5-HT may play a role in modulating embryonic AV cushion biomechanics.

The objectives of this study therefore were to characterize the remodeling capacity of TGFβ3 in AV cushions, and determine how TGFβ3 and 5-HT may act together to regulate cushion biomechanical remodeling. Chick AV cushion biomechanics, compaction, and candidate gene expression were quantified through implementation of an *ex vivo* cushion culture system. We determined that TGFβ3 induces AV valve stiffening through increases in cell proliferation, myofibroblastic differentiation, and collagen synthesis. 5-HT enhances the AV valve stiffening effect of TGFβ3 in a dose-dependent manner. Crosstalk between TGFβ3 and 5-HT signaling was investigated via molecular inhibition studies. The *ex vivo* results were then tested *in ovo* through an elevated 5-HT model. These results suggest that 5-HT may be an important potentiator of TGFβ3 signaling in embryonic valve morphogenesis and biomechanical stiffening.

Materials and Methods

Ethics Statement

Leghorn avian embryos from Hamburger-Hamilton stages (HH) 17–36 were utilized in this research. All procedures in this study followed the guidelines of Cornell University and NIH policy, which state that avian embryos of these stages are not considered vertebrate animals for the purposes of IACUC regulation.

AV cushion remodeling organ culture model

Fertilized leghorn chicken eggs were incubated until stage HH25 (Day 4.5). The AV cushions were isolated from their myocardial attachment in ice-cold sterile Earle's Balanced Salt Solution (EBSS; Quality Biological, Inc.). Single cushions were cultured in 20 μL hanging drops for 24 hours at 38°C in a 5% CO_2 environment. Control culture media consisted of Medium 199 (M199 w/phenol red and L-glutamine; Gibco) with 1% concentrations of penicillin/streptomycin (Gibco), Insulin-Trans-ferrin-Selenium (ITS, Gibco), and chick serum (Gibco). For experiments, control media was treated with one or more of the following reagents: human recombinant TGFβ3 (1 ng/ml, Sigma), serotonin hydrochloride (0.47–47 μM, Sigma), Cytochalasin D (1 μM, Sigma), 5-HT2a inhibitor MDL100,907 (0.01–1 μM, Axon Medchem BV), 5-HT2b inhibitor SB204741 (0.35–35 μM, Sigma), SERT inhibitor Fluoxetine (1–10 μM, Sigma) and Alk 4,5,&7 inhibitor SB431542 hydrate (0.26–26 μM, Sigma). TGFβ3 was reconstituted in 4 mM HCl solution containing 1 mg/ml BSA, all other reagents were dissolved in DMSO. The 470 nM 5-HT dose was considered physiological, based on HPLC measured concentrations in 10% fetal bovine serum media (~100 nM [44]). The 47 μM 5-HT dosage is similar to prior *in vitro/ex vivo* studies in postnatal valves [25,27,28,30,45], so we conservatively considered this dose high for our studies.

Micromechanical testing

Cushion mechanical properties were measured after 24 hour treatment in the *ex vivo* study and at HH25 in the *in ovo* study using the micromechanical pipette aspiration technique [22,46,47]. A glass micropipette (~70–100 μm in diameter) was placed adjacent to the cushion surface, and a small vacuum pressure was incrementally applied. The pressure source was a 200 μL pipetter calibrated with a custom manometer. Previous strain history was mitigated by preconditioning with ~20 cycles of low pressurization (<1 Pa). The tissue was then monotonically loaded with increasing static pressure loads, at which images were captured. Aspirated length L, measured as the length from the tip of the pipette to tip of the tissue furthest inside the pipette, was converted into an experimental "stretch ratio", $\lambda = \frac{L+r_p}{r_p}$, by normalizing to the pipette radius, r_p. The cushion was assumed to be an isotropic, incompressible, hyperelastic material with an exponential free energy law, $W = \frac{C}{2}\{\exp[\alpha(I_B-3)]-1\}$, where I_B is the first invariant of left Cauchy Green stretch tensor. AV cushion material isotropy at HH25 was supported by a lack of preferred matrix orientation as determined by ubiquitous protein stain 5-DTAF (50 μM Invitrogen; Figure S1). The ΔP vs. λ data was then fit to the axial stress equation of a uni-axially loaded bar of this exponential material, specifically, $\sigma_{axial} = \alpha C \exp\left[\alpha\left(\lambda^2 + \frac{2}{\lambda} - 3\right)\right]\left(\lambda^2 - \frac{1}{\lambda}\right)$. From previous analysis [22], the ΔP vs. λ curve differs from the uniaxial load expression by a scale factor, γ. This scale factor was numerically determined to be a function of only the material parameter α. Due to the nonlinear nature of the data, the mechanical testing data is presented as strain energy density. This was calculated as the area under the ΔP vs. λ curve fit from λ = 1–2 (Figure 1A), which from our assumed material model is $W_{1-2} = \frac{C^*}{2}\{\exp(2\alpha)-1\}$, where $C^* = \gamma C$.

Compaction & Opening Angle Assays

Compaction of the AV cushions was quantified as the ratio of cross-sectional area before (A_0) and after (A) 24 hours of culture in

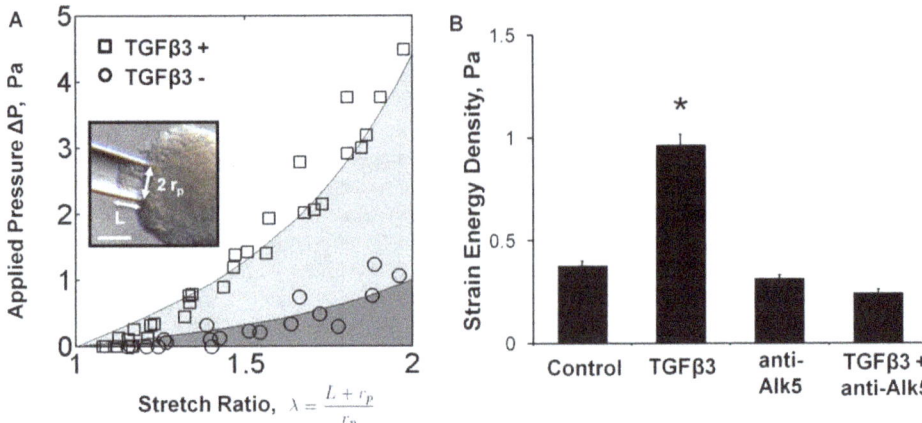

Figure 1. TGFβ3 treatment increases stiffness of AV cushions through Alk5 mediated pathway. A) Representative pipette test data for TGFβ3 (1 ng/ml, TGFβ3+) and control media (TGFβ3−) treated cushions, n = 4. Strain energy density was calculated from the shaded regions beneath the ΔP vs λ curves. Inset: image of aspirated HH25 AV cushion after 24 hours of culture. The pipette radius, r_p, and the aspirated length, L are indicated. Scale bar = 70 μm. **B)** AV cushion strain energy density increased with TGFβ3 treatment, but was blocked by Alk5 inhibition (SB431542, 2.6 μM). mean ± SEM, n≥7, *p<0.0001, 2-way ANOVA.

the different treatment conditions, denoted A/A_0. This ratio measures the combined biomechanical remodeling effects of cell traction, proliferation, and ECM synthesis. To isolate cell traction effects, we quantified the opening angles created by micro-slit incision in AV cushions after 24 hours of treatment. The incision was made along the centerline of the spherical cushion mass, extending approximately one radius into the cushion, and immediately created a pie-wedge with defined opening angle. Opening angles are an established indicator of tissue residual stress [48], which is primarily a function of cell traction forces in our culture system. Images were taken at 150× magnification using Zeiss Discovery v20 stereomicroscope (Spectra Services, Inc.) and QImaging Retiga 4000R Fast camera (Spectra Services, Inc). Cross-sectional area and opening angle were measured from calibrated images using NIH ImageJ image analysis software.

Immunohistochemistry (IHC)

Proliferation was assessed through bromodeoxyuridine (BrdU) incorporation into HH25 AV cushion hanging drops. BrdU reagent (Invitrogen) was added at 1:100 dilution in culture medium 6 hours prior to completion of 24 hour culture. AV cushions were then rinsed and fixed in 4% paraformeldehyde (PFA). BrdU incorporation was assessed via immunofluorescent antibody staining and confocal microscopy using anti-BrdU 488 (1:100, Invitrogen), with DRAQ5 (1:1000, Biostatus) as a DNA counterstain. Images were processed via ImageJ, and BrdU incorporation was quantified as the ratio of BrdU positive cells to total cell count. IHC was also used to label phosphorylated Smad2/3 (pSmad2/3) complex in HH25 cushions isolated from the systemic 5-HT *in ovo* model. Isolated cushions were fixed in 4% PFA and then stained via standard whole mount IHC protocol. The cushions were stained with primary pSmad2/3 polyclonal goat anti-human antibody (1:50, Santa Cruz) followed with 488 fluorescent secondary (1:100, Santa Cruz) and cell nuclei counter stain DRAQ5 (1:1000). pSmad2/3 was quantified as the number of cell nuclei with localized pSmad2/3 divided by the total number of cell nuclei.

PCR quantification of gene expression

At the end of 24 hour treatment, AV cushion mRNA was isolated and purified using RNEasy Isolation Kit (Qiagen). A set of 8–10 cushions were pooled per test sample. RNA integrity was determined by NanoDrop spectrometry, using A260/A280 ratio between 1.8 and 2.2 as quality control. cDNA synthesis was completed using SuperScript III first strand RT-PCR kit (Invitrogen) with oligo(dT) primers. Amplification reactions were as follows: (95°C 15 s), (54°C 15 s), (72°C 30 s). Power Syber Green (Applied Biosystems) replication indicator was read at the completion of each 72°C stage. Standard curves for all primers (listed in Table S1) were generated from HH34 brain mRNA and normalized to 18 s ribosomal RNA. Threshold cycle count, C(t), was used to calculate gene expression via the $\Delta\Delta Ct$ method using 18 s rRNA as a housekeeping reference gene [49].

5-HT administration in ovo

HH17 stage fertilized leghorn chicken eggs were windowed on their blunt side. Up to 1.0 mg of serotonin (Sigma) was diluted into 100 μL of PBS and dispensed directly onto the chorionic membrane at HH17, HH25, or HH31. The max 5-HT dosage was equivalent to 18 mg/kg which is comparable to other elevated 5-HT animal models (25 mg/kg and 75 mg/kg) [50,51]. After 5-HT treatment, chicks were then sealed and cultured at 55% humidity and 38°C until HH36 (Day 10). Preliminary experiments demonstrated that 5-HT treatment sometimes resulted in an ectopic heart, so additional embryos were alternatively subjected to a thoracotomy that mimicked an ectopic heart without serotonin administration as a control. Embryos were then dissected and analyzed for gross anatomical defects. Hearts with intact great artery connections were then removed, cleared, and analyzed with 3D confocal microscopy or serial section histology using Movat's pentachrome stain. Optical fluorescence tomography (OFT) of ventricular, valve, and outflow vessel anatomy was performed as previously described [52,53]. Briefly, HH36 hearts were freshly isolated and rinsed with 1% lidocaine in PBS buffer. Following rinse, hearts were perfused with fluorescein isothiocyanate–poly-L-lysine (Sigma) via micro injection and then fixed in 4% PFA. The poly-L-lysine binds to the negatively charged endothelial glycocalyx. Hearts were then cleared using Murray's

Clear, followed by deep tissue 3D imaging via fluorescence confocal microscopy. Hearts were screened for major defects, and valve morphometry were quantified from this using ImageJ. Valve measurements included leaflet length, average thickness, and minimal thickness with control n = 3 and 5-HT treatment n = 6. Average thickness (t_{avg}) was calculated as $t_{avg} = A_L/L$, where L is the annulus-tip length of the leaflet, and A_L is cross-sectional area of leaflet. The location of minimum thickness was generally the same for all specimens regardless of treatment.

Statistical Analyses

All data is presented as mean ± standard error of the mean for the number of samples reported. Statistical comparisons between groups were performed using ANOVA for data sets involving more than two groups, or two-tailed t test when only two groups were compared. Defect prevalence in the *in ovo* model was compared using a chi-squared statistical test. In all comparisons, differences between groups was considered statistically significant for p valves smaller than 0.05.

Results

TGFβ3 increases AV cushion stiffness

Ex vivo cultured AV cushions exhibited nonlinear mechanical behavior that was well described by the exponential constitutive model (Figure 1A). Administration of exogenous TGFβ3 (1 ng/ml) increased cushion stiffness 2.5 fold over controls ($W_{TGFβ3} = 0.965 \pm 0.051$ vs. $W_{Contr} = 0.378 \pm 0.021$, p<0.0001 Figure 1B). Inhibition of canonical TGFβ signaling via the TGFβ type 1 receptor Alk 5 (2.6 μM SB431542 [54]) blocked the increase in cushion stiffness ($W_{T+TI} = 0.245 \pm 0.043$ Figure 1B). The Alk5 inhibitor alone had no effect on cushion biomechanics. TGFβ3-treated cushions compacted less than controls, with compaction quantified as the ratio of cross-sectional area before and after treatment ($A/A_0 = 0.925 \pm 0.028$ vs. $A/A_0 = 0.508 \pm 0.017$, p<0.0001 Figure 2A). This was unexpected because the Cytochalasin D (CytD, 1 μM) results suggested that compaction and stiffness are directly related. CytD inhibited cytoskeletal actin polymerization which resulted in a 5.3 fold decrease in strain energy density of the AV cushions relative to control ($W_{CytD} = 0.072 \pm 0.016$, Figure S2A). Without actin polymerization the AV cushion cells did not compact the matrix, and the cushion did not remodel into the spherical configuration observed in all other treatments. Instead, the post treatment cushion area was significantly larger than initial area, suggesting a relaxation of pre-treatment actin forces ($A/A_0 = 1.60 \pm 0.03$, Figure S2B). The TGFβ3 results of stiffness increase with compaction decrease did not align with this trend. Alk5 inhibition did return compaction behavior to control levels ($A/A_0 = 0.570 \pm 0.035$ Figure S3), indicating that the stiffness and compaction results are both dependent on activation of canonical TGFβ3 signaling. To better understand the relationship between stiffness and compaction, cushion opening angles were quantified to approximate differences in cell traction forces. The opening angle of TGFβ3 cushions was 1.29 fold larger than controls ($74.6° \pm 2.0°$ vs. $57.7° \pm 1.4°$, p<0.001 Figure 2B), indicating that TGFβ3 treated cushions did indeed have higher cell traction forces. Together, these results demonstrate that TGFβ3 induces cushion stiffening through Alk5, but with a concurrent reduction in tissue compaction that suggests other processes are also affected.

TGFβ3 increases AV cushion proliferation and mesenchymal phenotype

Contractile phenotype markers αSMA and RhoA were significantly upregulated with TGFβ3 treatment, 5.3±0.4 and 2.1±0.3 fold (± SEM) respectively (Figure 3A), suggesting that TGFβ3 induced residual tension is partially due to an increased migratory/contractile phenotype of resident cushion mesenchyme. TGFβ3 treatment also upregulated mRNA expression of col1α2 mRNA (3.8±0.9, p<0.05) and cyclin b2 (3.9±0.7 fold, p<0.05), indicative of increased collagen I synthesis and cell proliferation, respectively. BrdU incorporation confirmed that TGFβ3 increased cushion cell proliferation 2.26±0.36 fold over controls (p<0.0001, Figure 3B). Collectively, these results strongly suggest that while TGFβ3 treated AV cushion mesenchyme are more migratory/contractile, concomitant increases in cell proliferation and matrix synthesis work to counteract aggregate matrix compaction. This explains how the TGFβ3 treated cushions are biomechanically stiffer, but appear minimally compacted. Furthermore, TGFβ3 treatment increased TGFβ3 transcription (2.2±0.6 fold, p<0.05), indicating a potential positive feedback loop for TGFβ3 control of AV cushion biomechanical remodeling.

5-HT potentiates TGFβ3 signaling through 5-HT2b receptor

The effect of 5-HT dose on biomechanical remodeling, independently and in combination with TGFβ3, was systematically evaluated through the stiffness and compaction metrics of the AV cushion organ culture system. 5-HT administration by itself had no statistically significant effect on cushion stiffness. Combined treatment of TGFβ3 with physiological 5-HT (470 nM) increased AV cushion stiffness ($W_{T+5-HT} = 1.136 \pm 0.035$), but high 5-HT dose (5-HT+ = 47 μM) eliminated any TGFβ3 induced stiffening effect ($W_{T+5-HT+} = 0.457 \pm 0.025$, Figure 4). Neither selective inhibition of the 5-HT2a (MDL100907 10 nM), 5-HT2b (SB204741 2.6 μM) receptors, nor the serotonin transporter SERT (Flouxetine 10 μM) alone affected cushion stiffness (Figure 4). Yet in combination with TGFβ3, the anti-5-HT2b treatment completely blocked TGFβ3 dependent stiffness and compaction behavior (Figure 4 & Figure S3). Inhibition of the 5-HT2a receptor or SERT had no measurable effect on TGFβ3 induced cushion biomechanics. The compaction and stiffness changes induced by 5-HT potentiated TGFβ3 followed the same trend of TGFβ3 treatment alone, with compaction decreasing as stiffness increased and vice versa (Figure 4 & Figure S3). The additional stiffening effect of 5-HT with TGFβ3 was also eliminated with Alk5 inhibition, as shown through the combined treatment of TGFβ3+5-HT+anti-Alk5 in Figure S4. This combined treatment generated a strain energy density similar to the TGFβ3+anti-Alk5 treatment (0.209±0.023 Pa vs 0.245±0.16 Pa, respectively), and further supported that the effects of 5-HT signaling on AV valve remodeling is dependent on canonical TGFβ signaling. Together, these findings suggest that exogenous 5-HT acts through the 5-HT2b receptor to augment or impair TGFβ3 induced cushion stiffening and compaction in a dose-dependent manner.

5-HT modulates TGFβ3 regulation of AV cushion mesenchyme phenotype

Exogenous 5-HT administration potentiated remodeling-relevant gene expression in organ cultured AV cushion mesenchyme. TGFβ3 mRNA transitioned from 1.9±0.1 fold upregulation over controls at physiological 5-HT to 0.40±0.16 downregulation at high 5-HT dose (Figure 5A). The physiological 5-HT dose had no

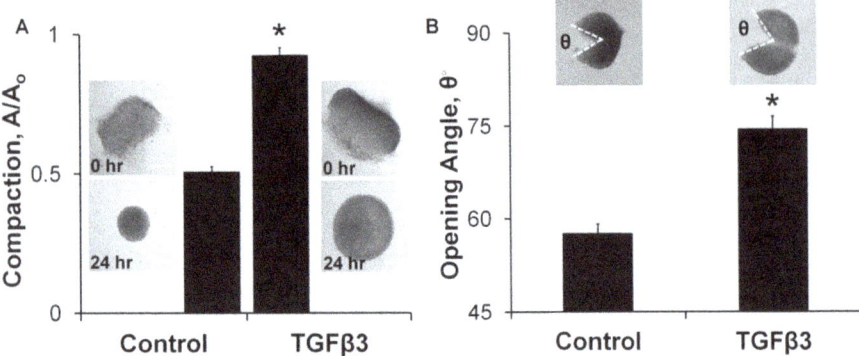

Figure 2. TGFβ3 treated cushions compact less than controls, but are under more residual tension. A) Bar graph of area ratios calculated from before and after images of 24 hour TGFβ3 treated cushions. Representative cushion images shown, scale bar = 100 μm. mean ± SEM, n≥12, *p<0.0001, t-test **B**) Opening angle of 24 hour TGFβ3 treated cushions is greater than control, indicating tissue is under greater residual tension. Inset shows representative images with opening angle, θ. mean ± SEM, n = 10–11, *p<0.001 t-test.

statistically significant effect on αSMA, col1α2, cyclin b2, and RhoA expression. In contrast, high 5-HT significantly decreased transcription of αSMA (0.18±0.09), collagen1α2 (0.22±0.07), and RhoA (0.46±0.11 Figure 5A). No effect on cyclin b2 expression was observed at either dose, suggesting proliferation was not directly regulated by 5-HT. Physiological 5-HT did not affect TGFβ3 induced gene expression (Figure 5B), but high dose 5-HT markedly reduced gene expression of TGFβ3 (0.86±0.20 vs. 2.2±0.6), αSMA (1.4±0.4 vs. 5.3±0.4), collagen1α2 (1.3±0.3 vs. 3.8±0.9), and RhoA (1.3±0.2 vs. 2.1±0.3) (Figure 5B). Proliferation-related gene cyclin b2 was not significantly affected by 5-HT in combination with TGFβ3. These results suggest that exogenous 5-HT potentiates TGFβ3 more likely through interaction with upstream activation points and/or TGFβ3 synthesis, rather than by interacting with TGFβ3 downstream targets directly.

We also analyzed the mRNA expression of intracellular 5-HT (i5-HT) related genes transglutaminase 2 (TGM2) and SERT. i5-HT transamidates small GTPases and matrix proteins, in a process called "serotonylation" [44]. TGM2 is an i5-HT binding partner which assists transamidation of RhoA [55] and fibronectin [56], altering tissue mechanics through GTPase activation and matrix protein cross-linking, respectively. SERT mRNA expres-

sion was significantly increased with 5-HT treatment (1.5±0.2 fold, p<0.05), but was downregulated with the 5-HT+ dose (0.46±0.12 fold, Figure S5A). TGFβ3 treatment stimulated a 4.0±1.0 fold increase in TGM2, but SERT transcription remained near control levels (0.70±0.11, Figure S5B). Addition of 5-HT with TGFβ3 significantly decreased SERT and TGM2 mRNA, regardless of 5-HT dose. Although TGFβ3 treatment did upregulate TGM2, the downregulation of SERT by 5-HT treatment and the lack of mechanical changes seen with the SERT inhibitor suggest that serotonylation is not a primary mechanism of stiffness increase in the *ex vivo* culture remodeling results.

Elevated 5-HT induces atrioventricular valvuloseptal defects in ovo

As the effects of TGFβ signaling on valve formation are well studied [17,18,57], we here test whether exogenous 5-HT administration *in ovo* alters valve morphogenesis. 5-HT administration *in ovo* at HH17 induced a spectrum of cardiac defects by HH36 (Day 10) as summarized in Table 1. Temporal and dosage dependant viability curves (Figure S6A) showed that a 0.7 mg dose

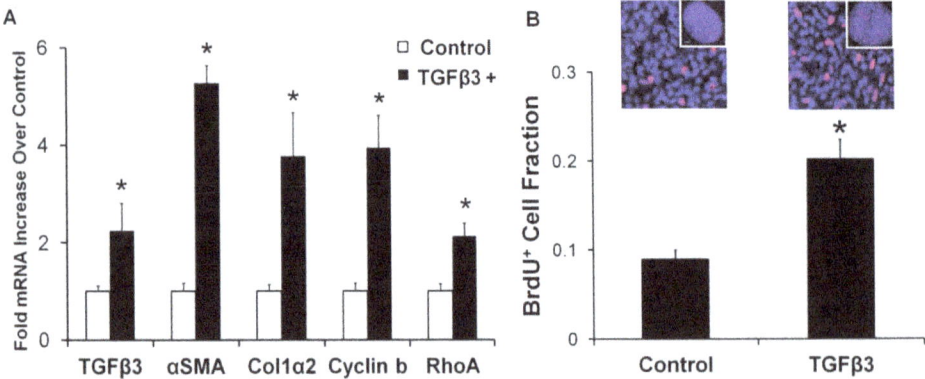

Figure 3. Remodeling behavior of TGFβ3 treated cushions is a balance of contractile differentiation, proliferation, and matrix synthesis. A) 24 hour TGFβ3 treated cushions upregulate contractile (αSMA, RhoA), proliferation (cyclin b), and extracellular matrix protein (col1α2) encoding genes. TGFβ3 administration also significantly stimulated its own production. mean ± SEM, n = 3–4 pooled samples of 8–10 cushions, *p<0.05, t-test. **B**) BrdU incorporation data (red) of TGFβ3 treated cushions normalized to DRAQ5 cell nuclei counter stain (blue). BrdU was administered 6 hours prior to completion of 24 hour treatment. Representative confocal images are shown above each bar, with a global view of cushion contained in the inset. mean ± SEM, n = 12, *p<0.0001, t-test.

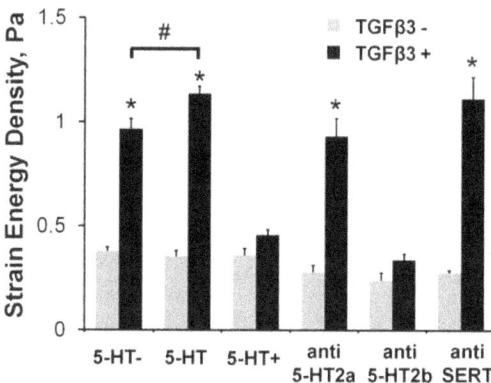

Figure 4. 5-HT signaling modulates TGFβ3 induced AV cushion stiffness. Physiological dosages of 5-HT (470 nM, *5-HT*) exacerbated TGFβ3 stiffening, while elevated dosages (47 μM, *5-HT+*) eliminated it. Molecular inhibition of the 5-HT2a receptor (MDL100907 10 nM, *anti-5-HT2a*) and the serotonin transporter (Fluoxetine 10 μM, *anti-SERT*) did not affect TGFβ3 mediated biomechanical stiffening. Inhibition of the 5-HT2b receptor (SB204741 35 μM, *anti-5-HT2b*) however eliminated the stiffening effect of TGFβ3. mean ± SEM, n≥6, *p<0.0001 t-test relative to control, #p<0.05 2-way ANOVA with Tukey post-hoc test.

was over 50% lethal at HH36, but administration of the same dose of 5-HT at HH25 or HH31 did not result in further lethality or defect formation (data not shown). The only gross malformations observed were localized to the heart and chest wall. Approximately 42% (24/57) of affected embryos exhibited an ectopic heart which protruded through an incomplete chest wall closure (Figure S6B). To confirm that interior defects resulted specifically from 5-HT exposure and not secondarily from the ectopia, an experimental thoracotomy was performed to model the ectopic condition. We found no statistically significant occurrence of any cardiac defects with experimental ectopia, supporting that 5-HT was responsible for the cardiac defects observed. A ventricular septal defect (VSD or SVSD) occurred in 42% (24/57) of the defective embryos. Approximately 18% (10/57) of the embryos exhibited double outlet right ventricle (DORV) defects. 5-HT administration also resulted in significantly enlarged atria with thinned walls in 35% (20/57) of the defective embryos (Table 1, Figure 6A). All of the embryos with DORV also exhibited highly stenotic or atretic atrioventricular (AV) valves (Figure 6B), with the normally muscular flap valve in the right AV canal appearing thin and fibrous like the left AV valve. Regardless of gross cardiac defect identified, the average (0.144±0.009 mm, mean ± SEM) and minimal (0.080±0.007 mm) thickness of the left AV septal leaflet was thinner in 5-HT treated embryos than controls (0.191±0.009 and 0.165±0.023 mm respectively, Figure 6C). No differences were found in mural leaflet thickness, or in the length of either leaflet. The reduction in AV valve thickness with 5-HT treatment indicated an increase in tissue compaction, and may possibly be a recapitulation of the migratory/contractile phenotype observed *ex vivo*.

Exogenous 5-HT increases AV cushion stiffness through TGFβ signaling in ovo

Systemic 5-HT treatment at HH17 resulted in a statistically significant 1.4±0.2 fold increase in AV cushion stiffness over control at stage HH25 (strain energy density of 0.43±0.06 Pa vs. 0.31±0.03 Pa, *p<0.05, Figure 7A). We next analyzed the mesenchymal gene expression patterns in this *in ovo* system. 5-HT significantly upregulated TGFβ3 (1.7±0.1), αSMA (1.5±0.1),

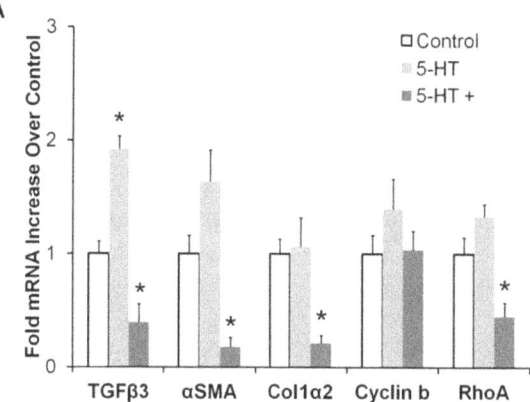

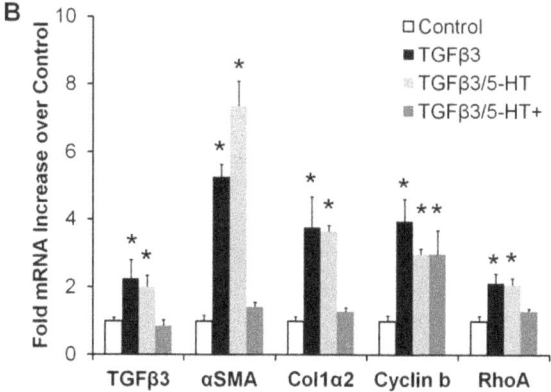

Figure 5. 5-HT treatment modulates TGFβ3 mediated gene expression. A) TGFβ3 mRNA transcripts increase with physiological 5-HT (470 nM, *5-HT*), but decrease at high dose (47 μM, *5-HT+*). αSMA, RhoA, and col1α2, were not affected by physiological 5-HT dose, but were significantly downregulated with high 5-HT treatment. **B**) High 5-HT treatment mitigates exogenous TGFβ3 induced contractile gene expression, while TGFβ3 induced proliferation was independent of 5-HT dose. mean ± SEM, n=3–5 pooled samples of 8–10 cushions, *p<0.05 via ANOVA comparisons with controls.

col1α2 (1.5±0.1), cyclin b (1.6±0.2), and RhoA (1.7±0.2) (*p<0.05, Figure 7B). Interestingly, the TGFβ3 mRNA expression was comparable to that observed in the *ex ovo* organ culture treatment of TGFβ3 alone (2.2±0.6), 5-HT alone (1.9±0.1), and TGFβ3+5-HT (2.0±0.3). αSMA and col1α2 mRNA were also upregulated *in ovo* with 5-HT, but less than with direct TGFβ3 administration in *ex vivo* culture (αSMA – 1.5 vs 5.7, RhoA – 1.7 vs 2.1). The similar mRNA profiles of the candidate genes in both models suggested that 5-HT also potentiates TGFβ signaling in AV cushions *in ovo*. To confirm that the 5-HT treatment was indeed modulating TGFβ signaling activity *in ovo*, we quantified nuclear pSmad2/3 expression in HH25 cushions with and without 5-HT treatment (Figure 8). 5-HT treatment increased the number of cell nuclei with localized pSmad2/3 expression 2.6±0.8 fold over control embryos (0.28±0.04 vs. 0.11±0.03, p<0.01). Together these results demonstrate that 5-HT potentiates TGFβ signaling in AV cushions to control contractile differentiation, proliferation, and biomechanical remodeling.

Discussion

In this study we implemented a quantitative organ culture assay that simultaneously interrogated the contributions of cellular and

Table 1. Cardiac Defect Summary of *in ovo* 5-HT Administration.

	Control	Serotonin	Thoracotomy[1]
# of embryos treated (HH17)	35	133	107
# of embryos survived (HH36)	34	60	49
# of defective embryos (HH36)	0	57*	27
Summary of Defects Represented in Survival Groups[2]			
Ectopic	-	24*	25*
VSD	-	5	-
SVSD	-	19*	1
DILV	-	3	-
DOLV	-	1	-
DORV	-	10*	-
Enlarged Atria	-	20*	3

[1]Thoracotomy control of ectopic heart condition was created by mechanically debriding the chest dermis and pericardium at HH17.
[2]Several embryos possessed more than one defect. VSD – ventricular septal defect; SVSD – *stenotic* VSD; DILV – double inlet left ventricle; DOLV – double outlet left ventricle; DORV – double outlet right ventricle.
*p<0.05 Chi-Squared test.

molecular signaling to drive cushion tissue-level remodeling and biomechanical strengthening. TGFβ3 stimulated a 2.5 fold increase in biomechanical stiffness (Figure 1), generated in part by an increase in cell traction. This contractile phenotype is a common outcome of TGFβ signaling in post-natal valve tissue. For

instance, porcine aortic valves express contractile marker αSMA when stimulated by TGFβ1 *in situ* [58]. Porcine aortic valve interstitial cells (VICs) embedded in collagen gels expressed αSMA in response to TGFβ1, and demonstrated significant gel compaction over untreated gels [59]. Similarly, TGFβ3 treated embryonic AV progenitors compacted collagen gels to 10% of initial area [23]. Yet in contrast to these reports, TGFβ3 induced contractility did not result in hyper-compacted AV cushions (Figure 2), but instead compacted less than controls. A key distinction between these two assays is that *in vitro* collagen gel cultures have much lower cell densities than our *ex vivo* system. The effect of proliferation on volume change is virtually undetectable in these gels, and cell traction dominates the compaction behavior. In native tissues, especially in the embryo, changes in cell proliferation and/or apoptosis have a significant impact on resulting tissue volume and apparent compaction. Hanging-drop culture of AV cushions enables precise control of the biochemical environment while maintaining the natural structural and cellular composition of the cushion. The lack of compaction with TGFβ3 treatment is therefore most likely due to a counterbalancing from increases in cell proliferation (Figure 3B) and ECM synthesis. This supports a mechanism of simultaneous tissue growth, matrix reorganization, and biomechanical stiffening during embryonic valve formation that is driven by a complex coordination of cell tractions, matrix synthesis, and cell proliferation. These findings underscore that embryonic valve mechanics, which is critical for proper valve function, cannot be inferred strictly from isolated compaction, proliferation, or matrix synthesis data, but is best measured directly.

The interplay of TGFβ3 and 5-HT signaling was most notably seen through the potentiation of TGFβ3 gene expression by 5-HT

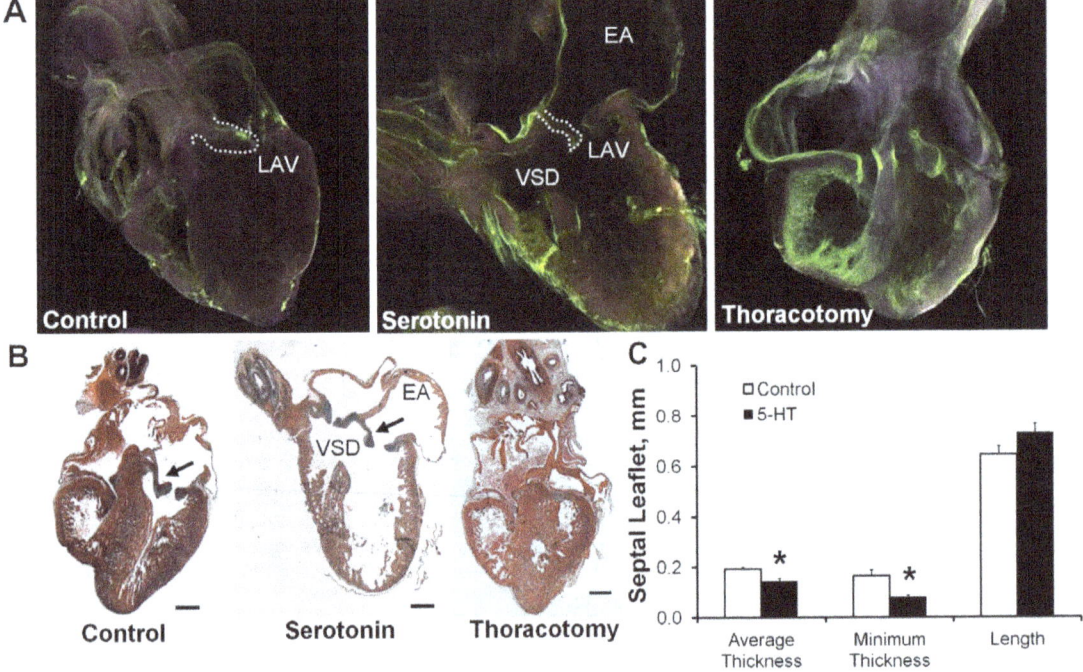

Figure 6. 5-HT administration *in ovo* induces cardiac defects. A) Representative virtual sections of control, 5-HT treated, and thoracotomy sham control hearts at HH36 via endopainting and confocal microscopy. **B**) Representative Movat's pentachrome stained sections of hearts with the same conditions. Prominent cardiac defects, including enlarged atria (EA) and ventricular septal defect (VSD), were associated with malformed and malfunctioning AV valves (arrows). 25×, scale bar = 500 μm. **C**) Left septal leaflet average thickness and minimum thickness are both statistically thinner in 5-HT treated leaflets than control. mean ± SEM, n = 3–6 hearts per treatment, *p<0.05, t-test.

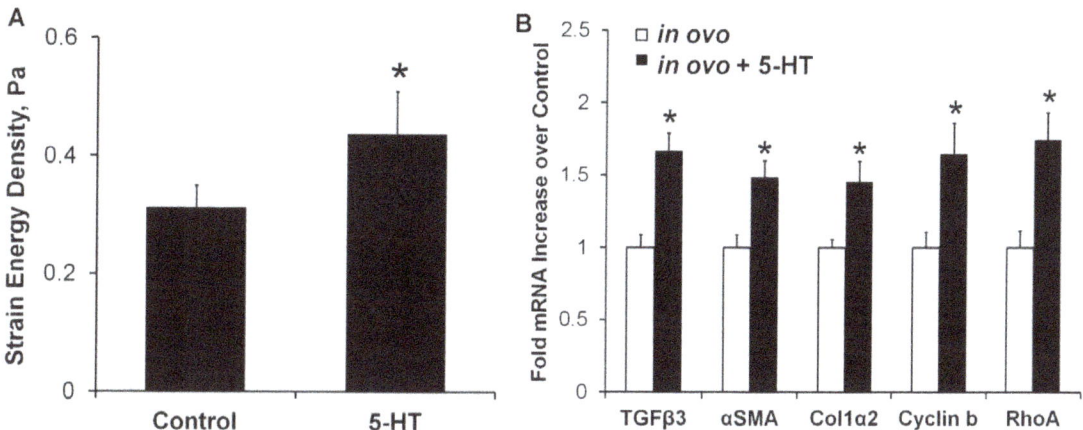

Figure 7. Exogenous 5-HT increases AV cushion stiffness and TGFβ related remodeling genes *in ovo*. A) The strain energy density (Pa) of HH25 cushions increased 1.4 fold with systemic 5-HT treatment *in ovo*, mean ± SEM, n = 8–10 cushion, *p<0.05, t-test. **B)** Gene expression levels of HH25 AV cushions isolated from embryos treated with 5-HT at HH17 (48 hours). mean ± SEM, n = 6–10 samples, each of 8–10 pooled HH25 cushions, *p<0.05, t-test.

dose (Figure 5). The physiological 5-HT concentration upregulated TGFβ3 expression, while the high concentration downregulated expression. Upregulation of TGFβ expression by 5-HT has been observed in several cardiac cells and tissues, though the molecular mechanism is still unclear. Adult aortic valve interstitial cells treated with 5-HT have increased TGFβ1 activity, predominantly through the 5-HT2a receptor [25,60]. Neo-natal rat cardiac fibroblasts treated with 5-HT and 5-HT2a agonists upregulated αSMA protein expression, which is a marker for fibroblast differentiation and a gene induced by TGFβ signaling [61]. Similarly, TGFβ1 and αSMA expression were elevated in SERT cre-lox KO mice hearts through heightened 5-HT2a signaling in late embryonic stage mice, purportedly due to excess 5-HT from SERT inhibition [43]. Other reports point to 5-HT2b as the key mechanism. 5-HT administration in adult rats increased 5-HT2b mRNA expression in both aortic and mitral valves, demonstrating a positive response to 5-HT treatment [50]. SERT mRNA was downregulated in these valves denoting a negative response to elevated 5-HT, which our results also demonstrate (Figure S5B). The 5-HT2b receptor, TGFβ receptor type I and II, and the TGFβ latent binding protein were all more expressed in canine myxomatous mitral valves than normal valves, suggesting a

coupling of these two pathways through 5-HT2b [26]. Long-term 5-HT treatment of rats generated valve-related echocardiographic and histology defects [62], but these defects did not occur in rats simultaneously treated with a 5-HT2b inhibitor [51]. This suggests that the 5-HT2b receptor may be a key pathway for cardiac and valve tissue remodeling. Cardiac fibroblast studies indicate that 5-HT upregulates TGFβ1 through a mutual transactivation of the epidermal growth factor (EGF) pathway and the 5-HT2b receptor [45,63]. Our results support a 5-HT2b dependant mechanism, as seen by 5-HT2b inhibition effectively blocking TGFβ3 stiffening. The TGFβ stiffening effect was independent of 5-HT2a and SERT. Although TGFβ3 upregulated TGM2 expression, 5-HT treatment mitigated this expression which suggests TGM2 activity does not contribute to the enhanced stiffening of TGFβ/5-HT signaling. High 5-HT also mitigated TGFβ3 stiffening, which may be due to desensitization of the 5-HT2b receptor by sustained high 5-HT exposure. 5-HT increased pSmad2/3 phosphorylation in cushion mesenchyme *in ovo*. This suggests that 5-HT signaling through 5HT2b may interact with Smad2/3 signaling, but further studies are warranted to clarify potential roles of other intermediate or downstream targets.

In our *in ovo* model, systemic 5-HT elevation induced severe heart defects, including failure of the ventricular septum to close, ballooned atria, DORV, and hyper-contracted AV valves. Variations of these defects have been observed in other TGFβ and 5-HT related studies. VSDs are the most prevalent congenital heart defects observed, occurring in approximately 50% of all clinical cardiac malformations [64,65]. Selective serotonin uptake inhibitors (SSRI) taken during the first trimester of pregnancy were associated with a statistical increase in VSD prevalence in newborns [66]. Our data supports elevated extracellular 5-HT as a possible cause of this correlation. Removal of TGFβ secondary messenger Smad4 causes VSDs and other lethal congenital defects, which are presumed to be the consequence of decreased TGFβ signaling [67]. Yet removal of TGFβ inhibitory messenger Smad7 also generates VSDs [68], indicating that exacerbated TGFβ signaling can also generate significant cardiac defects. The dilated atria observed in our model are not explicitly reported in other 5-HT studies, suggesting the defect may result from secondary effects, such as altered hemodynamics from valve incompetence. For instance, enlarged atria have been induced in zebrafish embryos through mechanical obstruction of the AV

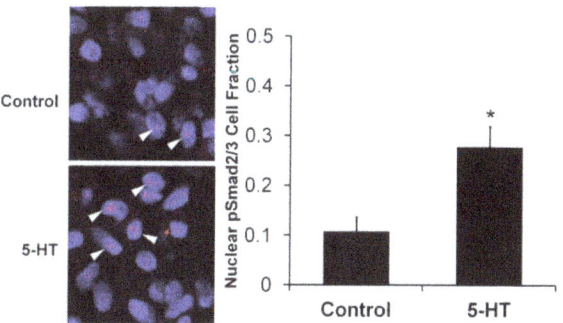

Figure 8. 5-HT increases AV cushion pSmad2/3 expression *in ovo*. A) Representative images of pSmad2/3 staining. Arrows indicate pSmad2/3 positive cells. Cell nuclei – blue, pSmad2/3 – red. **B)** Embryos treated with systemic 5-HT at HH17 have increased pSmad2/3 expression at HH25 indicating elevated TGFβ signaling. n = 6, mean ± SEM *p<0.01, t-test.

canal [69]. Our avian model exhibited a small (18%), but statistically significant, penetrance of DORV, which is a predominant congenital defect in TGFβ2 KO mice (87% penetrance) [17]. Collectively these defects highlight the morphogenetic potential of 5-HT in early cardiac development, and the similar spectrum of defects generated across 5-HT and TGFβ related animal models.

An interaction of TGFβ and 5-HT signaling was observed *in ovo* through the upregulation of TGFβ3 and contractile genes in the AV cushions (Figure 7B), the increase in pSmad2/3 expression (Figure 8), and the resulting thinned valve morphology (Figure 6C). While the pSmad2/3 and mRNA expression confirms that aspects of the *ex vivo* results occur *in ovo*, it is unclear whether elevated TGFβ signaling at HH25 is solely responsible for the thinned valve morphology observed at HH36. Hyperplastic and thickened AV valves occur in TGFβ2 KO (31% penetrance) [17,70], and TGFβ latent binding protein KO (81% penetrance) [57] animals, which supports this hypothesis. However, systemic 5-HT administration in adult rats generates thickened valves, with treatment duration dependent remodeling. Subcutaneous 5-HT injections for 7 days in adult rats produced thickened AV valves rich in GAGs [50], while 3-month treatment increased valve thickness, but consisted primarily of collagen [62]. Thickened, collagen-rich valves are also reported in adult SERT KO mice [71], and at late embryonic stage SERT KO pups [43]. Together these results indicate that elevated 5-HT signaling can instigate valvular remodeling *in vivo*, but changes in valve microstructure and morphology are clearly dependent on other factors such as treatment duration, specimen age, or secondary effects from accompanying congenital malformations. Altered hemodynamic loading can also generate defects, as evidenced through the serious malformations stimulated by mechanical perturbation [72,73]. Yet hemodynamic loading is simultaneously a consequence and stimulant of molecular signaling, interacting in a cyclical rather than a linear cause-effect manner. This again emphasizes the importance of direct assessment of mechanical stiffness, because it can distinguish the influence of these microstructure and microenvironment variations on valve performance.

Embryonic valve formation and maturation utilizes multiple TGFβ isoforms in spatially and temporally restricted ways that are also somewhat different between species [16,18]. We chose to focus on TGFβ3 over either TGFβ1 or TGFβ2 because of its principal role in cell invasion during chick cushion EMT [16], and confirmed increase in expression during post-EMT [23]. Our results establish a molecular mechanism for short-term (24 hours) TGFβ3 stimulation on AV cushion biomechanical remodeling, but the effects of prolonged signaling on biomechanical and morphological changes remain unclear. This could be addressed with a combined *in vivo*/*in vitro* experimentation over more time points using a system like the approach presented here. The *ex vivo* culture system contains both endocardial and mesenchymal cells, but the lack of chick reactive antibodies prohibited the determination of cell specific responses. Our *in ovo* exogenous 5-HT administration model data complements existing data on genetic mutant animal models of TGFβ and 5-HT related signaling in cardiac development [17,74]. Future studies will need to investigate whether the serotonin effects of TGFβ3 change with TGFβ3 dose.

In conclusion, tissue mechanics, cell phenotype, and molecular signaling all simultaneously direct and control tissue morphogenesis. Our results suggest that TGFβ is a potent stimulator of cushion stiffening, and that 5-HT is a key regulator of this stimulating effect. Connecting signaling networks with cell and tissue level responses will become increasingly important for understanding post-EMT valve remodeling and potentially other embryonic remodeling events. The quantitative experimental systems presented herein are an attractive approach for elucidating these multi-scale mechanisms and their downstream consequences.

Supporting Information

Table S1   RT-PCR Primer Sequences.

Figure S1   Minimal ECM organization in HH25 cushion supports use of an isotropic mechanical testing technique. A) Confocal image of a HH25 cushion with ECM labeled via 5-DTAF protein stain at 10× magnification. **B**) 40× magnification. Note the lack of matrix fiber density or preferential fiber orientation at this stage of development.

Figure S2   Compaction-related stiffness control. A) Molecular inhibition of actin polymerization (Cytochalasin D, 1 μM) caused an 80–85% reduction in effective modulus. mean ± SEM, n≥6 *p<0.0001, t-test **B**) Cushion area increased with actin inhibition, resulting in a 3 fold decrease in measured compaction compared to control. Insets: Representative images of AV cushions before and after treatment, scale bar = 100 μm. mean ± SEM, n≥12, *p<0.0001, t-test.

Figure S3   TGFβ3-induced decrease in compaction was blocked through inhibition of Alk5 (SB431542, 2.6 μM) or 5-HTR2b (SB204741 35 μM, *anti-5-HT2b*). Neither 5-HTR2a inhibitor (MDL100907 10 nM, *anti-5-HT2a*) nor serotonin transporter inhibitor (Fluoxetine 10 μM, *anti-SERT*) affected TGFβ3 compaction behavior. mean ± SEM, n≥7, *p<0.05, t-test with respect to untreated controls.

Figure S4   TGFβ3 and 5-HT stiffness generation is dependent on Alk5 signaling pathway. Strain energy density (Pa) of cushions treated with TGFβ3 (1 ng/ml) only, TGFβ3+Alk5 inhibitor (SB431542, 2.6 μM anti-Alk5), TGFβ3+5-HT (470 nM), and TGFβ3+5-HT+anti-Alk5. mean ± SEM, n≥8. Different letter pairings denotes statistically significant p<0.05, 2-way ANOVA.

Figure S5   Intracellular 5-HT uptake is modulated by 5-HT dose. A) 5-HT transporter (SERT) gene expression was downregulated via high 5-HT (47 μM, *5-HT+*) dose, while transglutaminase 2 (TGM2) was not affected. The physiological dose of 5-HT (470 nM, *5-HT*) had no effect on either SERT or TGM2 gene expression. **B**) TGFβ3 (1 ng/ml) stimulated 4-fold increase in TGM2, which was mitigated by either doses of 5-HT. TGFβ3 had no effect on SERT expression. mean ± SEM, n = 3–4, *p<0.05, t-test.

Figure S6   Characterization of *in ovo* 5-HT administration model. A) Plot of avian embryo viability as a function of time and 5-HT dose. 5-HT administration to the surface of HH17 chick embryos resulted in greater than 70% lethality at dosages above 0.75 mg. The majority of deaths occurred within 48 hours of incubation. Doses of 0.5 mg and below were over 80% viable with virtually no morphological defects. Doses administered at later incubation times (Day 5, Day 7) did not result in lethality or defects by HH36 (data not shown). 5-HT administration at the predicted 50% lethality dose (0.7 mg/100 μL) resulted in 55% lethality by Day 10. **B**) Representative image of ectopic heart (arrow) and unclosed chest (dashed line) observed with both 5-HT treatment and thoracotomy sham controls.

Acknowledgments

We thank Dr. Vladimir Mironov for helpful discussions on this work. We also thank Axon Medchem BV for the kind donation of reagent MDL100,907.

References

1. Butcher JT, Sedmera D, Guldberg RE, Markwald RR (2007) Quantitative volumetric analysis of cardiac morphogenesis assessed through micro-computed tomography. Dev Dyn 236(3): 802–809.
2. Hu N, Clark EB (1989) Hemodynamics of the stage 12 to stage 29 chick embryo. Circ Res 65(6): 1665–1670.
3. Keller BB, Hu N, Serrino PJ, Clark EB (1991) Ventricular pressure-area loop characteristics in the stage 16 to 24 chick embryo. Circ Res 68(1): 226–231.
4. Yalcin HC, Shekhar A, McQuinn TC, Butcher JT (2011) Hemodynamic patterning of the avian atrioventricular valve. Dev Dyn 240(1): 23–35.
5. Kruithof BP, Krawitz SA, Gaussin V (2007) Atrioventricular valve development during late embryonic and postnatal stages involves condensation and extracellular matrix remodeling. Dev Biol 302(1): 208–217.
6. Hinton RB,Jr, Lincoln J, Deutsch GH, Osinska H, Manning PB, et al. (2006) Extracellular matrix remodeling and organization in developing and diseased aortic valves. Circ Res 98(11): 1431–1438.
7. Person AD, Klewer SE, Runyan RB (2005) Cell biology of cardiac cushion development. Int Rev Cytol 243: 287–335.
8. Combs MD, Yutzey KE (2009) Heart valve development: Regulatory networks in development and disease. Circ Res 105(5): 408–421.
9. Butcher JT, Markwald RR (2007) Valvulogenesis: The moving target. Philos Trans R Soc Lond B Biol Sci 362(1484): 1489–1503.
10. Eisenberg LM, Markwald RR (1995) Molecular regulation of atrioventricular valvuloseptal morphogenesis. Circ Res 77(1): 1–6.
11. Attisano L, Wrana JL, Lopez-Casillas F, Massague J (1994) TGF-beta receptors and actions. Biochim Biophys Acta 1222(1): 71–80.
12. Massague J, Chen YG (2000) Controlling TGF-beta signaling. Genes Dev 14(6): 627–644.
13. Shi Y, Massague J (2003) Mechanisms of TGF-beta signaling from cell membrane to the nucleus. Cell 113(6): 685–700.
14. Potts JD, Runyan RB (1989) Epithelial-mesenchymal cell transformation in the embryonic heart can be mediated, in part, by transforming growth factor beta. Dev Biol 134(2): 392–401.
15. Boyer AS, Ayerinskas II, Vincent EB, McKinney LA, Weeks DL, et al. (1999) TGFbeta2 and TGFbeta3 have separate and sequential activities during epithelial-mesenchymal cell transformation in the embryonic heart. Dev Biol 208(2): 530–545.
16. Camenisch TD, Molin DG, Person A, Runyan RB, Gittenberger-de Groot AC, et al. (2002) Temporal and distinct TGFbeta ligand requirements during mouse and avian endocardial cushion morphogenesis. Dev Biol 248(1): 170–181.
17. Bartram U, Molin DG, Wisse LJ, Mohamad A, Sanford LP, et al. (2001) Double-outlet right ventricle and overriding tricuspid valve reflect disturbances of looping, myocardialization, endocardial cushion differentiation, and apoptosis in TGF-beta(2)-knockout mice. Circulation 103(22): 2745–2752.
18. Azhar M, Runyan RB, Gard C, Sanford LP, Miller ML, et al. (2009) Ligand-specific function of transforming growth factor beta in epithelial-mesenchymal transition in heart development. Dev Dyn 238(2): 431–442.
19. Potts JD, Vincent EB, Runyan RB, Weeks DL (1992) Sense and antisense TGF beta 3 mRNA levels correlate with cardiac valve induction. Dev Dyn 193(4): 340–345.
20. Norris RA, Moreno-Rodriguez RA, Sugi Y, Hoffman S, Amos J, et al. (2008) Periostin regulates atrioventricular valve maturation. Dev Biol 316(2): 200–213.
21. Butcher JT, McQuinn TC, Sedmera D, Turner D, Markwald RR (2007) Transitions in early embryonic atrioventricular valvular function correspond with changes in cushion biomechanics that are predictable by tissue composition. Circ Res 100(10): 1503–1511.
22. Buskohl PR, Gould RA, Butcher JT (2012) Quantification of embryonic atrioventricular valve biomechanics during morphogenesis. J Biomech 45(5): 895–902.
23. Chiu YN, Norris RA, Mahler G, Recknagel A, Butcher JT (2010) Transforming growth factor beta, bone morphogenetic protein, and vascular endothelial growth factor mediate phenotype maturation and tissue remodeling by embryonic valve progenitor cells: Relevance for heart valve tissue engineering. Tissue Eng Part A 16(11): 3375–85.
24. Norris RA, Potts JD, Yost MJ, Junor L, Brooks T, et al. (2009) Periostin promotes a fibroblastic lineage pathway in atrioventricular valve progenitor cells. Dev Dyn 238(5): 1052–1063.
25. Jian B, Xu J, Connolly J, Savani RC, Narula N, et al. (2002) Serotonin mechanisms in heart valve disease I: Serotonin-induced up-regulation of transforming growth factor-beta1 via G-protein signal transduction in aortic valve interstitial cells. Am J Pathol 161(6): 2111–2121.
26. Disatian S, Orton EC (2009) Autocrine serotonin and transforming growth factor beta 1 signaling mediates spontaneous myxomatous mitral valve disease. J Heart Valve Dis 18(1): 44–51.
27. El-Hamamsy I, Balachandran K, Yacoub MH, Stevens LM, Sarathchandra P, et al. (2009) Endothelium-dependent regulation of the mechanical properties of aortic valve cusps. J Am Coll Cardiol 53(16): 1448–1455.
28. Warnock JN, Gamez CA, Metzler SA, Chen J, Elder SH, et al. (2010) Vasoactive agents alter the biomechanical properties of aortic heart valve leaflets in a time-dependent manner. J Heart Valve Dis 19(1): 86–95; discussion 96.
29. Roth BL, Willins DL, Kristiansen K, Kroeze WK (1998) 5-Hydroxytryptamine2-family receptors (5-hydroxytryptamine2A, 5-hydroxytryptamine2B, 5-hydroxytryptamine2C): Where structure meets function. Pharmacol Ther 79(3): 231–257.
30. Balachandran K, Hussain S, Yap CH, Padala M, Chester AH, et al. (2011) Elevated cyclic stretch and serotonin result in altered aortic valve remodeling via a mechanosensitive 5-HT(2A) receptor-dependent pathway. Cardiovasc Pathol.
31. Hafizi S, Taylor PM, Chester AH, Allen SP, Yacoub MH (2000) Mitogenic and secretory responses of human valve interstitial cells to vasoactive agents. J Heart Valve Dis 9(3): 454–458.
32. Oyama MA, Levy RJ (2010) Insights into serotonin signaling mechanisms associated with canine degenerative mitral valve disease. J Vet Intern Med 24(1): 27–36.
33. Lauder JM (1988) Neurotransmitters as morphogens. Prog Brain Res 73: 365–387.
34. Levin M, Buznikov GA, Lauder JM (2006) Of minds and embryos: Left-right asymmetry and the serotonergic controls of pre-neural morphogenesis. Dev Neurosci 28(3): 171–185.
35. Moiseiwitsch JR, Lauder JM (1995) Serotonin regulates mouse cranial neural crest migration. Proc Natl Acad Sci U S A 92(16): 7182–7186.
36. Fukumoto T, Blakely R, Levin M (2005) Serotonin transporter function is an early step in left-right patterning in chick and frog embryos. Dev Neurosci 27(6): 349–363.
37. Sadler TW (2011) Selective serotonin reuptake inhibitors (SSRIs) and heart defects: Potential mechanisms for the observed associations. Reprod Toxicol 32(4): 484–9.
38. Lauder JM, Wilkie MB, Wu C, Singh S (2000) Expression of 5-HT(2A), 5-HT(2B) and 5-HT(2C) receptors in the mouse embryo. Int J Dev Neurosci 18(7): 653–662.
39. Choi DS, Ward SJ, Messaddeq N, Launay JM, Maroteaux L (1997) 5-HT2B receptor-mediated serotonin morphogenetic functions in mouse cranial neural crest and myocardiac cells. Development 124(9): 1745–1755.
40. Millan FA, Denhez F, Kondaiah P, Akhurst RJ (1991) Embryonic gene expression patterns of TGF beta 1, beta 2 and beta 3 suggest different developmental functions in vivo. Development 111(1): 131–143.
41. Yavarone MS, Shuey DL, Tamir H, Sadler TW, Lauder JM (1993) Serotonin and cardiac morphogenesis in the mouse embryo. Teratology 47(6): 573–584.
42. Nakajima Y, Miyazono K, Kato M, Takase M, Yamagishi T, et al. (1997) Extracellular fibrillar structure of latent TGF beta binding protein-1: Role in TGF beta-dependent endothelial-mesenchymal transformation during endocardial cushion tissue formation in mouse embryonic heart. J Cell Biol 136(1): 193–204.
43. Pavone LM, Spina A, Rea S, Santoro D, Mastellone V, et al. (2009) Serotonin transporter gene deficiency is associated with sudden death of newborn mice through activation of TGF-beta1 signalling. J Mol Cell Cardiol 47(5): 691–697.
44. Watts SW, Priestley JR, Thompson JM (2009) Serotonylation of vascular proteins important to contraction. PLoS One 4(5): e5682.
45. Jaffre F, Bonnin P, Callebert J, Debbabi H, Setola V, et al. (2009) Serotonin and angiotensin receptors in cardiac fibroblasts coregulate adrenergic-dependent cardiac hypertrophy. Circ Res 104(1): 113–123.
46. Aoki T, Ohashi T, Matsumoto T, Sato M (1997) The pipette aspiration applied to the local stiffness measurement of soft tissues. Ann Biomed Eng 25(3): 581–587.
47. Zhao R, Sider KL, Simmons CA (2011) Measurement of layer-specific mechanical properties in multilayered biomaterials by micropipette aspiration. Acta Biomater 7(3): 1220–1227.
48. Fung YC (1991) What are the residual stresses doing in our blood vessels? Ann Biomed Eng 19(3): 237–249.
49. Bookout AL, Mangelsdorf DJ (2003) Quantitative real-time PCR protocol for analysis of nuclear receptor signaling pathways. Nucl Recept Signal 1: e012.

Author Contributions

Conceived and designed the experiments: PRB RPT JTB. Performed the experiments: PRB MLS RTP JTB. Analyzed the data: PRB MLS JTB. Contributed reagents/materials/analysis tools: JTB RPT. Wrote the paper: PRB JTB.

50. Elangbam CS, Job LE, Zadrozny LM, Barton JC, Yoon LW, et al. (2008) 5-hydroxytryptamine (5HT)-induced valvulopathy: Compositional valvular alterations are associated with 5HT2B receptor and 5HT transporter transcript changes in sprague-dawley rats. Exp Toxicol Pathol 60(4–5): 253–262.

51. Hauso O, Gustafsson BI, Loennechen JP, Stunes AK, Nordrum I, et al. (2007) Long-term serotonin effects in the rat are prevented by terguride. Regul Pept 143(1–3): 39–46.

52. Miller CE, Thompson RP, Bigelow MR, Gittinger G, Trusk TC, et al. (2005) Confocal imaging of the embryonic heart: How deep? Microsc Microanal 11(3): 216–223.

53. Kern CB, Norris RA, Thompson RP, Argraves WS, Fairey SE, et al. (2007) Versican proteolysis mediates myocardial regression during outflow tract development. Dev Dyn 236(3): 671–683.

54. Inman GJ, Nicolas FJ, Callahan JF, Harling JD, Gaster LM, et al. (2002) SB-431542 is a potent and specific inhibitor of transforming growth factor-beta superfamily type I activin receptor-like kinase (ALK) receptors ALK4, ALK5, and ALK7. Mol Pharmacol 62(1): 65–74.

55. Guilluy C, Rolli-Derkinderen M, Tharaux PL, Melino G, Pacaud P, et al. (2007) Transglutaminase-dependent RhoA activation and depletion by serotonin in vascular smooth muscle cells. J Biol Chem 282(5): 2918–2928.

56. Liu Y, Wei L, Laskin DL, Fanburg BL (2010) Role of protein transamidation in serotonin-induced proliferation and migration of pulmonary artery smooth muscle cells. Am J Respir Cell Mol Biol 44(4): 548–55.

57. Todorovic V, Finnegan E, Freyer L, Zilberberg L, Ota M, et al. (2011) Long form of latent TGF-beta binding protein 1 (Ltbp1L) regulates cardiac valve development. Dev Dyn 240(1): 176–187.

58. Merryman WD, Lukoff HD, Long RA, Engelmayr GC Jr, Hopkins RA, et al. (2007) Synergistic effects of cyclic tension and transforming growth factor-beta1 on the aortic valve myofibroblast. Cardiovasc Pathol 16(5): 268–276.

59. Walker GA, Masters KS, Shah DN, Anseth KS, Leinwand LA (2004) Valvular myofibroblast activation by transforming growth factor-beta: Implications for pathological extracellular matrix remodeling in heart valve disease. Circ Res 95(3): 253–260.

60. Xu J, Jian B, Chu R, Lu Z, Li Q, et al. (2002) Serotonin mechanisms in heart valve disease II: The 5-HT2 receptor and its signaling pathway in aortic valve interstitial cells. Am J Pathol 161(6): 2209–2218.

61. Yabanoglu S, Akkiki M, Seguelas MH, Mialet-Perez J, Parini A, et al. (2009) Platelet derived serotonin drives the activation of rat cardiac fibroblasts by 5-HT2A receptors. J Mol Cell Cardiol 46(4): 518–525.

62. Gustafsson BI, Tommeras K, Nordrum I, Loennechen JP, Brunsvik A, et al. (2005) Long-term serotonin administration induces heart valve disease in rats. Circulation 111(12): 1517–1522.

63. Monassier L, Laplante MA, Ayadi T, Doly S, Maroteaux L (2010) Contribution of gene-modified mice and rats to our understanding of the cardiovascular pharmacology of serotonin. Pharmacol Ther 128(3): 559–567.

64. Hoffman JI, Kaplan S (2002) The incidence of congenital heart disease. J Am Coll Cardiol 39(12): 1890–1900.

65. Reller MD, Strickland MJ, Riehle-Colarusso T, Mahle WT, Correa A (2008) Prevalence of congenital heart defects in metropolitan atlanta, 1998–2005. J Pediatr 153(6): 807–813.

66. Merlob P, Birk E, Sirota L, Linder N, Berant M, et al. (2009) Are selective serotonin reuptake inhibitors cardiac teratogens? echocardiographic screening of newborns with persistent heart murmur. Birth Defects Res A Clin Mol Teratol 85(10): 837–841.

67. Qi X, Yang G, Yang L, Lan Y, Weng T, et al. (2007) Essential role of Smad4 in maintaining cardiomyocyte proliferation during murine embryonic heart development. Dev Biol 311(1): 136–146.

68. Chen Q, Chen H, Zheng D, Kuang C, Fang H, et al. (2009) Smad7 is required for the development and function of the heart. J Biol Chem 284(1): 292–300.

69. Hove JR, Koster RW, Forouhar AS, Acevedo-Bolton G, Fraser SE, et al. (2003) Intracardiac fluid forces are an essential epigenetic factor for embryonic cardiogenesis. Nature 421(6919): 172–177.

70. Azhar M, Brown K, Gard C, Chen H, Rajan S, et al. (2011) Transforming growth factor Beta2 is required for valve remodeling during heart development. Dev Dyn 240(9): 2127–2141.

71. Mekontso-Dessap A, Brouri F, Pascal O, Lechat P, Hanoun N, et al. (2006) Deficiency of the 5-hydroxytryptamine transporter gene leads to cardiac fibrosis and valvulopathy in mice. Circulation 113(1): 81–89.

72. Yalcin HC, Shekhar A, Nishimura N, Rane AA, Schaffer CB, et al. (2010) Two-photon microscopy guided femtosecond-laser photoablation of avian cardiogenesis: Noninvasive creation of localized heart defects. Am J Physiol Heart Circ Physiol.

73. Sedmera D, Pexieder T, Rychterova V, Hu N, Clark EB (1999) Remodeling of chick embryonic ventricular myoarchitecture under experimentally changed loading conditions. Anat Rec 254(2): 238–252.

74. Nebigl CG, Hickel P, Messaddeq N, Vonesch JL, Douchet MP, et al. (2001) Ablation of serotonin 5-HT(2B) receptors in mice leads to abnormal cardiac structure and function. Circulation 103(24): 2973–2979.

7

Identification of Functional Mutations in GATA4 in Patients with Congenital Heart Disease

Erli Wang[1,2,9], **Shuna Sun**[3,9], **Bin Qiao**[4], **Wenyuan Duan**[4], **Guoying Huang**[3], **Yu An**[3,5], **Shuhua Xu**[1], **Yufang Zheng**[2], **Zhixi Su**[2], **Xun Gu**[2], **Li Jin**[1,2]*, **Hongyan Wang**[2,5]*

1 Chinese Academy of Sciences Key Laboratory of Computational Biology, Chinese Academy of Sciences and Max Planck Society (CAS-MPG) Partner Institute for Computational Biology, Shanghai Institutes for Biological Sciences, Chinese Academy of Sciences, Shanghai, China, 2 The State Key Laboratory of Genetic Engineering and MOE Key Laboratory of Contemporary Anthropology, School of Life Sciences, Fudan University, Shanghai, China, 3 Children's Hospital of Fudan University, Shanghai, China, 4 Institute of Cardiovascular Disease General Hospital of Jinan Military Region, Jinan, China, 5 The Institutes of Biomedical Sciences, Fudan University, Shanghai, China

Abstract

Congenital heart disease (CHD) is one of the most prevalent developmental anomalies and the leading cause of noninfectious morbidity and mortality in newborns. Despite its prevalence and clinical significance, the etiology of CHD remains largely unknown. GATA4 is a highly conserved transcription factor that regulates a variety of physiological processes and has been extensively studied, particularly on its role in heart development. With the combination of TBX5 and MEF2C, GATA4 can reprogram postnatal fibroblasts into functional cardiomyocytes directly. In the past decade, a variety of GATA4 mutations were identified and these findings originally came from familial CHD pedigree studies. Given that familial and sporadic CHD cases allegedly share a basic genetic basis, we explore the GATA4 mutations in different types of CHD. In this study, via direct sequencing of the *GATA4* coding region and exon-intron boundaries in 384 sporadic Chinese CHD patients, we identified 12 heterozygous non-synonymous mutations, among which 8 mutations were only found in CHD patients when compared with 957 controls. Six of these non-synonymous mutations have not been previously reported. Subsequent functional analyses revealed that the transcriptional activity, subcellular localization and DNA binding affinity of some mutant GATA4 proteins were significantly altered. Our results expand the spectrum of GATA4 mutations linked to cardiac defects. Together with the newly reported mutations, approximately 110 non-synonymous mutations have currently been identified in GATA4. Our future analysis will explore why the evolutionarily conserved GATA4 appears to be hypermutable.

Editor: Mathias Toft, Oslo University Hospital, Norway

Funding: This work was supported by grants from the National Science Fund for Distinguished Young Scholars (81025003), the 973 Program (2010CB529601), the Program for Innovative Research Team in University (IRT1010), Doctoral Fund of Ministry of Education of China (20110071110026), and the Commission for Science and Technology of Shanghai Municipality (10JC1401300, 11XD1400900) to HYW. The funders had no role in study design, data collection and analysis, decision to publish, or preparation of the manuscript.

Competing Interests: The authors have declared that no competing interests exist.

* E-mail: wanghy@fudan.edu.cn (HYW); ljin007@gmail.com (LJ)

⑨ These authors contributed equally to this work.

Introduction

Congenital heart disease (CHD) is a widespread birth defect that occurs in approximately 1~5% of newborns and accounts for approximately one-tenth of all infant deaths [1–4]. During the past decade, remarkable progress has been made in elucidating the etiology of CHD, but the precise mechanisms involved in the majority of patients remain unknown.

In vertebrates, cardiogenesis is a very complex process that requires the accurate spatial and temporal cooperation of various regulatory factors. Disordered transcription factor interactions, altered hemodynamics, signal defects and microRNA dysfunction could all result in CHD [1]. The GATA4 zinc finger protein belongs to an evolutionarily conserved GATA family that consists of six members. It recognizes the nucleotide consensus sequence WGATAR in the promoter region of its downstream target genes [5]. Through interaction with specific cofactors, GATA4 regulates different physiological processes and integrates many signaling

pathways [6–9]. GATA4 plays an especially critical role during several stages of cardiogenesis, from formation of the primitive heart tube to maturation of the four-chambered heart [10]. A recent study showed that in the presence of MEF2C and TBX5, GATA4 can induce cardiomyocyte differentiation and directly reprogram endogenous cardiac fibroblasts into cardiomyocytes by activating cardiac gene expression [11].

The accumulating evidences have shown that genetic defects in GATA4 play a vital role in the pathogenesis of CHD. Since the year it was identified as a genetic cause of septal defects [12], *GATA4* has been extensively screened for CHD-specific variations. All function-proved variations would help us in understanding the mechanisms underlying both the familial and sporadic non-syndrome cardiac defects. In this study, we conducted a population-based mutation screening of *GATA4* in 384 Chinese sporadic non-syndrome CHD patients and 760 matched controls. A total of twelve heterozygous non-synonymous mutations were found. Eight of these mutations were found exclusively in CHD patients, and six of them have not been previously reported. The functional analyses demonstrated that the GATA4 mutants A66T, A353T, E360G and a previously reported mutant T280M significantly changed the transcriptional activity of *ANF* luciferase reporter, and the C-terminal mutants A353T, E360G, G375R, S377G and A442V were partially located at the cytoplasm besides the nucleus. Gel shift assay showed that the DNA binding affinity of mutants A74D, G150W (*de novo*) and T280M reduced significantly compared to wild type GATA4.

According to published reports and the dbSNP database, there have been approximately 110 GATA4 non-synonymous mutations identified, including those identified in our study. Approximately 80% of these mutations are found in patients with septal defects. The functionally impaired GATA4 mutants identified in this study should contribute to the progress being made in the early diagnosis and prevention of congenital heart defects.

Materials and Methods

Ethics Statement

Protocols used in this study were reviewed and approved by the Ethics Committee of the School of Life Sciences, Fudan University. Written consent was obtained from the parents or guardians of the children patients prior to the study's commencement.

Study Subjects

Samples of the 384 CHD patients (185 males and 199 females) and 760 (362 males and 398 females) controls used in this study were consecutively recruited between August 2008 and February 2011 from the Cardiovascular Disease Institute of Jinan Military Command (Jinan, Shandong Province, China) and Children's Hospital of Fudan University (Shanghai, China). CHD patients who were diagnosed with other syndromes or had a positive family history of CHD in a first-degree relative (parents, siblings and children) were excluded. If available, samples from the unaffected parents of the CHD patients were also collected. The controls were non-CHD outpatients from the same geographic area and

during the same time period. The controls were also matched to the affected individuals in age and sex. The ethnicity of all the subjects is Han Chinese and they are genetically unrelated to each other.

We classified each of the 384 CHD cases into four broad categories as previously described [13]. Specifically, 34 (8.9%) had conotruncal defects, 275 (71.6%) had septation defects, 14 (3.6%) had right ventricular outflow tract obstruction, and 61 (15.9%) had other CHD defects (Table 1).

Approximately 3–5 ml peripheral blood was collected from each test subject. Genomic DNA of each test subject was isolated from peripheral blood using conventional reagents.

Sequencing and Genotyping of Human *GATA4*

The human *GATA4* gene (NM_002052.3), mapped to 8p23.1, consists of 6 exons that encode a 442 amino acid protein. For each of the collected 384 CHD cases, all exons and the intron-exon flanking regions of *GATA4* were amplified by polymerase chain reaction (PCR) for a mutation screen by sequencing. PCR primers were designed by the online software Primer3 and are listed in Table S1 (the reaction conditions are available upon request). PCR products were individually pretreated with a mixture of 1 unit ExoI and 1 unit SAP (TAKARA). Direct dye terminator sequencing of the purified PCR products was conducted using the ABI Prism BigDye system following the manufacturer's instructions (ABI, Foster City, CA). Precipitation was done by 75% alcohol after second purification by 1 unit SAP. HiDi formamide was used in the subsequent denaturation, and finally the samples were subjected to sequencing using an ABI 3730XL sequencer. The results were analyzed by the Sequence Scanner and DNASTAR software.

The GATA4 mutations identified were confirmed by reverse sequencing of the independent PCR amplifications using the mutation carrier case DNA samples. The available DNA samples of the parents of CHD children carrying the identified mutations were also amplified and sequenced.

The 1000 Genomes Project data (http://www.1000genomes. org), which contains 197 Han Chinese people, was used as a phase one control to exclude benign GATA4 mutations. The first round CHD-specific GATA4 mutations identified with no record in the 1000 Genomes Project database were then genotyped in the 760 control samples using the SNaPshot method (ABI, Foster City, CA), and the results were analyzed by the Peak Scanner software. The CHD case specific mutations of GATA4 were finally identified after the comparison with the mixed controls (197+760).

Plasmid Construction and Site Directed Mutagenesis

The construction of rat ANF-Luc has been previously reported [5,14–16]. By pairwise sequence alignment, we confirmed the locations of the GATA4 binding sites in the human *ANF* (*NPPA*, NM 006172.3) promoter region. A 679 bp fragment of the human *ANF* promoter from −644 to +35 was PCR-amplified using pfu ultra (Stratagene, La Jolla, CA). The PCR products were cloned into the *Mlu*I and *Bgl*II restriction sites of the pGL3-Basic vector (Promega) to produce ANF-Luc.

The full-length human *GATA4* cDNA was constructed and cloned into the Myc-tagged pCMV mammalian expression vector. Mutated complementary primers were designed, and PCR was performed using the full-length pCMV-Myc-GATA4 wild type plasmid as a template and the KOD polymerase enzyme (TOYOBO). After treating with *Dpn*I, the products were used to transform *E.coli* DH5α competent cells to select mutant GATA4.

To assess the impact of mutations in the C-terminal region on the structural and functional properties of GATA4, wild-type

Table 1. Phenotypes of study subjects with congenital heart defects.

Classification	Number	Frequency (%)
CHD classification I		
Conotruncal defects	34	8.9
Septation defects	275	71.6
RVOTO	14	3.6
Other CHDs	61	15.9
CHD classification II		
Isolated CHD	324	84.4
Non-isolated CHD	60	15.6
Isolated CHD phenotype		
ASD	48	12.5
VSD	162	42.1
PDA	27	7.0
TOF	23	6.0

RVOTO, right ventricular outflow tract obstruction; ASD, atrial septal defect; VSD, ventricular septal defect; PDA, paten ductus arteriosus; TOF, tetralogy of Fallot.

Table 2. GATA4 non-synonymous variations only identified in 384 CHD patients.

Location	Nucleotide change	Amino acid change	Number	Cardiac defects	Parents carriers	New mutations/ reported
Exon 1	c.196G>A	p.A66T	1	VSD, PDA	Father	[37]
	c.221C>A	p.A74D	1	PS	NA	Novel
	c.448G>T	p.G150W	1	TOF	De novo	Novel
Exon 2	c.628G>A	p.D210N	1	unknown	NA	Novel
	c.749T>A	p.I250N	1	VSD	Mother	Novel
Exon 5	c.1057G>A	p.A353T	1	TOF	Father	Novel
	c.1079A>G	p.E360G	1	VSD	NA	Novel
Exon 6	c.1325C>T	p.A442V	1	VSD	Mother	[25]

(Detailed clinical information for D210N was unclear, and "NA" means samples of the relative parents were unavailable.).

pEGFP-C1-GATA4 and mutated types were generated using the same method.

Cell Culture and Luciferase Assay

Hela cells were cultured in Dulbecco's minimum essential medium (DMEM,Gibco) supplemented with 10% fetal bovine serum (FBS,Gibco) and seeded in 24-well plates (1×10^5) before transfection. Eighteen hours after plating, the cells were cotransfected with 200 ng of pGL3-ANF luciferase reporter, 200 ng of pCMV-Myc-GATA4 wild-type or mutant-type plasmids and 1 ng of pRL-TK (Promega) internal control plasmid using Lipofectamine^{TM} 2000 (Invitrogen, Carlsbad, CA). Forty-eight hours after transfection, cells were collected and luciferase reporter levels were measured using the Dual-Luciferase Reporter Assay System according to the manufacturer's instructions (Promega). The relative reporter activity was determined by normalizing the firefly activity to the *Renilla* activity. Protein expression levels were confirmed by western blot analysis, and each experiment was performed in triplicate for three times. The student's *t*-test was used for statistical comparisons, and differences were considered to be significant if the *P*-value <0.05.

Immunohistochemistry

Human cardiac myocytes cells (HCM, ScienCell) were cultured in cardiac myocyte medium (CMM). Forty-eight hours after the transient transfection of pEGFP-C1-GATA4 wild-type or mutant plasmids using Lipofectamine^{TM} 2000, HCM cells were fixed with 4% formaldehyde/PBS, permeabilized with 0.2% Triton X-100/PBS, and stained with DAPI. Fixed cells were washed with $1 \times$ PBS 3 times for 5 minutes at the end of each step. A Laser Scanning Confocal Microscope was used to observe the results.

Electrophoretic Mobility Shift Assay (EMSA)

We extracted nuclear proteins using Thermo Scientific NE-PER Nuclear and Cytoplasmic Extraction Reagents. The endogenous GATA4 expression of 293T, COS7, Hela and H1299 cells was detected by western blot using human GATA4-Specific Polyclonal antibody (Proteintech, Chicago, IL 60612, USA). Expression of GATA4 in Hela cells transfected with pCMV-Myc-GATA4 wild type and mutants were also detected using western blot.

Annealed oligonucleotides (5′-GCAGTTAACTGATAATGA-CACTGTG-3′) of human *dHAND* which correspond to the GATA element upstream of mouse *dHAND* used in previous studies were labelled with biotin [12,17,18]. EMSA was performed using LightShift Chemiluminescent EMSA kit (Pierce, Rockford, 1L 61101, USA). Binding reactions contained ddH$_2$O, 2 ul of 10×binding buffer, 1μg of poly (dI-dC) and 2 μl of nuclear extracts. The reaction was incubated for 10 min at room temperature before 2ul (1 pmol) of biotin-labelled oligonucleotides were added. For competition analysis, 100-fold unlabled specific competitor or non-specific competitor was included in the binding reaction. A total of 20 ul reaction mix was incubated at room temperature for 20 minutes. The samples were loaded on a 6% nondenaturing polyacrylamide gel in 0.5×TBE.

Results

Identification of Human *GATA4* Mutations

By direct sequencing of the *GATA4* coding region, we identified 12 heterozygous non-synonymous mutations in 14 individuals out of the 384 patients with diverse forms of CHD (Table 2 and Table 3). None of these mutations were found in the 1000 Genomes Project sequencing results in the Chinese Han from

Table 3. GATA4 non-synonymous variations found in both CHD and control population.

Location	Nucleotide change	Amino acid change	Heterogeneity rate		Cardiac defects
			Patients(n = 384)	Controls(n = 760+197)	
Exon 1	c.487C>T	p.P163S	0.005 (2/384)	0.017 (13/957)	VSD,PS
Exon 3	c.799G>A	p.V267M	0.005 (2/384)	0.005 (4/957)	VSD,PDA
Exon 5	c.1123G>A	p.G375R	0.003 (1/384)	0.003 (2/957)	VSD
	c.1129A>G	p.S377G	0.003 (1/384)	0.005 (4/957)	VSD

Table 4. Synonymous and intronic variations identified in *GATA4*.

Location	Nucleotide change	Amino acid change	Number	Cardiac defects
Exon 1	c.99G>T	p.A33A	20/384	ASD,VSD, PDA, etc
	c.132G>T	p.V44V	1/384	VSD
	c.531C>A	p.A177A	1/384	VSD,PH
Intron 1	c.617-64G>A		1/384	
	c.617-16C>T		1/384	
Exon 2	c.678G>A	p.P226P	1/384	VSD
	c.723C>T	p.C241C	1/384	VSD
	c.744C>T	p.N248N	1/384	ASD,VSD
Intron 3	c.910-58T>A		17/384	
Exon 4	c.975G>A	p.L325L	1/384	ASD
Intron 5	c.1147-107A>G		1/384	
	c.1147-76C>A		1/384	
Exon 6	c.1326G>A	p.A442A	1/384	ASD

Beijing (CHB) and Chinese Han from South (CHS) populations. In addition, we also found 8 synonymous mutations and 5 intronic variations in the flanking regions (Table 4).

Four of these 12 CHD mutations (out of the first round compared with the 1000 Genomes Project data) (P163S, V267M, G375R and S377G) were also found in control individuals (Table 3), and had been previously reported (Table S2). Among the 8 mutations exclusively found in CHD patients, 6 of them (A74D, G150W, D210N, I250N, A353T and E360G) have not been previously reported, while the other 2 mutations (A66T and A442V) were reported in either previous studies or the dbSNP database. GATA4 G150W was a *de novo* mutation that was absent in both parents (Table 2).

We summarized all the non-synonymous mutations of GATA4, and found that currently, approximately 110 non-synonymous mutations have been identified in CHD cases within the coding region spanning the 3rd residue Gln to the 442nd residue Ala (Figure S1). These findings suggest that GATA4 is a hypermutable protein in CHD patients. To determine whether GATA4 is selectively constrained in the Chinese population, we calculated the nucleotide diversity π and sequence-based neutrality tests Tajima's D using the public sequencing data of CHB and CHS from the 1000 Genomes Project [19]. *GATA4* is an essential gene;

Table 5. The Pi value and Tajimas' D of GATA4 compared with 1475 essential genes based on the Han Chinese population data from the 1000 Genomes.

Regions	Population	N(Pi)	Pi value	N(Tajimas' D)	Tajimas' D
Transcript region	CHB	792	0.0007241	390	−0.24
	CHS	792	0.0007330	391	−0.34
Coding region	CHB	792	0.0008428	149	−0.75
	CHS	792	0.0008486	149	−0.53

(N means the number of essential genes that have larger Pi value or Tajimas' D than GATA4).

therefore, we restricted our comparison to 1475 essential genes [20]. The statistical analysis did not provide strong evidence showing that GATA4 is under positive or purifying selection in the Han Chinese population (Table 5).

As previously described, GATA4 contains two independent transcriptional activation domains in the N-terminal region, two highly conserved zinc finger domains, the interval basic domains and the C-terminal domain [3,21–23]. The locations of the 12 mutations identified in this study are indicated in the GATA4 structural diagram in Figure 1A. Multiple sequence alignments indicate that among the 8 CHD specific mutations, only the residues 210, 250, 360 and 442 are highly conserved across species (Figure 1B). Even though these residues are highly conserved, it has been reported that the Glu located at residue 360 could be substituted by Gln or Gly, and that the Ala located at residue 442 could be substituted by Gly, Val or Thr (Table S2).

Biochemical Analysis of GATA4 Mutations

GATA4 is a nucleic transcription factor that has been reported to localize entirely in the nucleus [12,18]. Five non-synonymous mutations A353T, E360G, G375R, S377G and A442V located in C-terminal region are adjacent to the nuclear localization signal (NLS) [21]. To determine whether these GATA4 mutants affect normal protein trafficking, which would then prevent GATA4 from properly functioning, immunofluorescence staining for GFP-tagged GATA4 was conducted in human cardiac myocytes cells. The results showed that wild-type pEGFP-GATA4 was exclusively located in the nucleus. The NLS adjacent mutants A353T, E360G, G375R, S377G and A442V, however, had partially abnormal localization patterns. A small amount of these GATA4 mutants appeared to be located in the cytoplasm (Figure 2). Similar results were also found in H1299 cells (data not shown). These results suggest that mutations adjacent to the NLS of hGATA4 impede normal nuclear localization.

The human *ANF* gene promoter region contains two highly conserved GATA binding elements (Figure 3A) and is activated in a dose dependent manner by GATA4. The *in vitro* luciferase reporter assays showed that A66T and A353T significantly increased the ANF promoter activity; while T280M, a previously reported mutation identified in a Chinese CHD family [24], and E360G decreased the ANF-Luc reporter activity when compared

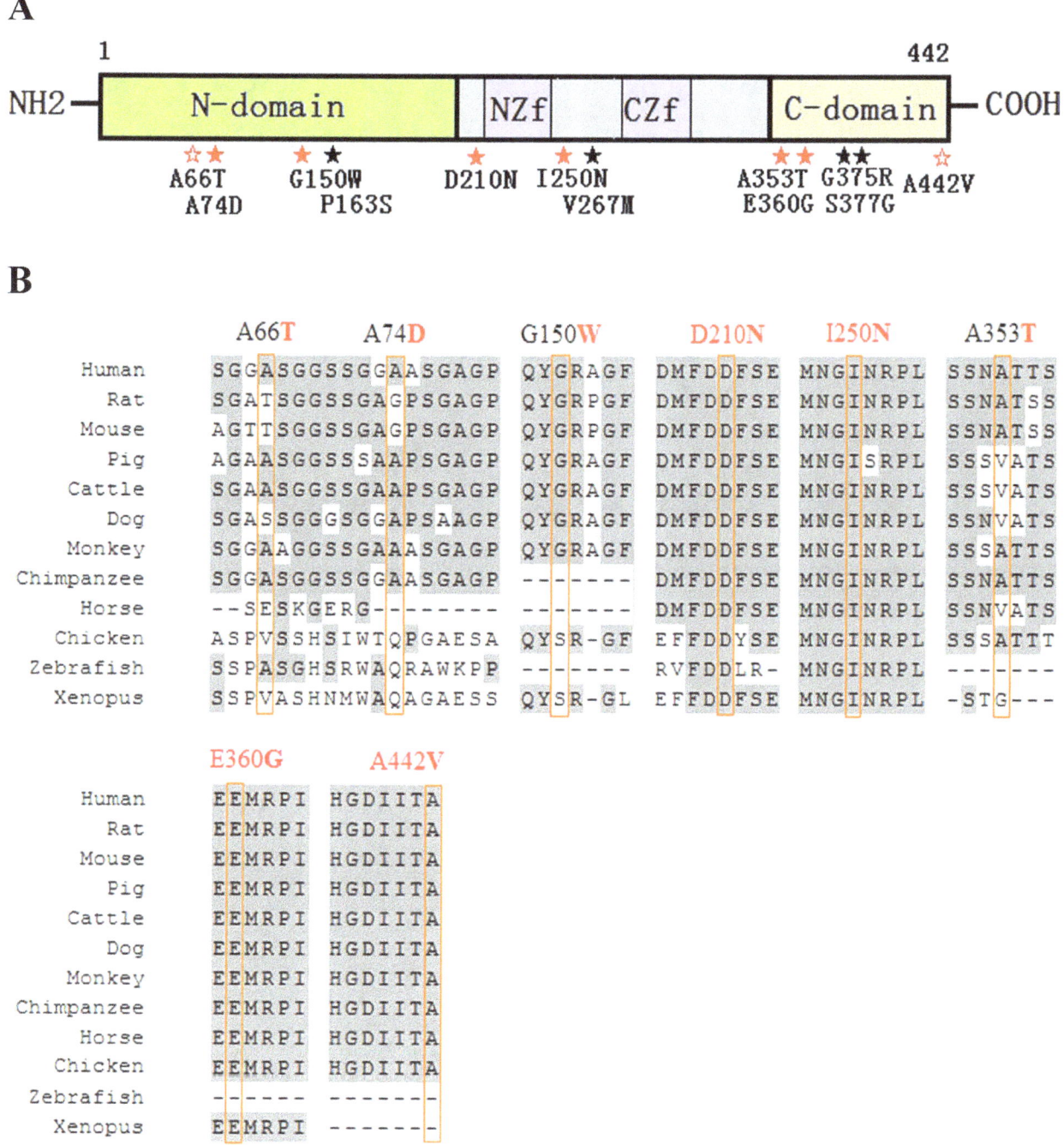

Figure 1. Distribution of the identified GATA4 mutations and multiple sequence alignment across species. (A) A schematic diagram of the GATA4 protein and the locations of the 12 non-synonymous mutations identified in this study (solid red star indicates a mutation that has not been previously reported; empty red star indicates a CHD-specific mutation that has been previously reported; solid black star indicates a mutation that is also found in controls). N-domain, N terminal domain; NZf, N terminal zinc finger domain; CZf, C terminal zinc finger domain; C-domain, C terminal domain. (B) Multiple sequence alignment of the GATA4 protein across different species. The result shows that residues 210 and 250 are highly evolutionarily conserved, and residues 360 and 442 are conserved in mammals.

with wild-type GATA4 (Student's t-test: $P<0.05$). The other mutations tested did not significantly change the luciferase activity (Figure 3B). To further test the DNA binding affinity of GATA4 mutants, EMSA was performed with the GATA cis element upstream of human *dHAND*. Western blot result showed that GATA4 could not be detected in the nuclear extraction of the cells transfected with pCMV-Myc empty vector (Figure 4A). Expression of GATA4 in Hela cells transfected with pCMV-Myc-GATA4 wild type and mutants were kept equivalent (Figure 4B). The EMSA result showed that the DNA binding affinity of mutants A74D, G150W and T280M was clearly reduced compared to wild type GATA4 (Figure 4C).

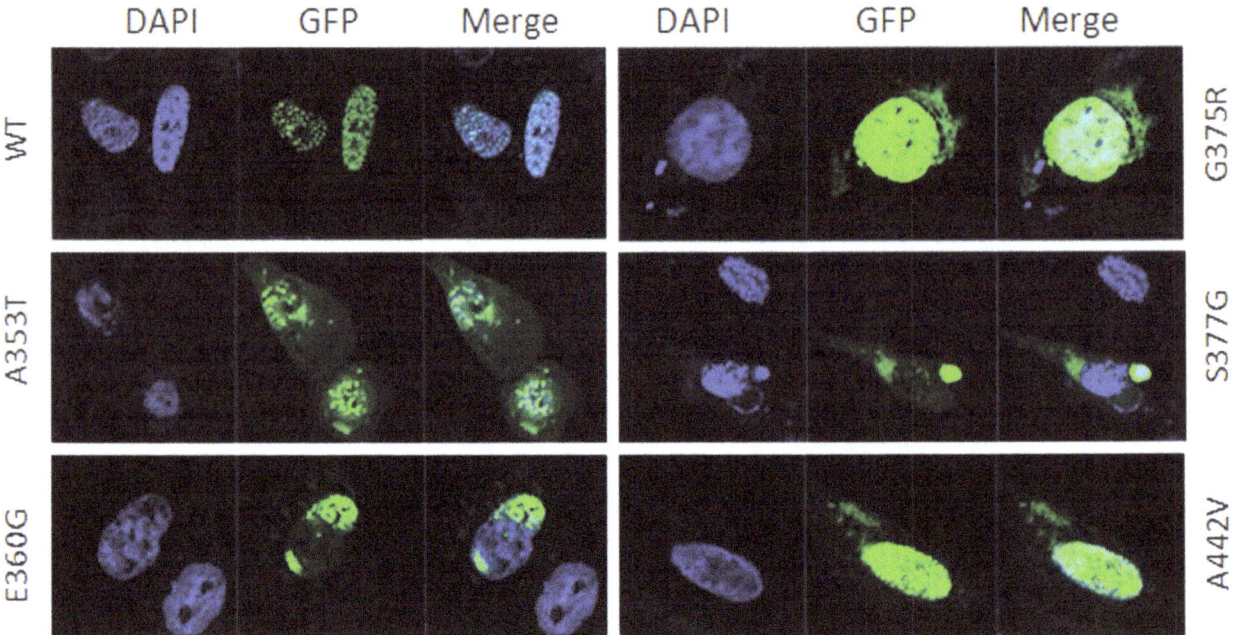

Figure 2. Subcellular location of GATA4 wild type and mutant proteins. GFP (green) represents the over expressed GATA4 protein, and DAPI (blue) represents the location of the nucleus. The subcellular localization of pEGFP-GATA4 wild-type (WT) and mutant-type proteins shows that wild-type GATA4 completely localized to the nucleus, while mutated GATA4 proteins were partially distributed in the cytoplasm besides the nucleus.

Discussion

GATA4 is essential for normal heart development, and a variety of mutations in this gene have been found in many cardiac defects. We found 12 heterozygous GATA4 mutations in a large panel of 384 sporadic CHD patients and 8 of them were found exclusively in CHD patients. Of these 8 mutations, 6 have not been previously reported. The prevalent frequency of GATA4 non-synonymous mutations specifically identified in sporadic CHD patients in our study is approximately 2.1% (8/384). These results are consistent with the 2.5% GATA4 mutation prevalence found in a previous study on 486 Chinese CHD patients [25]. The GATA4 mutation prevalence in Chinese CHD patients, however, is noticeably different from the 0.8% GATA4 mutation prevalence found in 628 American CHD patients [26]. Altogether, these results suggest that GATA4 non-synonymous mutations contribute to CHD differently between different ethnic populations (Table S2).

Even though GATA4 is a highly evolutionarily conserved protein that plays an essential role in normal heart development, the numerous mutations found indicate that GATA4 is a hypermutable protein in CHD patients. These findings appear to be in contrast to previously published data suggesting that GATA4 is a hypomutable protein [26–29]. Currently, approximately 110 non-synonymous mutations have been found in the GATA4 protein, including the mutations identified in this study. Approximately one third of the identified mutations are highly evolutionarily conserved, and 16 mutations are located in the well-conserved zinc finger domains (Figure S1). Some of the functionally important substitutions have even been detected several times in CHD cases (Table S2). For example, the mutation Cys292Arg located in the C terminal zinc finger domain of GATA4 was found in 31 DNA samples isolated from 68 formalin fixed malformed hearts with septal defects [23]. All of this evidence suggests that GATA4 mutations are frequently observed in CHD groups.

Our immunostaining results showed that wild-type GATA4 localized to the nucleus, while the GATA4 mutants A353T, E360G, G375R, S377G and A442V were partially detected in the cytoplasm, which suggests that these mutants do not properly localize to the nucleus. The alternative conformation or misfolding of these mutants may impede GATA4 protein transportation and trafficking. These mutations are not located in the previously identified NLS region [21], but they do affect the distribution of the protein. Similarly, mutations located outside of the identified NLS of TBX5 also impede nuclear localization [30,31]. These results suggest that the nuclear localization of these transcription factors is affected by a wider region of the protein that is not limited to the traditional NLS region.

The luciferase assay revealed that the mutants A66T and A353T up-regulated transcriptional activity, but the increased activation ability could not be explained by DNA binding affinity (Figure 4C). The mutation A66T is located in the TAD1 domain (amino acids 1–77) of GATA4 [21], but it is not evolutionarily conserved (Figure 1B, Figure S2). Mutants A74D and G150W, which located in the TAD1 and TAD2 (amino acids 130–177) domains separately [21], did not change the transcriptional activity significantly but the DNA binding affinity were obviously changed (Figure 4C). The loss-of-function effect observed in the T280M mutant may be because this mutation affects the structural stability of the zinc finger and thus impairs the protein's transcriptional activity and DNA binding affinity (Figure 3B and Figure 4C). The mutations A353T and E360G are located in the nascent C-terminal domain of the GATA4 protein, but they have an opposite effect on the regulation of ANF expression. The 353rd residue changes from a hydrophobic, nonpolar Ala to a hydrophilic polar Thr, while the 360th residue changes from an acidic, polar Glu to a neutral, nonpolar Gly. These changes in residue properties may be responsible for the different regulatory effects observed for these mutants. Furthermore, GATA4 always regulates ANF expression synergistically with other cofactors,

A

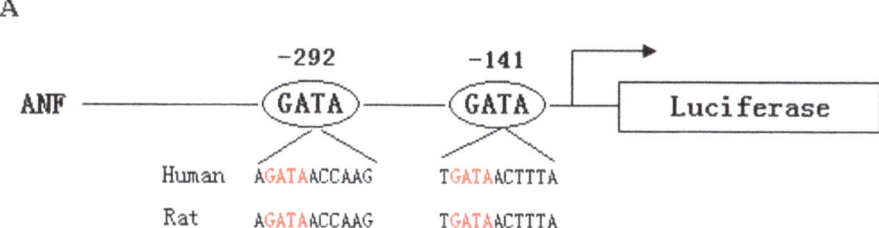

B

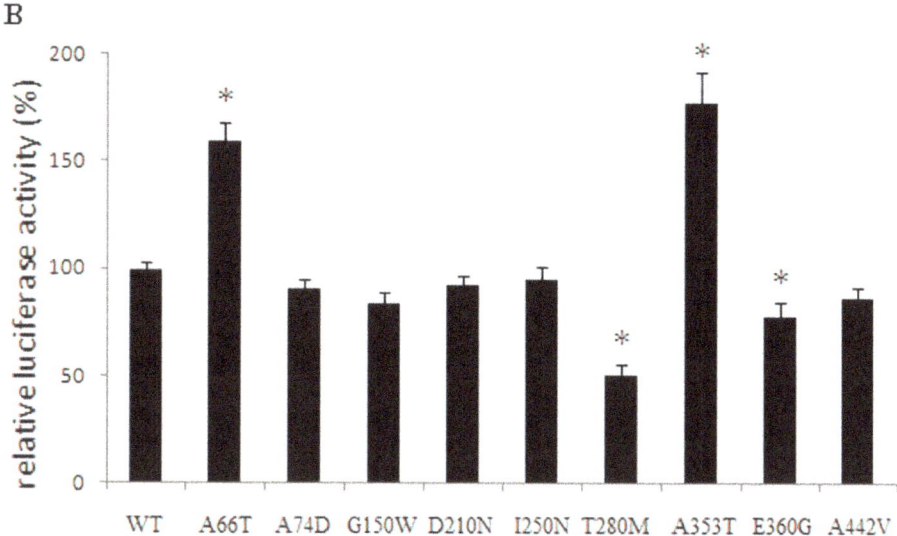

Figure 3. Relative luciferase activity of GATA4 wild type and mutant proteins in Hela cells. (A) Schematic of the human ANF-Luc. The region from the proximal −300 to −130 shows the conserved GATA transcription factor binding sites involved in regulating ANF expression. Two consensus GATA4 binding sites are highlighted in red. (B) Relative luciferase activity of wild type (WT) and CHD specific GATA4 mutant expression constructs that were co-transfected with ANF-Luc in Hela cells. Mean±SD are shown in the histogram. The relative luciferase activity for the A66T mutant was 160±8%, for the T280M mutant was 51±5%, for the A353T mutant was 178±14%, and for the E360G mutant was 78±6%. Student t-test was performed and four mutants caused significant transcriptional activation difference compared with wild-type GATA4 (*, $P<0.05$). Other mutants did not change the ANF-Luc activation significantly.

such as GATA6, TBX5, NKX2-5, or SP1 [12,32–35]. In this study, we ignored the influence of other factors and only focused on the effect of GATA4 mutations. Therefore, the *in vitro* results may not precisely reflect the *in vivo* regulation of ANF expression.

The relationship between the phenotypes of CHD and the genotypes of the GATA4 mutations is very complex, although it is interesting to note that GATA4 mutations are frequently associated with septal defects,such as ASD, VSD and AVSD (Table S2). Periodically, a mutation will be specifically associated with one type of CHD. For example, it has been reported that S52F and S358Del are only associated with ASD, one of the most common types of CHD [35,36]. However, the same CHD phenotype may be caused by different GATA4 mutations, and the same GATA4 mutation may result in different phenotypes in different individuals, even individuals belonging to the same family [12]. We also observed that an affected child could inherit the same mutation from his or her unaffected parents. The different CHD cases, however, may be the result of several factors, such as epigenetic regulation, genetic and environmental factors, and even the personalized genetic signature or age difference. In our study, the questionnaire data collected from the parents of children with CHD revealed that the mothers of these children may have caught a cold, had a fever, lived in a newly decorated house, or worked in an unclean environment, such as an electronics factory. We cannot exclude the possibility that these types of factors may influence the

probability of offspring inheriting CHD, but we are unable to make accurate correlations at this time because these data have no matched control.

Finally, we need to address the hypermutable and hypomutable characteristics found in the GATA4 mutations. The large number of GATA4 non-synonymous mutation count historically identified in CHD patients suggests that it looks like a hypermutable protein. Moreover, most of the genetic results from CHD studies are based on blood samples (Table S2). This strategy, however, may not detect all of the disease associated mutations [4], especially the severe lethal mutations. Therefore, these results may not reveal all of the genetic alterations. But the general ratio of the identified GATA4 mutations in CHD patients is less than 3% as discussed before, which suggests that it is a hypomutable protein. So we further compared the mutation ratio of GATA4 with other essential genes using the Han Chinese population data from the 1000 Genomes Project and the results did not provide strong evidence that GATA4 is under positive or purifying selection in the Han Chinese population. Thus the hypermutable or hypomutable feature is a relative term based on different circumstances. The hypomutable feature is defined based on the mutation ratio, while the hypermutable feature comes from the large number of GATA4 mutations identified in CHD patients.

Why GATA4 mutations are enriched in CHD patients obviously is an interesting question. We first needed to determine

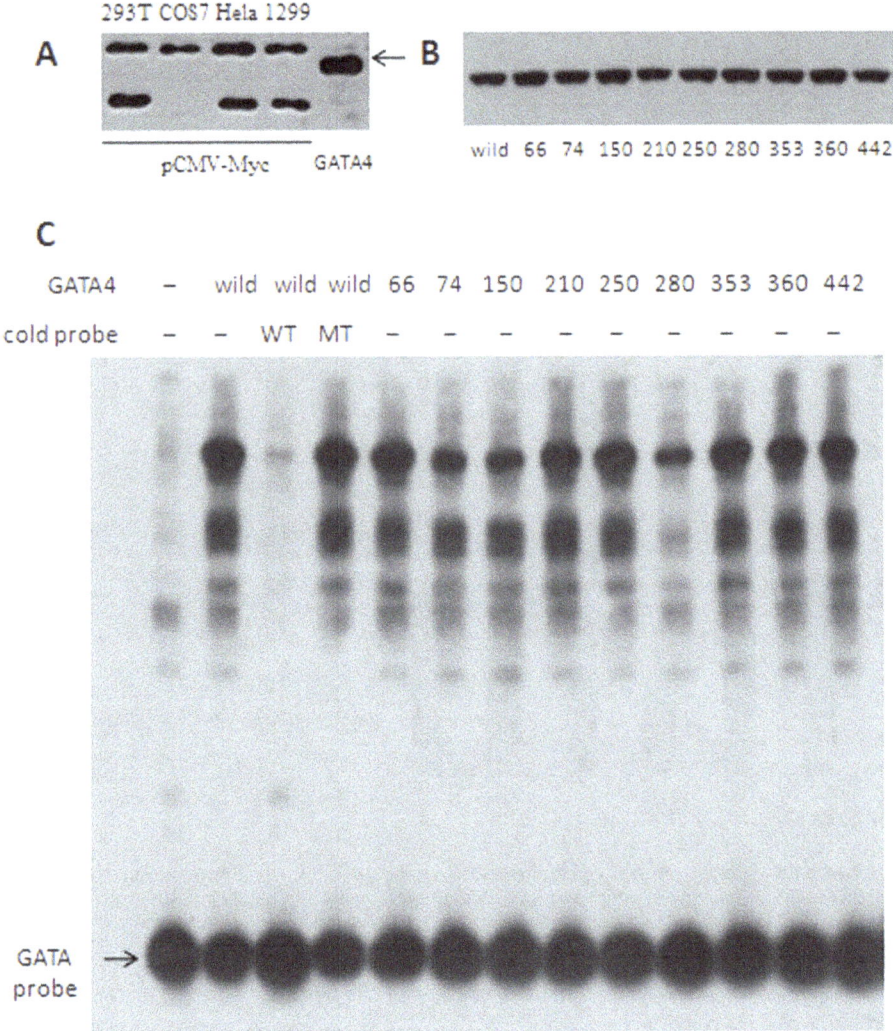

Figure 4. DNA binding affinity of GATA4 wild type and mutants. (A) Detection of the endogenous expression of GATA4 in 293T, COS7, Hela and H1299 cells transfected with pCMV-Myc empty vector. (B) Protein levels of nuclear extracts were kept equivalent between pCMV-Myc-GATA4 wild type and each mutant. (C) GATA4 A74D, G150W and T280M mutant proteins demonstrated abnormal DNA binding affinity compared to wild type GATA4 by using electromobility shift assay of biotin-labelled GATA binding element. 100-fold wild type cold oligonucleotides (WT) could compete for GATA4 binding while 100-fold cold mutant oligonucleotides (MT) failed to compete.

whether the frequency of GATA4 mutations is higher than the frequency of mutations in other essential genes, which may help in explaining the phenomenon of enrichment. The results indicate that there is no difference in the mutation frequency for GATA4 compared with other essential genes (Table 5). This finding does not support the possibility that the hypermutable GATA4 is the result of a higher mutation frequency. If there were correlations between the more severe CHD symptoms and the more conserved or functionally important GATA4 mutations, then it would be reasonable for us to conclude that the conserved GATA4 gene mutations will result in a severe phenotype, such as CHD, and that many CHD patients will have several GATA4 mutations. It is difficult to make these correlations, however, because the classifications/manifestations of CHD are complex and only limited sample sizes have been reported.

The transcriptional regulatory pathways involved in cardiac morphogenesis are extremely complex, and the effects exerted by the critical genetic transcriptional factors participating in these

networks are still being elucidated. From a clinical perspective, the identification of novel and functional GATA4 mutations could be potentially useful as risk predictors in the molecular diagnosis of CHD.

Supporting Information

Figure S1 Geogrphical distribution of GATA4 mutations and conservation analysis.

Figure S2 Multiple sequence alignment of GATA 4, 5, 6 across species.

Table S1 GATA4 primers used in PCR amplification.

Table S2 Detailed information of the identified GATA4 mutations so far.

Acknowledgments

We sincerely thank all the participants in this study and the clinicians who helped in the identification and collection of the CHD samples.

Author Contributions

Designed the study: EW. Drafted the initial manuscript: EW. Added the EMSA experiment: SS. Did the clinical related works: WD BQ. Offered the samples: WD BQ GH. Revised the initial manuscript: YA XG. Compared GATA4 with other essential genes (Table 4): SX. Revised the later versions of the manuscript: YZ. Alignmented GATA4,5,6 across species (Figure S1): ZS. Conceived the study: LJ. Revised the manuscript: LJ HW. Designed the experiments: HW. Performed the experiments: EW.

References

1. Bruneau BG (2008) The developmental genetics of congenital heart disease. Nature 451: 943–948.
2. Hoffman JIE, Kaplan S (2002) The Incidence of Congenital Heart Disease. J Am Coll Cardiol 39: 1890–1900.
3. Nemer G, Fadlalah F, Usta J, Nemer M, Dbaibo G, et al. (2006) A novel mutation in the GATA4 gene in patients with Tetralogy of Fallot. Hum Mutat 27: 293–294.
4. Reamon-Buettner SM, Borlak J (2005) Genetic analysis of cardiac-specific transcription factors reveals novel insights into molecular causes of congenital heart disease. Future Cardiol 1: 355–361.
5. Molkentin JD, Kalvakolanu DV, Markham BE (1994) Transcription factor GATA-4 regulates cardiac muscle-specific expression of the alpha-myosin heavy-chain gene. Mol Cell Biol 14: 4947–4957.
6. Agnihotri S, Wolf A, Munoz DM, Smith CJ, Gajadhar A, et al. (2011) A GATA4-regulated tumor suppressor network represses formation of malignant human astrocytomas. J Exp Med 208: 689–702.
7. Belaguli NS, Zhang M, Rigi M, Aftab M, Berger DH, et al. (2007) Cooperation between GATA4 and TGF-β signaling regulates intestinal epithelial gene expression. Am J Physiol Gastrointest Liver Physiol 292: G1520–1533.
8. FANTOM C, Suzuki H, Forrest AR, van Nimwegen E, Daub CO, et al. (2009) The transcriptional network that controls growth arrest and differentiation in a human myeloid leukemia cell line. Nat Genet 41: 553–562.
9. Selvetella G, Hirsch E, Notte A, Tarone G, Lembo G (2004) Adaptive and maladaptive hypertrophic pathways : points of convergence and divergence. Cardiovasc Res 63: 373–380.
10. Nemer M (2008) Genetic insights into normal and abnormal heart development. Cardiovasc Pathol 17: 48–54.
11. Ieda M, Fu JD, Delgado-Olguin P, Vedantham V, Hayashi Y, et al. (2010) Direct Reprogramming of Fibroblasts into Functional Cardiomyocytes by Defined Factors. Cell 142: 375–386.
12. Garg V, Kathiriya IS, Barnes R, Schluterman MK, King IN, et al. (2003) GATA4 mutations cause human congenital heart defects and reveal an interaction with TBX5. Nature 424: 443–447.
13. Botto LD, Lin AE, Riehle-Colarusso T, Malik S, Correa A (2007) Seeking causes: Classifying and evaluating congenital heart defects in etiologic studies. Birth Defects Res A Clin Mol Teratol 79: 714–727.
14. Grepin C, Dagnino L, Robitaille L, Haberstroh L, Antakly T, et al. (1994) A Hormone-Encoding Gene Identifies a Pathway for Cardiac but Not Skeletal Muscle Gene Transcription. Mol Cell Biol 14: 3115–3129.
15. Seidman CE, Wongt DW, Jarcho JA, Bloch KD, Seidman JG (1988) Cis-acting sequences that modulate atrial natriuretic factor gene expression. Proc Natl Acad Sci U S A 85: 4104–4108.
16. Sprenkle AB, Murray SF, Glembotski CC (1995) Involvement of multiple cis elements in basal- and alpha-adrenergic agonist-inducible atrial natriuretic factor transcription. Roles for serum response elements and an SP-1-like element. Circ Res 77: 1060–1069.
17. McFadden DG, Charit J, Richardson JA, Srivastava D, Firulli AB, et al. (2000) A GATA-dependent right ventricular enhancer controls dHAND transcription in the developing heart. Development 5341: 5331–5341.
18. Schluterman MK, Krysiak AE, Kathiriya IS, Abate N, Chandalia M, et al. (2007) Screening and Biochemical Analysis of GATA4 Sequence Variations Identified in Patients With Congenital Heart Disease. Am J Med Genet A 143A: 817–823.
19. The 1000 Genomes Project Consortium (2010) A map of human genome variation from population-scale sequencing. Nature 467: 1061–1073.
20. Liao BY, Scott NM, Zhang J (2006) Impacts of gene essentiality, expression pattern, and gene compactness on the evolutionary rate of mammalian proteins. Mol Biol Evol 23: 2072–2080.
21. Morrisey EE, Ip HS, Tang Z, Parmacek MS (1997) GATA-4 activates transcription via two novel domains that are conserved within the GATA-4/5/6 subfamily. J Biol Chem 272: 8515–8524.
22. Molkentin J (2000) The zinc finger-containing transcription factors GATA-4, -5, and -6. Ubiquitously expressed regulators of tissue-specific gene expression. J Biol Chem 275: 38949–38952.
23. Reamon-Buettner SM, Borlak J (2005) GATA4 zinc finger mutations as a molecular rationale for septation defects of the human heart. J Med Genet 42: e32.
24. Chen Y, Mao J, Sun Y, Zhang Q, Cheng HB, et al. (2010) A novel mutation of GATA4 in a familial atrial septal defect. Clinica Chimica Acta 411: 1741–1745.
25. Zhang W, Li X, Shen A, Jiao W, Guan X, et al. (2008) GATA4 mutations in 486 Chinese patients with congenital heart disease. Eur J Med Genet 51: 527–535.
26. Tomita-Mitchell A, Maslen CL, Morris CD, Garg V, Goldmuntz E (2007) GATA4 sequence variants in patients with congenital heart disease. J Med Genet 44: 779–783.
27. Posch MG, Perrot A, Schmitt K, Mittelhaus S, Esenwein E-m, et al. (2008) Mutations in GATA4, NKX2.5, CRELD1, and BMP4 are infrequently found in patients with congenital cardiac septal defects. Am J Med Genet A 146A: 251–253.
28. Reamon-Buettner SM, Cho S-h, Borlak J (2007) Mutations in the 3'-untranslated region of GATA4 as molecular hotspots for congenital heart disease (CHD). BMC Med Genet 8: 38.
29. Zhang L, Tümer Z, Jacobsen JR, Andersen PS, Tommerup N, et al. (2006) Screening of 99 Danish Patients with Congenital Heart Disease for GATA4 Mutations. Genet Test 10: 277–280.
30. Collavoli A, Hatcher CJ, He J, Okin D, Deo R, et al. (2003) TBX5 nuclear localization is mediated by dual cooperative intramolecular signals. J Mol Cell Cardiol 35: 1191–1195.
31. Fan C, Liu M, Wang Q (2006) Functional analysis of TBX5 missense mutations associated with Holt-Oram syndrome. J Biol Chem 278: 8780–8785.
32. Charron F, Nemer M (1999) GATA transcription factors and cardiac development. Semin Cell Dev Biol 10: 85–91.
33. Durocher D, Charron F, Warren R, Schwartz R, Nemer M (1997) The cardiac transcription factors Nkx2.5 and GATA-4 are mutual cofactors. EMBO J 16: 5687–5696.
34. Hu X, Li T, Zhang C, Liu Y, Xu M, et al. (2011) GATA4 regulates ANF expression synergistically with Sp1 in a cardiac hypertrophy model. J Cell Mol Med 15: 1865–1877.
35. Hirayama-Yamada K, Kamisago M, Akimoto K, Aotsuka H, Nakamura Y, et al. (2005) Phenotypes with GATA4 or NKX2.5 mutations in familial atrial septal defect. J Med Genet A 135: 47–52.
36. Okubo A, Miyoshi O, Baba K, Takagi M, Tsukamoto K, et al. (2004) A novel GATA4 mutation completely segregated with atrial septal defect in a large Japanese family. J Med Genet 41: e97.
37. Chen M, Pang Y, Guo Y, Pan J, Liu B, et al. (2009) GATA4 Mutations in Chinese Patients with Congenital Cardiac Septal Defects. Pediatr Cardiol 31: 85–89.

8

Jun is Required in *Isl1*-Expressing Progenitor Cells for Cardiovascular Development

Tao Zhang[1], Junchen Liu[2], Jue Zhang[3], Eldhose B. Thekkethottiyil[1], Timothy L. Macatee[4], Fraz A. Ismat[5], Fen Wang[2], Jason Z. Stoller[1]*

1 Division of Neonatology, Department of Pediatrics, Perelman School of Medicine at the University of Pennsylvania, Children's Hospital of Philadelphia, Philadelphia, Pennsylvania, United States of America, 2 Center for Cancer and Stem Cell Biology, Institute of Biosciences and Technology, Texas A & M Health Science Center, Houston, Texas, United States of America, 3 Morgridge Institute for Research, Madison, Wisconsin, United States of America, 4 Department of Pathology and Laboratory Medicine, Perelman School of Medicine at the University of Pennsylvania, Philadelphia, Pennsylvania, United States of America, 5 Division of Cardiology, Department of Pediatrics, Perelman School of Medicine at the University of Pennsylvania, Children's Hospital of Philadelphia, Philadelphia, Pennsylvania, United States of America

Abstract

Jun is a highly conserved member of the multimeric activator protein 1 transcription factor complex and plays an important role in human cancer where it is known to be critical for proliferation, cell cycle regulation, differentiation, and cell death. All of these biological functions are also crucial for embryonic development. Although all *Jun* null mouse embryos die at mid-gestation with persistent truncus arteriosus, a severe cardiac outflow tract defect also seen in human congenital heart disease, the developmental mechanisms are poorly understood. Here we show that murine Jun is expressed in a restricted pattern in several cell populations important for cardiovascular development, including the second heart field, pharyngeal endoderm, outflow tract and atrioventricular endocardial cushions and post-migratory neural crest derivatives. Several genes, including *Isl1*, molecularly mark the second heart field. *Isl1* lineages include myocardium, smooth muscle, neural crest, endocardium, and endothelium. We demonstrate that conditional knockout mouse embryos lacking Jun in *Isl1*-expressing progenitors display ventricular septal defects, double outlet right ventricle, semilunar valve hyperplasia and aortic arch artery patterning defects. In contrast, we show that conditional deletion of Jun in *Tie2*-expressing endothelial and endocardial precursors does not result in aortic arch artery patterning defects or embryonic death, but does result in ventricular septal defects and a low incidence of semilunar valve defects, atrioventricular valve defects and double outlet right ventricle. Our results demonstrate that Jun is required in *Isl1*-expressing progenitors and, to a lesser extent, in endothelial cells and endothelial-derived endocardium for cardiovascular development but is dispensable in both cell types for embryonic survival. These data provide a cellular framework for understanding the role of Jun in the pathogenesis of congenital heart disease.

Editor: Maurizio Pesce, Centro Cardiologico Monzino, Italy

Funding: This work was supported by the National Institutes of Health (NIH, www.nih.gov), American Heart Association (AHA, www.heart.org) and the Cancer Prevention and Research Institute of Texas (CPRIT, www.cprit.state.tx.us). JZ was supported by the AHA (2010130). FW was supported by the NIH (R01-2R01CA096824) and the CPRIT (RP110555). JZS was supported by the NIH (K08-HL086633) and AHA (11BGIA7370043). The funders had no role in study design, data collection and analysis, decision to publish, or preparation of the manuscript.

Competing Interests: FAI is currently employed by Bristol-Myers Squibb. The contributions of FAI related to this manuscript occurred while employed at the Children's Hospital of Philadelphia and prior to employment at Bristol-Myers Squibb.

* E-mail: stoller@email.chop.edu

Introduction

Jun (a.k.a. c-Jun) is a highly conserved member of the multimeric activator protein 1 (AP-1) transcription factor complex [1]. The AP-1 protein complexes are a heterogeneous group of transcriptionally active dimers and include members of the Jun family (Jun, Jund, Junb), Fos family (c-Fos, Fosb, Fosl1, Fosl2) and other transcription factor families such as ATF and Maf [2]. Several *Jun* mutant mice have been generated to study AP-1 function. While *Jun* heterozygous mice are normal [3], all *Jun* null embryos die between E12.5 and E14.5 with persistent truncus arteriosus (PTA) [3,4,5]. PTA is a severe developmental cardiac abnormality seen in many patients as an isolated finding or as part of a syndrome such as DiGeorge/22q11 deletion syndrome. Jun proteins can form homo- or heterodimers to differentially regulate transcription [1]. Examination of the promiscuity of these dimer protein-protein interactions has revealed that as part of a DNA-binding complex, Jun is critical for multiple biological processes including cell proliferation, apoptosis, cell cycle progression and differentiation [6,7,8,9]. Although these cellular phenomena are critical for mammalian development and for diseases such as cancer, data regarding the role of Jun during embryogenesis is limited.

The cardiac outflow tract (OFT) incorporates the lineages of multiple cardiac progenitors and its development is dependent upon the complex interaction of several cell types. Neural crest (NC) cells migrate from the dorsal neural tube to the developing aorticopulmonary septation complex to mediate septation of the truncus arteriosus into the main pulmonary artery and aorta [10]. These NC cells contribute to the OFT endocardial cushion mesenchyme which is also comprised of endothelial-derived endocardial cells [11]. Second heart field (SHF) progenitors contribute to the OFT myocardium and smooth muscle [12,13] while endothelial progenitors give rise to the mature endothelial cells and semilunar valves of the OFT [14,15]. Defects seen in *Jun* null embryos are striking and may be mediated by Jun function in one or more of these cell populations involved in OFT development. Here we show that murine Jun is expressed in a restricted pattern in several cell populations important for cardiovascular development, including the SHF, pharyngeal endoderm, OFT endocardial cushions, atrioventricular (AV) endocardial cushions and post-migratory NC derivatives. Using tissue-specific conditional deletion studies in mice, we demonstrate that Jun is required in *Isl1*-expressing progenitors and, to a lesser extent, in endothelial cells and endothelial-derived endocardium for cardiovascular development but is dispensable in both cell types for embryonic survival.

Results

Jun is Detected during Mid-gestation in Restricted Cell Populations

Several cell populations are important for normal OFT development and septation. The 100% incidence of PTA in *Jun* null embryos indicates that Jun is clearly required in one or more of these cell populations. An overview of *Jun's* spatial and temporal expression pattern during embryonic development in the mouse is lacking in the literature, particularly prior to E14.5. In limited expression analyses by *in situ* hybridization and Northern blot, it has been reported that *Jun* mRNA is expressed in the developing heart, cartilage, gut, central nervous system, lung, kidney, adrenal gland and placenta of the developing mouse [16,17,18,19,20]. To determine the specific cell populations in which Jun might be functioning to regulate cardiac morphogenesis, we examined the expression of *Jun* by *in situ* hybridization and immunohistochemistry at several stages of embryonic development between E8.5 and E15.5. Our Jun expression analysis revealed expression in multiple tissues important for heart development and aortic arch artery remodeling. At E8.5, Jun was expressed in the pharyngeal endoderm, dorsal aortae, common atrial chamber, endocardial cushions and in regions populated by SHF mesoderm (Fig. 1A). The anterior SHF expression was stronger than the posterior SHF (Fig. 1A). The expression of *Jun* in the SHF was also evident at E9.5 by whole mount *in situ* hybridization (Fig. 1B, C). This is consistent with our previous observation of Jun expression in SHF-derived OFT myocardium [21]. At E9.5, *Jun* was expressed in the otic vesicle, telencephalon, somites, and aortic arch arteries (Fig. 1B, C). The expression in the telencephalon, somites and pharyngeal arches is consistent with publically available *in situ* hybridization data at E11 (http://goo.gl/DoJro) [22]. At E10.5, Jun was highly expressed in the OFT endocardial cushions, AV endocardial cushions and cranial nerve IX (Fig. 1D). The high levels of Jun expression in the OFT endocardial cushions persists until E11.5 (Fig. 1E), where expression in pericardium (Fig. 1E) and dorsal root ganglia (data not shown) was also evident. At E15.5, Jun was broadly expressed in the myocardium and both the semilunar and AV valves (Fig. S1).

Conditional Deletion of *Jun* in *Isl1*-expressing Progenitors Results in Severe Cardiovascular Malformations

Jun is expressed in the SHF (Fig. 1) and SHF-derived myocardium (Fig. S1) [21]. The SHF comprises a specialized subset of cardiac progenitor cells derived from early splanchnic mesoderm [13]. These progenitors are marked by the expression of genes such as *Isl1* [13,23,24] and play a critical role in the

development of the right ventricle and OFT. To determine if Jun is expressed in *Isl1*-positive cells, we examined the expression of Jun and Isl1 at E8.5 using immunohistochemistry. Our analysis using confocal microscopy revealed co-localization of Jun and Isl1 in the anterior SHF mesoderm (Fig. 2A, C–F) and pharyngeal endoderm (Fig. 2A, B).

To determine if Jun is required in *Isl1*-expressing progenitors, we performed a conditional deletion of *Jun* using *Isl1*$^{Cre/+}$ knock-in mice [25,26]. There are several mutant mice expressing Cre recombinase in *Isl1*–expressing lineages [25,26,27,28]. To avoid the variable Cre activity observed with the *Isl1*-IRES-Cre mice (*Isl1*$^{tm1(cre)Tmj}$) [25,27], we utilized the *Isl1*$^{Cre/+}$ knock-in mice [25] which have been extensively characterized and shown to drive Cre recombinase expression as early as E8-8.5 [25,26]. *Jun* conditional knockout mice (*Jun*$^{flox/flox}$) [7] have been validated through tissue-specific deletion in liver [7,29], neuroepithelial cells [30], keratinocytes [31,32] and notochord and sclerotome [33]. To determine if Jun was deleted in the *Isl1* lineage, we performed Jun immunostaining of E10.5 *Isl1*$^{Cre/+}$; *Jun*$^{flox/flox}$; *mT/mG* and control embryos. Cre-mediated recombination in mT/mG embryos [34] indelibly marks *Isl1*-derived progenitors with GFP expression. Confocal microscopy of *Isl1*$^{Cre/+}$; *Jun*$^{flox/flox}$ and control embryonic sections revealed that Jun was efficiently deleted in derivatives of *Isl1*-expressing progenitors residing in the OFT (Fig. 3).

Isl1$^{Cre/+}$; *Jun*$^{flox/flox}$ embryos were present at the expected Mendelian ratios (E14.5-P0, n = 23, 100% of predicted; Table 1) and thus survived longer than *Jun* null embryos [3,4,5]. This suggests that Jun function in *Isl1*-expressing cells is not responsible for the embryonic mortality seen in *Jun* null embryos and supports the hypothesis of Hilberg and Eferl et al. that the embryonic death in *Jun* nulls is attributable to impaired hepatogenesis [3,5] rather to the cardiac defects. We examined E14.5 to P0 *Isl1*$^{Cre/+}$; *Jun*$^{flox/flox}$ and control embryos for cardiac defects. Upon careful examination, we found that 32% of *Isl1*$^{Cre/+}$; *Jun*$^{flox/flox}$ conditional mutant embryos (n = 22) showed aortic arch artery remodeling defects (Fig. 4B, B′; Table 2). These defects included interrupted aortic arch (IAA) type B, hypoplasia of the B segment of the aortic arch and aberrant retro-esophageal right subclavian artery. OFT defects were observed in 88% of conditional mutant embryos (n = 8) and included ventricular septal defect (VSD), double outlet right ventricle, and semilunar valve hyperplasia (Fig. 4F, K–N; Table 2). Although there is some evidence that Isl1 progenitors may contribute to the mature AV valves [35], we observed very few GFP-expressing cells derived from *Isl1*-expressing progenitors cells in the developing AV cushions (Fig. 3A, F). Consistent with this observation, we did not observe any AV valve defects in *Isl1*$^{Cre/+}$; *Jun*$^{flox/flox}$ embryos (Fig. 4G, H; Table 2).

Because *Isl1*$^{Cre/+}$ is a loss-of-function allele [25], we looked for evidence of a genetic interaction between *Isl1* and *Jun*. Neither *Isl1*$^{+/-}$ nor *Isl1*$^{Cre/+}$ mice have discernible cardiac defects [23,25,36], thus heterozygosity of *Isl1* from the Cre knock-in could not account for the phenotype in *Isl1*$^{Cre/+}$; *Jun*$^{flox/flox}$ mutants. We observed a single *Isl1*$^{Cre/+}$; *Jun*$^{flox/+}$ embryo (1 of 22) with IAA type B. No other OFT or aortic arch abnormalities were noted among *Isl1*$^{Cre/+}$; *Jun*$^{flox/+}$ embryos. While this suggests a subtle genetic interaction, it does not account for the significantly higher incidence of defects observed in *Isl1*$^{Cre/+}$; *Jun*$^{flox/flox}$ embryos.

Given Jun's role in proliferation and apoptosis [6,7], we investigated whether an alteration in one or both of these cellular processes may contribute to the OFT defects observed in *Jun* mutant mice. Using phospho-histone H3 (pHH3) and TUNEL as markers of cell proliferation and apoptosis, we could not detect any

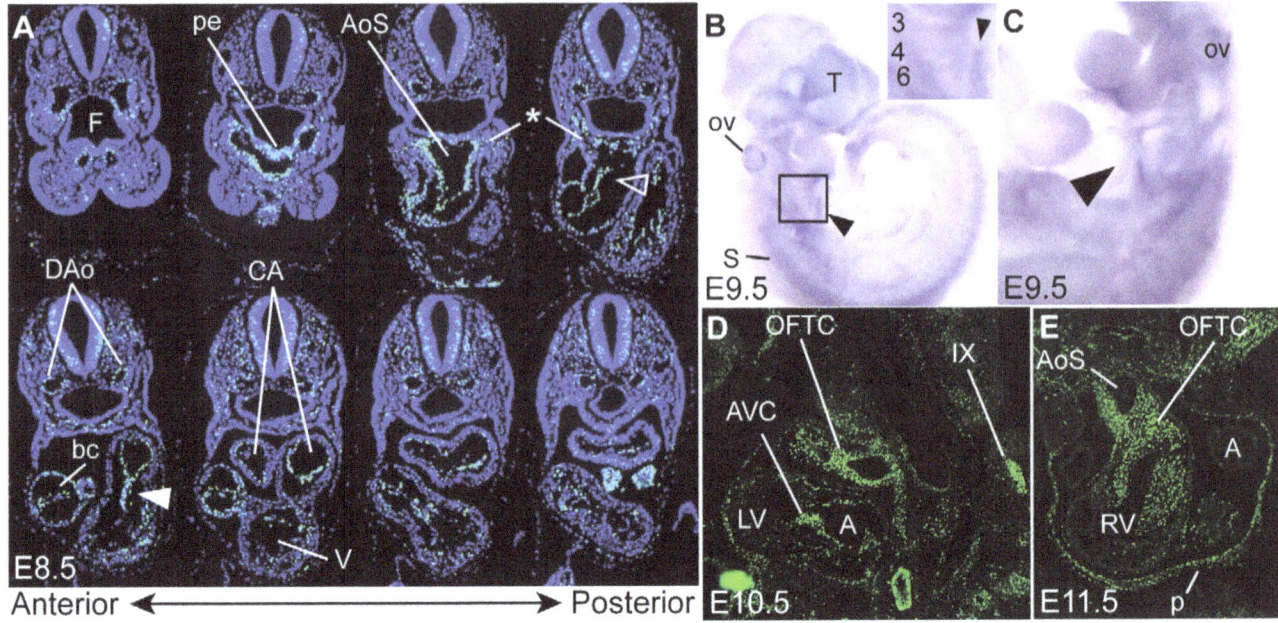

Figure 1. Jun is expressed in cell populations known to contribute to cardiogenesis. (A) Transverse sections along the full anteroposterior axis showing Jun immunostaining (green) in the pharyngeal endoderm (pe), SHF mesoderm (*), OFT cushions (open arrowhead), AV cushions (closed arrowhead), dorsal aortae (DAo) and common atrial chamber (CA). **(B, C)** Whole mount *in situ* hybridization of *Jun* expression in the SHF (arrowhead), somites (S), otic vesicle (ov) and telencephalon (T). Inset is a higher power image of the area shown in the black box in panel B showing *Jun* expression in aortic arch arteries 3, 4 and 6. Parasagittal **(D)** and transverse **(E)** sections showing Jun expression in endocardial cushions, and cranial nerve IX. A, atrium; AoS, aortic sac; AVC, atrioventricular cushion; bc, bulbus cordis; F, foregut; LV, left ventricle; OFTC, outflow tract cushion p, pericardium; RV, right ventricle; V, ventricle.

statistically significant differences in the percent of pHH3- or TUNEL-positive cells in serial sections of the OFT of E10.5 $Isl1^{Cre/+}$; $Jun^{flox/flox}$, $Isl1^{Cre/+}$; $Jun^{flox/-}$ and control littermates (Fig. 5A–E). Although the differences were not statistically significant, there was a trend toward a decrease in proliferating cells and an increase in apoptosis in the OFT of mutant embryos. These findings suggest that the observed OFT defects may not be solely the result of altered proliferation or apoptosis, but raises the possibility that in combination, these alterations could contribute to the phenotype.

Endothelial progenitors, contributing to the developing OFT endocardial cushion mesenchyme, and cardiac NC cells play an important role in the development of the OFT [10,11,14,15]. We used NFATc1 as an endocardial marker [14,37] and Tfap2a (a.k.a. AP-2α) as a marker of migrating NC cells (and ectoderm) [36,38] to determine if conditional deletion of Jun in *Isl1*-expressing progenitors affected the developing endocardium or NC cells. We could not detect any significant differences in NFATc1 or Tfap2a expression in E10.5 $Isl1^{Cre/+}$; $Jun^{flox/-}$ embryos compared with control littermates (Fig. 5F–I). These findings suggest that the defects observed in *Isl1* conditional *Jun* mutant embryos are not attributable to a failure of endocardial formation or cardiac NC migration.

Jun is Required in the Endocardium and Endothelial Progenitors for Valve and Ventricular Septum Formation but not for Aortic Arch Artery Remodeling

Although *Isl1*-expressing progenitors populate the SHF mesoderm, *Isl1* lineages also include other cell populations such as the endocardium and scattered endothelial cells in the aortic arch arteries [13,23,24,26,39]. Endothelial cells, giving rise to the endocardium, undergo an epithelial-to-mesenchymal transforma-

tion to contribute to the OFT cushion mesenchymal tissue during OFT septation [11]. The endocardial cushions subsequently give rise to the valves of the mature heart [14,15]. Our finding that Jun was strongly expressed in the OFT endocardial cushion mesenchyme (Fig. 1D, E) together with the prominent endocardial cushions noted in *Jun* null embryos [5] suggests that Jun may be required in the endothelial progenitors giving rise to endocardial cushion mesenchyme. Hence, we performed fate-mapping studies of endothelial cells in *Jun* mutant embryos. Endothelial cells and endothelial-derived endocardium were marked with ß-galactosidase or GFP expression by crossing transgenic *Tie2-Cre* mice with R26R or mT/mG Cre reporter mice [34,40,41]. *Tie2-Cre* mice have been extensively characterized and shown to drive expression specifically in the embryonic endothelium and endocardium as early as E7.5 [41]. In global *Jun* nulls at E10.5 (Fig. 6D, E), and in endothelial-specific conditional mutants at E15.5 (Fig. 6F), we observed the contribution of *Tie2*-expressing endothelial progenitors to the endothelial cushion mesenchyme and endothelial lining of the truncus arteriosus and aortic sac and to the semilunar valves in a pattern similar to control embryos (Fig. 6A–C). Although these fate mapping experiments suggest that Jun is not required in *Tie2*-expressing endothelial progenitors, it remains possible that the loss of Jun in the endocardium results in a functional defect resulting in cardiac defects or aortic arch artery remodeling defects.

To determine if Jun was required for OFT development and aortic arch artery remodeling, we performed a conditional deletion of *Jun* in endothelium and endothelial-derived endocardium by crossing $Jun^{flox/flox}$ mice with transgenic *Tie2-Cre* mice. To ensure that *Tie2-Cre* was efficiently deleting Jun in endothelial progenitors we performed co-immunostaining for Jun, the endothelial marker, CD31 (Pecam1) and the smooth muscle cell marker, α-smooth

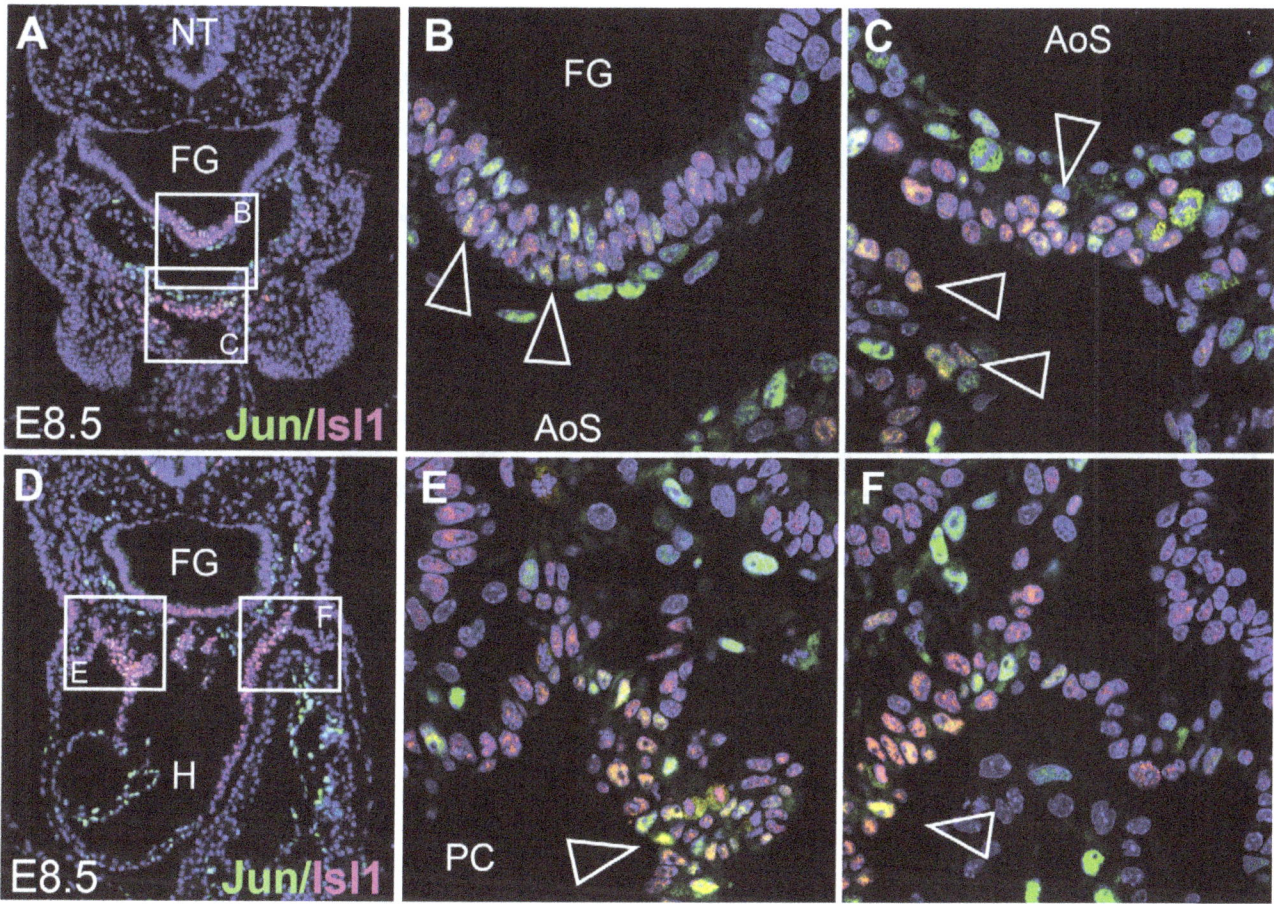

Figure 2. Jun and Isl1 are co-expressed in a subset of cells in the developing outflow tract. (A, D) Transverse sections of an E8.5 wild-type embryo showing Jun (green) and Isl1 (pink) immunostaining in anterior SHF mesoderm and pharyngeal endoderm. Sections were co-stained with DAPI to illustrate nuclei. **(B, C, E, F)** Higher power confocal images of the areas indicated by white boxes in panels A and D. Cell populations co-expressing Jun and Isl1 are indicated by the open arrowheads. AoS, aortic sac; FG, foregut; H, heart; NT, neural tube; PC, pericardial cavity.

muscle actin (SMA). Confocal microscopy of $Jun^{flox/flox}$ and $Tie2$-$Cre; Jun^{flox/flox}$ embryonic sections revealed that Jun was efficiently deleted in endothelial cells (Fig. 7J) whereas expression in smooth muscle cells was unaffected (Fig. 7J, T).

We analyzed embryonic and neonatal $Tie2$-$Cre; Jun^{flox/flox}$ mutants for a recapitulation of the cardiac phenotype observed in the Jun null and $Isl1$ conditional Jun mutant embryos. We quantified the incidence of embryonic death, aortic arch remodeling defects, and cardiac defects and found that, similar to the $Isl1^{Cre/+}; Jun^{flox/flox}$ embryos, the endothelial-specific knockouts of Jun survive until late gestation or even until birth. $Tie2$-$Cre; Jun^{flox/flox}$ embryos were present at the expected Mendelian ratios (E15.5-P0; Table 1). We examined E15.5 to P0 $Tie2$-$Cre; Jun^{flox/flox}$ and control embryos for cardiac defects. Upon careful examination, we did not observe any $Tie2$-$Cre; Jun^{flox/flox}$ conditional mutant embryos (n = 10) with aortic arch artery remodeling defects (Table 2). 43% of conditional mutant embryos had a perimembranous VSD and 14% had double outlet right ventricle, mitral or pulmonary valve hyperplasia (Fig. 8A, C; Table 2). We also noted thinning of the compact myocardium of the right ventricle (Fig. 8A) in 43% (n = 3/7) of $Tie2$-$Cre; Jun^{flox/flox}$ embryos. This phenotype is similar to that previously described in the global Jun null embryos [5]. To determine if these defects were due to a cell non-autonomous effect on NC cell migration, we performed Tfap2a immunostaining of $Tie2$-Cre conditional Jun

mutant and control embryos. We observed a similar pattern of Tfap2a expression in the developing OFT and pharyngeal arches in E10.5 $Tie2$-$Cre; Jun^{flox/-}$ embryos compared with controls (Fig. 6G–J) suggesting that defects observed in $Tie2$ conditional Jun mutant embryos are not attributable to a failure of cardiac NC cell migration. Thus, Jun is not required in endothelial cells and endothelial-derived endocardial cushions for aortic arch artery remodeling or embryonic survival, but is required for the formation of the ventricular septum, compact myocardium and to a lesser extent for formation of the OFT and valves.

Discussion

Congenital heart disease (CHD) is the most commonly occurring major birth defect in humans with an incidence of 6 per 1000 live births [42]. OFT malformations, including PTA, constitute the largest class of life-threatening CHD. It has been more than a decade since it was recognized that the global loss of Jun in mice uniformly results in PTA [5]. Information regarding Jun expression in cardiac progenitors during critical stages of heart development has been poorly described and thus it has remained unclear in what cell populations Jun may regulate transcription. We show that Jun is expressed in a restricted pattern in several cell populations including the SHF, pharyngeal endoderm, OFT and

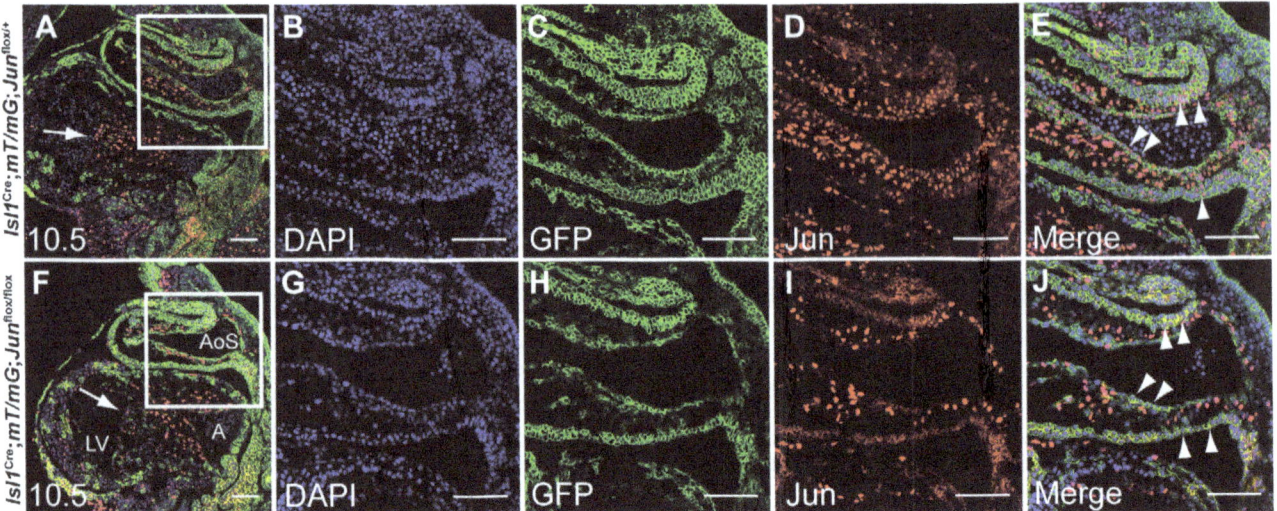

Figure 3. Jun is efficiently deleted in derivatives of *Isl1*-expressing cells in the outflow tract. Saggital sections of E10.5 *Isl1*^Cre/+; *mT/mG*; *Jun*^flox/+ (**A**) and *Isl1*^Cre/+; *mT/mG*; *Jun*^flox/flox (**F**) embryos co-immunostained with anti-GFP (green) and anti-Jun (red) and analyzed by confocal microscopy showing nuclear Jun expression. *Isl1*^Cre/+-expressing progenitors were marked with GFP expression using the mT/mG double-fluorescent Cre reporter mice. Sections were co-stained with DAPI to illustrate nuclei. (**B–E, G–J**) Higher power images of the areas indicated by white boxes in panels A, F. Jun is efficiently deleted in derivatives of *Isl1*-expressing progenitors located in the OFT (arrowheads) whereas AV cushion cells (arrows), not derived from *Isl1*-expressing progenitors, express Jun in both control (**E**) and mutant embryos (**J**). A, atrium; AoS, aortic sac; LV, left ventricle. Scale bar: 100 μm.

AV endocardial cushions and post-migratory NC derivatives such as cranial nerve IX and the dorsal root ganglia.

Although *Jun* null embryos die with PTA, we did not observe PTA in conditional *Jun* mutants. There are at least two explanations for this finding. There may be functional redundancy among Jun proteins and/or Jun may be required in other cardiac progenitors not expressing *Isl1*. There is evidence to suggest some degree of functionally redundancy among Jun proteins, such as Jun, Junb and Jund, during heart development. *Jund*^−/− mice have no cardiac defects [43] and *Junb*^−/− null embryos die at E8.5-E10 due to multiple defects in extra-embryonic tissues [44]. Wagner et al. have generated mice in which either *Junb* or *Jund* is knocked-in to the *Jun* locus to test whether Junb or Jund, under the control of the endogenous Jun regulatory elements, can rescue the *Jun* null phenotype [20,45]. While both of these knock-in mice rescue the mortality at E13 seen in *Jun*^−/− embryos [20,45], the rescue of the cardiac defects is not as straightforward. *Jun*^Junb/Junb embryos survive to E18.5 in Mendelian ratios but continue to have PTA (similar to *Jun*^−/− embryos [20]) and VSDs. The same authors then tested whether overexpression of Junb, with *Junb* transgenic mice under the control of human ubiquitin C promoter [46] were able to rescue the *Jun* null phenotype. *Junb*-Tg; *Jun*^−/− embryos are born with no cardiac defects demonstrating redundancy that is dependent on gene dosage [20]. *Jun*^Jund/Jund embryos survive to E18.5 in Mendelian ratios but also display PTA similar to *Jun*^−/− embryos [45], suggesting that Jund is not functionally redundant for Jun during cardiac development. The rescue of embryonic lethality but not heart defects indicates that different developmental processes have different sensitivities to Jun dosage. It is unclear whether Jund overexpression can rescue the cardiac defects see in *Jun* null embryos. Future studies to test whether decreasing the dosage of Jund or Junb will uncover functional redundancy during heart development may include the analysis of heart defects in *Isl1*^Cre/+; *Jun*^flox/flox; *Junb*^+/− or *Isl1*^Cre/+; *Jun*^flox/flox; *Jund*^+/− mutants.

Jun transcriptional activity is dependent on Jun N-terminal kinase (JNK) phosphorylation [47,48]. This JNK-dependent Jun phosphorylation is dispensable for embryonic development, including for cardiogenesis. Behrens et al. demonstrated this by generating mice in which the *Jun* locus was mutated to prevent JNK phosphorylation (*JunAA*) [49]. *JunAA* homozygous mice, unlike *Jun*^−/− mice, are born in Mendelian ratios and are healthy and fertile, without heart defects, as adults. The notion that JNK-dependent phosphorylation is not essential for heart development is further supported by the observation that *Jnk* mutant mice survive without heart defects [50].

An alternative explanation for the PTA seen in *Jun* null embryos but not in the conditional mutants is that Jun may have roles in multiple cell populations involved in regulating OFT septation. The proximal portion of the OFT cushions (conus) becomes the subpulmonary infundibulum and failure of this structure to form properly results in VSDs. The distal OFT cushions (truncus) gives rise to the semilunar valves and intrapericardial portions of the aorta and pulmonary artery. More distally, the dorsal wall of the aortic sac becomes the aorticopulmonary septum. In humans, defects in this structure result in an aorticopulmonary window [51,52]. A failure of septation in both the distal OFT and the aortic sac-derived portion of the great arteries results in PTA which usually, but not always [53], is associated with VSDs. The PTA in *Jun* null embryos [5] together with our observation of VSDs in the absence of both PTA and a common truncal valve, supports a model in which "conal" septation, regulated by Jun in *Isl1*-progenitors, is mechanistically separate from both "truncal" and aorticopulmonary septation. Jun may play a role in a non-*Isl1*-expressing domain to regulate "truncal" and aorticopulmonary septation.

Heart development is dependent upon the complex interaction and contribution of several cell types. There are multiple lines of evidence supporting the notion that within the early mesoderm, there is a common cardiovascular progenitor that gives rise to myocardial, smooth muscle and endothelial lineages [54]. Within

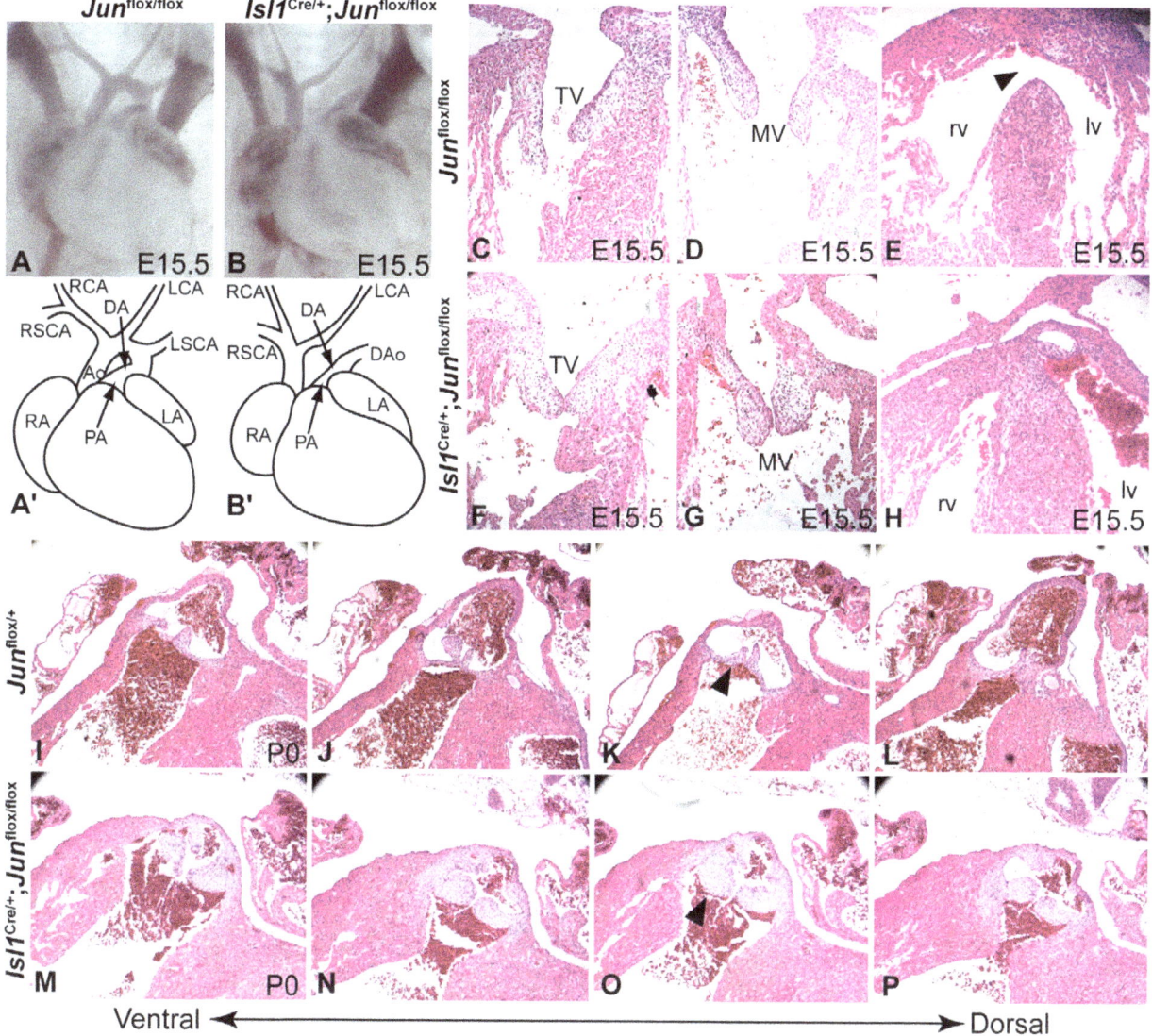

Figure 4. *Isl1*-specific deletion of *Jun* results in cardiovascular defects. Compared to control embryos (**A, A′, C–E, I–L**), the loss of *Jun* in *Isl1*-expressing precursors results in IAA (**B, B′**), VSD (arrowhead, **E**), and enlarged and hyperplastic pulmonary valve leaflets (arrowhead, **O**). The atrioventricular valves are unaffected (**C, D, F, G**). Ao, aorta; CA, carotid artery; DA, ductus arteriosus; DAo, descending aorta; LA, left atrium; lv, left ventricle; MV, mitral valve; PA, pulmonary artery; RA, right atrium; rv, right ventricle; SCA, subclavian artery; TV, tricuspid valve.

the splanchnic mesoderm, the SHF, a group of cardiovascular precursors destined to give rise to the right ventricle and OFT, is molecularly marked by the expression of *Tbx1*, a *Mef2c* regulatory module, and by *Isl1* [13,23,55,56,57]. Data from both murine

Table 1. Summary of genotypes for *Jun* conditional mutants.

Genotype (E14.5-P0)	n (%)	Genotype (E15.5-P0)	n (%)
Isl1^Cre/+; *Jun*^flox/+	23 (25%)	*Tie2*-Cre; *Jun*^flox/+	12 (24%)
Isl1^Cre/+; *Jun*^flox/flox	23 (25%)	*Tie2*-Cre; *Jun*^flox/flox	10 (20%)
Jun^flox/+	26 (28%)	*Jun*^flox/+	15 (31%)
Jun^flox/flox	20 (22%)	*Jun*^flox/flox	12 (24%)
χ²	p = 0.94	χ²	p = 0.92

models and from humans suggest that *ISL1* plays a role in heart development and possibly human CHD. There is a report of a diabetic patient who harbors an *ISL1* mutation [58], but there have been none described in patients with CHD. Despite this, there is evidence to suggest that common *ISL1* single nucleotide polymorphisms (SNPs) are associated with human CHD [59]. It remains to be determined if these SNPs are causative or if they are linked to an associated causative locus. The current study provides data to support a possible role for JUN in ISL1 progenitors and thus adds to the likelihood that this association may be causative. Multipotent Isl1-positive progenitors, when isolated and cultured from either mouse or human embryonic hearts, are capable of differentiating into each of these three lineages [24,60]. This has also been demonstrated using a potentially overlapping population of Nkx2.5-positive progenitor cells [61]. This *ex vivo* data is consistent with *in vivo* fate-mapping studies, using an *Isl1* inducible Cre, showing the contribution of *Isl1* derivatives to the same three lineages [28]. Recent evidence suggests that some *Isl1*-expressing

Table 2. Cardiovascular abnormalities in late gestation *Jun* conditional mutants.

E14.5–P0	*Jun*flox/+ or *Jun*flox/flox	*Isl1*Cre/+; *Jun*flox/flox	*Tie2-Cre*; *Jun*flox/flox
Aortic arch artery remodeling defects	0% (0/46)	32% (7/22)	0% (0/10)
Ventricular septal defect	0% (0/9)	88% (7/8)	43% (3/7)
Double outlet right ventricle	0% (0/9)	88% (7/8)	14% (1/7)
Mitral valve defect	0% (0/9)	0% (0/8)	14% (1/7)
Tricuspid valve defect	0% (0/9)	0% (0/8)	0% (0/7)
Pulmonary valve defect	0% (0/9)	88% (7/8)	14% (1/7)
Aortic valve defect	0% (0/9)	75% (6/8)	0% (0/7)

progenitor cells may also be of a NC lineage (discussed below) [62].

Our analysis of mutants lacking Jun in the endothelial lineage reveals that Jun is required for heart development in some, but not all, *Tie2*-derived endothelial cells and endothelial-derived endo-

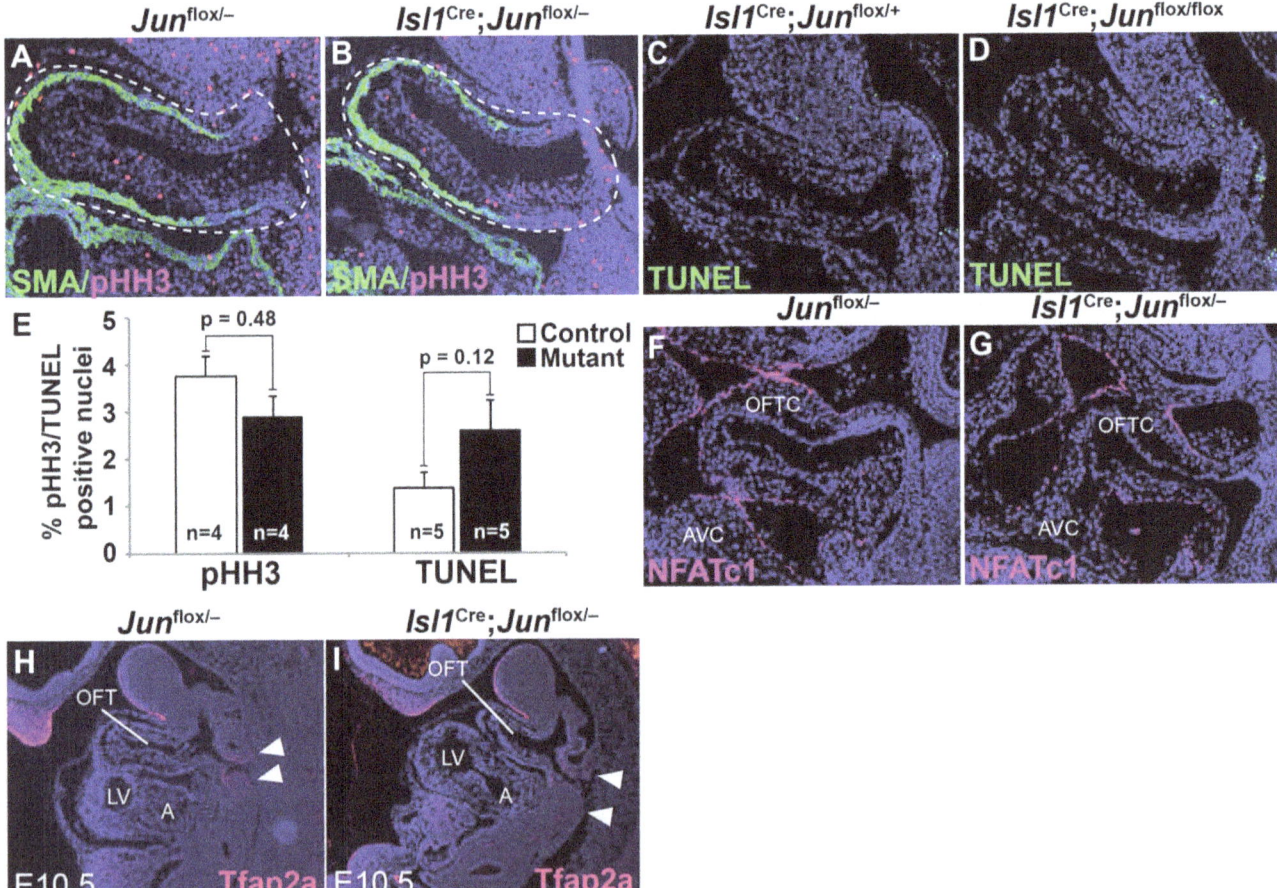

Figure 5. Effect of the loss of Jun in *Isl1*-expressing progenitors on proliferation, apoptosis, cardiac neural crest cells and the endocardium. Sagittal sections of E10.5 mutant (**B, D, G**) and control (**A, C, F**) embryos analyzed by pHH3 and NFATc1 immunostaining and by TUNEL assay. pHH3 immunostaining (pink) reveals similar proliferation rates in mutant and control OFT cells (**A, B**). Dotted lines show representative areas used for cell counting with ImageJ software. TUNEL assay reveals similar numbers of TUNEL-positive (green) OFT cells in mutant and control embryos (**C, D**). (**E**) Quantitative analysis of the percentage of pHH3- and TUNEL-positive OFT cells in serial sections showing a statistically insignificant trend toward less proliferation and more apoptosis in conditionally deleted embryos at E10.5. Results are expressed as mean ± SEM of the percent positive nuclei. The statistical significance of differences between groups was analyzed by the Student's t-test. (**F, G**) Expression of the endocardial marker NFATc1 (pink), is not significantly different between conditional mutant and control embryos. Saggital sections of anti-Tfap2a immunostained *Jun*flox/− (**H**) and *Isl1*Cre/+; *Jun*flox/− (**I**) embryos showing no significant difference in Tfap2a-expressing neural crest cells (arrowheads) at E10.5. Sections were co-stained with DAPI to illustrate nuclei. A, atrium; AVC, atrioventricular cushion; LV, left ventricle; OFT, outflow tract; OFTC, outflow tract cushion; SMA, smooth muscle actin.

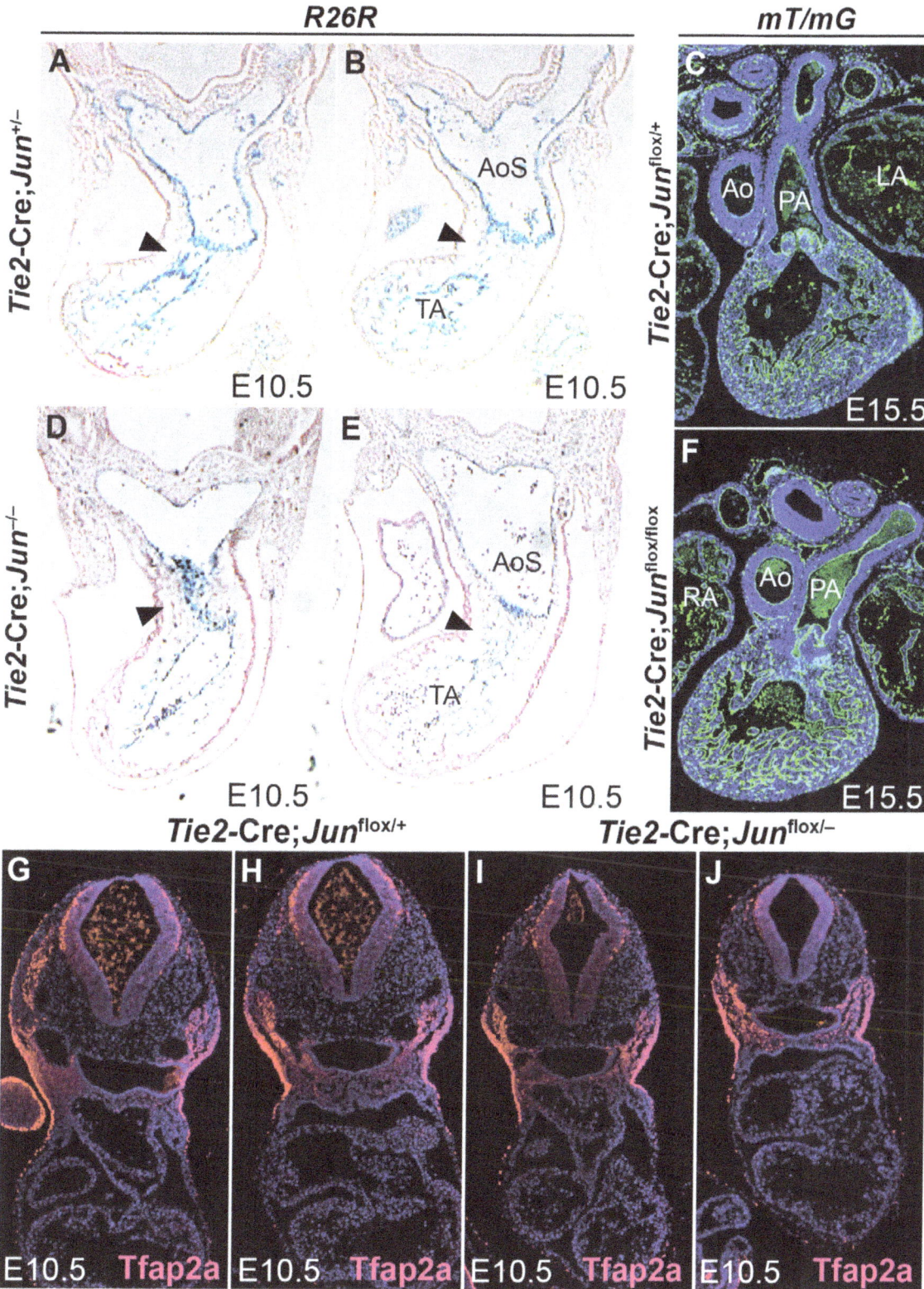

Figure 6. Loss of *Jun* does not alter the fate of *Tie2*-expressing endothelial derivatives or cardiac neural crest cells in the developing OFT. Transverse sections of X-gal stained *Jun*$^{+/-}$; *Tie2-Cre;R26R* (**A, B**) and *Jun*$^{-/-}$; *Tie2-Cre; R26R* (**D, E**) embryos showing no significant difference in endothelial derivatives (blue) populating the OFT endocardial cushion mesenchyme (arrowheads) at E10.5. Transverse sections of anti-GFP immunostained *Tie2-Cre; Jun*$^{flox/+}$; *mT/mG* (**C**) and *Tie2-Cre; Jun*$^{flox/flox}$; *mT/mG* (**F**) embryos showing no significant difference in endothelial derivatives (green) populating the semilunar valves, heart and blood vessels at E15.5. Transverse sections of anti-Tfap2a immunostained *Tie2-Cre; Jun*$^{flox/+}$ (**G, H**) and *Tie2-Cre; Jun*$^{flox/-}$ (**I, J**) embryos showing no significant difference in Tfap2a-expressing neural crest cells at E10.5. Sections were co-stained with DAPI to illustrate nuclei. Ao, aorta; AoS, aortic sac; LA, left atrium; PA, pulmonary artery; RA, right atrium; TA, truncus arteriosus.

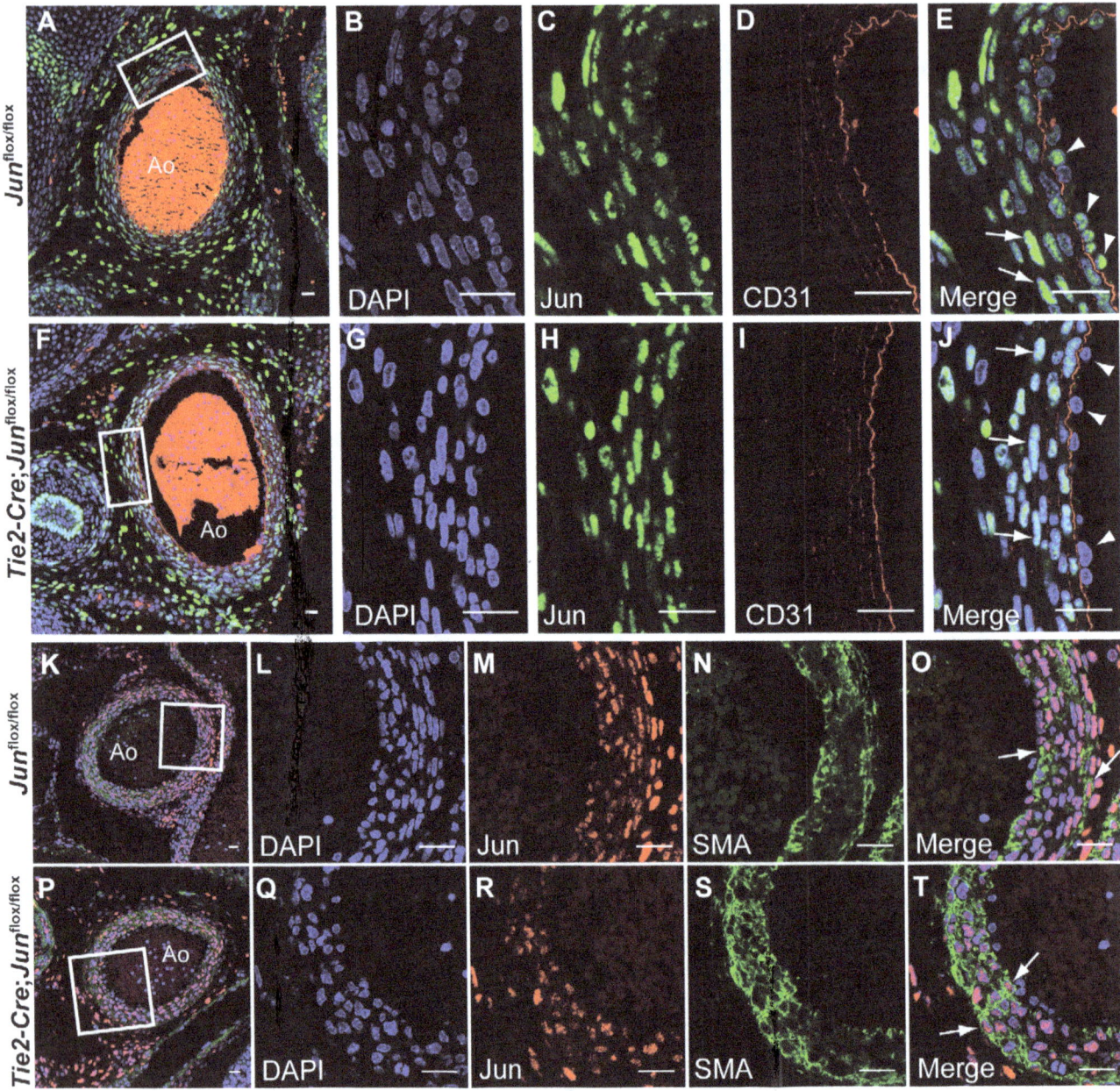

Figure 7. Jun is efficiently deleted in *Tie2*-expressing endothelial derivatives. Cross sections of E15.5 *Jun*flox/flox (**A, K**) and *Tie2-Cre; Jun*flox/flox (**F, P**) embryos co-immunostained with anti-CD31, anti-SMA and anti-Jun analyzed by confocal microscopy. Sections were co-stained with DAPI to illustrate nuclei. (**B–E, G–J**) Higher power images of the areas indicated by white boxes in panels A, F. Smooth muscle cells (arrows) express Jun (green) in control (**E**) and mutant embryos (**J**) whereas Jun is efficiently deleted in endothelial cells (arrowheads). (**L–O, Q–T**) Higher power images of the area indicated by white boxes in panels K, P. Jun (red) is expressed in SMA-positive smooth muscle cells (green; arrows) in control (**K**) and mutant embryos (**P**). Ao, aorta. Scale bar: 20 μm.

cardium. The thinning of the compact myocardium of the right ventricle observed in the *Tie2* conditional *Jun* mutants suggests a model in which there is signaling from the endocardium to regulate the differentiation of primitive myocardial epithelium into compact myocardium. Pathways involved in reciprocal paracrine signaling between the endocardium and myocardium include Neuregulin-1, EphrinB2, Notch, Neurofibromin 1, VEGF, Angiopoietin-1, and Fgf [63,64,65,66,67]. The role of endocardial Jun in one of these pathways or in a parallel pathway remains to be determined. It is intriguing that there was no compact zone thinning of the left ventricle suggesting that endocardial Jun is not

required for the differentiation of *all* primitive myocardial epithelium. Our findings of VSDs in both *Isl1* and *Tie2* conditional *Jun* mutants also support this paracrine model although we cannot conclude from our data whether or not the critical subset of *Tie2*-derived cells is descended from Isl1-positive progenitors. Currently available techniques do not allow us to conditionally delete *Jun* in *Tie2/Isl1*-positive progenitors *in vivo* while leaving *Jun* unaltered in *Tie2*-positive *Isl1*-negative progenitors. Thus, it remains to be tested if Jun is dispensable in the *Isl1*-negative endothelial lineage. Alternatively, the VSDs we observed may be a common phenotype resulting from independent requirement for Jun in

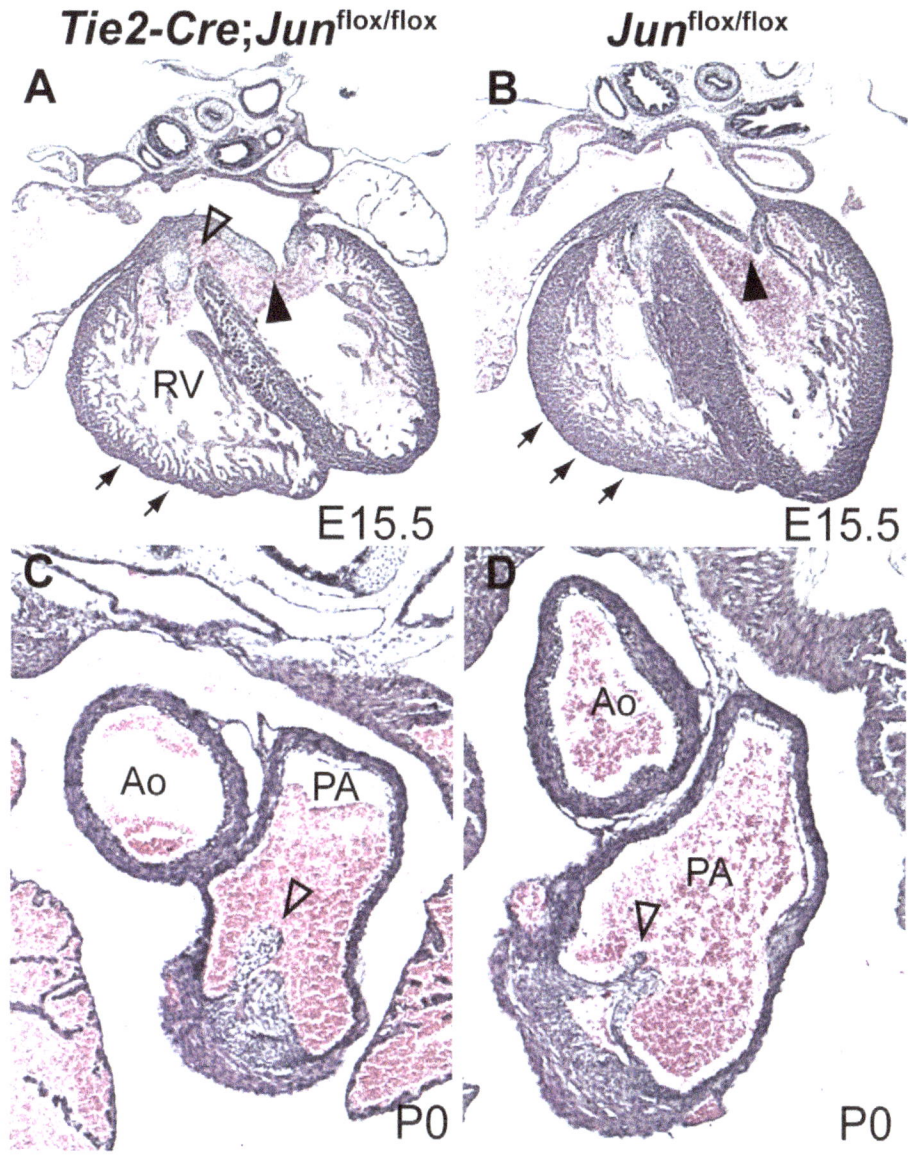

Figure 8. *Tie2*-specific deletion of *Jun* results in cardiovascular defects. Compared to control embryos (**B, D**), the loss of *Jun* in *Tie2*-expressing precursors results in VSD (open arrowhead, **A**), thinned RV (arrows, **A**) and thickened and hyperplastic mitral valve (closed arrowhead, **A**) and pulmonary valve leaflets (open arrowhead, **C**). Ao, aorta; PA, pulmonary artery; RV, right ventricle.

both *Isl1*-negative endothelial/endocardial cells and *Tie2*-negative *Isl1* progenitors.

Our finding of aortic arch artery patterning defects in *Isl1*-specific *Jun* deleted embryos raises the possibility of a cell autonomous effect of Jun in an *Isl1*-derived smooth muscle lineage or alternatively a cell non-autonomous effect on another cell population such as NC. There are other examples of genetic alterations in the SHF affecting a tissue-tissue interaction with NC cells. We have shown that deletion of Notch in the SHF using *Isl1*^Cre or *Mef2c*-AHF-Cre results in severe NC-related cardiac defects including PTA and IAA [36], defects identical to those seen in our *Isl1*^Cre/+; *Jun*^flox/flox embryos and in *Jun* null embryos [5]. Further tissue-restricted deletion studies are required to determine the relative requirement for Jun specifically in the smooth muscle or myocardial lineages.

Our expression analysis indicates that Jun is expressed in post-migratory NC derivatives. NC cells are a specialized subset of

neuroepithelial cells in the dorsal neural tube that migrate ventrally and contribute to a diverse array of tissues. Raivich et al. have previously reported that Jun is expressed in neuroepithelial cells [68] yet deletion of Jun in neuroepithelial cells with *Nestin*-Cre did not result in congenital heart defects [30,69]. It is unclear if *Nestin*-Cre is expressed in a cardiac NC subset of neuroepithelial cells. Cardiac NC cells, originating between the mid-otic placode and the third somite, invade the pharyngeal arches and encompass the aortic arch arteries around E10. By E10.5 they populate the cardiac OFT as two columns of cells subsequently forming a portion of the mesenchymal tissue in the OFT endocardial cushions. Notably, these cushions are abnormal in *Jun* null embryos [5]. Ultimately, descendants of this subset of NC cells contribute to the aorticopulmonary septum, dividing the truncus arteriosus into the aorta and pulmonary artery [10,70,71]. Although there is evidence that the complete loss of *Jun* does not globally affect the fate of NC cells, by E12.5 there are fewer connexin43-labeled cardiac NC cells populating the right ventricular OFT of *Jun* null embryos [5]. In contrast, our findings suggest that the defects observed in *Isl1* and *Tie2* conditional *Jun* mutant embryos are not attributable to a cell non-autonomous defect of cardiac NC migration. In the global *Jun* null embryo, it is unknown whether the fewer connexin43-labeled cells is due to a secondary cell non-autonomous mechanism affecting NC as the result of a loss of Jun function in another tissue such as SHF or pharyngeal endoderm. This is further complicated by the recent observation that some *Isl1*-expressing progenitor cells may be of a NC lineage [62]. This novel and surprising data raises the possibility that the defects observed in *Isl1*-conditional *Jun* mutants may reflect a cell autonomous defect of NC. The effect of conditional deletion of *Jun* in *Isl1*-expressing progenitors on NC cell differentiation was not determined in the current study but is an important area for future investigation. Tissue-restricted deletion studies using *Wnt1*-Cre or *Pax3*$^{Cre/+}$ mice [72,73] are required to determine the requirement for Jun specifically in NC derivatives.

Jun, as part of the AP-1 transcription factor complex, is a positive regulator of cell proliferation [7,8,32] and positively regulates cell cycle progression through p19, p53, cyclin D1 and cyclin A pathways [6,8,29,74,75,76,77]. It regulates the differentiation of varied cell populations such as hematopoietic cells and keratinocytes [6,9] and has also been shown to regulate apoptosis in such cells as fibroblasts, hepatocytes and neurons [6,8,78,79]. Although these pleiotropic cellular functions are likely to be important for all progenitors, our observation that *Isl1*- and *Tie2*-specific *Jun* knockouts survive embryogenesis in Mendelian ratios indicates that Jun is dispensable in these progenitors for overall embryonic survival. Though Jun is not required for formation or maintenance of the blood vessels (at least after the time of *Tie2*-Cre-mediated recombination), it is not completely dispensable in endothelial precursors as they display a low incidence of cardiac defects. Out data do not exclude the possibility of subtle defects in endothelial cell function in these *Jun* mutant embryos.

The molecular mechanisms by which Jun functions during heart development, in *Isl1*-expressing cells and other cells remains to be determined. In the embryonic human heart, ISL1 is strongly expressed in highly proliferative SHF-derived cell populations in the arterial and venous poles [80]. We observed a statistically insignificant trend toward a decrease in proliferating cells and an increase in apoptosis in the OFT of mutant embryos. These individual differences were modest when compared with controls, but in combination these two alterations may contribute to defects in OFT septation or complete formation of the ventricular septum. There are several transcriptional networks and signaling pathways known to regulate proliferation in the SHF. These include *Nkx2.5*, Wnt/ß-catenin, Notch, Fgf, Shh, *Isl1*, and *Tbx1* signaling pathways (reviewed in [13]). *TBX1* is a molecular marker of the SHF and accruing evidence points to a causative role for this transcription factor in the pathogenesis of DiGeorge syndrome (DGS). It has been proposed that the loss of *TBX1* in patients with DGS results in defective proliferation in the SHF [81,82], although little mechanistic data have yet been published to support this notion. Cardiac defects observed in patients with DGS and in *Tbx1* mutant mice are strikingly similar to those seen in *Jun* mutant mouse embryos [83,84,85] and to mice in which NC has been disrupted [10]. Despite the similarity with NC mutants and reports of a disruption in the distribution of NC-derived cells in *Tbx1* nulls, *Tbx1* is not expressed in NC [86]. One hypothesis is that Jun and Tbx1 could be acting in concert to regulate the proliferation of SHF progenitors and subsequently affect interactions with other tissues such as NC. Future studies are required to determine if Jun may function in a Tbx1-dependent pathway and to further elucidate cell autonomous and cell non-autonomous mechanisms of Jun function during heart development.

Materials and Methods

Ethics Statement

Animal studies were conducted in accordance with the National Institutes of Health National Research Council Guide for the Care and Use of Laboratory Animals and were approved by the Children's Hospital of Philadelphia Research Institute Institutional Animal Care and Use Committee (No. 2008-6-840; Department of Health and Human Services Animal Welfare Assurance #A3442-01).

X-Gal Staining

Whole mount embryos were stained for ß-galactosidase activity using previously described methods [87].

Confocal Microscopy

Confocal images were acquired with the Zeiss LSM 510/NLO META confocal microscope using 20x, 0.8 NA Plan-Apochromat air immersion and 63x, 1.4 NA Plan-Apochromat oil immersion objectives.

Mutant Mice and Genotyping

All mouse strains used are previously described and listed here: *Jun*$^{flox/flox}$ is *Jun*^{tm4Wag} [7], *Isl1*$^{Cre/+}$ is *Isl1*$^{tm1(cre)Sev}$ [25], *Tie2*-Cre is Tg(Tek-cre)1Ywa [41], R26R is *Gt(ROSA)26Sor*^{tm1Sor} [40], mT/mG is *Gt(ROSA)26Sor*$^{tm4(ACTB-tdTomato,-EGFP)Luo}$ [34], and *Jun*$^{+/-}$ is *Jun*^{tm1Pa} [4]. The last four lines were obtained from the Jackson Laboratory (Bar Harbor, ME). Mouse genotyping was performed using real-time quantitative polymerase chain reaction (qPCR) techniques. Genomic DNA was isolated with the Extract-N-Amp Tissue PCR kit (Sigma-Aldrich, St. Louis, MO) according to the manufacturer's recommended protocol. PrimeTime qPCR assays (Integrated DNA Technologies, Coralville, IA) consisting of the primer and probe sequences listed in Table S1 were used. The mouse GAPD TaqMan Gene Expression Assay (Life Technologies, Carlsbad, CA) was used as the endogenous control.

Immunohistochemistry

Immunofluorescence (IF) and horseradish peroxidase (HRP) immunostaining were performed as described previously [88] using rabbit monoclonal anti-Jun 60A8 (1:100 IF; Cell Signaling Technology, Danvers, MA), rat monoclonal anti-CD31 MEC13.3 (Pecam1; 1:100; BD Pharmingen, Franklin Lakes, NJ), mouse monoclonal anti-Isl-1 39.4D5 (1:25 IF; Developmental Studies Hybridoma Bank, Iowa City, IA), rabbit polyclonal anti-GFP (1:200 IF, Life Technologies), mouse monoclonal anti-SMA 1A4 (1:200 IF, Life Technologies), rabbit polyclonal phospho-histone H3 Ser10 (1:200 IF, Cell Signaling Technology), mouse monoclonal AP-2 alpha (Tfap2a) 3B5 (1:4 IF, Developmental Studies Hybridoma Bank) and mouse monoclonal NFATc1 7A6 (1:25 IF, Developmental Studies Hybridoma Bank). TUNEL assays were performed using the In Situ Cell Death Detection Kit (Roche, Indianapolis, IN) according to the manufacturer's recommended protocol. Images were quantified by using the Image-based Tool for Counting Nuclei (ITCN) plug-in (http://goo.gl/fPQ6B) for ImageJ (NIH, Bethesda, MD). The mean and SEM were calculated based on three independent sections per embryo.

Whole Mount in situ Hybridization

Whole mount *in situ* hybridization was performed as described [89] with modifications. Digoxigenin-UTP-labeled RNA probes were generated from plasmid template containing mouse *Jun* (IMAGE clone 3493248; GenBank accession number BC002081) by *Xma*I restriction digestion and transcription with T7 RNA polymerase. Embryos were fixed in 4% PFA overnight, then dehydrated in a graded series of methanol in PBST. The embryos were serially rehydrated to PBST. Embryos were permeabilized in RIPA buffer thrice for 5 minutes at room temperature. Embryos were refixed in 4% PFA/0.2% glutaraldehyde in PBS for 20 minutes, washed and hybridized overnight at 70°C in hybridization solution containing 1 µg probe/mL. Embryos were washed and hybridized with alkaline phosphatase conjugated anti-digoxigenin antibody (Roche) overnight at 4°C, washed for 24 hours and developed in BM purple (Roche).

Supporting Information

Figure S1   Jun is broadly expressed in the late gestation mouse heart. (**A, E**) Transverse sections of an E15.5 wild-type mouse heart showing nuclear Jun immunostaining (green) in the myocardium and valves. (**B–D**) Higher power images of the areas shown in the white boxes in panel A showing Jun expression in the myocardium and atrioventricular valves. (**F**) Higher power image of the area shown in the white box in panel E showing Jun expression in the right ventricular outflow tract myocardium and pulmonary valve. Sections were co-stained with DAPI to illustrate nuclei. Ao, aorta; IVS, interventricular septum; LA, left atrium; LV, left ventricle; MV, mitral valve; PA, pulmonary artery; PV, pulmonary valve; RA, right atrium; RV, right ventricle; TV, tricuspid valve.

Table S1   qPCR Genotyping Assays. Primer and probe sequences used for mouse genotyping. Mouse GAPD was used as the endogenous control.

Acknowledgments

We would like to thank Axel Behrens and Sylvia Evans for providing *Jun*^{flox/flox} and Isl1^{Cre/+} mice.

Author Contributions

Conceived and designed the experiments: FAI JZS. Performed the experiments: TZ JL JZ EBT TLM JZS. Analyzed the data: TZ JL JZ FAI FW JZS. Contributed reagents/materials/analysis tools: TZ EBT TLM FAI JZS. Wrote the paper: FAI JZS.

References

1. Mechta-Grigoriou F, Gerald D, Yaniv M (2001) The mammalian Jun proteins: redundancy and specificity. Oncogene 20: 2378–2389.
2. Eferl R, Wagner EF (2003) AP-1: a double-edged sword in tumorigenesis. Nat Rev Cancer 3: 859–868.
3. Hilberg F, Aguzzi A, Howells N, Wagner EF (1993) c-jun is essential for normal mouse development and hepatogenesis. Nature 365: 179–181.
4. Johnson RS, van Lingen B, Papaioannou VE, Spiegelman BM (1993) A null mutation at the c-jun locus causes embryonic lethality and retarded cell growth in culture. Genes Dev 7: 1309–1317.
5. Eferl R, Sibilia M, Hilberg F, Fuchsbichler A, Kufferath I, et al. (1999) Functions of c-Jun in liver and heart development. J Cell Biol 145: 1049–1061.
6. Hess J, Angel P, Schorpp-Kistner M (2004) AP-1 subunits: quarrel and harmony among siblings. J Cell Sci 117: 5965–5973.
7. Behrens A, Sibilia M, David JP, Mohle-Steinlein U, Tronche F, et al. (2002) Impaired postnatal hepatocyte proliferation and liver regeneration in mice lacking c-jun in the liver. EMBO J 21: 1782–1790.
8. Wisdom R, Johnson RS, Moore C (1999) c-Jun regulates cell cycle progression and apoptosis by distinct mechanisms. EMBO J 18: 188–197.
9. Szabo E, Preis LH, Brown PH, Birrer MJ (1991) The role of jun and fos gene family members in 12-O-tetradecanoylphorbol-13-acetate induced hemopoietic differentiation. Cell Growth Differ 2: 475–482.
10. Stoller JZ, Epstein JA (2005) Cardiac neural crest. Semin Cell Dev Biol 16: 704–715.
11. Snarr BS, Kern CB, Wessels A (2008) Origin and fate of cardiac mesenchyme. Dev Dyn 237: 2804–2819.
12. Evans SM, Yelon D, Conlon FL, Kirby ML (2010) Myocardial lineage development. Circ Res 107: 1428–1444.
13. Vincent SD, Buckingham ME (2010) How to make a heart: the origin and regulation of cardiac progenitor cells. Curr Top Dev Biol 90: 1–41.
14. DeLaughter DM, Saint-Jean L, Baldwin HS, Barnett JV (2011) What chick and mouse models have taught us about the role of the endocardium in congenital heart disease. Birth defects research Part A, Clinical and molecular teratology 91: 511–525.
15. de Lange FJ, Moorman AF, Anderson RH, Manner J, Soufan AT, et al. (2004) Lineage and morphogenetic analysis of the cardiac valves. Circulation research 95: 645–654.
16. Wilkinson DG, Bhatt S, Ryseck RP, Bravo R (1989) Tissue-specific expression of c-jun and junB during organogenesis in the mouse. Development 106: 465–471.
17. Carrasco D, Bravo R (1995) Tissue-specific expression of the fos-related transcription factor fra-2 during mouse development. Oncogene 10: 1069–1079.
18. Ryder K, Nathans D (1988) Induction of protooncogene c-jun by serum growth factors. Proc Natl Acad Sci U S A 85: 8464–8467.
19. Foletta VC, Sonobe MH, Suzuki T, Endo T, Iba H, et al. (1994) Cloning and characterisation of the mouse fra-2 gene. Oncogene 9: 3305–3311.
20. Passegue E, Jochum W, Behrens A, Ricci R, Wagner EF (2002) JunB can substitute for Jun in mouse development and cell proliferation. Nat Genet 30: 158–166.
21. Zhang J, Chang JY, Huang Y, Lin X, Luo Y, et al. (2010) The FGF-BMP Signaling Axis Regulates Outflow Tract Valve Primordium Formation by Promoting Cushion Neural Crest Cell Differentiation. Circ Res 107: 1209–1219.
22. Magdaleno S, Jensen P, Brumwell CL, Seal A, Lehman K, et al. (2006) BGEM: an in situ hybridization database of gene expression in the embryonic and adult mouse nervous system. PLoS Biol 4: e86.
23. Cai CL, Liang X, Shi Y, Chu PH, Pfaff SL, et al. (2003) Isl1 identifies a cardiac progenitor population that proliferates prior to differentiation and contributes a majority of cells to the heart. Developmental Cell 5: 877–889.
24. Bu L, Jiang X, Martin-Puig S, Caron L, Zhu S, et al. (2009) Human ISL1 heart progenitors generate diverse multipotent cardiovascular cell lineages. Nature 460: 113–117.
25. Yang L, Cai CL, Lin L, Qyang Y, Chung C, et al. (2006) Isl1Cre reveals a common Bmp pathway in heart and limb development. Development 133: 1575–1585.
26. Park EJ, Ogden LA, Talbot A, Evans S, Cai CL, et al. (2006) Required, tissue-specific roles for Fgf8 in outflow tract formation and remodeling. Development 133: 2419–2433.
27. Srinivas S, Watanabe T, Lin C, William C, Tanabe Y, et al. (2001) Cre reporter strains produced by targeted insertion of EYFP and ECFP into the ROSA26 locus. BMC Dev Biol 1: 4.
28. Sun Y, Liang X, Najafi N, Cass M, Lin L, et al. (2007) Islet 1 is expressed in distinct cardiovascular lineages, including pacemaker and coronary vascular cells. Developmental biology 304: 286–296.
29. Stepniak E, Ricci R, Eferl R, Sumara G, Sumara I, et al. (2006) c-Jun/AP-1 controls liver regeneration by repressing p53/p21 and p38 MAPK activity. Genes Dev 20: 2306–2314.
30. Raivich G, Bohatschek M, Da Costa C, Iwata O, Galiano M, et al. (2004) The AP-1 transcription factor c-Jun is required for efficient axonal regeneration. Neuron 43: 57–67.
31. Zenz R, Eferl R, Scheinecker C, Redlich K, Smolen J, et al. (2008) Activator protein 1 (Fos/Jun) functions in inflammatory bone and skin disease. Arthritis Res Ther 10: 201.
32. Zenz R, Scheuch H, Martin P, Frank C, Eferl R, et al. (2003) c-Jun regulates eyelid closure and skin tumor development through EGFR signaling. Dev Cell 4: 879–889.
33. Behrens A, Haigh J, Mechta-Grigoriou F, Nagy A, Yaniv M, et al. (2003) Impaired intervertebral disc formation in the absence of Jun. Development 130: 103–109.
34. Muzumdar MD, Tasic B, Miyamichi K, Li L, Luo L (2007) A global double-fluorescent Cre reporter mouse. Genesis 45: 593–605.
35. Ma Q, Zhou B, Pu WT (2008) Reassessment of Isl1 and Nkx2-5 cardiac fate maps using a Gata4-based reporter of Cre activity. Developmental biology 323: 98–104.
36. High FA, Jain R, Stoller JZ, Antonucci NB, Lu MM, et al. (2009) Murine Jagged1/Notch signaling in the second heart field orchestrates Fgf8 expression and tissue-tissue interactions during outflow tract development. J Clin Invest 119: 1986–1996.

37. Wu B, Wang Y, Lui W, Langworthy M, Tompkins KL, et al. (2011) Nfatc1 coordinates valve endocardial cell lineage development required for heart valve formation. Circulation research 109: 183–192.

38. Zhang J, Lin Y, Zhang Y, Lan Y, Lin C, et al. (2008) Frs2alpha-deficiency in cardiac progenitors disrupts a subset of FGF signals required for outflow tract morphogenesis. Development 135: 3611–3622.

39. Ishii Y, Langberg J, Rosborough K, Mikawa T (2009) Endothelial cell lineages of the heart. Cell and tissue research 335: 67–73.

40. Soriano P (1999) Generalized lacZ expression with the ROSA26 Cre reporter strain. Nat Genet 21: 70–71.

41. Kisanuki YY, Hammer RE, Miyazaki J, Williams SC, Richardson JA, et al. (2001) Tie2-Cre transgenic mice: a new model for endothelial cell-lineage analysis in vivo. Dev Biol 230: 230–242.

42. Hoffman JI, Kaplan S (2002) The incidence of congenital heart disease. J Am Coll Cardiol 39: 1890–1900.

43. Thepot D, Weitzman JB, Barra J, Segretain D, Stinnakre MG, et al. (2000) Targeted disruption of the murine junD gene results in multiple defects in male reproductive function. Development 127: 143–153.

44. Schorpp-Kistner M, Wang ZQ, Angel P, Wagner EF (1999) JunB is essential for mammalian placentation. EMBO J 18: 934–948.

45. Meixner A, Karreth F, Kenner L, Penninger JM, Wagner EF (2010) Jun and JunD-dependent functions in cell proliferation and stress response. Cell death and differentiation 17: 1409–1419.

46. Schorpp M, Jager R, Schellander K, Schenkel J, Wagner EF, et al. (1996) The human ubiquitin C promoter directs high ubiquitous expression of transgenes in mice. Nucleic acids research 24: 1787–1788.

47. Derijard B, Hibi M, Wu IH, Barrett T, Su B, et al. (1994) JNK1: a protein kinase stimulated by UV light and Ha-Ras that binds and phosphorylates the c-Jun activation domain. Cell 76: 1025–1037.

48. Kyriakis JM, Banerjee P, Nikolakaki E, Dai T, Rubie EA, et al. (1994) The stress-activated protein kinase subfamily of c-Jun kinases. Nature 369: 156–160.

49. Behrens A, Sibilia M, Wagner EF (1999) Amino-terminal phosphorylation of c-Jun regulates stress-induced apoptosis and cellular proliferation. Nature genetics 21: 326–329.

50. Kuan CY, Yang DD, Samanta Roy DR, Davis RJ, Rakic P, et al. (1999) The Jnk1 and Jnk2 protein kinases are required for regional specific apoptosis during early brain development. Neuron 22: 667–676.

51. Anderson RH, Cook A, Brown NA, Henderson DJ, Chaudhry B, et al. (2010) Development of the outflow tracts with reference to aortopulmonary windows and aortoventricular tunnels. Cardiology in the young 20 Suppl 3: 92–99.

52. Webb S, Qayyum SR, Anderson RH, Lamers WH, Richardson MK (2003) Septation and separation within the outflow tract of the developing heart. J Anat 202: 327–342.

53. Thiene G, Bortolotti U (1980) Truncus arteriosus communis with intact ventricular septum. Br Heart J 43: 605–606.

54. Sturzu AC, Wu SM (2011) Developmental and regenerative biology of multipotent cardiovascular progenitor cells. Circulation research 108: 353–364.

55. Huynh T, Chen L, Terrell P, Baldini A (2007) A fate map of Tbx1 expressing cells reveals heterogeneity in the second cardiac field. Genesis 45: 470–475.

56. Chen L, Fulcoli FG, Tang S, Baldini A (2009) Tbx1 regulates proliferation and differentiation of multipotent heart progenitors. Circ Res 105: 842–851.

57. Verzi MP, McCulley DJ, De Val S, Dodou E, Black BL (2005) The right ventricle, outflow tract, and ventricular septum comprise a restricted expression domain within the secondary/anterior heart field. Dev Biol 287: 134–145.

58. Shimomura H, Sanke T, Hanabusa T, Tsunoda K, Furuta H, et al. (2000) Nonsense mutation of islet-1 gene (Q310X) found in a type 2 diabetic patient with a strong family history. Diabetes 49: 1597–1600.

59. Stevens KN, Hakonarson H, Kim CE, Doevendans PA, Koeleman BP, et al. (2010) Common variation in ISL1 confers genetic susceptibility for human congenital heart disease. PLoS ONE 5: e10855.

60. Moretti A, Caron L, Nakano A, Lam JT, Bernshausen A, et al. (2006) Multipotent embryonic isl1+ progenitor cells lead to cardiac, smooth muscle, and endothelial cell diversification. Cell 127: 1151–1165.

61. Wu SM, Fujiwara Y, Cibulsky SM, Clapham DE, Lien CL, et al. (2006) Developmental origin of a bipotential myocardial and smooth muscle cell precursor in the mammalian heart. Cell 127: 1137–1150.

62. Engleka KA, Manderfield LJ, Brust RD, Li L, Cohen A, et al. (2012) Islet1 derivatives in the heart are of both neural crest and second heart field origin. Circulation research 110: 922–926.

63. Grego-Bessa J, Luna-Zurita L, del Monte G, Bolos V, Melgar P, et al. (2007) Notch signaling is essential for ventricular chamber development. Developmental cell 12: 415–429.

64. Rentschler S, Zander J, Meyers K, France D, Levine R, et al. (2002) Neuregulin-1 promotes formation of the murine cardiac conduction system. Proceedings of the National Academy of Sciences of the United States of America 99: 10464–10469.

65. Gitler AD, Zhu Y, Ismat FA, Lu MM, Yamauchi Y, et al. (2003) Nf1 has an essential role in endothelial cells. Nat Genet 33: 75–79.

66. Smith TK, Bader DM (2007) Signals from both sides: Control of cardiac development by the endocardium and epicardium. Seminars in cell & developmental biology 18: 84–89.

67. Tian Y, Morrisey EE (2012) Importance of myocyte-nonmyocyte interactions in cardiac development and disease. Circulation research 110: 1023–1034.

68. Raivich G, Behrens A (2006) Role of the AP-1 transcription factor c-Jun in developing, adult and injured brain. Prog Neurobiol 78: 347–363.

69. Sclafani AM, Skidmore JM, Ramaprakash H, Trumpp A, Gage PJ, et al. (2006) Nestin-Cre mediated deletion of Pitx2 in the mouse. Genesis 44: 336–344.

70. Hutson MR, Kirby ML (2007) Model systems for the study of heart development and disease. Cardiac neural crest and conotruncal malformations. Semin Cell Dev Biol 18: 101–110.

71. Jiang X, Rowitch DH, Soriano P, McMahon AP, Sucov HM (2000) Fate of the mammalian cardiac neural crest. Development 127: 1607–1616.

72. Danielian PS, Muccino D, Rowitch DH, Michael SK, McMahon AP (1998) Modification of gene activity in mouse embryos in utero by a tamoxifen-inducible form of Cre recombinase. Curr Biol 8: 1323–1326.

73. Engleka KA, Gitler AD, Zhang M, Zhou DD, High FA, et al. (2005) Insertion of Cre into the Pax3 locus creates a new allele of Splotch and identifies unexpected Pax3 derivatives. Dev Biol 280: 396–406.

74. Verde P, Casalino L, Talotta F, Yaniv M, Weitzman JB (2007) Deciphering AP-1 function in tumorigenesis: fra-ternizing on target promoters. Cell Cycle 6: 2633–2639.

75. Zenz R, Wagner EF (2006) Jun signalling in the epidermis: From developmental defects to psoriasis and skin tumors. Int J Biochem Cell Biol 38: 1043–1049.

76. Katabami M, Donninger H, Hommura F, Leaner VD, Kinoshita I, et al. (2005) Cyclin A is a c-Jun target gene and is necessary for c-Jun-induced anchorage-independent growth in RAT1a cells. J Biol Chem 280: 16728–16738.

77. Shaulian E, Karin M (2002) AP-1 as a regulator of cell life and death. Nat Cell Biol 4: E131–136.

78. Bossy-Wetzel E, Bakiri L, Yaniv M (1997) Induction of apoptosis by the transcription factor c-Jun. EMBO J 16: 1695–1709.

79. Ameyar M, Wisniewska M, Weitzman JB (2003) A role for AP-1 in apoptosis: the case for and against. Biochimie 85: 747–752.

80. Sizarov A, Ya J, de Boer BA, Lamers WH, Christoffels VM, et al. (2011) Formation of the building plan of the human heart: morphogenesis, growth, and differentiation. Circulation 123: 1125–1135.

81. Zhang Z, Huynh T, Baldini A (2006) Mesodermal expression of Tbx1 is necessary and sufficient for pharyngeal arch and cardiac outflow tract development. Development 133: 3587–3595.

82. Parisot P, Mesbah K, Theveniau-Ruissy M, Kelly RG (2011) Tbx1, subpulmonary myocardium and conotruncal congenital heart defects. Birth Defects Res A Clin Mol Teratol 91: 477–484.

83. Liao J, Kochilas L, Nowotschin S, Arnold JS, Aggarwal VS, et al. (2004) Full spectrum of malformations in velo-cardio-facial syndrome/DiGeorge syndrome mouse models by altering Tbx1 dosage. Hum Mol Genet 13: 1577–1585.

84. Lindsay EA, Botta A, Jurecic V, Carattini-Rivera S, Cheah YC, et al. (1999) Congenital heart disease in mice deficient for the DiGeorge syndrome region. Nature 401: 379–383.

85. Scambler PJ (2010) 22q11 deletion syndrome: a role for TBX1 in pharyngeal and cardiovascular development. Pediatr Cardiol 31: 378–390.

86. Vitelli F, Morishima M, Taddei I, Lindsay EA, Baldini A (2002) Tbx1 mutation causes multiple cardiovascular defects and disrupts neural crest and cranial nerve migratory pathways. Hum Mol Genet 11: 915–922.

87. Brown CB, Feiner L, Lu MM, Li J, Ma X, et al. (2001) PlexinA2 and semaphorin signaling during cardiac neural crest development. Development 128: 3071–3080.

88. Stoller JZ, Degenhardt KR, Huang L, Zhou DD, Lu MM, et al. (2008) Cre reporter mouse expressing a nuclear localized fusion of GFP and beta-galactosidase reveals new derivatives of Pax3-expressing precursors. Genesis 46: 200–204.

89. Barnes JD, Crosby JL, Jones CM, Wright CV, Hogan BL (1994) Embryonic expression of Lim-1, the mouse homolog of Xenopus Xlim-1, suggests a role in lateral mesoderm differentiation and neurogenesis. Developmental biology 161: 168–178.

9

Outlier-Based Identification of Copy Number Variations using Targeted Resequencing in a Small Cohort of Patients with Tetralogy of Fallot

Vikas Bansal[1,2,9], **Cornelia Dorn**[1,3,9], **Marcel Grunert**[1], **Sabine Klaassen**[4,5,6], **Roland Hetzer**[7], **Felix Berger**[6,8], **Silke R. Sperling**[1,3]*

1 Department of Cardiovascular Genetics, Experimental and Clinical Research Center, Charité - Universitätsmedizin Berlin and Max Delbrück Center (MDC) for Molecular Medicine, Berlin, Germany, **2** Department of Mathematics and Computer Science, Free University of Berlin, Berlin, Germany, **3** Department of Biology, Chemistry, and Pharmacy, Free University of Berlin, Berlin, Germany, **4** For the National Register for Congenital Heart Defects, Berlin, Germany, **5** Experimental and Clinical Research Center, Charité - Universitätsmedizin Berlin and Max Delbrück Center (MDC) for Molecular Medicine, Berlin, Germany, **6** Department of Pediatric Cardiology, Charité - Universitätsmedizin Berlin, Berlin, Germany, **7** Department of Cardiac Surgery, German Heart Institute Berlin, Berlin, Germany, **8** Department of Pediatric Cardiology, German Heart Institute Berlin, Berlin, Germany

Abstract

Copy number variations (CNVs) are one of the main sources of variability in the human genome. Many CNVs are associated with various diseases including cardiovascular disease. In addition to hybridization-based methods, next-generation sequencing (NGS) technologies are increasingly used for CNV discovery. However, respective computational methods applicable to NGS data are still limited. We developed a novel CNV calling method based on outlier detection applicable to small cohorts, which is of particular interest for the discovery of individual CNVs within families, *de novo* CNVs in trios and/or small cohorts of specific phenotypes like rare diseases. Approximately 7,000 rare diseases are currently known, which collectively affect ~6% of the population. For our method, we applied the Dixon's Q test to detect outliers and used a Hidden Markov Model for their assessment. The method can be used for data obtained by exome and targeted resequencing. We evaluated our outlier- based method in comparison to the CNV calling tool CoNIFER using eight HapMap exome samples and subsequently applied both methods to targeted resequencing data of patients with Tetralogy of Fallot (TOF), the most common cyanotic congenital heart disease. In both the HapMap samples and the TOF cases, our method is superior to CoNIFER, such that it identifies more true positive CNVs. Called CNVs in TOF cases were validated by qPCR and HapMap CNVs were confirmed with available array-CGH data. In the TOF patients, we found four copy number gains affecting three genes, of which two are important regulators of heart development (*NOTCH1, ISL1*) and one is located in a region associated with cardiac malformations (*PRODH* at 22q11). In summary, we present a novel CNV calling method based on outlier detection, which will be of particular interest for the analysis of *de novo* or individual CNVs in trios or cohorts up to 30 individuals, respectively.

Editor: Chunyu Liu, University of Illinois at Chicago, United States of America

Funding: This work was supported by the European Community's Seventh Framework Programme contracts ("CardioGeNet") 2009-223463 and ("CardioNet") People-2011-ITN-289600 (all to SRS), a Marie Curie PhD fellowship to VB, a PhD scholarship to CD by the Studienstiftung des Deutschen Volkes, and the German Research Foundation (Heisenberg professorship and grant 574157 to SRS). This work was also supported by the Competence Network for Congenital Heart Defects funded by the Federal Ministry of Education and Research (BMBF), support code FKZ 01GI0601. The funders had no role in study design, data collection and analysis.

Competing Interests: The authors have declared that no competing interests exist.

* E-mail: silke.sperling@charite.de

9 These authors contributed equally to this work.

Introduction

Many genomic studies have revealed a high variability of the human genome, ranging from single nucleotide variations and short insertions or deletions to larger structural variations and aneuploidies. Structural variations include copy number variations (CNVs), which cause gains (duplications) or losses (deletions) of genomic sequence. These copy number changes are usually defined to be longer than ~500 bases, including large variations with more than 50 kilobases [1,2]. Recent studies have identified CNVs associated with a number of complex diseases such as

Crohn's disease, intellectual disability and congenital heart disease [3–6].

Congenital heart disease (CHD) are the most common birth defect in human with an incidence of around 1% in all live births [7,8]. They comprise a heterogeneous group of cardiac malformations that arise during heart development. The most common cyanotic form of CHD is Tetralogy of Fallot (TOF), which accounts for up to 10% of all heart malformations [9]. TOF is characterized by a ventricular septal defect with an overriding aorta, a right ventricular outflow tract obstruction and a right ventricular hypertrophy [10]. It is a well-recognized subfeature of syndromic disorders such as DiGeorge syndrome (22q11 deletion),

Down syndrome, Holt-Oram syndrome and Williams-Beuren syndrome [11]. Deletions at the 22q11 locus account for up to 16% of TOF cases [12] and copy number changes at other loci were identified in several syndromic TOF patients [13–15]. However, the majority of TOFs are isolated, non-syndromic cases caused by a multifactorial inheritance with genetic-environmental interactions, which is also the situation for the majority of CHDs [16]. Using SNP arrays, three recent studies also identified CNVs in large cohorts of non-syndromic TOF patients [17–19]. Observing the overlap between these studies with hundreds of cases revealed only one locus (1q21.1) affected in 11 patients (Figure 1), which underlines the heterogeneous genetic background of non-syndromic TOF.

As an alternative to the conventional SNP arrays, next-generation sequencing (NGS) technologies have been widely used to detect single or short sequence variations. The obtained sequence data can also be used to find larger CNVs. Depending on the sequencing technologies, there are different computational approaches for detecting copy numbers from NGS data. For exome sequencing or targeted resequencing, the read-depth or depth of coverage approach is widely used. It assumes that the mapped reads are randomly distributed across the reference genome or targeted regions. Based on this assumption, the read-depth approach analyses differences from the expected read distribution to detect duplications (higher read depth) and deletions (lower read depth) [20]. Applying this approach, several tools have been developed to identify CNVs from exome sequencing data, such as FishingCNV, CONTRA, ExomeCNV, ExomeDepth, XHMM, CoNVEX and CoNIFER [21–27].

Here, we aimed to identify copy number alterations in a small cohort of non-syndromic TOF patients based on targeted resequencing data. Assuming a heterogeneous genetic background with individual disease-relevant CNVs, we developed a novel CNV calling method based on outlier detection using Dixon's Q test and assessment of outliers using a Hidden Markov Model (HMM). For evaluation, we applied our method to a small cohort of HapMap samples and compared it to results obtained with ExomeDepth and CoNIFER. Subsequently, our method and CoNIFER were used to detect CNVs in the TOF patients. Two copy number gains were identified by both methods and are duplications in the *PRODH* gene located at the 22q11 locus. In addition, our outlier-based method found a gain in *NOTCH1* as well as in *ISL1*. All four CNVs could be validated by quantitative real-time PCR.

Materials and Methods

Ethics Statement

Studies on TOF patients were performed according to institutional guidelines of the German Heart Institute in Berlin, with approval of the ethics committee of the Charité Medical Faculty and informed written consent of patients and/or parents, kin, caretakers, or guardians on the behalf of the minors/children participants involved in our study.

TOF Samples and DNA Targeted Resequencing

Targeted resequencing was performed for eight TOF patients, which are unrelated sporadic cases with a well-defined coherent

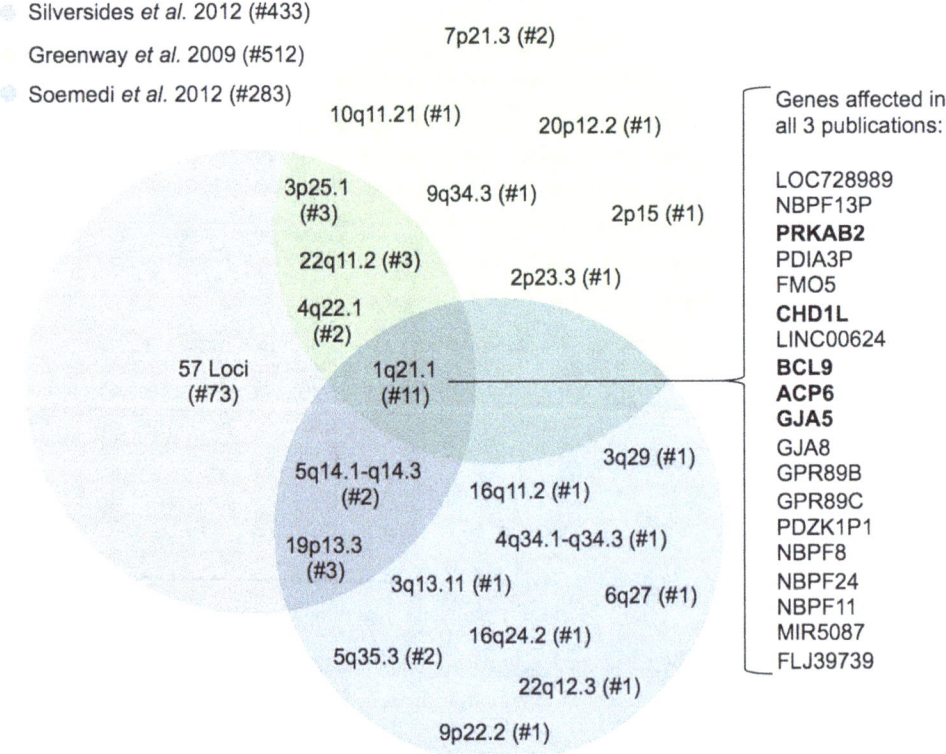

Figure 1. Overlap of three recent CNV studies in TOF patients. All three studies are based on SNP arrays. Loci with detected CNVs are depicted according to their respective cytoband. For 1q21.1, which was identified in all three studies, the RefSeq genes that are affected in at least one patient in each of the publications are listed in the order of their genomic position. Genes that are expressed in mouse heart development (E8.5–E12.0, Mouse Atlas of Gene Expression at http://www.mouseatlas.org/mouseatlas_index_html) are marked in bold. # denotes the number of individuals.

Table 1. Number and quality of 36 bp paired-end reads obtained from targeted resequencing in TOF patients using Illumina's Genome Analyzer IIx platform.

| Sample | Number of reads | Number of read pairs | Captured regions | | | |
			Phred quality score	Median coverage	Mean coverage	Target bases with ≥10x coverage
TOF-01	31,942,782	15,971,391	33.3	40	47	93.85%
TOF-02	26,970,680	13,485,340	32.7	66	76	97.70%
TOF-18	25,476,308	12,738,154	35.4	71	80	98.35%
TOF-23	20,885,192	10,442,596	35.0	60	69	97.41%
TOF-24	25,483,166	12,741,583	34.7	51	58	96.72%
TOF-25	30,551,674	15,275,837	34.6	84	92	98.91%
TOF-26	27,878,750	13,939,375	34.7	75	84	98.34%
TOF-27	24,118,022	12,059,011	34.6	78	90	98.00%

phenotype and no further anomalies. Blood samples (TOF-23, TOF-24, TOF-25, TOF-26, TOF-27) and cardiac tissue from the right ventricle (TOF-01, TOF-02, TOF-18) were collected in collaboration with the German Heart Institute in Berlin and the National Registry of Congenital Heart Disease in Berlin and used for the extraction of genomic DNA. 3–5 μg of genomic DNA were used for Roche NimbleGen sequence capturing using 365 K arrays. For array design, 867 genes and 167 microRNAs (12,910 exonic targets representing 4,616,651 target bases) were selected based on knowledge gained in various projects [28–30]. DNA enriched after NimbleGen sequence capturing was sequenced using the Illumina Genome Analyzer (GA) IIx (36 bp paired-end reads). Sequencing was performed by Atlas Biolabs (Berlin) according to manufacturers' protocols.

On average, sequencing resulted in 13,331,661 read pairs per sample (Table 1). Average read depths of 75× and base quality

scores of 34 (Phred scores) were reached in the captured regions over all samples (Table 1 and Figure 2).

HapMap Samples

We used exome sequencing data from eight HapMap individuals (NA18507, NA18555, NA18956, NA19240, NA12878, NA15510, NA18517, NA19129). The exomes were captured using Roche NimbleGen EZ Exome SeqCap Version 1 and sequencing was performed using an Illumina HiSeq 2000 platform with 50 bp paired-end reads. The exome sequence data are available from the Short Read Archive at the NCBI (SRA039053). The reads were further trimmed to 36 bp.

Outlier-based CNV Calling Method

Our CNV calling method was developed for exome or targeted resequencing data of small sets of samples (at least 3 and at most 30) assuming that the bias in the captured regions is similar in all samples enriched and sequenced with the same technology. Based on a heterogeneous genetic background in the cohort, it was further assumed that a unique disease-related copy number change is only present in very few samples.

First, read mapping and calculation of copy number values were performed for each sample separately. The sequenced reads were mapped to the targeted regions of the reference genome using BWA v 0.5.9 in paired-end mode ('sampe') with default parameters [31]. Up- and downstream, the targeted regions (usually exons) were extended by 35 bp (read length minus one base pair) to correctly capture the coverage at the start and end of a region. After mapping, the extended regions with their mapped reads were joined chromosome-wise and the tool mRCaNaVaR v0.34 [32] was used to split the joined regions into non-overlapping windows of 100 bp in length. The copy number value C for each window $W \in \{1,...,n\}$ of a sample $S \in \{1,...,n\}$ was then calculated by mRCaNaVaR using the following formula:

$$C_W^S = \frac{\text{Number of reads mapped to W}}{\text{Average number of reads mapped over all windows}} \times 2,$$

with additional GC correction [32] (Figure 3A). Reads spanning the border of two windows were assigned to the left window. In general, our method calculates a copy number value using

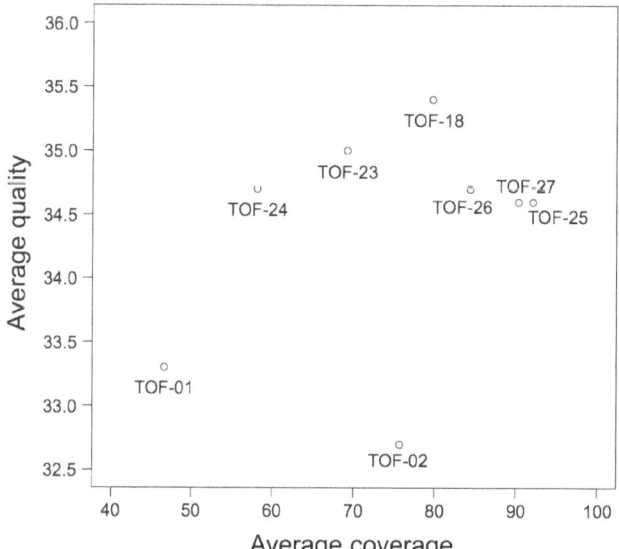

Figure 2. Base qualities versus coverage values. Scatterplot indicates the average base qualities (Phred scores) and depths of coverage for samples targeted resequenced by Illumina's Genome Analyzer IIx platform (36 bp paired-end reads).

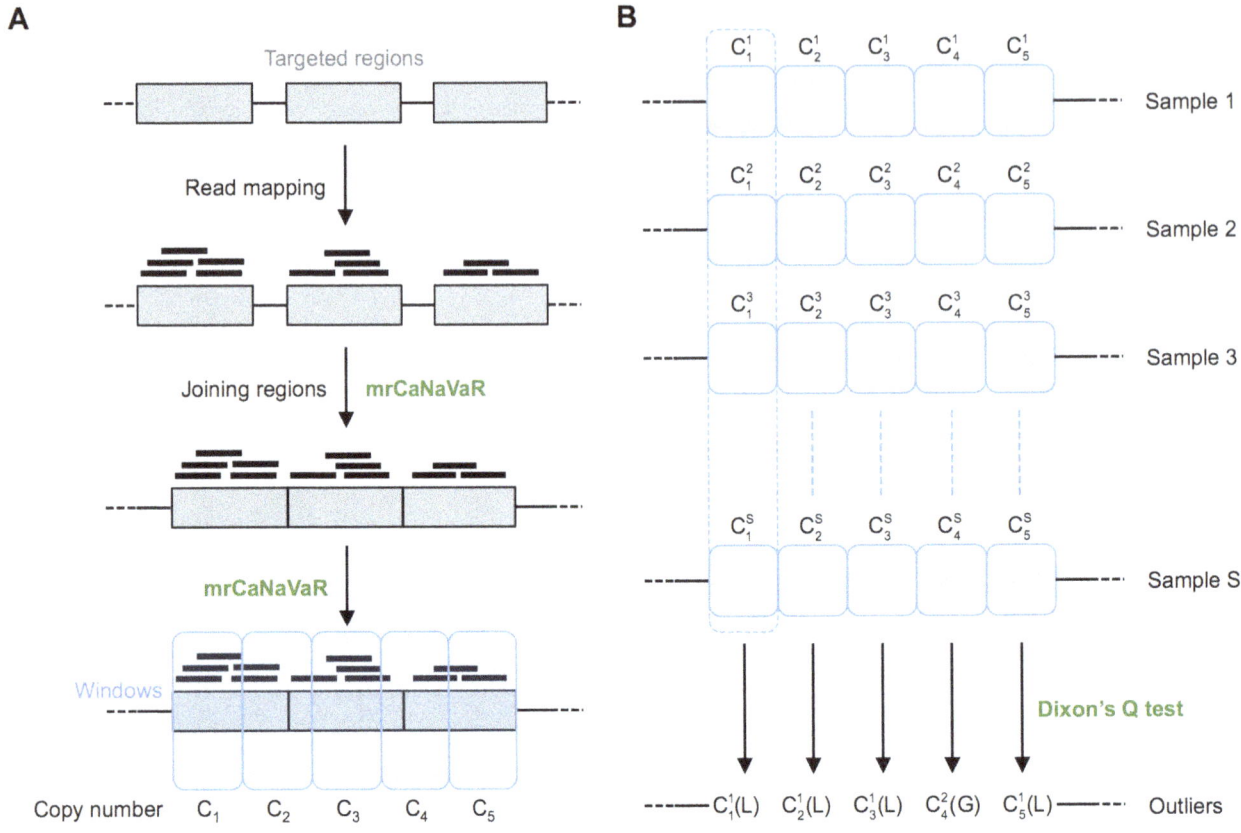

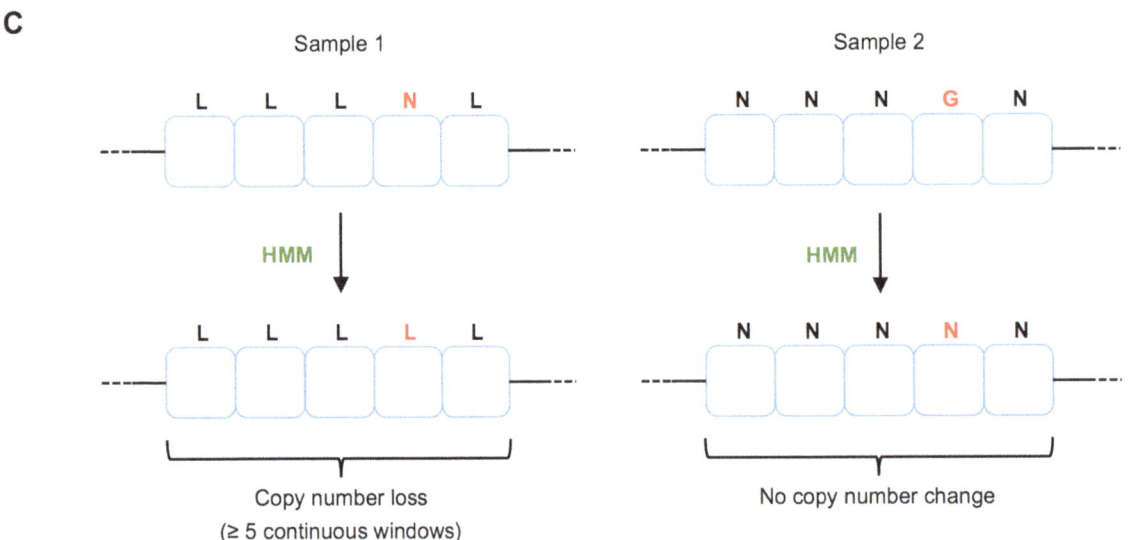

Figure 3. Outlier-based CNV calling method. (A) Read mapping and calculation of copy number value per window. Reads are mapped to extended targeted regions, which are then joined chromosome-wise. mrCaNaVaR is used to split the joined regions into windows. For each window, its copy number value is calculated by mrCaNaVaR, where C_W^S represents the value for window W in sample S. (B) Dixon's Q test is applied for each window over all samples to identify outliers. Here, sample 1 represents an outlier (loss, L) for the first, second, third and fifth window, while sample 2 represents an outlier (gain, G) for the fourth window. (C) Assessment of outliers using a Hidden Markov Model (HMM). In the given example, the fourth window of sample 1 is considered as normal (N). After applying the HMM, it will also be considered as a loss. Similarly, the fourth window of sample 2 is considered as normal after applying the HMM. A region is called as a copy number alteration, if at least five continuous windows show the same kind of change, i.e. either gain or loss.

mrCaNaVaR, which can accurately predict CNVs with at least 4x coverage [32].

Second, Dixon's Q test was applied for each window at the same position over all samples to identify gains or losses considered

Table 2. Exome sequencing-based CNV calls in HapMap samples.

Method	Number of CNVs	Validation dataset	Number of overlapping CNVs	Positive predictive value	Sensitivity
Outlier-based calling method with type10	40	3,330 arrayCGH calls	37	93%	1.1%
Outlier-based calling method with type20 including type10	65		55	85%	1.7%
CoNIFER	32		26	81%	0.8%
ExomeDepth	1,555		253	16%	7.6%

as outliers (Figure 3B). This test was introduced in 1950 for the analysis of extreme values and for the rejection of outlying values [33]. We used the formulas for r_{10} and r_{20} [34], also known as type10 and type20 in the R package 'outliers' v0.14 (http://www.R-project.org). Type10 (recommended for 3–7 samples) can only detect a single outlying window at the same genomic position over all samples, while type20 (recommended for 8–30 samples) can identify exactly two outlying windows, meaning the Q test will not detect outliers if more than 2 outliers are present. For each window, we first applied type20, however, if no two significant outliers (samples) were found, type10 was used to detect at most one outlier. Note that our method can also be applied using type10 and type20 independently. Outliers were regarded as significant with a p-value of less than or equal to 0.01. In general, the higher the p-value cutoff, the higher the number of detected outliers but also the number of false positives, i.e. the p-value is a tuning parameter for sensitivity of our method.

In the third and final step, the samples were again considered separately. For each sample, a Hidden Markov Model [35] was applied to get the most likely state of each window (i.e. gain, loss or normal). The initial transition and emission probabilities of the HMM are given in Table S1 and the values were recomputed using the Baum-Welch algorithm [36] implemented in the R package 'HMM' v1.0. The most likely sequence of the hidden states was then found by the Viterbi algorithm [37] also implemented in the R package 'HMM'. Finally, a region was called as copy number gain or loss if at least five continuous windows were considered as a gain or loss, respectively (Figure 3C). This results in a minimum size of 500 bp for detectable CNVs.

We have included a script, written in R 2.15.1 (http://www.R-project.org), for our CNV calling method based on outlier detection in exome and/or targeted resequencing data (Script S1).

CNV Validation

Genomic DNA was extracted from whole blood or cardiac biopsies using standard procedures. Quantitative real-time PCR was carried out using GoTaq qPCR Master Mix (Promega) on an ABI PRISM 7900HT Sequence Detection System (Applied Biosystems) according to the manufacturer's instructions and with normalization to the *RPPH1* gene. Primer sequences are available on request. As a reference, genomic DNA from the HapMap individual NA10851 was obtained from the Coriell Cell Repositories (New Jersey, USA).

Results and Discussion

We applied our outlier-based CNV calling method to eight HapMap control samples and intersected our exome-based calls from five of the samples with previously generated calls from high-resolution microarray-based comparative genomic hybridization (array-CGH) [2]. In addition to our method, we used the two publicly available tools ExomeDepth and CoNIFER [23,27]. Other tools such as CONTRA, FishingCNV, CoNVEX and ExomeCNV could not be applied to this dataset since they need either matched or non-matched controls.

CoNIFER (copy number inference from exome reads) is a method that combines the read-depth approach with singular value decomposition (SVD) normalization to identify rare and common copy number alterations from exome sequencing data [27]. Applying our method with type10 Dixon's Q test (assuming at most one outlier), we found 40 CNVs over the five HapMap controls (Table S2), out of which 37 regions were also identified in the array-CGH data, showing a high positive predictive value of 93%. With type20 (assuming at most two outliers), we found 65 copy number changes (Table S3), out of which 55 regions are present in the array-CGH data, resulting in a positive predictive value of 85%. Using CoNIFER, 32 CNVs were identified in the

Table 3. Targeted resequencing-based CNV calls in TOF patients.

Method	Type of variation	Position (hg19)	Length in bp	Gene	Sample
Outlier-based calling method with type20 including type10	Gain	chr5:50,689,340–50,689,940	601	*ISL1*	TOF-23
	Gain	chr9:139,402,477–139,404,228	1,752	*NOTCH1*	TOF-01
	Gain	chr22:18,900,412–18,901,127	716	*PRODH*	TOF-02
	Gain	chr22:18,910,691–18,918,575	7,885	*PRODH*	TOF-02
CoNIFER	Gain	chr22:18,900,414–18,905,939	5,526	*PRODH*	TOF-02
	Gain	chr22:18,910,575–18,923,866	13,292	*PRODH*	TOF-02

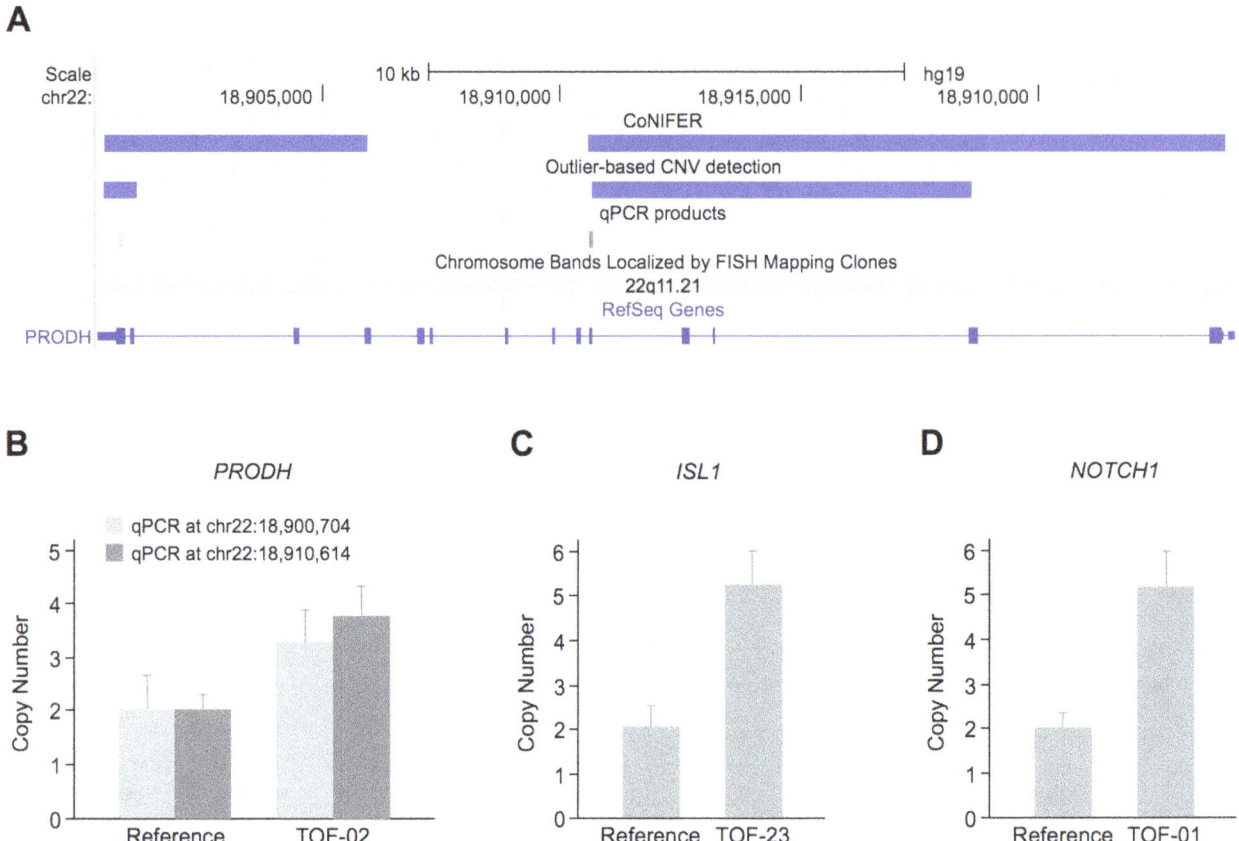

Figure 4. CNVs in TOF patients. (A) CNVs detected in *PRODH* by CoNIFER and our outlier-based CNV calling method. The duplications are depicted in the UCSC Genome Browser as blue bars. The positions of the two quantitative real-time PCR products selected for validation are shown as light and dark grey bars, respectively. (B) Quantitative real-time PCR validation of *PRODH* copy number gains. Measurement was performed at two different positions (light and dark grey bars, respectively) and normalized to the *RPPH1* gene. The HapMap individual NA10851 was used as a reference. The plot shows a representative of two independent measurements, which were each performed in triplicates. (C–D) Validation of copy number gains in *ISL1* and *NOTCH1*, respectively, that were only identified by our outlier-based CNV calling method.

five HapMap exome controls and only 26 of these regions are also present in the array-CGH data [27], which corresponds to a positive predictive value of 81% (Table 2). Comparing our results to those obtained from CoNIFER, we found that with type10 16 out of 40 regions (40%) are overlapping with regions called by CoNIFER by at least one base pair. Vice versa, 11 out of 32 regions (34%) overlap with our calls. With type20, 24 out of our 65 called regions (37%) overlap with those from CoNIFER and oppositely, 47% of the regions (15 out of 32) overlap with our calls. In general, CNV regions identified by CoNIFER are longer than those found by our method, meaning that regions called by CoNIFER can correspond to more than one of our CNVs, which explains the different overlap proportions.

Overall, our method was able to detect more copy number changes and has a higher proportion of true positives compared to CoNIFER. However, there is still a large number of CNVs observed in the array-CGH data, which were identified by neither of the two exome-based methods (Table 2). This can for example be explained by their location in segmental duplications and polymorphic but not duplicated regions [27].

ExomeDepth uses a beta-binomial model for the read count data to identify CNVs from exome sequencing data [24]. We applied ExomeDepth with default parameters to the eight HapMap samples and intersected the found CNVs from five of the samples with previously generated calls from array-CGH. In

summary, ExomeDepth found 1,555 CNVs in the five samples (median number of 286 CNVs per sample). Out of these, only 253 CNVs overlapped with 3,330 array-CGH calls, which suggest a positive predictive value of 16% and sensitivity of 7.6% (Table 2).

Interestingly, all the five rare CNVs in the five HapMap samples (see Krumm *et al.* 2012, Table S2 [27]) were found by our method, CoNIFER and ExomeDepth. Moreover, ExomeDepth identified more CNVs as compared to CoNIFER and to our method (Table 2), however; the positive predictive value is very low. Therefore, we decided not to use ExomeDepth for detecting CNVs in the TOF patients.

To identify copy number alterations in TOF patients, we applied our outlier-based method as well as CoNIFER to targeted resequencing data of our eight cases. Using our method, we found four copy number gains in three genes, namely *ISL1*, *NOTCH1* and *PRODH*. CoNIFER only identified two gains in *PRODH*, which overlap with the two regions found by our method (Table 3 and Figure 4A). We further validated all four regions identified by our method using quantitative real-time PCR (Figure 4B–D). ISL1 is a homeobox transcription factor that marks cardiovascular progenitors [38] and is known to be associated with human congenital heart disease [39]. NOTCH1 is a transmembrane receptor involved in the NOTCH signaling pathway, which plays a crucial role in heart development [40]. Mutations in *NOTCH1* are associated with a spectrum of congenital aortic valve anomalies

[41,42] and a copy number loss was identified in a patient with TOF [17] (locus 9q34.3, Figure 1). The mitochondrial protein PRODH catalyzes the first step in proline degradation and is located in the 22q11.2 locus. Deletions in this region are associated with the DiGeorge syndrome and 80% of cases harbor cardiovascular anomalies [43]. A copy number gain and two losses in the 22q11.2 locus overlapping *PRODH* were also identified in sporadic TOF patients [17,18] (Figure 1).

In summary, we developed an outlier-based CNV calling method for a small cohort size of up to 30 individuals. The exploration of the human phenotype and its genetic and molecular background is the challenge of the next century and it is already clear that more precise phenotyping will lead to smaller cohort sizes. Here, novel approaches will be of exceptional relevance. Moreover, analyzing small patient cohorts is of special interest for rare diseases with only few available patient samples. Approximately 7,000 rare diseases are currently known and together affect about 6% of the population [44]. Our method is based on the assumption that individual CNVs (outliers) are disease-relevant and can be applied to exome as well as targeted resequencing data. Both sequencing techniques achieve a high read coverage over the targeted regions. Nevertheless, there are non-uniform patterns in the read depth resulting mainly from repetitive regions. Thus, the detection of copy number alterations is limited in these genomic regions, which is shown by the high number of false negatives compared to array-CGH [27].

We evaluated our method using publicly available data of eight HapMap samples and subsequently applied it to a small number of TOF patients. Compared to CoNIFER we identified more CNVs in both the HapMap samples as well as in our TOF cohort. In general, our method assumes a uniform read distribution over all exons of all individuals enriched and sequenced with the same technology to compare read counts between all samples to detect outliers. In contrast, CoNIFER considers the read depth across all individuals after SVD normalization. This difference is also reflected by the overlap of their calls in the eight HapMap samples. Although the general overlap is relatively low, we were able to identify all rare CNVs detected by CoNIFER. In addition to searching for rare CNVs, we also found a subset of common CNVs called by CoNIFER. This might be explained by variations present in only one or two of the eight individuals, but defined as common based on their frequency in a larger population.

In our TOF cohort comprising eight cases, we found four copy number gains in three patients, while CoNIFER only detected two

of the gains in one patient. All four gains could be validated and in addition, the three genes affected by the CNVs are important regulators of heart development (*NOTCH1*, *ISL1*) or are located in a region associated with cardiac malformations (*PRODH*). Two of the variations also overlap with copy number alterations in TOF patients previously identified by array-CGH [17,18]. Taken together, this illustrates the advantage of using an outlier-based detecting method in a small cohort with a heterogeneous genetic background. Thus, our method is of special interest for small cohorts of specific phenotypes like rare diseases. Moreover, it can be used for the discovery of individual CNVs within families and *de novo* CNVs in trios.

Supporting Information

Table S1   Initial transition and emission probabilities of the HMM.

Table S2   CNVs found in the five HapMap samples using type10 Dixon's Q test in the outlier-based CNV calling method.

Table S3   CNVs found in the five HapMap samples using type20 Dixon's Q test in the outlier-based CNV calling method.

Script S1   R script for CNV calling.

Acknowledgments

We are deeply grateful to the TOF patients and families for their cooperation. We thank the German Heart Institute Berlin (Berlin, Germany) and the National Registry of Congenital Heart Disease (Berlin, Germany) for sample contribution. We further thank Ilona Dunkel for sample preparation. We also thank Biostar (www.biostars.org) and Cross Validated Stack Exchange (www.stats.stackexchange.com) for providing supporting discussion platforms.

Author Contributions

Conceived and designed the experiments: SRS. Performed the experiments: CD. Analyzed the data: VB MG. Contributed reagents/materials/analysis tools: FB RH SK SRS. Wrote the paper: CD MG VB.

References

1. Feuk L, Carson AR, Scherer SW (2006) Structural variation in the human genome. Nat Rev Genet 7: 85–97. doi:10.1038/nrg1767.

2. Conrad DF, Pinto D, Redon R, Feuk L, Gokcumen O, et al. (2010) Origins and functional impact of copy number variation in the human genome. 464: 704–712. Available: http://eutils.ncbi.nlm.nih.gov/entrez/eutils/elink. fcgi?dbfrom = pubmed&id = 19812545&retmode = ref&cmd = prlinks.

3. Fellermann K, Stange DE, Schaeffeler E, Schmalzl H, Wehkamp J, et al. (2006) A chromosome 8 gene-cluster polymorphism with low human beta-defensin 2 gene copy number predisposes to Crohn disease of the colon. 79: 439–448. Available: http://eutils.ncbi.nlm.nih.gov/entrez/eutils/elink. fcgi?dbfrom = pubmed&id = 16909382&retmode = ref&cmd = prlinks.

4. de Vries BBA, Pfundt R, Leisink M, Koolen DA, Vissers LELM, et al. (2005) Diagnostic genome profiling in mental retardation. 77: 606–616. Available: http://eutils.ncbi.nlm.nih.gov/entrez/eutils/elink. fcgi?dbfrom = pubmed&id = 16175506&retmode = ref&cmd = prlinks.

5. Thienpont B, Mertens L, de Ravel T, Eyskens B, Boshoff D, et al. (2007) Submicroscopic chromosomal imbalances detected by array-CGH are a frequent cause of congenital heart defects in selected patients. Eur Heart J 28: 2778–2784. doi:10.1093/eurheartj/ehl560.

6. Erdogan F, Larsen LA, Zhang L, Tümer Z, Tommerup N, et al. (2008) High frequency of submicroscopic genomic aberrations detected by tiling path array comparative genome hybridisation in patients with isolated congenital heart disease. J Med Genet 45: 704–709. doi:10.1136/jmg.2008.058776.

7. Hoffman JIE, Kaplan S (2002) The incidence of congenital heart disease. J Am Coll Cardiol 39: 1890–1900.

8. Reller MD, Strickland MJ, Riehle-Colarusso T, Mahle WT, Correa A (2008) Prevalence of congenital heart defects in metropolitan Atlanta, 1998–2005. J Pediatr 153: 807–813. doi:10.1016/j.jpeds.2008.05.059.

9. Ferencz C, Rubin JD, McCarter RJ, Brenner JI, Neill CA, et al. (1985) Congenital heart disease: prevalence at livebirth. The Baltimore-Washington Infant Study. American journal of epidemiology 121: 31–36. Available: http:// eutils.ncbi.nlm.nih.gov/entrez/eutils/elink. fcgi?dbfrom = pubmed&id = 3964990&retmode = ref&cmd = prlinks.

10. Apitz C, Webb G (2009) ScienceDirect.com - The Lancet - Tetralogy of Fallot. Available: http://www.sciencedirect.com/science/article/pii/s0140-6736(09)60657-7.

11. Fahed AC, Gelb BD, Seidman JG, Seidman CE (2013) Genetics of congenital heart disease: the glass half empty. Circ Res 112: 707–720. doi:10.1161/ CIRCRESAHA.112.300853.

12. Goldmuntz E, Clark BJ, Mitchell LE, Jawad AF, Cuneo BF, et al. (1998) Frequency of 22q11 deletions in patients with conotruncal defects. J Am Coll Cardiol 32: 492–498.

13. Cuturilo G, Menten B, Krstic A, Drakulic D, Jovanovic I, et al. (2011) 4q34.1-q35.2 deletion in a boy with phenotype resembling 22q11.2 deletion syndrome. 170: 1465–1470. Available: http://eutils.ncbi.nlm.nih.gov/entrez/eutils/elink. fcgi?dbfrom = pubmed&id = 21833498&retmode = ref&cmd = prlinks.

14. Luo H, Xie L, Wang S-Z, Chen J-L, Huang C, et al. (2012) Duplication of 8q12 encompassing CHD7 is associated with a distinct phenotype but without duane anomaly. 55: 646–649. Available: http://eutils.ncbi.nlm.nih.gov/entrez/eutils/elink.fcgi?dbfrom = pubmed&id = 22902603&retmode = ref&cmd = prlinks.

15. Luo C, Yang Y-F, Yin B-L, Chen J-L, Huang C, et al. (2012) Microduplication of 3p25.2 encompassing RAF1 associated with congenital heart disease suggestive of Noonan syndrome. 158A: 1918–1923. Available: http://eutils. ncbi.nlm.nih.gov/entrez/eutils/elink. fcgi?dbfrom = pubmed&id = 22786616&retmode = ref&cmd = prlinks.

16. Nora JJ (1968) Multifactorial inheritance hypothesis for the etiology of congenital heart diseases. The genetic-environmental interaction. Circulation 38: 604–617.

17. Greenway SC, Pereira AC, Lin JC, DePalma SR, Israel SJ, et al. (2009) De novo copy number variants identify new genes and loci in isolated sporadic tetralogy of Fallot. Nat Genet 41: 931–935. doi:10.1038/ng.415.

18. Silversides CK, Lionel AC, Costain G, Merico D, Migita O, et al. (2012) Rare copy number variations in adults with tetralogy of Fallot implicate novel risk gene pathways. PLoS Genet 8: e1002843. doi:10.1371/journal.pgen.1002843.

19. Soemedi R, Wilson IJ, Bentham J, Darlay R, Töpf A, et al. (2012) Contribution of Global Rare Copy-Number Variants to the Risk of Sporadic Congenital Heart Disease. The American Journal of Human Genetics 91: 489–501. doi:10.1016/j.ajhg.2012.08.003.

20. Alkan C, Coe BP, Eichler EE (2011) Genome structural variation discovery and genotyping. Nat Rev Genet 12: 363–376. doi:10.1038/nrg2958.

21. Shi Y, Majewski J (2013) FishingCNV: a graphical software package for detecting rare copy number variations in exome-sequencing data. Bioinformatics 29: 1461–1462. doi:10.1093/bioinformatics/btt151.

22. Li J, Lupat R, Amarasinghe KC, Thompson ER, Doyle MA, et al. (2012) CONTRA: copy number analysis for targeted resequencing. Bioinformatics 28: 1307–1313. doi:10.1093/bioinformatics/bts146.

23. Sathirapongsasuti JF, Lee H, Horst BAJ, Brunner G, Cochran AJ, et al. (2011) Exome sequencing-based copy-number variation and loss of heterozygosity detection: ExomeCNV. 27: 2648–2654. Available: http://eutils.ncbi.nlm.nih. gov/entrez/eutils/elink. fcgi?dbfrom = pubmed&id = 21828086&retmode = ref&cmd = prlinks.

24. Plagnol V, Curtis J, Epstein M, Mok KY, Stebbings E, et al. (2012) A robust model for read count data in exome sequencing experiments and implications for copy number variant calling. Bioinformatics 28: 2747–2754. doi:10.1093/bioinformatics/bts526.

25. Fromer M, Moran JL, Chambert K, Banks E, Bergen SE, et al. (2012) Discovery and statistical genotyping of copy-number variation from whole-exome sequencing depth. Am J Hum Genet 91: 597–607. doi:10.1016/j.ajhg.2012.08.005.

26. Amarasinghe KC, Li J, Halgamuge SK (2013) CoNVEX: copy number variation estimation in exome sequencing data using HMM. BMC Bioinformatics 14 Suppl 2: S2. doi:10.1186/1471-2105-14-S2-S2.

27. Krumm N, Sudmant PH, Ko A, O'Roak BJ, Malig M, et al. (2012) Copy number variation detection and genotyping from exome sequence data. 22: 1525–1532. Available: http://eutils.ncbi.nlm.nih.gov/entrez/eutils/elink. fcgi?dbfrom = pubmed&id = 22585873&retmode = ref&cmd = prlinks.

28. Kaynak B, Heydebreck von A, Mebus S, Seelow D, Hennig S, et al. (2003) Genome-wide array analysis of normal and malformed human hearts. Circulation 107: 2467–2474. Available: http://eutils.ncbi.nlm.nih.gov/entrez/ eutils/elink. fcgi?dbfrom = pubmed&id = 12742993&retmode = ref&cmd = prlinks.

29. Toenjes M, Schueler M, Hammer S, Pape UJ, Fischer JJ, et al. (2008) Prediction of cardiac transcription networks based on molecular data and complex clinical phenotypes. Mol Biosyst 4: 589–598. Available: http://eutils.ncbi.nlm.nih.gov/ entrez/eutils/elink. fcgi?dbfrom = pubmed&id = 18493657&retmode = ref&cmd = prlinks.

30. Schlesinger J, Schueler M, Grunert M, Fischer JJ, Zhang Q, et al. (2011) The cardiac transcription network modulated by Gata4, Mef2a, Nkx2.5, Srf, histone modifications, and microRNAs. PLoS Genet 7: e1001313. doi:10.1371/journal.pgen.1001313.

31. Li H, Durbin R (2009) Fast and accurate short read alignment with Burrows-Wheeler transform. 25: 1754–1760. Available: http://eutils.ncbi.nlm.nih.gov/ entrez/eutils/elink. fcgi?dbfrom = pubmed&id = 19451168&retmode = ref&cmd = prlinks.

32. Alkan C, Kidd JM, Marques-Bonet T, Aksay G, Antonacci F, et al. (2009) Personalized copy number and segmental duplication maps using next-generation sequencing. Nat Genet 41: 1061–1067. doi:10.1038/ng.437.

33. Dixon WJ (1950) Analysis of extreme values. Available: http://www.jstor.org/stable/10.2307/2236602.

34. Rorabacher DB (1991) Statistical treatment for rejection of deviant values: critical values of Dixon's 'Q' parameter and related subrange ratios at the 95% confidence level - Analytical Chemistry (ACS Publications). Available: http://pubs.acs.org/doi/abs/10.1021/ac00002a010.

35. Rabiner LR (1989) A tutorial on hidden Markov models and selected applications in speech recognition. 77: 257–286. Available: http://ieeexplore. ieee.org/lpdocs/epic03/wrapper.htm?arnumber = 18626.

36. Baum LE, Petrie T, Soules G, Weiss N (1970) A maximization technique occurring in the statistical analysis of probabilistic functions of Markov chains. Available: http://www.jstor.org/stable/10.2307/2239727.

37. Viterbi A (1967) Error bounds for convolutional codes and an asymptotically optimum decoding algorithm. Available: http://ieeexplore.ieee.org/xpls/abs_all.jsp?arnumber = 1054010.

38. Bu L, Jiang X, Martin-Puig S, Caron L, Zhu S, et al. (2009) Human ISL1 heart progenitors generate diverse multipotent cardiovascular cell lineages. 460: 113–117. Available: http://pubget.com/site/paper/19571884?institution = .

39. Stevens KN, Hakonarson H, Kim CE, Doevendans PA, Koeleman BPC, et al. (2009) Common Variation in ISL1 Confers Genetic Susceptibility for Human Congenital Heart Disease. 5: e10855–e10855. Available: http://pubget.com/site/paper/20520780?institution = .

40. Nemir M, Pedrazzini T (2008) Functional role of Notch signaling in the developing and postnatal heart. 45: 10–10. Available: http://pubget.com/site/paper/18410944?institution = .

41. Garg V, Muth AN, Ransom JF, Schluterman MK, Barnes R, et al. (2005) Mutations in NOTCH1 cause aortic valve disease. Nature 437: 270–274. doi:10.1038/nature03940.

42. Mohamed SA, Aherrahrou Z, Liptau H, Erasmi AW, Hagemann C, et al. (2006) Novel missense mutations (p.T596M and p.P1797H) in NOTCH1 in patients with bicuspid aortic valve. 345: 1460–1465. Available: http://eutils.ncbi.nlm. nih.gov/entrez/eutils/elink. fcgi?dbfrom = pubmed&id = 16729972&retmode = ref&cmd = prlinks.

43. Momma K (2010) Cardiovascular anomalies associated with chromosome 22q11.2 deletion syndrome. Am J Cardiol 105: 1617–1624. doi:10.1016/j.amjcard.2010.01.333.

44. Humphreys G (2012) Coming together to combat rare diseases. Bull World Health Organ 90: 406–407. doi:10.2471/BLT.12.020612.

10

Two Heterozygous Mutations in *NFATC1* in a Patient with Tricuspid Atresia

Zahi Abdul-Sater[1], Amin Yehya[1], Jean Beresian[1], Elie Salem[1], Amina Kamar[1], Serine Baydoun[1], Kamel Shibbani[1], Ayman Soubra[1], Fadi Bitar[2]*, Georges Nemer[1]*

1 Department of Biochemistry and Molecular Genetics, American University of Beirut, Beirut, Lebanon, 2 Department of Pediatrics and Adolescent Medicine, American University of Beirut, Beirut, Lebanon

Abstract

Tricuspid Atresia (TA) is a rare form of congenital heart disease (CHD) with usually poor prognosis in humans. It presents as a complete absence of the right atrio-ventricular connection secured normally by the tricuspid valve. Defects in the tricuspid valve are so far not associated with any genetic locus, although mutations in numerous genes were linked to multiple forms of congenital heart disease. In the last decade, Knock-out mice have offered models for cardiologists and geneticists to study the causes of congenital disease. One such model was the *Nfatc1*$^{-/-}$ mice embryos which die at mid-gestation stage due to a complete absence of the valves. NFATC1 belongs to the Rel family of transcription factors members of which were shown to be implicated in gene activation, cell differentiation, and organogenesis. We have previously shown that a tandem repeat in the intronic region of *NFATC1* is associated with ventricular septal defects. In this report, we unravel for the first time a potential link between a mutation in *NFATC1* and TA. Two heterozygous missense mutations were found in the *NFATC1* gene in one indexed-case out of 19 patients with TA. The two amino-acids changes were not found neither in other patients with CHDs, nor in the control healthy population. Moreover, we showed that these mutations alter dramatically the normal function of the protein at the cellular localization, DNA binding and transcriptional levels suggesting they are disease-causing.

Editor: Osman El-Maarri, University of Bonn, Institut of experimental hematology and transfusion medicine, Germany

Funding: This work was supported by a grant from the Lebanese National Council for Scientific Research (LNCSR Grant# 114170 522296). The funders had no role in study design, data collection and analysis, decision to publish, or preparation of the manuscript.

Competing Interests: The authors have declared that no competing interests exist.

* E-mail: gn08@aub.edu.lb (GN); fadi.bitar@aub.edu.lb (FB)

Introduction

Cardiac valvulogenesis refers to the formation of valves in the heart, an evolutionary conserved mechanism in vertebrates that occurs at mid-gestation and results in the unidirectional flow of blood throughout the heart. Both the semilunar (aortic and pulmonary), and atrioventricular valves (tricuspid and mitral) are thought to arise from endocardial cells that undergo multiple processes governed by an array of growth factors, transcription factors, and extracellular proteins [1,2,3].

Endocardial cells destined to become valves undergo an epithelial to mesenchymal transformation (EMT) upon their stimulation by the TGFβ and BMP2/4 growth factors secreted from the underlying myocardium [2]. This process of transformation is dependent on two signaling pathways from within the endocardial cells, specifically the Wnt and NOTCH pathways [4]. The mesenchymal cells will invade the cardiac jelly composed mainly of hyaluronic acid. These cells will undergo proliferation and subsequent differentiation into mature valves, a process that is subject to tight regulation by growth factors amongst which the vascular endothelial growth factor (VEGF). The final valve structure is made up of at least 2 leaflets (mitral has 2 while tricuspid has 3) composed mainly of endocardially-derived cells. The involvement of neural crest cells in semilunar but not atrioventricular valves formation is supported by conditional

knock-outs although neither myocardial nor neural crests cells are detected in the mature valves [2,3,5]. The final process of remodeling is governed mainly by apoptosis. Defects in any of the steps involved in valvulogenesis lead to the valvular congenital heart disease including Mitral and Tricuspid Atresia (MA and TA). These two conditions, which account for 1–2% of all congenital heart disease in humans, are still difficult to treat [6,7]

Some of the molecular pathways involved in valve formation have been unraveled through the unexpected phenotype encountered in mice lacking the *Nfatc1* gene [8,9]. NFATC1 (Nuclear Factor for Activated T-Cells) belongs to the Rel/NF-kB family of transcription factors that were first described as being key regulators of T-cells' activation. Five members (NFATC1-5) are found in mammals; all playing different non-redundant roles during embryonic and postnatal development [10,11,12,13]. All five members share a conserved DNA-binding domain at the C-terminus of the protein that binds specifically to the consensus (A/T)GGAAA sequence [14]. In addition, they harbor at the N-terminal region a series of conserved serine-proline residues (S/P) that when dephosphorylated unmasked a nuclear localization signal allowing the translocation of NFATC proteins from the cytoplasm to the nucleus [15,16,17,18]. All NFATC proteins except NFATC5 are dephosphorylated by the calcium dependent phosphatase calcineurin (PPP3CA/PPP3CB) at the N-terminus triggering the translocation process. Although NFATC proteins are weak transactivators, their transcriptional potency is boosted through their interactions with different classes of transcription factors mainly the AP-1 family members, c-Fos and Jun, the MADS family, and the GATA zinc finger proteins [19,20,21,22,23].

NFATC1 was shown to be expressed in numerous cell types including lymphocytes, osteoclasts, neurons, and myotubes [17,24,25,26,27]. The first *in vivo* assessment of the role of the gene came however from the inactivation of the gene in mice. Two independent reports showed that *Nfatc1−/−* mice die at mid-gestation stage (e14.5) due to lack of EC growth and remodeling [8,9]. While Ranger AM et al showed a selective defect in the semilunar valves, the *Nfatc1−/−* embryos generated by de la Pompa Jl et al had severe defects in both atrioventricular and semilunar valves. Although this discrepancy might be linked to the genetic background and/or knock-out strategy, the fact that in both phenotypes the endocardial cushions are hypoplastic do point out to a major role for NFATC1 in endocardial cushion formation and proliferation. This role is even highlighted by the inactivation of PPP3CB, which encodes the calcineurin regulatory subunit, specifically in the endocardium and that results in a mirror-image phenotype identical to that of the *Nfatc1−/−* knock-out [28,29]. This intrinsic requirement for endocardial expression of NFATC1 in endocardial cushion formation is dispensable for endocardial-mesenchymal transformation since in both *Ppp3cb−/−* and *Nfatc1−/−* embryos, mesenchymal cells are found in the cardiac jelly. The Calcineurin/NFAT pathway is however required in myocardial cells to control EMT through the repression of secreted VEGF.

Given the fact that NFATC1 is at the center of valve formation in mammals, we hypothesize that mutations in the gene encoding it would be associated with valve malformations in humans. We have previously shown that a tandem repeat in the intronic region of *NFATC1* is associated with ventricular septal defects but with no valvular phenotype [30]. We therefore screened for such mutations in patients with different valve diseases registered at the congenital heart disease genetics program at the American University of Beirut Medical Center. Results showed 2 novel missense (P66L, I701L) single nucleotide polymorphisms (SNPs) in only one patient with tricuspid atresia. Functional analyses of the mutated protein do show a defect in its cellular localization, transcriptional activities and DNA binding patterns suggesting that the mutations are disease causing.

Materials and Methods

Subject Recruitment and DNA extraction

Blood was extracted from registered patients at the Children's Cardiac Registry Center at the American University of Beirut Medical Center (AUB-MC) after signing a consent form approved by the IRB (Protocol Number: Bioch.GN01). Patients included in the study, were evaluated by a pediatric cardiologist. The diagnosis was confirmed at least by echocardiography. Patients with known syndromes (I,e Noonan, DiGeorge, Holt-Oram, Marfan, Alagille, and Char) were excluded from the study. EDTA tubes were used for blood collection and DNA extraction was carried out as previously described [31,32]. The obtained DNA was quantified at 260 nm and DNA concentration was in the range [400 ng/µl–800 ng/µl].

Cell Lines

HEK 293T cells (Human Embryonic Kidney cells) and HeLa cells (human cervical cancer cells) were cultured and maintained in Dulbecco's Modified Eagle Media (DMEM) supplemented with 10% Fetal Bovine Serum (PAA) (FBS), 1% Penicillin/Streptomy-

cin and 1% Sodium pyruvate. Incubation was carried out in a humid atmosphere 5% CO2 at 37°C as previously described [31].

Generation of NFATC1 mutants by PCR-mediated site-directed mutagenesis

After identifying each mutant gene sequence, an oligonucleotide (forward primer) harboring the desired mutation was synthesized in a way to complement the human NFATC1 cDNA (Addgene) subcloned in the pCEP4 expression vector (Invitrogen). The second primer (reverse) was designed in a way that it starts from the same start site of the first primer but extends to the opposite direction. Primers were then phosphorylated and PCR was performed using Site-Directed Mutagenesis kit from FINN-ZYMES (product code: F-541). The resultant amplicon was ligated and transformed into XL-1 Blue competent bacteria. The generated plasmid was extracted and sequenced to make sure the mutation was incorporated. The primers used for generating the mutants are as follows: 5′ CGGCGCACTC-CACCCTGC T GGCCCCGTGC 3′ an its reverse complement for the first mutation , and 5′ CAACGGTAACGCC C TCTTTC-TAACCG 3′ and its reverse complement for the second mutation.

Immunofluorescence

Hela cells were plated in 12-well Costar culture plates on cover slips with 100,000 cells/well. Tranfections were done on the second day of plating using polyethylenimine (PEI) transfecting reagent. Briefly, 2 µg of DNA per well were diluted in 150 µL of NaCl (150 mM, culture grade) in an eppendorf tube, vortexed and then 6 µL of PEI (ratio 1:3 of DNA to PEI) were added on the mixture of DNA/NaCl, vortexed for 3 seconds and then incubated for 20 minutes at room temperature. The prepared mixture was applied on the cells gently and the medium was replaced on the second day.

Then, immunofluorescence was performed on transfected Hela cells. The cells were first washed for 3 times with PBS 1× (phosphate buffered saline), and then fixed with 4% paraformaldehyde for 20 minutes. Fixed cells were blocked with 3% BSA/PBT (bovine serum albumin/phosphate buffer saline Tween) for 1 hour. The primary antibodies Mouse anti-flag (Flag M2 from Sigma Aldrich) and rabbit anti-HA (Santa Cruz) were used for assessment of subcellular localization of PPP3CA, NFATC1 and its mutants. The primary antibodies were diluted in BSA/PBT and added to the cells with an overnight incubation at 4°C. The cells were then washed in PBT 3 times, and the secondary antibody horse anti-mouse biotinylated or donkey anti-rabbit biotinylated (General Electric) were diluted 1:500 in BSA/PBT. They were added to the cells for 1 hour at RT with shaking. After washing 3 times with PBT, cells were incubated with Streptavidin Texas red or anti-mouse/anti-rabbit FITC for 1 hour at RT. Staining for the Nuclei was done using the Hoechst dye. The cells were mounted on a rectangular slide containing an anti-fading agent (DABCO), and the slides were examined using an Olympus BH-2 microscope. The nuclear versus cytoplasmic staining was conducted on 3 independent experiments and by assessing a total of 10 fields/per experiment with a total of 125 cells for each mutant and wild type protein.

Luciferase Assay

HeLa cells were transfected with the 1.4 kbp human DEGS1 or CCND1 promoter coupled to luciferase, the NFATC1 cDNA encoding the different proteins (Wt, P66L, I701L, and P66L/ I701L) and/or the constitutively activated PPP3CA and/or GATA5 (Generous gifts from Drs J. Molkentin and M. Nemer) and/or HAND2. Both the DEGS1 and CCND1 promoters were

Table 1. Number and Phenotypes of the Lebanese Subjects Enrolled in this Study.

TA	19
CoA	14
PA	9
MA	4
AS	5
PS (Valvular)	63 (9)
VSD	21
Control subjects	100

amplified using specific primers and subcloned into the PGL3 Luciferase vector (Invitrogen). The 1.4 Kbp DEGS1 promoter harbors a conserved NFATC1 binding site at −914 bp (5′ TCTTTA**GGAAA**GTCATCTGGTCTGC 3′) in addition to multiple GATA *cis* elements. After 24 hours, cells were washed with PBS (1X) and then lysed with 1X lysis buffer and left on the shaker for 20 minutes at RT. Luciferin (Promega, Cat # E 1501) was prepared according to the manufacturer's protocol. The lysed cells were transferred to a 96 well plate (Costar) to which luciferin was added and the signal was read immediately using the Ascent Fluoroscan in the Molecular Biology Core Facility at AUB.

Protein over-expression and Western Blots

For over expression experiments, transfections were done using calcium phosphate. Briefly, HEK293T cells were first plated in 100 mm culture plates (Corning) with 70% confluency. On the second day, 20 µg DNA was added to an eppendorf tube; water was added till 200 µl total volume. 400 µl of HBS (Hepes Buffer Sulfate) is added to a tube. Then the mixture of DNA and water is

added to the tube. Bubbles are created to promote more DNA precipitation. The mixture is left for 20 minutes at room temperature. The mixture was then applied on cells and after 4 hours the media was replaced. Nuclear protein extracts from HEK293T cells were obtained as previously described. 30 µL aliquots were stored at −80°C . For Western blots, equal amounts of nuclear cell extracts (10 µg protein) were resuspended in 5X laemmli buffers. The samples were boiled for 3 minutes and run on a denaturing SDS-PAGE for 1.5 hours then transferred to a PVDF membrane (Amersham). The membrane was blocked for 45 minutes in 2% non-fat dry milk . After blocking, the membrane was incubated with the primary antibody, Anti- Flag (against NFATC1) or/and anti-HA (against PPP3CA). The antibody was diluted 1:1000 in 1% non-fat dry milk and the incubation was carried out overnight at 4°C. The membrane was afterwards incubated with the secondary antibody conjugated with horseradish-peroxidase, anti-mouse or anti-rabbit- HRP, diluted 1:40000. Revelation was done using the Western Lightening Chemiluminescence Kit (Perkin Elmer, Cat # NEL 103). The protein bands were visualized by autoradiography.

Electrophoretic Mobility Shift Assay (EMSA)

For probe synthesis, two pairs of primers were designed corresponding to the NFAT consensus region 5′ CGCCCAAA-GA**GGAAA**ATTTGTTTCATA 3′ (Santa Cruz). The single stranded primers were annealed and labeled with P32 in presence of T4 Kinase. The labeled probe was then run on a nondenaturing 12% Bis-Acrylamide gel (Acrylamide: Bis (38:2), 1.6%APS, TEMED, water and 1X TBE) at 125 volts for 30 minutes. The gel was exposed to a XOMAT film and the bands corresponding to a double stranded probe were cut accordingly and purified using Costar Spin-X columns (Costar, Cat # 8161) according to the manufacturer's protocol. The probe was then used in gel shift assay experiments.

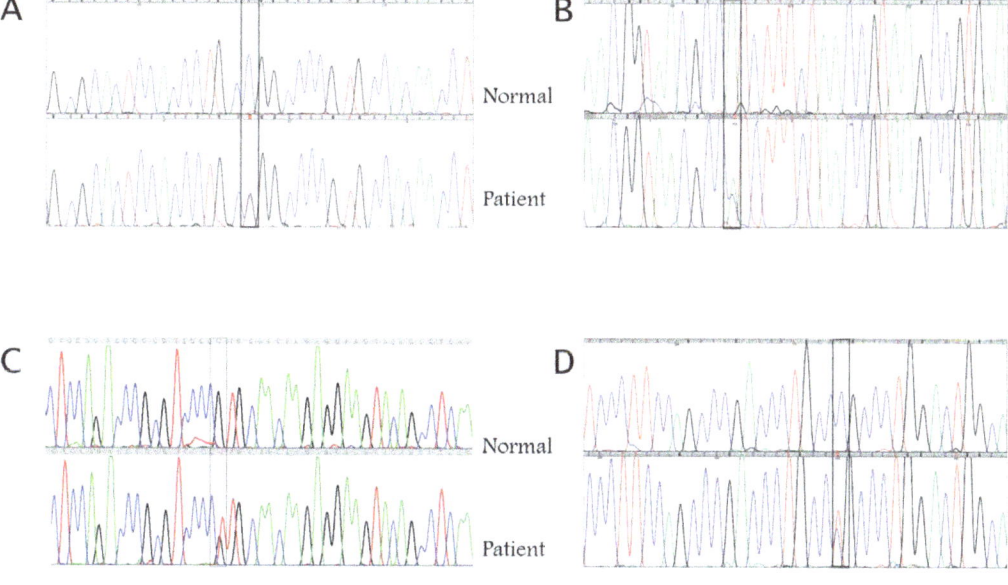

Figure 1. Sequencing results showing the different NFATC1 SNPs. Representative chromatograms of the different missense SNPs in exons 2 and 8 (A and B respectively) and synonymous SNPs in exon 2 and 3 (C and D respectively).The boxed region indicates the place of the polymorphisms in the patient as compared to a normal sequence. In all cases, the SNPs occur on one allele as visualized by overlapping peaks at the indicated position inside the box. In (A) a cytosine is substituted by a thymine, in (B) an adenine is substituted by a cysteine, in (C) a guanine is substituted by a thymine, and in (D) a cytosine is substituted by a thymine.

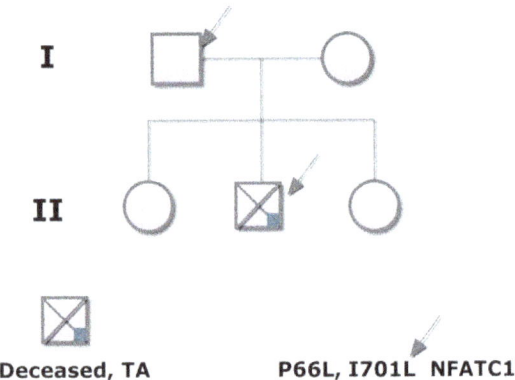

Figure 2. Mendelian inheritance of the different NFATC1 SNPs. Genotype-phenotype correlations showed that in addition to the indexed patient with tricuspid atresia who died at 17 years of age, his "healthy" father carried the four different SNPs. None of the siblings, nor the mother who all are healthy have any of these SNPs.

The nuclear extracts were run on a 6% non-denaturing polyacrylamide gel (Acrylamide: Bis (29:1), 1.6%APS, TEMED, water and 0.25X TBE) in 0.25X TBE buffer at 200 volts. The reaction consisted of 10 μg of extracts, 4 μl binding buffer (20 mM Tris pH 7.9, 120 mM KCl, 2 mM EDTA, 25 mM MgCl2 and 25% glycerol), 1 μl poly dI/dC (General Electric) and 1 μl of the probe. The reaction was completed to 20 μl with water. After

incubation for 20 minutes the samples were loaded and the gel was run for 2.5 hours. The gel was then dried using the BioRad gel dryer (Model 583) for 2 hours at 80°C followed by exposition to a PhosphoImager screen. The results were visualized using the STORM scanner (General Electric). Quantification of the bands was done using TotalLab2010 (General Electric).

Statistical Analysis

The significance of the luciferase transcriptional assays was analyzed using the one-way Anova single test ($p<0.05$).

Bioinformatics

The NFATC1 secondary structures were predicted and visualized by the Discovery Studio program (Acclerys Inc.). Briefly, the human NFATC1 protein sequence was imported from the SWISS database and the secondary amino acid structure was predicted based on the nature and structure of the composing amino acids using already validated approaches by the Discovery Studio. The mutated amino acids were introduced to the same sequence, and the prediction of the structure was carried on using the same approach.

Results

Patients with various heart valve defects were recruited as part of the ongoing study on the genetics of CHD in the Lebanese population. The subjects' list included a total of 135 patients and 100 control healthy individuals. The distribution of valvular CHDs among patients was as follows: tricuspid atresia (19 patients), pulmonary stenosis (63 patients, 9 of which are strictly valvular),

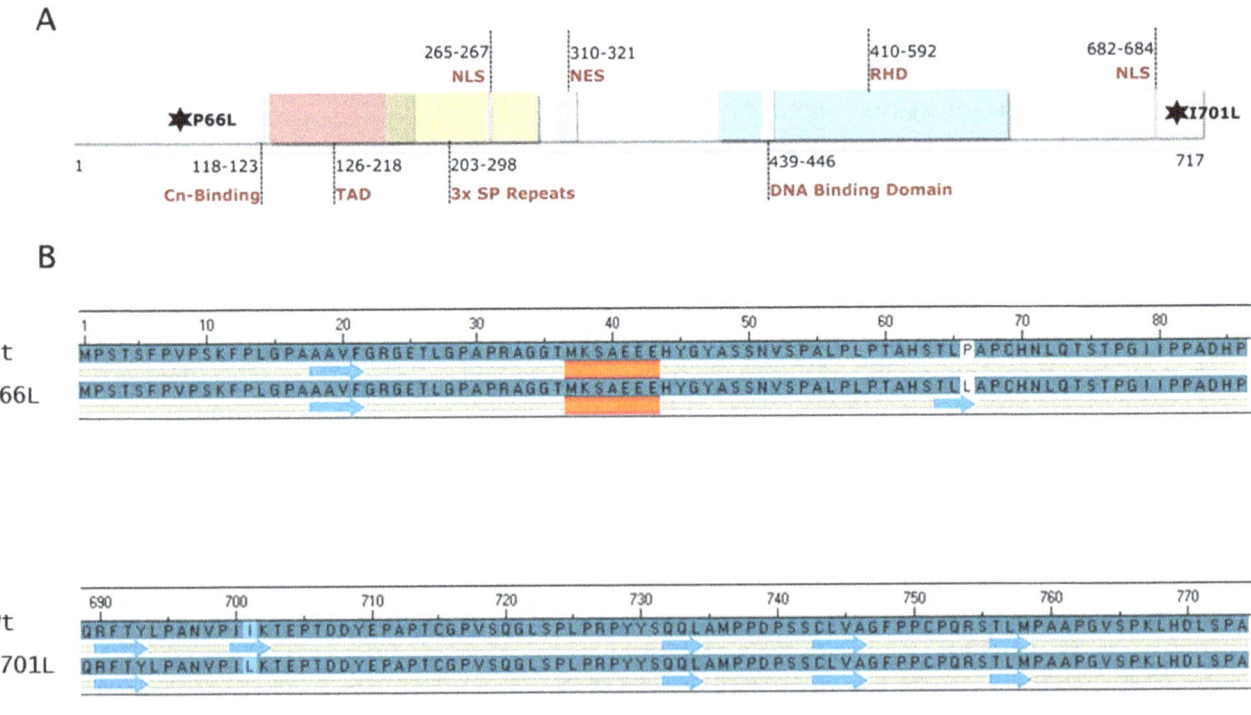

Figure 3. Effects of the two missense SNPs on the structure of the NFATC1 protein. A- The missense SNPs lead to a P66L substitution at the N-terminal region of the protein near the calcineurin-docking site (Cln binding), and to a I701L substitution at the C-terminal region downstream of the Rel Homolgy Domain (RHD). The schematic represents isoform A, the most abundant NFATC1 protein with 717 amino acids, a transactivation domain (TAD) at the N-terminus, and a DNA binding domain at the C-terminus. (NLS = nuclear localization signal, NES = nuclear export signal, and SP = Serine-Proline). B- The NFATC1 secondary structures were predicted and visualized by the Discovery Studio program (Acclerys Inc.). The results demonstrate the formation of a new beta-sheet in the P66L mutant and a deletion of a beta-sheet in the I701L mutant as compared to the wild type protein.

Table 2. Frequency of the NFATC1 mutations according to the Exome Sequencing Project (ESP).

rsID	Alleles	EA Allele#	AA Allele#	All Allele#	MAF(%) (EA/AA/All)	Amino Acid Position	Polyphen Prediction
rs148104245	T/C	T = 0 C = 8598	T = 3 C = 4403	T = 3 C = 13001	0.0/0.0681/0.0231	LEU,PRO 66/7171	Probably Damaging
rs113736099	C/A	C = 10 A = 8590	C = 12 A = 4392	C = 22 A = 12982	0.1163/0.2725/0.1692	LEU,ILE 701/717	Unknown

rs ID
dbSNP reference SNP identifier.
EA Allele Count
The observed allele counts for the listed alleles in European American population. (delimited by /).
AA Allele Count
The observed allele counts for the listed alleles in African American population. (delimited by /).
Allele Count
The observed allele counts for the listed alleles in all populations. (delimited by /).
MAF (%) (EA/AA/All):
the minor-allele frequency in percent listed in the order of European American (EA), African American(AA) and all populations (All). (delimited by /).

aortic stenosis (5 patiens), pulmonary atresia (9 patients), and mitral atresia (4 patients). In addition, 21 cases of ventricular septal defect and 14 cases of coarctation of the aorta (14 patients) were included (Table 1).

Heterozygous SNPs in exon 2 and 8 of NFATC1 in one patient with TA

We screened all 8 coding exons of the *NFATC1* gene for the 135 patients. Only one patient (#120) suffering from Tricuspid Atresia

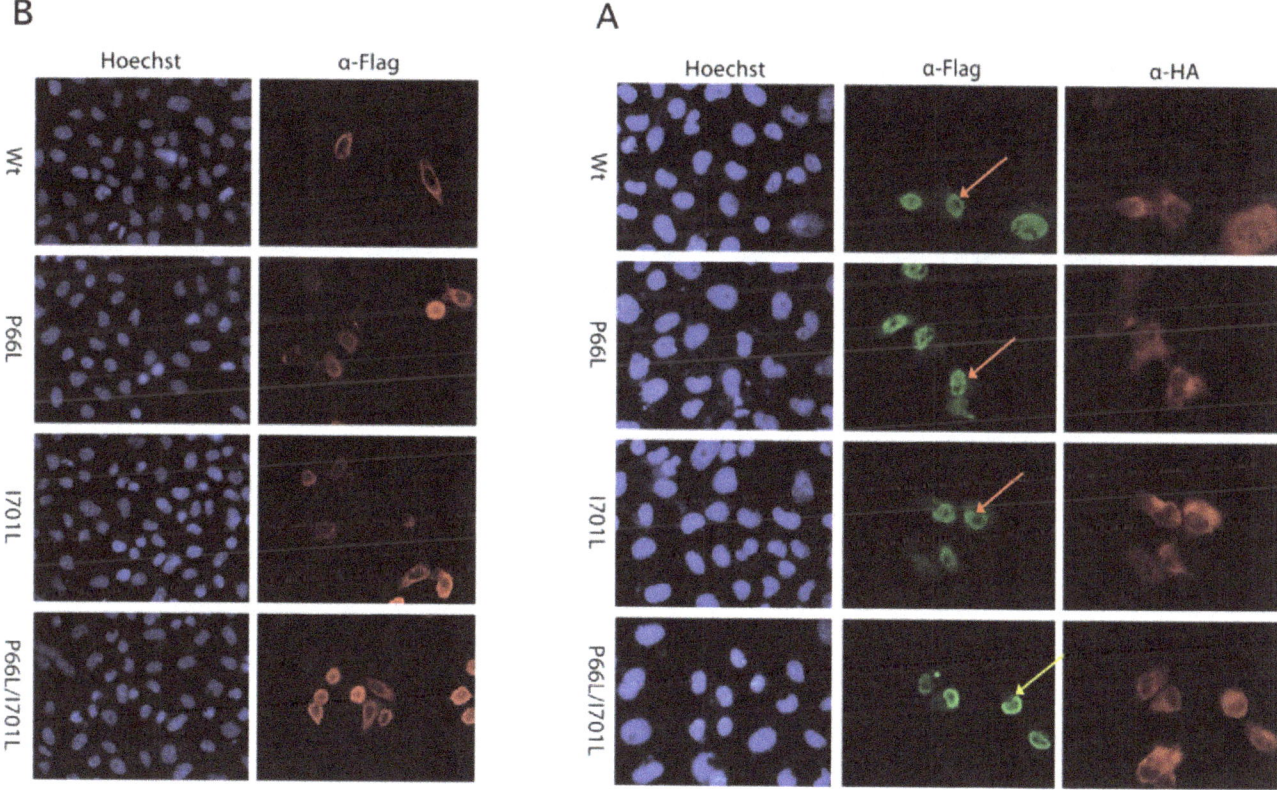

Figure 4. Effect of the NFATC1 missense SNPs on the cellular localization of the protein. A- Immunofluorescence of HeLa cells transfected with plasmids encoding for the Wt NFATC1 and NFATC1 Mutants (P66L, I701L, P66L/I701L). The localization of NFATC1 was visualized using an anti-Flag antibody. Nuclei of cells were visualized using the Hoechst dye (blue color). Wt and NFATC1 mutants localized to the cytoplasm in the absence of PPP3CA (red color). (Magnification ×40). B- Immunofluorescence of HeLa cells transfected with plasmids encoding for the Wt NFATC1 and NFATC1 Mutants (P66L, I701L, P66L/I701L) co-transfected with PP3CA. The localization of NFATC1 was visualized using an anti-Flag antibody (red color) while PP3CA was visualized using anti-HA antibody (green color). Nuclei of cells were visualized using Hoechst dye (blue color). Most of the cells co-transfected with the double NFATC1 mutant were retained in the cytoplasm around the nuclear membrane, whereas in the other cases, the protein was totally translocated to the nucleus. (Magnification ×40). Yellow arrows indicate cytoplasmic (peri-nuclear) staining, while red arrows indicate nuclear staining.

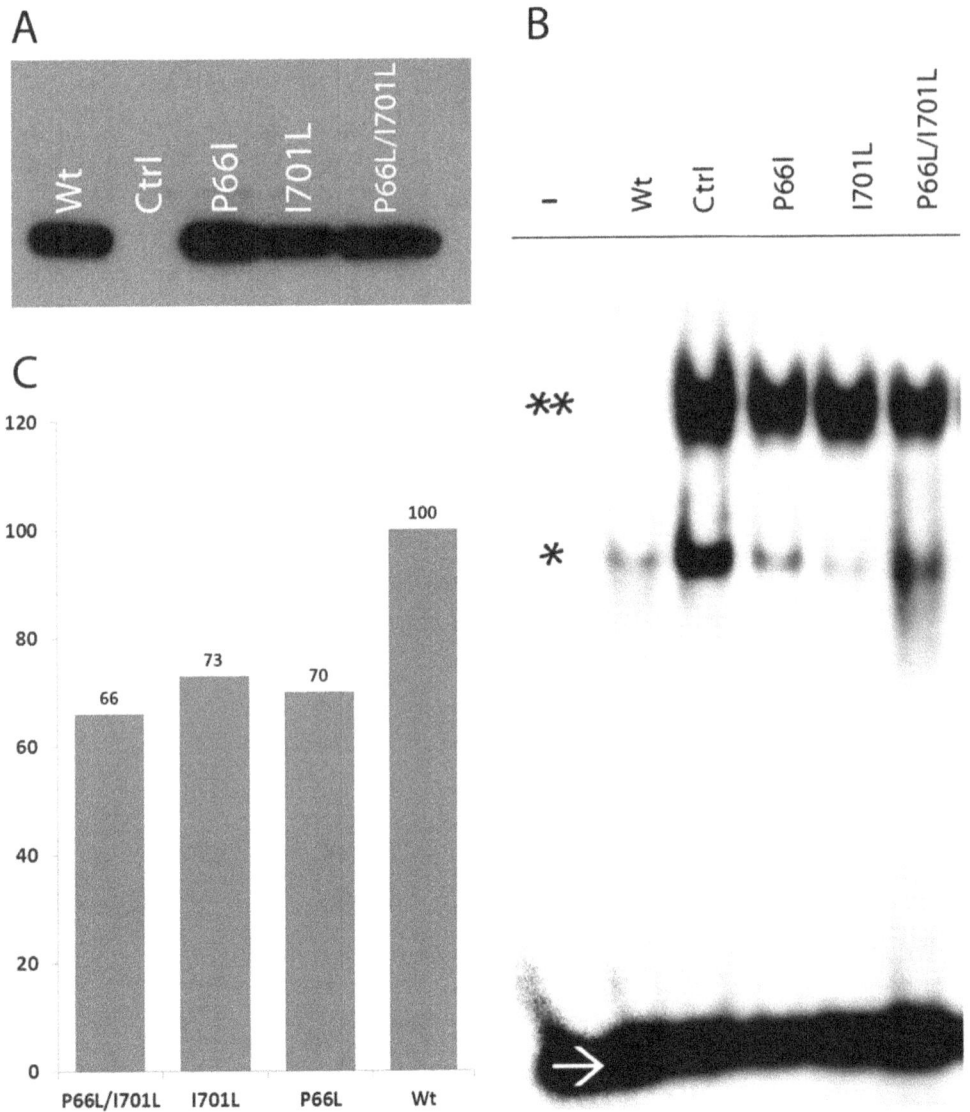

Figure 5. DNA binding affinity of the mutated NFATC1 proteins. A- NFATC1 extracts from HEK 293 cells transfected with Wt NFATC1 and Mutants (P66L – I701L – P66L/I701L) were resolved on an SDS-PAGE prior to gel shift assays. Western blots showed equal amounts of expressed proteins as depicted by the anti-Flag antibody. (Ctrl refers to nuclear extracts from mock-transfected cells). B- EMSA was performed using equal amounts of the overexpressed NFATC1 proteins from HEK 293 cells transfected with Wt NFATC1 and NFATC1 mutants (P66L, I701L, P66L/I701L) and NFAT-consensus binding site as a probe. – ve sign indicates absence of nuclear extracts/* indicates NFATC1 monomer/** indicates NFATC1 Dimer/→ refers to the ^{32}P labeled free DNA probe. C- Quantification of the NFATC1 dimers in the EMSA using the TotalLab2010 software from Amersham shows a 30% decrease in DNA binding affinity of the single and double mutant as compared to the wild type NFATC1 protein.

was found to have two missense heterozygous SNPs in exons 2 and 8 respectively (Figure 1 A,B). Additional silent SNPs were found in various exons in many patients (data not shown) including patient 120 (Figure 1 C,D). The patient presented to the clinic at the American University of Beirut Medical Center at sixteen years of age with severe hypoxemia probably due to complications of his undiagnosed tricuspid atresia problem over the years. The echocardiography at that stage showed in addition to TA, a D-TGA (transposition of the great arteries), atrial septal defect (ASD), hypoplasia of the aortic arch, and severe pulmonary hypertension. The patient died shortly after hospital admission. Family members of the patient (Figure 2) were screened to check for a Mendelian inheritance of the missense SNPs. Surprisingly the father who is "healthy" with no cardiac phenotype was also found to carry the

same SNPs. All other family members including the mother and two siblings were genotypically normal. The T/C nucleotide SNP in exon 2 leads to a Leucine instead of a Proline at position 66 and the A/C nucleotide SNP in exon 8 generates a Leucine instead of Isoleucine at position 701 (Figure 3A). The screening of 100 healthy control individuals didn't show the presence of these SNPs, suggesting they might be disease-causing. Both SNPs were however found in the dbSNP database with the following rsID: rs1481042045 and rs113736099 for the P66L and I701L respectively. The minor allele frequency (MAF) is considerably very low especially for rs1481042045, and *in silico* prediction, using Polyphen-2 shows that this particular SNP is potentially damaging for the protein (Table 2).

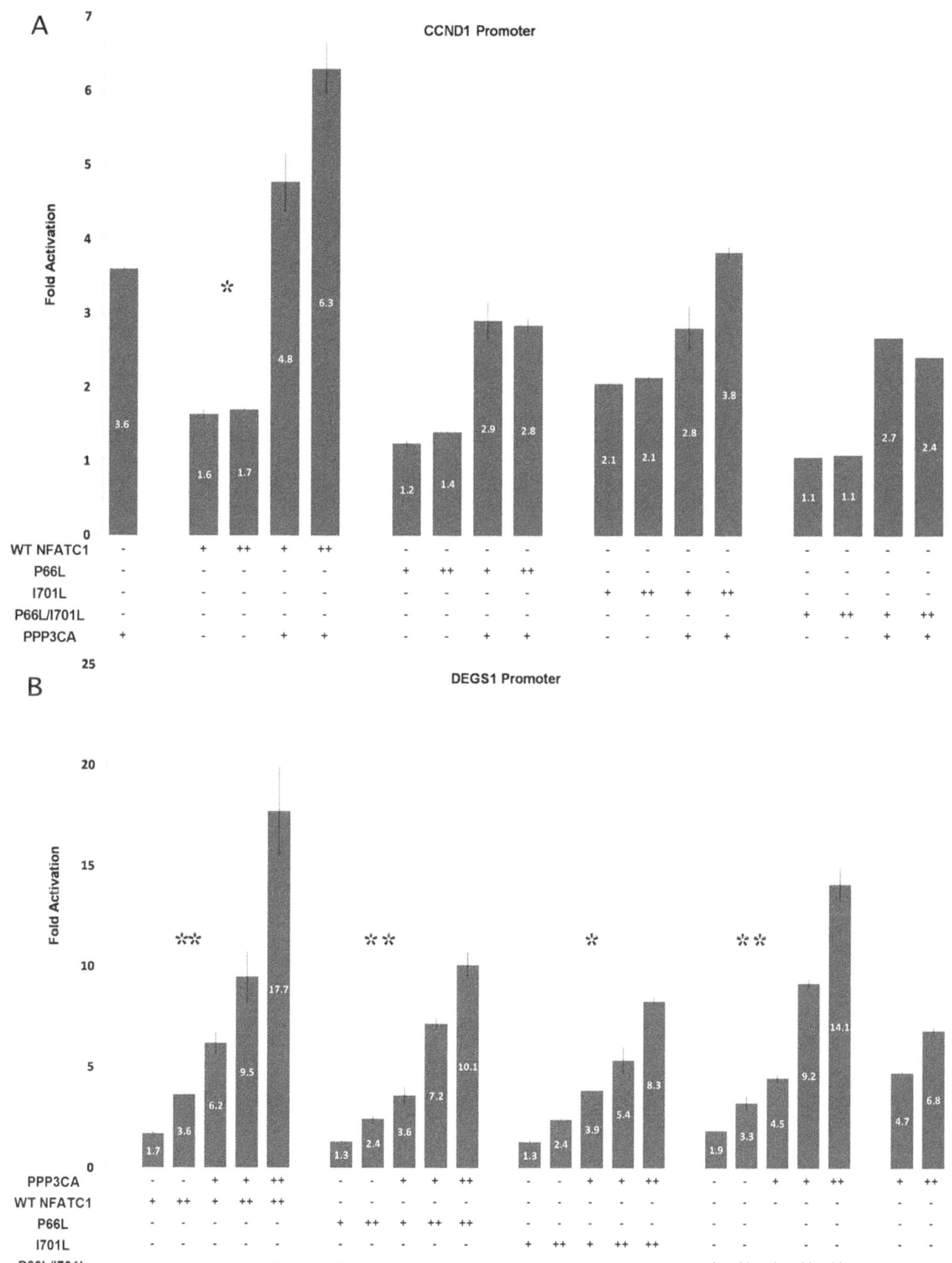

Figure 6. Transcriptional activity of the mutated NFATC1 proteins. A- Wt NFATC1 or NFATC1 Mutants (P66L, I701L, P66L/I701L) were cotransfected with the human CCND1 promoter coupled luciferase reporter construct in the presence or absence of activated calcineurin (PPP3CA) in Hela cells. Six hours post transfection, media was changed and cells were harvested for luciferase assay after 36 hours. Relative luciferase activities are represented as fold activation. The data are the mean of three independent experiments done in duplicates +/− standard deviation. Significance (p<0.05) was assessed using the one-way Anova test. (* p<0.01, ** p<0.05) B- Wt NFATC1 or NFATC1 Mutants (P66L, I701L, P66L/I701L) were cotransfected with the human DEGS1 promoter coupled luciferase reporter construct in the presence or absence of activated calcineurin (PPP3CA) in Hela cells. Six hours post transfection, media was changed and cells were harvested for luciferase assay after 36 hours. Relative luciferase activities are represented as fold activation. The data are the mean of three independent experiments done in duplicates +/− standard deviation. Significance (p<0.05) was assessed using the one-way Anova test. (* p<0.01, ** p<0.05).

Disruption of the secondary structure of the P66L and I701L NFATC1 proteins

Bioinformatics secondary structure prediction tools were used to assess the effect of the mutations on the secondary structure of NFATC1 protein. Upon substitution of P with L at position 66, a new beta sheet was formed in comparison with the Wt NFATC1 while a beta sheet was removed at position 701 upon substitution of I with L (Figure 3B). This confirms the *in silico* predictions done by the Polyphen-2 software used by the Exome Variant Server (EVS) database to predict the effect of amino acid substitution on protein function (http://evs.gs.washington.edu/EVS/).

The NFATC1 double mutant protein is partially retained in the cytoplasm

In order to assess the impact of the P66L and I701L mutations on NFATC1 structural and functional properties, site directed mutagenesis was done on a human *NFATC1* cDNA (Isoform A, NP_765978.1) cloned in an expression vector. Three vectors were generated harboring P66L alone (P66L), I701L alone (I701L) and both mutations together (P66L/I701L). The generated plasmids were transfected into HeLa cells to study the cellular localization of the mutated protein. Immunostaining revealed that Wt NFATC1 and NFATC1 mutants are located in the cytoplasm in absence of PPP3CA(Figure 4A). Wt NFATC1, P66l, and I701L translocated to the nucleus when cotransfected with the activated form of PPP3CA (Figure 4B). However, NFATC1 double mutant P66L/I701L failed to translocate to the nucleus in more than 80% of co-transfected cells (Figure 4B).

Attenuated DNA binding affinity of the mutant NFATC1 mutant proteins

Gel shift assays were carried out to assess the binding affinity of the mutated NFATC1 proteins to an NFAT consensus binding sites. Equal amounts of overexpressed proteins were verified by western blots (Figure 5A), and used for DNA-binding activity. Multiple assays with different amounts of proteins showed a consistent decrease in DNA binding affinity of around 30% for all mutant proteins as compared to the wild type NFATC1 (Figure 5, B,C).

NFATC1 mutations hampered Calcineurin induced transcriptional activity

In order to assess the impact of the mutations on the regulatory function of NFATC1 protein, transactivation assays using the cyclin D1 (CCND1), and the Degenerative Spermatocyte Homolog 1 (DEGS1) promoter fused to luciferase were performed. HeLa cells were transfected with 1 μg of (DEGS1/luc)/well and increasing concentration of Wt NFATC1 and NFATC1 mutants with or without constitutively activated PPP3CA. The DEGS1 promoter harbors a consensus NFAT binding site at −914 bp in addition to multiple GATA binding sites. The results showed that the Wt NFATC1 is a moderate activator of the DEGS1 promoter with a maximum fold increase of 1.7 (Figure 6A). Upon co-

transfection with PPP3CA, the activation of DEGS1 promoter increased to reach 6.2 without attaining a synergistic threshold. This synergy is however observed when the amount of Wt NFATC1 was increased (Figure 6 A). In comparison, the different mutant NFATC1 proteins have a decreased transcriptional activity alone or in combination with PPP3CA.

The same approach was adopted to assess NFATC1 regulation of CCND1 promoter, a recently described *bona fide* target of NFATC1 [33]. The Wt protein showed a dose dependent activation of the promoter that was increased in presence of PPP3CA. NFATC1 mutants (P66l, I701L, and P66L/I701L) showed decreased activation of the promoter that was more significant in the case of the double mutant P66L/I701L (Figure 6 B).

The NFATC1 double mutant is unable to functionally interact with both GATA5 and HAND2

Interaction of GATA5 and NFATC1 on DEGS1 promoter was studied based on previous data implicating both proteins in having physical and functional interaction over the endothelin promoter [19]. Hela cells were transfected with GATA5 alone, PPP3CA alone, Wt NFATC1 alone or NFATC1 mutants, a combination of each two, or a combination of the three together. Wt NFATC1 alone, PPP3CA alone, and GATA5 alone resulted in 1.8, 11.4 and 21.5 times fold activation respectively. Wt NFATC1 cotransfected with GATA5 caused a synergistic activation of 35 fold, while transfection of Wt NFATC1 with PPP3CA and GATA5 caused even a stronger synergy reaching 68 fold (Figure 7A). The combination of GATA5 with either the P66L or I701L NFATC1 mutants still yield a synergistic activation of the DEGS1 though at a much reduced magnitude as compared to the Wt. Only the double NFATC1 mutant failed to synergistically interact with GATA5.

On the contrary, the interaction of NFATC1 and HAND2, a recently identified pathway implicated in chronic hypoxia, was totally disrupted over the DEGS1 promoter when any of the NFATC1 mutation was introduced (Figure 7B).

Discussion

Congenital heart diseases are still the leading cause of death in newborns in addition to being the most frequent congenital diseases in humans [6]. The genetic mechanisms underlying such diseases however, are being unraveled slowly in the last decade because of the tremendous work done on understanding the molecular mechanisms governing cardiac development in numerous organisms [34]. These mechanisms include the collaborative interaction between transcription factors and their occupancy of conserved *cis* regulatory elements on different cardiac-specific promoters. The cloning and functional characterization of the genes encoding these transcription factors have successfully led to the formulation of hypotheses that mutations in these genes could cause heart malformations in humans. More importantly, the available data on genes such as *GATA4*, *NKX2-5* and *TBX5* do

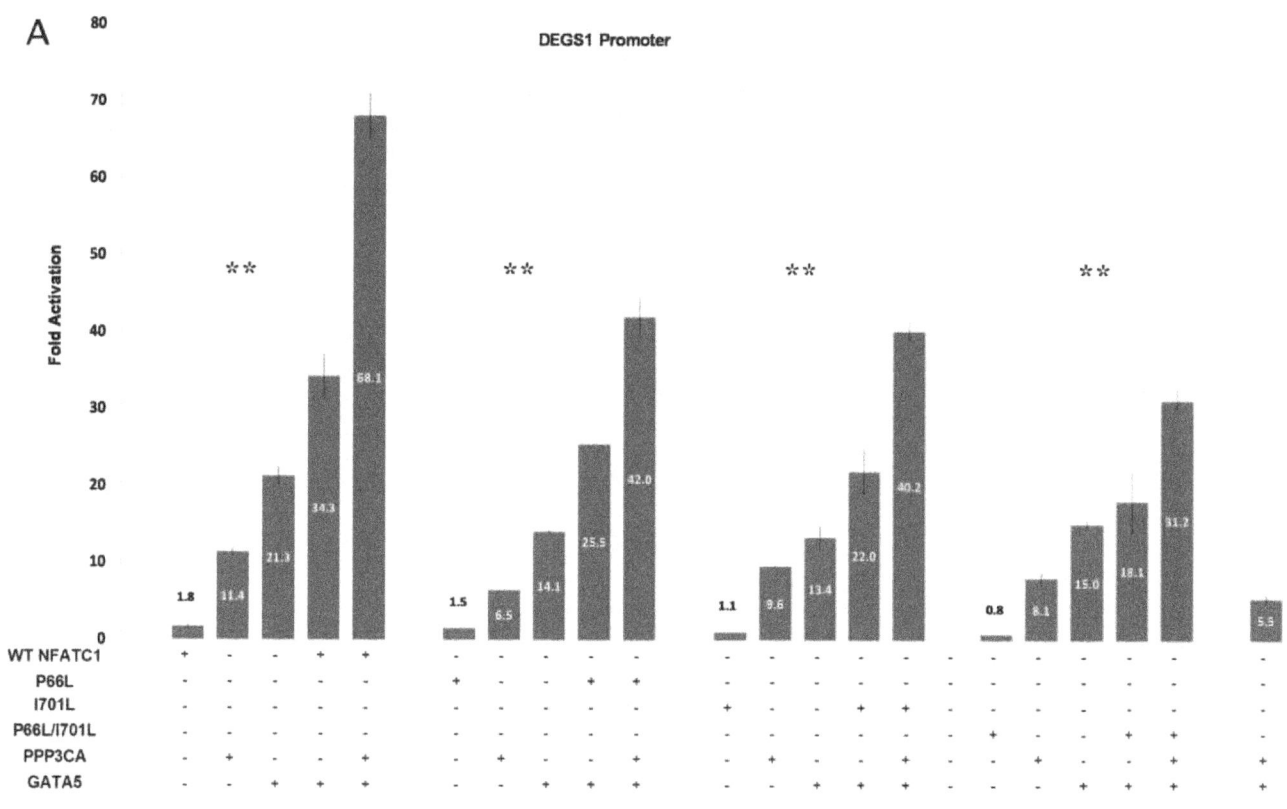

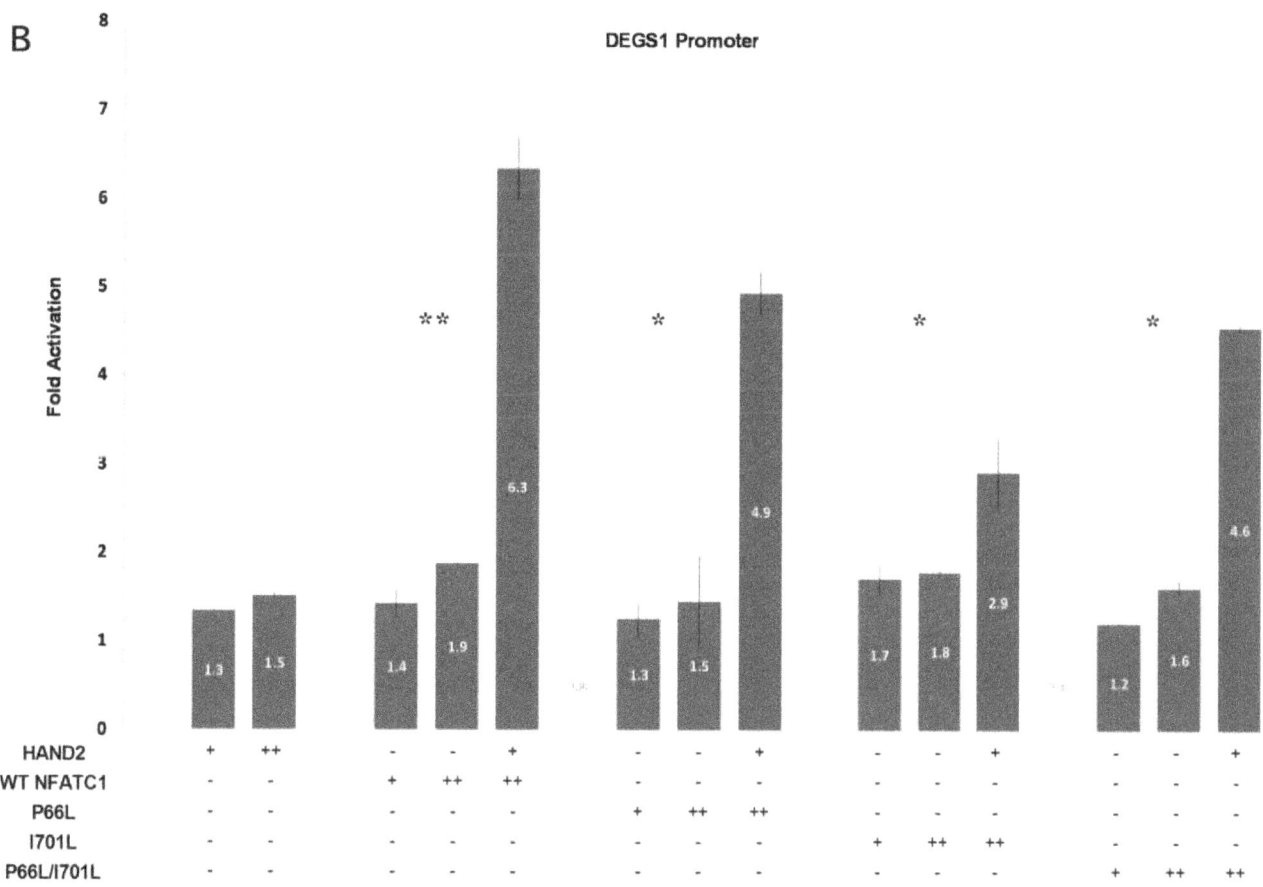

Figure 7. NFATC1 mutations impair functional interactions with GATA5 and HAND2. A- Wt NFATC1 or NFATC1 Mutants (P66L, I701L, P66L/I701L) were transfected with/without HAND2 and the DEGS1 promoter coupled to luciferase reporter construct in Hela cells. Six hours post transfection, media was changed and cells were harvested for luciferase assay after 36 hours. Relative luciferase activities are represented as fold activation. The data are the mean of three independent experiments done in duplicates +/− standard deviation. Wt NFATC1 and HAND2 synergistically activate DEGS1 promoter. This synergy was abrogated in all NFATC1 mutants. Significance (p<0.05) was assessed using the one-way Anova test. (* p<0.01, ** p<0.05) B- Wt NFATC1 or NFATC1 Mutants (P66L, I701L, P66L/I701L) were transfected with/without PPP3CA and with/ without GATA5 to assess their combinatorial regulation of the DEGS1 promoter in HeLa cells. Six hours post transfection, media was changed and cells were harvested for luciferase assay after 36 hours. Relative luciferase activities are represented as fold activation. The data are the mean of three independent experiments done in duplicates +/− standard deviation. Wt NFATC1 cotransfected with GATA5 caused a synergistic activation of 35 fold, while transfection of Wt NFATC1 with PPP3CA and GATA5 caused even a stronger synergy reaching 68 fold. The synergestic activation was maintained in all mutants except for P66L/I701L double mutant where the synergy was totally lost. Significance (p<0.05) was assessed using the one-way Anova test. (* p<0.01, ** p<0.05).

point to a dose-dependent genotype-phenotype correlation whereby haploinsufficiency is by itself diseases-causing [31,35,36,37,38]. Our results go along with what is published in that regard by adding the *NFATC1* gene to the list of mutated genes linked to congenital heart disease in humans, particularly valve diseases.

NFATC1 haploinsufficiency and Tricupid Atresia

We have shown two heterozygous mutations on one allele of the NFATC1 gene in one patient with tricuspid atresia out of 19. The fact that the double mutation is also found in the father who has a normal phenotype argues for incomplete penetrance, a phenomenon seen in other genes encoding transcription factors involved in cardiac and non-cardiac congenital diseases. One such example is the Arg25Cys mutation, which was shown to abrogate the transcriptional activity of the NKX2-5 protein and yet has reduced penetrance depending on the population study groups [39,40]. In mice, the Holt-Oram syndrome recreated with the heterozygous Tbx5 model is the best example of a dosage dependent phenotype-genotype correlation. In fact, null mice for both Tbx5 alleles showed a very severe cardiac phenotype leading to early embryonic lethality, while mice carrying only one Tbx5 allele display a spectrum of phenotypes recapitulating the ones observed in humans [41]. Unfortunately, in our case the indexed-patient was evaluated for the first time at the age of 16 years at our center when he presented with severe cyanosis and complications of his condition which was not well taken care of at earlier stages and had led to the his death few days after his admission to the hospital. Exon by exon sequencing of different genes encoding transcription factors, including *GATA4,5,6*, *TBX5,20*, *NKX2-5*, *PITX2*, and *NFATC1* was carried out on the whole family and none except *NFATC1* showed polymorphisms that could be disease causing. We cannot exclude however, that other not tested gene(s) could also be mutated and carried on the maternally inherited allele, and that the combination of such mutations is responsible for the observed phenotype. Alternatively, we could postulate that the father who is phenotypically normal carries the two mutations on separate alleles and that during spermatogenesis a cross-over did occur leaving the two mutations on one allele inherited by the patient, and another normal inherited by the other children. Structurally, the two mutations leading to amino acids substitution at both the N and C terminal of the protein were predicted to be pathogenic, and in our *in vitro* analysis we did show that the double mutation affects both the transcriptional activity and the localization of the protein. At the subcellular localization level, most of the NFATC1 double mutant proteins failed to translocate to the nucleus when co-expressed with constitutively active calcineurin. Although the mutation is not within the calcineurin docking site, we do suggest that the distorted structure of the protein doesn't allow proper dephosphorylation of its N-terminal domain [16,42,43]. This is supported by the results obtained in gel

shift experiments whereby the DNA binding activity was significantly reduced by 30–40% although the same amount of overrepresed proteins was used for both wild type and mutant NFATC1. On the other hand, the structure function analysis done on the most expressed isoform, Isoform A, does also mask a possible effect the mutation I701L could have on the sumolation process on isoform C which occurs on K702 [44].

The NFATC1 P66L/I701L double mutant: an orphan partner?

NFATC1 is a weak transcription factor although it has a specific and strong DNA affinity. Its activity is however enhanced by its interaction with ubiquitously and/or tissue-specific transcription factors like members of the AP-1 and GATA families [21,45]. GATA5 was previously shown to be a strong partner of NFATC1 and its recent inactivation in mice did show that the embryos develop aortic stenosis one of the most frequent valve abnormalities [19,46]. The observed phenotype in mice involves the formation of a bicuspid aortic valve instead of a tricuspid one suggesting a role of GATA5 similar to that of NFATC1 in the proliferation of valve precursors and final remodeling part. Our results go in parallel with this suggested role, since the interaction of GATA5 and NFATC1 is relatively hampered by the double mutation. In fact, the functional synergy between both proteins was reduced by 50% over the DEGS1 promoter, which was recently shown by our group to be directly regulated by NFAT and HAND2 in chronic hypoxia, a mouse model mimicking cyanotic CHD including Tricuspid Atresia (unpublished data). The HAND2/NFATC1 interaction is also severely affected by the double mutation suggesting a combinatorial interaction between GATA5/NFATC1/HAND2 in a common pathway regulating endocardial cushion formation and valve maturation. One could argue however, that the fact the double mutant is trapped in the cytoplasm might cause the observed inhibition. Nevertheless even with higher doses of transfected mutant vectors, the observed synergy with the wild type protein couldn't be recapitulated. Our hypothetical model would involve regulation of downstream target genes like cyclin D1, which was previously shown to be a direct target for GATA and NFATC1 proteins in the early phases of endocardial cushion proliferation (Figure 8). In fact, in human pulmonary valve endothelial cells, NFATC1 activates in vitro endothelial-specific genes ultimately leading to their proliferation [47]. Furthermore, NFATC1 promotes cell cycle progression in 3T3-L1 cells showing altered expression of cell cycle genes including high levels of cyclin D1 [48]. On the other hand, DEGS1 would be ideal factor involved in valve maturation whereby apoptosis is a key event. In fact, DEGS1 is known to be involved in *de novo* ceramide production, an obligate path leading to apoptosis.

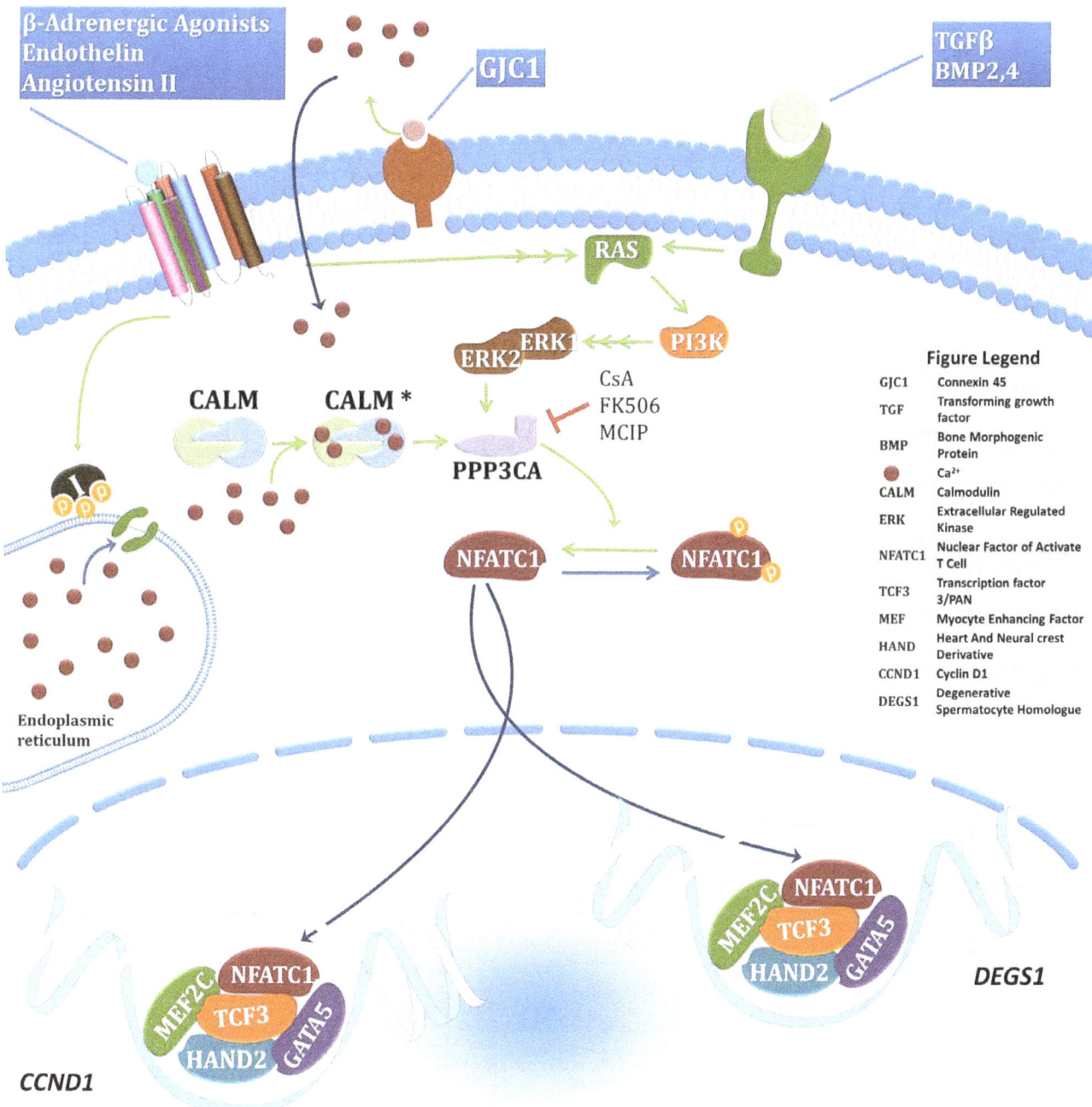

Figure 8. Hypothetical pathway involving NFATC1 in endocardial cushion proliferation and valve maturation.

This hypothetical pathway needs to be supported however by an *in vivo* knock-in model for NFATC1 and a cardiac/endocardial conditional knock-out for DEGS1.

Acknowledgments

The authors would like to thank Mr. Nehme El-Hachem and Miss Theresa Farhat for the Bioinformatics and Biostatistics help, and Mrs Inaam El-Rassy from the Molecular Core Facility at AUB for DNA sequencing. This work was supported by a grant from the Lebanese National Council for Research (LNCSR).

Author Contributions

Conceived and designed the experiments: GN. Performed the experiments: AY ZA KS AS AK JB ES SB. Analyzed the data: GN ZA FB. Contributed reagents/materials/analysis tools: FB GN. Wrote the paper: GN ZA.

References

1. Wirrig EE, Yutzey KE (2011) Transcriptional regulation of heart valve development and disease. Cardiovasc Pathol 20: 162–167.

2. Chakraborty S, Combs MD, Yutzey KE (2010) Transcriptional regulation of heart valve progenitor cells. Pediatr Cardiol 31: 414–421.

3. Armstrong EJ, Bischoff J (2004) Heart valve development: endothelial cell signaling and differentiation. Circ Res 95: 459–470.

4. Beis D, Bartman T, Jin SW, Scott IC, D'Amico LA, et al. (2005) Genetic and cellular analyses of zebrafish atrioventricular cushion and valve development. Development 132: 4193–4204.

5. Jain R, Engleka KA, Rentschler SL, Manderfield LJ, Li L, et al. (2011) Cardiac neural crest orchestrates remodeling and functional maturation of mouse semilunar valves. J Clin Invest 121: 422–430.

6. Hoffman JI, Kaplan S (2002) The incidence of congenital heart disease. J Am Coll Cardiol 39: 1890–1900.

7. Nabulsi MM, Tamim H, Sabbagh M, Obeid MY, Yunis KA, et al. (2003) Parental consanguinity and congenital heart malformations in a developing country. Am J Med Genet A 116A: 342–347.

8. de la Pompa JL, Timmerman LA, Takimoto H, Yoshida H, Elia AJ, et al. (1998) Role of the NF-ATc transcription factor in morphogenesis of cardiac valves and septum. Nature 392: 182–186.

9. Ranger AM, Grusby MJ, Hodge MR, Gravallese EM, de la Brousse FC, et al. (1998) The transcription factor NF-ATc is essential for cardiac valve formation. Nature 392: 186–190.

10. Northrop JP, Ho SN, Chen L, Thomas DJ, Timmerman LA, et al. (1994) NF-AT components define a family of transcription factors targeted in T-cell activation. Nature 369: 497–502.

11. Park J, Takeuchi A, Sharma S (1996) Characterization of a new isoform of the NFAT (nuclear factor of activated T cells) gene family member NFATc. J Biol Chem 271: 20914–20921.

12. Horsley V, Pavlath GK (2002) NFAT: ubiquitous regulator of cell differentiation and adaptation. J Cell Biol 156: 771–774.

13. Crabtree GR, Olson EN (2002) NFAT signaling: choreographing the social lives of cells. Cell 109 Suppl: S67–79.

14. Crabtree GR (1999) Generic signals and specific outcomes: signaling through Ca2+, calcineurin, and NF-AT. Cell 96: 611–614.

15. Rao A, Luo C, Hogan PG (1997) Transcription factors of the NFAT family: regulation and function. Annu Rev Immunol 15: 707–747.

16. Masuda ES, Liu J, Imamura R, Imai SI, Arai KI, et al. (1997) Control of NFATx1 nuclear translocation by a calcineurin-regulated inhibitory domain. Mol Cell Biol 17: 2066–2075.

17. Chin ER, Olson EN, Richardson JA, Yang Q, Humphries C, et al. (1998) A calcineurin-dependent transcriptional pathway controls skeletal muscle fiber type. Genes Dev 12: 2499–2509.

18. Molkentin JD, Lu JR, Antos CL, Markham B, Richardson J, et al. (1998) A calcineurin-dependent transcriptional pathway for cardiac hypertrophy. Cell 93: 215–228.

19. Nemer G, Nemer M (2002) Cooperative interaction between GATA5 and NF-ATc regulates endothelial-endocardial differentiation of cardiogenic cells. Development 129: 4045–4055.

20. Wada H, Hasegawa K, Morimoto T, Kakita T, Yanazume T, et al. (2002) Calcineurin-GATA-6 pathway is involved in smooth muscle-specific transcription. J Cell Biol 156: 983–991.

21. Wisniewska M, Pyrzynska B, Kaminska B (2004) Impaired AP-1 dimers and NFAT complex formation in immature thymocytes during in vivo glucocorticoid-induced apoptosis. Cell Biol Int 28: 773–780.

22. Ikeda F, Nishimura R, Matsubara T, Tanaka S, Inoue J, et al. (2004) Critical roles of c-Jun signaling in regulation of NFAT family and RANKL-regulated osteoclast differentiation. J Clin Invest 114: 475–484.

23. Olson EN, Williams RS (2000) Remodeling muscles with calcineurin. Bioessays 22: 510–519.

24. Asagiri M, Sato K, Usami T, Ochi S, Nishina H, et al. (2005) Autoamplification of NFATc1 expression determines its essential role in bone homeostasis. J Exp Med 202: 1261–1269.

25. Negishi-Koga T, Takayanagi H (2009) Ca2+-NFATc1 signaling is an essential axis of osteoclast differentiation. Immunol Rev 231: 241–256.

26. Kulkarni RM, Greenberg JM, Akeson AL (2009) NFATc1 regulates lymphatic endothelial development. Mech Dev 126: 350–365.

27. Hernandez-Ochoa EO, Contreras M, Cseresnyes Z, Schneider MF (2007) Ca2+ signal summation and NFATc1 nuclear translocation in sympathetic ganglion neurons during repetitive action potentials. Cell Calcium 41: 559–571.

28. Chang CP, Neilson JR, Bayle JH, Gestwicki JE, Kuo A, et al. (2004) A field of myocardial-endocardial NFAT signaling underlies heart valve morphogenesis. Cell 118: 649–663.

29. Schulz RA, Yutzey KE (2004) Calcineurin signaling and NFAT activation in cardiovascular and skeletal muscle development. Dev Biol 266: 1–16.

30. Yehya A, Souki R, Bitar F, Nemer G (2006) Differential duplication of an intronic region in the NFATC1 gene in patients with congenital heart disease. Genome 49: 1092–1098.

31. Nemer G, Fadlalah F, Usta J, Nemer M, Dbaibo G, et al. (2006) A novel mutation in the GATA4 gene in patients with Tetralogy of Fallot. Hum Mutat 27: 293–294.

32. Yamak AA, Bitar F, Karam P, Nemer G (2007) Exclusive cardiac dysfunction in familial primary carnitine deficiency cases: a genotype-phenotype correlation. Clin Genet 72: 59–62.

33. Karpurapu M, Wang D, Van Quyen D, Kim TK, Kundumani-Sridharan V, et al. (2010) Cyclin D1 is a bona fide target gene of NFATc1 and is sufficient in the mediation of injury-induced vascular wall remodeling. J Biol Chem 285: 3510–3523.

34. Olson EN (2006) Gene regulatory networks in the evolution and development of the heart. Science 313: 1922–1927.

35. Schott JJ, Benson DW, Basson CT, Pease W, Silberbach GM, et al. (1998) Congenital heart disease caused by mutations in the transcription factor NKX2-5. Science 281: 108–111.

36. Reamon-Buettner SM, Borlak J (2004) TBX5 mutations in non-Holt-Oram syndrome (HOS) malformed hearts. Hum Mutat 24: 104.

37. Pehlivan T, Pober BR, Brueckner M, Garrett S, Slaugh R, et al. (1999) GATA4 haploinsufficiency in patients with interstitial deletion of chromosome region 8p23.1 and congenital heart disease. Am J Med Genet 83: 201–206.

38. Mori AD, Bruneau BG (2004) TBX5 mutations and congenital heart disease: Holt-Oram syndrome revealed. Curr Opin Cardiol 19: 211–215.

39. Elliott DA, Kirk EP, Yeoh T, Chandar S, McKenzie F, et al. (2003) Cardiac homeobox gene NKX2-5 mutations and congenital heart disease: associations with atrial septal defect and hypoplastic left heart syndrome. J Am Coll Cardiol 41: 2072–2076.

40. Akcaboy MI, Cengiz FB, Inceoglu B, Ucar T, Atalay S, et al. (2008) The effect of p.Arg25Cys alteration in NKX2-5 on conotruncal heart anomalies: mutation or polymorphism? Pediatr Cardiol 29: 126–129.

41. Bruneau BG, Nemer G, Schmitt JP, Charron F, Robitaille L, et al. (2001) A murine model of Holt-Oram syndrome defines roles of the T-box transcription factor Tbx5 in cardiogenesis and disease. Cell 106: 709–721.

42. Rodriguez A, Roy J, Martinez-Martinez S, Lopez-Maderuelo MD, Nino-Moreno P, et al. (2009) A conserved docking surface on calcineurin mediates interaction with substrates and immunosuppressants. Mol Cell 33: 616–626.

43. Martinez-Martinez S, Redondo JM (2004) Inhibitors of the calcineurin/NFAT pathway. Curr Med Chem 11: 997–1007.

44. Nayak A, Glockner-Pagel J, Vaeth M, Schumann JE, Buttmann M, et al. (2009) Sumoylation of the transcription factor NFATc1 leads to its subnuclear relocalization and interleukin-2 repression by histone deacetylase. J Biol Chem 284: 10935–10946.

45. Musaro A, McCullagh KJ, Naya FJ, Olson EN, Rosenthal N (1999) IGF-1 induces skeletal myocyte hypertrophy through calcineurin in association with GATA-2 and NF-ATc1. Nature 400: 581–585.

46. Laforest B, Andelfinger G, Nemer M (2011) Loss of Gata5 in mice leads to bicuspid aortic valve. J Clin Invest 121: 2876–2887.

47. Johnson EN, Lee YM, Sander TL, Rabkin E, Schoen FJ, et al. (2003) NFATc1 mediates vascular endothelial growth factor-induced proliferation of human pulmonary valve endothelial cells. J Biol Chem 278: 1686–1692.

48. Neal JW, Clipstone NA (2003) A constitutively active NFATc1 mutant induces a transformed phenotype in 3T3-L1 fibroblasts. J Biol Chem 278: 17246–17254.

11

Deficient Signaling via Alk2 (Acvr1) Leads to Bicuspid Aortic Valve Development

Penny S. Thomas[1], Somyoth Sridurongrit[1¤], Pilar Ruiz-Lozano[2], Vesa Kaartinen[1]*

1 Department of Biologic and Materials Sciences, University of Michigan, Ann Arbor, Michigan, United States of America, 2 Department of Pediatrics, Stanford University School of Medicine, Stanford, California, United States of America

Abstract

Bicuspid aortic valve (BAV) is the most common congenital cardiac anomaly in humans. Despite recent advances, the molecular basis of BAV development is poorly understood. Previously it has been shown that mutations in the *Notch1* gene lead to BAV and valve calcification both in human and mice, and mice deficient in *Gata5* or its downstream target *Nos3* have been shown to display BAVs. Here we show that tissue-specific deletion of the gene encoding Activin Receptor Type I (*Alk2* or *Acvr1*) in the cushion mesenchyme results in formation of aortic valve defects including BAV. These defects are largely due to a failure of normal development of the embryonic aortic valve leaflet precursor cushions in the outflow tract resulting in either a fused right- and non-coronary leaflet, or the presence of only a very small, rudimentary non-coronary leaflet. The surviving adult mutant mice display aortic stenosis with high frequency and occasional aortic valve insufficiency. The thickened aortic valve leaflets in such animals do not show changes in Bmp signaling activity, while Map kinase pathways are activated. Although dysfunction correlated with some pro-osteogenic differences in gene expression, neither calcification nor inflammation were detected in aortic valves of *Alk2* mutants with stenosis. We conclude that signaling via Alk2 is required for appropriate aortic valve development in utero, and that defects in this process lead to indirect secondary complications later in life.

Editor: Saverio Bellusci, Childrens Hospital Los Angeles, United States of America

Funding: This study was financially supported by the National Institutes of Health RO1 grant number HL074862 (http://www.nih.gov). The funders had no role in study design, data collection and analysis, decision to publish, or preparation of the manuscript.

Competing Interests: The authors have declared that no competing interests exist.

* E-mail: vesa@umich.edu

¤ Current address: Department of Anatomy, Mahidol University, Bangkok,Thailand

Introduction

Bicuspid aortic valve (BAV) is the most common cardiac malformation affecting 1–2% people worldwide [1–3]. While those with BAV often remain asymptomatic for years, almost all will eventually require surgical intervention [3]. The molecular mechanisms underlying BAV formation are still poorly elucidated. In humans, mutations in the *NOTCH1* gene have been shown to lead to BAV [4]. An increased incidence of BAV has also been found in in mice deficient in the transcription factor Nkx2-5 [5], endothelium-specific nitric oxide synthase *Nos3* [6] and, most recently, transcription factor Gata5, which is proposed to positively regulate *Nos3* expression and affect the Notch signaling pathway [7].

An initial key event in cardiac valve development is formation of endocardial cushions [8], which starts with a regional increase of cardiac jelly, a hyaluronic acid-rich extracellular matrix (ECM), between the myocardial and endocardial cell layers at the sites of the future atrio-ventricular junction (AVJ) and outflow tract (OFT) [9]. This is followed by transformation of a subset of the overlying endocardial cells to mesenchymal cells (EMT) [10] which migrate into the underlying ECM to populate the cushions. In the OFT, the proximal cushion mesenchyme is so derived from the endocardium, and much of the more distal cushion mesenchyme is of cranial neural crest origin [11]. Before OFT septation, four ridge-like cushions spiral around the internal circumference of the

OFT lumen; two larger (septal and parietal) and, between them, two smaller (anterior and posterior intercalated). The two larger cushions fuse across the midline of the OFT lumen, creating separate outlet lumens connecting the left and right ventricles to their respective arterial valves (aortic and pulmonary). Around each of these, further cushion growth from each of the larger (fused) cushions and the intercalated cushion forms the three arterial valve leaflet precursors for each truncal valve (aortic and pulmonary) [12]. After further development, the right and left coronary arteries connect to the aortic valve sinuses in characteristic positions immediately downstream of the right and left coronary leaflet precursors respectively [13]. The remaining leaflet, the 'non-coronary', is the one arising from the intercalated cushion position. These cushions undergo characteristic morphogenesis to form three flexible apposing leaflets and adjacent sinuses [14]. Normal function of these leaflets requires that they are sufficiently apart during ventricular systole, and appose each other to prevent backflow during diastole, otherwise aortic stenosis and insufficiency respectively will result. A critical distinctive extracellular matrix arrangement is required to maintain these properties throughout life [15–17]. With time, or if the leaflets are abnormal in shape or number, the leaflets are more likely to fail mechanically and develop abnormal structure and function [18,19]. From examination of human examples, a reduction in effective leaflet number to form a bicuspid (two leaflet, or bifoliate) aortic valve

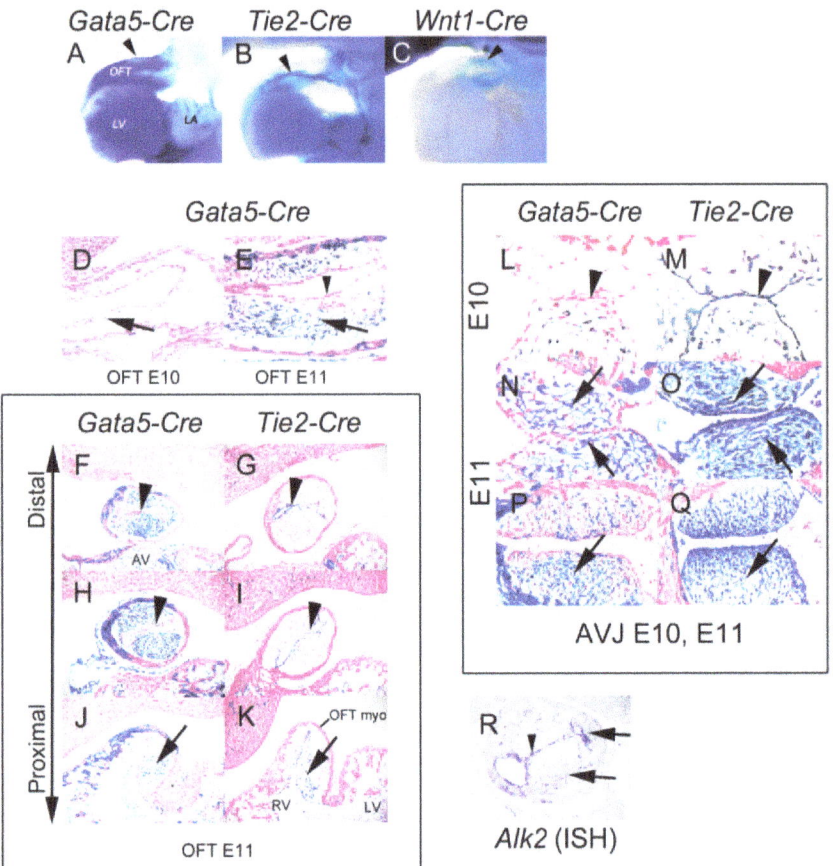

Figure 1. The *Gata5-Cre* transgene induces recombination in the endocardial cushion mesenchyme after EMT. Comparison of areas of *Gata5-Cre (A)*, *Tie2-Cre* (B) and *Wnt1-Cre* (C) recombination (blue) in OFT region (arrowhead) at E11.5 (wholemount *R26R*-driven βgal stain, viewed from the left side, distal OFT to the right). βgal staining of sagittal sections at E10 (D) and at E11 (E) shows extensive *Gata5-Cre*-induced recombination in OFT cushion mesenchyme by E11 (arrow), but not in endocardium (arrowhead). Comparison of *Gata5-Cre* (F, H and J) and *Tie2-Cre* (G, I and K) recombination patterns (*R26R*-driven β-gal stain in blue) at three levels of the OFT, from proximal (J, K) to distal (F, G). *Tie2-Cre* (arrowheads, G, I) but not *Gata5-Cre* (arrowheads F, H) drives recombination (blue) in endocardium; recombined mesenchymal cells (blue) in both lines (arrows, J, K) only in proximal OFT. Comparison of *Gata5-Cre* and (L, N and P) *Tie2-Cre* (M, O and Q) recombination at AV junction: sagittal sections (L–O) at E10 (L, M) and E11 (N, O) and transverse sections at E11 (P, Q). At E10 (L, M) endocardium (arrowhead) recombined (blue) by *Tie2-Cre* but not *Gata5-Cre*. At E11 (N–P) AV mesenchymal cells (arrows) recombined (blue) by both *Tie2-Cre* and *Gata5-Cre*. R, In situ hybridization for *Alk2* RNA showing expression (blue) in OFT cushion mesenchyme (black arrows) and endocardium (arrowhead) at E11.5. LV, left ventricle; RV, right ventricle; OFT myo, OFT myocardium; AV, AV cushion; AVJ, atrioventricular junction.

(BAV) has been proposed to arise to from fusion of two leaflets, including before birth at the 'cushion' stage, rather than the presence of only two leaflet cushions per arterial valve at the outset.

In humans, anatomical classification of BAVs indicates all combinations of leaflet fusion can be found, the two most common being right- with non-coronary leaflets (R-N), and right with left-coronary leaflets (R-L) [3,20]. A recent comparative study of the *Nos3* knockout mouse (R-L) and inbred Syrian hamster (R-L) bicuspid models demonstrates that the etiologies of these phenotypes are different [21]. Given that patients with R-N leaflet fusion develop different clinical phenotypes from those of patients with R-L leaflet fusion, mechanistic understanding of aortic valve development at both morphological and molecular levels is of critical importance [22,23].

Bmp signaling has been shown to play a critical role during cardiac valve development. Several studies have shown that Bmp2 is able to induce EMT both in vitro and in vivo [24,25]. Both Bmp type I receptor Alk3 (Bmpr1a) and Activin type I receptor (Alk2; Acvr1) are expressed in the endocardium, and epithelium-specific

deletion of these receptors leads to EMT defects in both OFT and AV cushions [25–28]. The importance of Alk2-mediated signaling in human cardiac disease is highlighted by recent studies, which demonstrate that mutations in the *ALK2* gene are also responsible for cardiac defects in humans [29,30].

While the role of *Alk2* in endothelial EMT is well-established [26], very little is known about Alk2-mediated Bmp signaling in subsequent stages of valve development. In this study we examined the role of Alk2 in cardiac valve development by deleting *Alk2* function in the cushion mesenchyme after EMT using the *Gata5-Cre* driver line. Most of the resulting *Alk2* mutant mice developed aortic valve defects characterized as 'functional' BAV as they consisted of only two, apposed, morphologically functional aortic leaflets (or their precursors), even if other structures were present, prior to birth. A subset of mutant mice that survived to adulthood developed aortic insufficiency and/or stenosis associated with some markers of a pro-osteogenic phenotype: attenuated *Sox9* expression, increased *osteopontin (Spp1)* expression and activated Erk1/2 but did not develop calcification. These results suggest that signaling via Alk2 is required for normal aortic valve development and that defects in this process lead an increased incidence of aortic insufficiency and/or stenosis and formation of a bicuspid aortic valve phenotype commonly found in humans.

Results

Gata5-Cre drives an efficient recombination in the endocardial cushion mesenchyme

The *Gata5-Cre* transgenic mouse line was originally designed as an epicardium-specific driver line [31]. When analyzing recombination patterns in these mice, we noticed that in addition to epicardial cells and occasional myocardial cells, efficient recombination could also be detected in endocardial cushion mesenchyme at both the OFT and AV junction at E11 (Figure 1). Unlike the *Wnt1-Cre* and *Tie2-Cre* drivers, which induce recombination in neural crest (NC) cells including the distal cushion mesenchyme, and in endothelial cells and endocardium-derived proximal cushion mesenchyme, respectively, *Gata5-Cre*-induced recombination occurred in mesenchyme the entire length of the OFT cushions (Figure 1A–C). Recombination occurred soon after mesenchyme cell formation or arrival (E11) in OFT and AV cushions (Figure 1D–Q), but did not start in the overlying endocardial cells until E12 (data not shown). We have previously shown that, in addition to endocardial cells, *Alk2* is strongly expressed in the newly formed AV cushion mesenchyme [26]. Similarly, *Alk2* is expressed in the OFT endocardium, as well as in the NC-derived and endocardium-derived OFT cushion mesenchyme (Figure 1R).

Deletion of Alk2 in the post-EMT cushion mesenchyme leads to valve and septal defects

To investigate roles for Alk2 in mesenchyme during valve formation and maturation following EMT we deleted *Alk2* function there using the *Gata5-Cre* driver line. A role in these events for Alk2 expressed in other cell types in which *Gata5-Cre*-induced recombination occurs (epicardium and patches of differentiated myocardium) can be largely ignored as key epicardium-dependent events were not affected when *Alk2* function was deleted using the epicardial driver *Tbx18-Cre* (Figure S1) or in the working myocardium [26].

At E11, OFT cushions in *Alk2/Gata5-Cre* mutants contained numerous mesenchymal cells arranged in characteristic cushions indistinguishable from those of *Alk2/Gata5-Cre⁻* controls despite efficient recombination of the *Alk2* gene as shown by the RT PCR assay using primers flanking exon 7 which is deleted in the recombined allele [32] (Figure 2), and reduced downstream signaling: a 50% reduction in Smad1,5,8 phosphorylation levels in OFT cushion tissues harvested at E12.

By E14, *Alk2/Gata5-Cre* mutants had developed abnormal cardiac phenotypes that showed high penetrance (Table 1). Seven out of nine mutant embryos displayed essentially bicuspid (two leaflet or bifoliate) aortic valves (BAVs) and/or perimembranous ventricular septal defects (VSDs) (Table 1). In all controls (*Alk2^{FXWT}/Gata5-Cre⁻*) examined, fusion events to complete the ventricular septum had occurred and the aortic valves had three normal leaflets. No abnormal pulmonary valves, or defects in great artery development were found in controls or mutants.

Detailed histological examination (representative examples shown in Figure 3) were undertaken to define the morphology of the mutant aortic valves at E14 and E17, and to enable comparison with established rodent models of BAV [22] and bicuspid human aortic valves [33]. The abnormal valve phenotype was manifest as two large leaflet cushions and one much smaller, less developed, leaflet cushion in the non-coronary position at E14

(Figure 3F), and functionally bicuspid aortic valves (i.e. morphological evidence that the function of preventing backflow was being performed by only two, large apposing leaflets) at E17 (Figure 3K, L). By this later stage, a spectrum of abnormal right and non-coronary leaflet development was found, ranging from apparent fusion (as implied by the presence of a raphe, for example: Figure 3N) to the presence of a small, poorly developed cushion in the non-coronary position but slightly proximal to the level of apposition of the two, functional, leaflets (Figure 3O, R). Position and number of coronary orifices was normal in all mutants examined (Figure 3A, B, G–I) and these and the relative position of the pulmonary valve enabled the position of the abnormal/'missing' valve cushion to be consistently identified. Thus the bicuspid phenotype here more closely resembled the mouse BAV models in which *Gata5* or *Nos3* are deficient, as the hamster model involves common or fused right- and left-, and not non-coronary, leaflets. It was also notable that, even in E18 control valves, the right and non-coronary leaflet cushions had not yet become separated more proximally to form an 'interleaflet triangle', unlike the other leaflet pairs (Figure 3M,P). This maintained proximity may contribute to or reflect the mechanism by which this class of bicuspid valve persists into postnatal life.

45% of *Alk2/Gata5-Cre* mutants survived to 3 weeks postnatally (n = 53). In surviving postnatal mutants at two months and older, 3 of 22 examined had a functionally bicuspid aortic valve (Figure 3T) of the same pattern as identified prenatally. Overall, a spectrum of aortic valve phenotypes was present, including tricuspid, tricuspid with a smaller non-coronary leaflet, and functionally bicuspid with a very small third sinus and thickened non-coronary leaflet only revealed by sectioning (data not shown). Valves identified as functionally stenotic had irregularly thickened leaflets on sectioning whether bi or tri-cuspid (see the results below and data not shown).

The VSD phenotype found in 7 of 9 mutant hearts at E14 was detectable in only 2 out of 6 mutants at E18, suggesting earlier VSDs likely represented a subtle delay in fusion that could still could be 'rescued' during the last four gestational days. Besides the aortic valves, *Alk2/Gata5-Cre* mutants also displayed abnormally short and muscular right atrioventricular valve leaflets at E18 when compared to corresponding control littermates, while the left atriocentricular valves appeared grossly normal (Figure 4).

Cushion mesenchyme deficient in Alk2 showed reduced cell proliferation and altered gene expression

Maturation of cushion morphology is tightly coordinated with growth by cell proliferation and remodeling by programmed cell death. A 20–25% reduction in mesenchymal cell proliferation has previously been reported in *Gata5*-deficient BAV model mice [7], so we looked for differences in these processes between *Alk2/Gata5-Cre* mutants and controls. At E11 and E12, a period of rapid cushion growth, *Alk2/Gata5-Cre* mutant OFT cushions showed a 40% reduction in proliferation when compared to controls (Figure 5), but no detectable changes in apoptosis at E12 (data not shown).

Transcription factors and ECM components have been proposed to contribute to cushion morphogenesis. Sox9 and Tbx20 have been reported as positive regulators of cushion mesenchyme proliferation and Bmp2, a possible ligand for Alk2, shown to induce *Tbx20* expression indirectly in vitro [23,24,25] so we examined their expression by in situ hybridization (ISH). There was no difference in staining pattern in cushion endocardium for either RNA between control and mutant, including areas of higher expression (Figure 6I,J). In cushion mesenchymal cells, expression of both genes was easily detected in both control and mutant

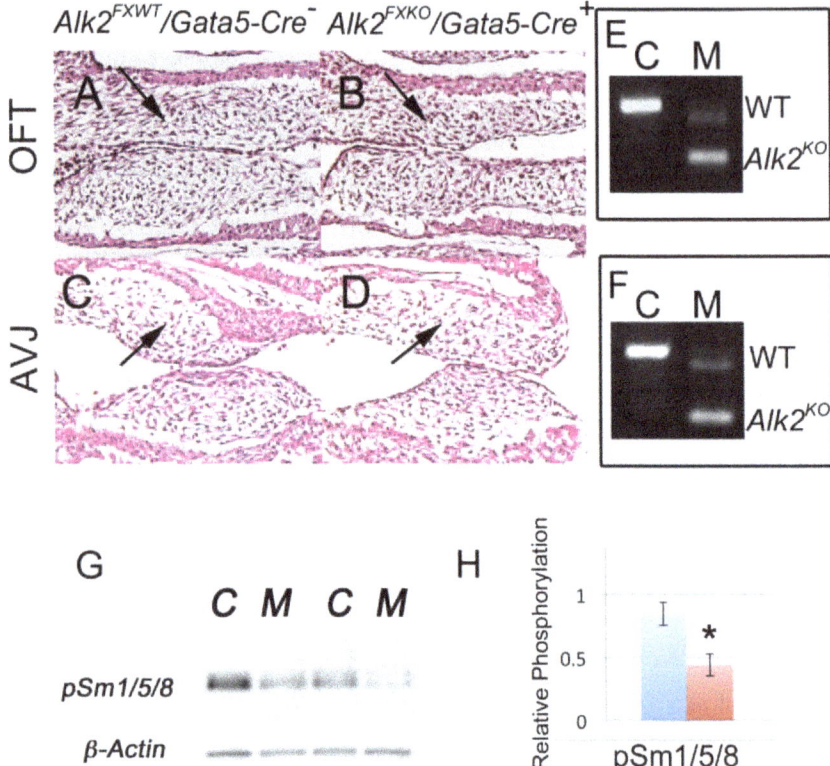

Figure 2. The overall cushion morphology is unaffected in *Alk2/Gata5-Cre* mutants at E11. H&E-stained sagittal sections through OFT cushions (A, B) and AV cushions (C, D) show plentiful mesenchymal cells in controls (A, C) and *Alk2/Gata5-Cre* mutants (B, D). Black arrows in A–D point to cushion mesenchyme. E–F, RT-PCR analysis of mRNAs from OFT (E) and AVJ (F) tissues at E11.5. C *Alk2^{FXWT}/Gata5-Cre^−* control; M *Alk2^{FXKO}/Gata5-Cre^+* mutant. The shorter amplification product (*Alk2^{KO}*) predominant in mutant tissues confirms an efficient Cre-induced recombination. G, *Gata5-Cre*-induced recombination leads to reduction in Smad 1/5/8 phosphorylation in mutant (M) relative to control (C) E12.5 OFT tissue protein lysates analyzed by immunoblotting. H, Bar graph shows relative quantification of phospho-Smad1/5/8 in control (blue) and mutant (red) OFT tissues at E12.5 (normalized to β-actin; n = 3). Error bars, SEM; *p<0.05.

cushions (Figure 6A–J) suggesting no simple dependence on Alk2 function. A more detailed examination of the relative stain intensities within the same section showed variation amongst adjacent mesenchyme cells in the same cushion. While some of this may be attributable to cells cut by sectioning there are areas where all the cells appear less stained (for *Tbx20* in mutant OFT cushion: Figure 6H; the same regional pattern was obtained on a sister section (data not shown).

It was recently shown that proteolytic cleavage of versican, a large extracellular matrix proteoglycan, is an important step in the regulation of late embryonic valve development and that a failure in this process leads to formation of thick myxomatous valves [34]. While versican protein levels were comparable between *Alk2/Gata5-Cre* mutants and controls (Figure 6K–L), immunostaining also detected less cleaved versican in mutant AV, but not OFT,

cushions (Figure 7). In addition, immunostaining for the extra-cellular matrix glycoprotein, tenascin-C, expression of which has been shown to be associated with areas undergoing major structural changes during OFT morphogenesis in the chick [35], was reduced in both OFT cushions and in developing AV valves (Figure 6Q–T). These results imply that Alk2-mediated signaling is involved in regulation of extracellular matrix deposition and/or remodeling. However, the lack of differences in anti-DPEAAE-positive immunostaining between *Alk2* mutant and control OFT cushions argues that Adamts-induced versican cleavage here is not involved in development of the aortic valve phenotype observed in *Alk2/Gata5-Cre* mutants.

Despite a reduced proliferation rate in OFT mesenchyme at E11 and 12, sufficient mesenchymal cells were present in time for both AV and OFT septation to occur in mutants, However, other cushion-related abnormalities occurred subsequently, so subtle defects in expression and processing of molecules such as those discussed above might still leave *Alk2/Gata5-Cre* mutants more vulnerable to morphological abnormalities and environmental or epigenetic effects.

Expression of key regulators associated with BAVs or valve maturation

It has previously been shown that defective function of *Notch1, Gata5* or *Nos3* leads to BAV development, and that, where

Table 1. BAV and VSD in *Alk2/Gata5-Cre* mutants.

Stage	Genotype	Total	BAV (percentage)	VSD (percentage)
E14	Alk2^{KOFX}/Gata5-Cre+	9	7 (78%)	7 (78%)
E17–E18	Alk2^{KOFX}/Gata5-Cre+	6	5 (83%)	2 (33%)

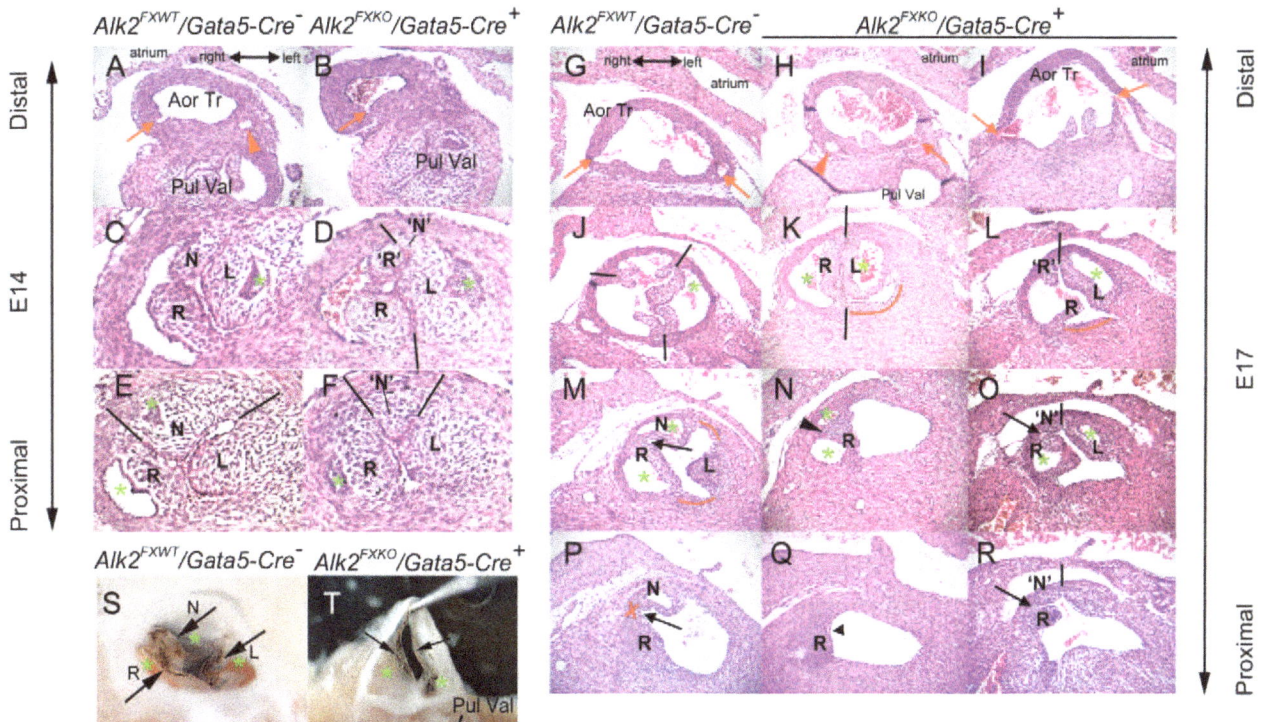

Figure 3. *Gata5-Cre*-induced deletion of *Alk2* function leads to defective development of aortic valves. A–F: Histological comparison of representative control (A, C, E) and mutant (B, D, F) aortic valves at E14; approximately transverse sections of the same valves at three levels. A, B: lower magnification at the level of coronary orifices (red arrow; coronary vessel: red arrowhead), where formed, distal to aortic valve leaflets showing normal development and relationship of aortic-side structures relative to pulmonary valve. All three control aortic leaflet cushions show evidence of excavation forming sinuses (green *): left (L) in panel C, right (R) and non-coronary (N) in panel E. N cushion occupies a similar segment of the circumference (black lines) as each of R and L (in E). In mutant valve, L (in D) and R (in F) leaflet cushions show normal excavation. Cushion 'R', although in the same position as N in control, is continuous with tissue R (panel D), not simply apposed as in control (in C). Nearer the base of the leaflet cushions (in E, F), mutant R is larger than control R. A small cushion ('N') is present between L and 'R' (in D, F), but shows no evidence of excavation and occupies a much smaller segment of the circumference (black lines in F) than N in control, so the valve is functionally bicuspid (bifoliate), with two excavating leaflet cushions, L and R/'R', apposing one another distally (in D). **G–R**: Histological comparison of representative control (A, J, M, P) and two functionally bicuspid mutant (H, K, N, Q and I, L, O, R) aortic valves at E17; approximately transverse sections of the same valves at four levels. G-I, at the level of coronary orifices showing their consistent position above right and left coronary leaflets, and consistent positioning of the leaflets in relation to adjacent tissues, in control and mutants. All three control aortic leaflet walls lie adjacent to well-developed sinuses (green *) left (L) in panel J, right (R) and non-coronary (N) in panel M. N leaflet occupies a similar segment of the circumference (black lines) as R and L (in J). Two examples of functionally bicuspid mutant valves are shown to illustrate key details of their morphology at this stage. The example in H, K, N, Q has features consistent with a fusion of R and N leaflets. Distally (K), only two leaflets, R and L, appose each other, with no small leaflet between them in the non-coronary position, each occupying about half the circumference (black lines). More proximally, the sinus of the R leaflet is divided into two (green *) by a raphe (black arrowhead) in N, but the leaflet does not then divide into two separate bases (arrowhead, Q). Distally the mutant valve shown in I, L, O, R also consists of two leaflets (in panel L; as R and 'R' are joined more proximally) that are not separated by a small cushion, but more proximally, one ('N') present. An area representing an interleaflet triangle (red curved line) can be identified between L and R leaflets in control (in M) and mutant (K, L) valves, and between L and N (control, in M) but the bases of the R and N leaflets even in control remain adjacent (in P, red X, black arrow) though not continuous (unlike Q). **S,T**: 6 month old adult control aortic valve with normal left (L) right (R) and non-coronary (N) leaflets (black arrows) and three sinuses (green*), and partially dissected functionally bicuspid aortic valve in *Alk2/Gata5-Cre* mutant, demonstrating two leaflets (black arrows) which appose only with each other across the entire lumen, and two sinuses (green *). Aor Tr, Aortic trunk; Pul Val, Pulmonary Valve.

investigated, the abnormal morphology was already detectable as early as E11.5 [7]. To examine whether abnormal expression of these genes was part of the mechanism underlying our model we therefore compared the mRNA expression patterns of using ISH (*Notch1*, *Gata5*) or immunofluorescence (Nos3) at E11, and at several levels of the OFT to ensure that regional defects in expression, perhaps associated specifically with the future intercalated cushion development, were not missed. In both control and mutant sections, the expression of all three genes was detected in AV and OFT endocardium, and in a somewhat similar, non-uniform, way both along the length of the OFT and around its lumen (Figure 7). *Notch1* and Nos3 were detected in most if not all OFT endocardial cells but staining was stronger (or

appeared sooner) more distally, and in lateral areas between adjacent cushions and where the intercalated cushions were developing. *Gata5* endocardial expression was harder to detect but present in endocardium adjacent to rather than over the two main cushions at distal and mid-levels, the same areas in which *Notch1* and Nos3 staining was also higher (Figure 7G–L). They were all detected in endocardium over the proximal cushion as it extends into the ventricle (Figure 7M–R). We also examined expression of *Notch1* target genes *Hey1* and *Hey2* (Figure S2). In OFT endocardial cells, *Hey1* expression was highly restricted, principally to the endocardium between the main cushions, similar to that of *Gata5* (see above). *Hey2* expression was detected in most OFT endocardial cells, in a pattern very similar to that of *Notch1*. In AV

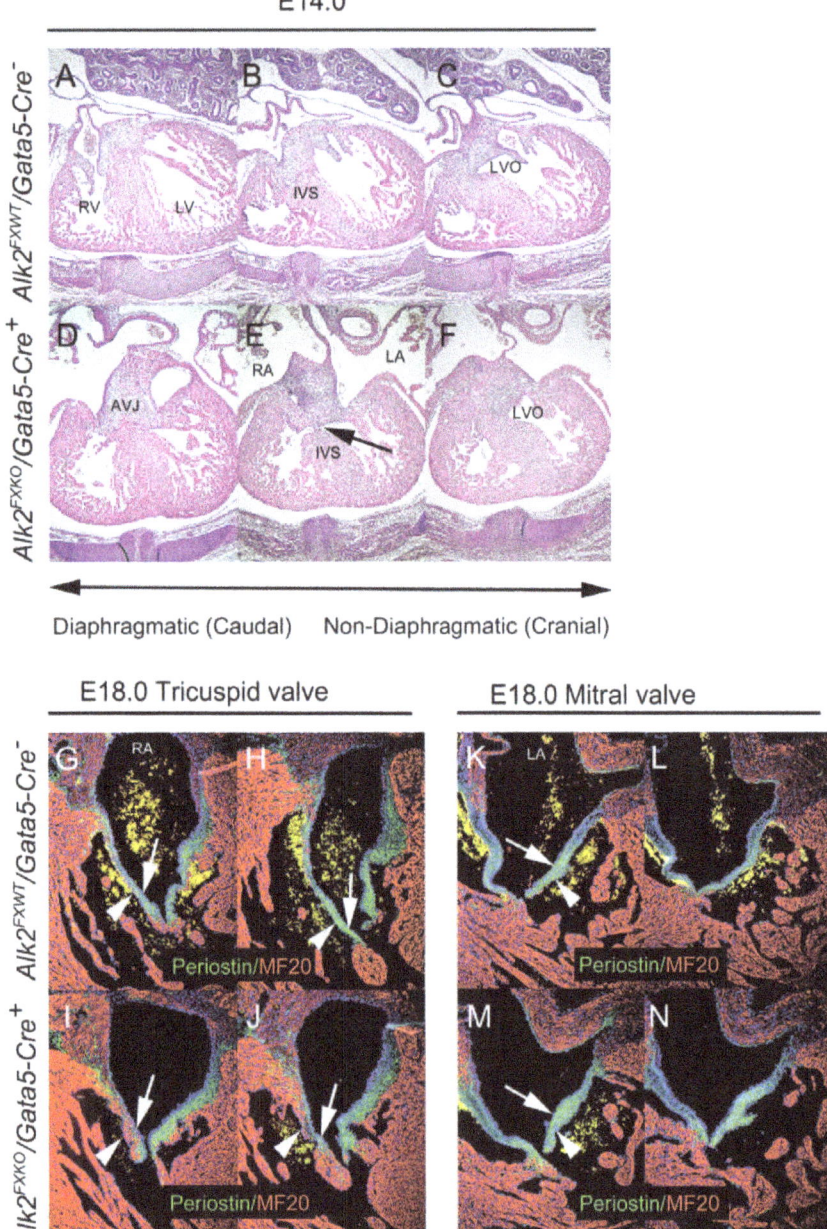

Figure 4. Ventricular septal defect and abnormal right atrioventricular valve leaflets in *Alk2/Gata5-Cre* mutants. H&E-stained sections of control (A–C) and *Alk2/Gata5-Cre* mutant (D–F) at three different levels showing perimembranous VSD in mutant (black arrow in E) but not control. Right (G–J) and left (K–N) atrioventricular valves from control (G, H, K, L) and *Alk2/Gata5-Cre* mutant (I, J, M, N) samples. Representative immunostained sections from two levels from each heart are shown: periostin (green), MF20 (red). Postero-inferior leaflet (G–J) shorter with less periostin-positive tissue (green) in mutant (I, J) than control (G, H) (arrows) and more myocardium (red: arrowheads). Control (K, L) and mutant (M, N) left AV valve leaflets do not differ (arrows, arrowheads). AVJ posterior side of atrioventricular junction; IVS muscular part of ventricular septum; LA, left atrium; LV, left ventricle; LVO, outlet part of LV leading to aortic valve; RA, right atrium; RV, right ventricle.

endocardium, expression of both these genes appeared in only a small subset of *Notch1*-positive cells, *Hey1* being almost completely undetected. Again we could demonstrate no consistent differences in expression between control and mutant tissues.

Levels of mesenchymal staining present in sections probed for these genes were too low to interpret and compare (Figure 7, Figure S2 and data not shown). Nos3 expression was not detected above background in mesenchyme cells by immunofluorescence. In non-endocardial cells, *Gata5* and *Hey1* expressions were

detected in overlapping domains of second heart field cells of the distal OFT, *Hey1* expression in atrial appendage myocardium and a regional population of epicardial cells, *Hey2* in ventricular wall myocardium and Gata5 weakly in AV and some OFT myocardium (Figure 7, Figure S2 and data not shown).

From this detailed examination of expression of genes previously associated with BAV, we conclude that although there were regional differences in gene expression within the OFT consistent with a role for these genes in the development of the

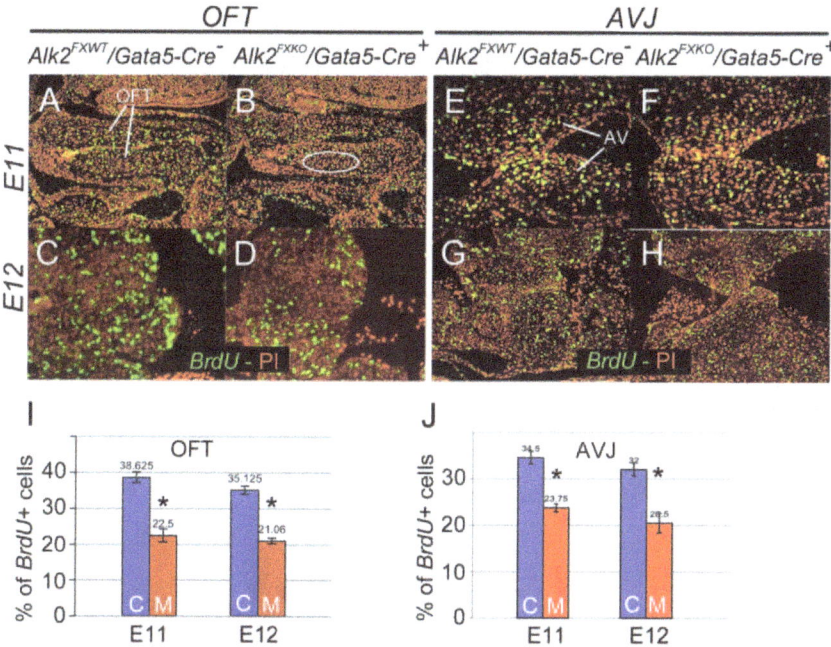

Figure 5. Less proliferation in endocardial cushion mesenchyme in *Alk2/Gata5-Cre* mutants. Representative images of anti-BrdU immunostaining (green-yellow) of control (A, C, E, G) and *Alk2/Gata5-Cre* mutant (B, D, F, H) sagittal sections at E11 (A, B, E, F) and E12 (C, D, G, H). A–D, OFT cushions; E–H, AV cushions. Mutant OFT cushion shows patchy incidence of BrdU- labeled nuclei (e.g., less in myocardium-adjacent region ringed by white ellipse). Bar graphs (I, J) illustrate differences in proportion of BrdU-labeled nuclei in the OFT (I) and AVJ (J) mesenchyme at E11 (left columns) and E12 (right columns) (n = 3) OFT, Outflow tract cushions; AV, atrioventricular cushions; C, control; M, mutant; Error bars, SEM; *p<0.05.

intercalated cushions, there were no differences in these patterns between control and mutant samples. Despite the similarity of bicuspid phenotype (R-N fusion) with that reported in *Gata5* and *Nos3* mutants, these results provide no evidence that Alk2-mediated signaling leads to mis-expression of genes known to be associated with BAV, suggesting that the pathogenetic mechanism leading to BAV in these Alk2 mutants is novel or acting downstream of these genes.

Functional defects in adult Alk2/Gata5-Cre mutants

As mentioned above, 45% of mutant mice survived to adulthood. We analyzed aortic valve function in 22 of these mice at 3–18 months using echocardiography (Figure 8A–C). Hemodynamic evaluation of *Alk2/Gata5-Cre* mutant and age/sex-matched control mice (see methods) demonstrated an increased velocity gradient across the aortic valve of 6 mutant mice consistent with aortic stenosis (Figure 8D). In addition, two of the six mice with stenosis displayed regurgitation indicative of aortic insufficiency (Figure 8B). Subsequently, the mice were euthanized and aortic valve tissues further analyzed grossly, then histologically (as also reported above) or for gene expression by real-time quantitative RT-PCR (below). Histological analyses showed that mutant valve leaflets were irregularly thickened and hypercellular when compared to corresponding controls (Figure 8E–F) typical of stenotic valve leaflets, though elevated cell proliferation was not detected (Figure S3B). Such features might be expected at least to compromise flexibility, resulting in stenosis, as well as efficient apposition, resulting in insufficiency.

We harvested aortic valve tissue from three functionally abnormal *Alk2* mutants and three functionally normal age/sex-matched controls and analyzed them for expression of selected genes associated with osteogenic differentiation or inflammation implicated in human valve disease [36]. The results imply that inflammatory pathways were not involved in the pathogenesis as there were no genotype-consistent changes in *Alox5* or *Cd68* expression between mutant and control tissues (Figure S3). In contrast, mutant tissues showed a clear tendency for higher *osteopontin (Spp1, p = 0.054)* and lower *Sox9* (p = 0.057) expression when compared to corresponding control tissues (Figure 8I). Moreover, the *Spp1* and *Sox9* expression levels were inversely related to one another (Figure S3A), consistent with the recent model proposed by Peacock et al [37]. Since reduced levels of *Sox9* have been shown to be causally related to valve ossification [37], the observed differences are consistent with a model in which affected valve tissues in *Alk2* mutants with aortic stenosis and insufficiency display pro-osteogenic changes. However, expression of the key osteogenic transcription factor *Runx2* was consistently lower in mutant valve tissues than in controls, and valve calcification was not detected by von Kossa or Alizarin Red staining (Figure 8G–H). We also analyzed activation of Bmp Smads (Smads1/5/8), Erk1/2 and p38 Mapk using Western blotting and probing with phospho-specific antibodies. Phosphorylation levels of Bmp Smads were very low and did not show detectable differences between mutants and controls. In contrast, the samples harvested from *Alk2* mutants that showed both stenosis and insufficiency showed consistent, robust increase in Erk1/2 phosphorylation, and a less pronounced increase in p38-Mapk phosphorylation (Figure 8J–K). Prolonged Erk1/2 activation has been shown to lead to calcification in valve interstitial cell cultures *in vitro* [38]. Although the limited sample number (n = 2) does not allow us to establish statistical significance, these experiments suggest that the increase in Erk1/2 phosphorylation we observe contributes to pro-osteogenic expression pattern shown in Figure 8I.

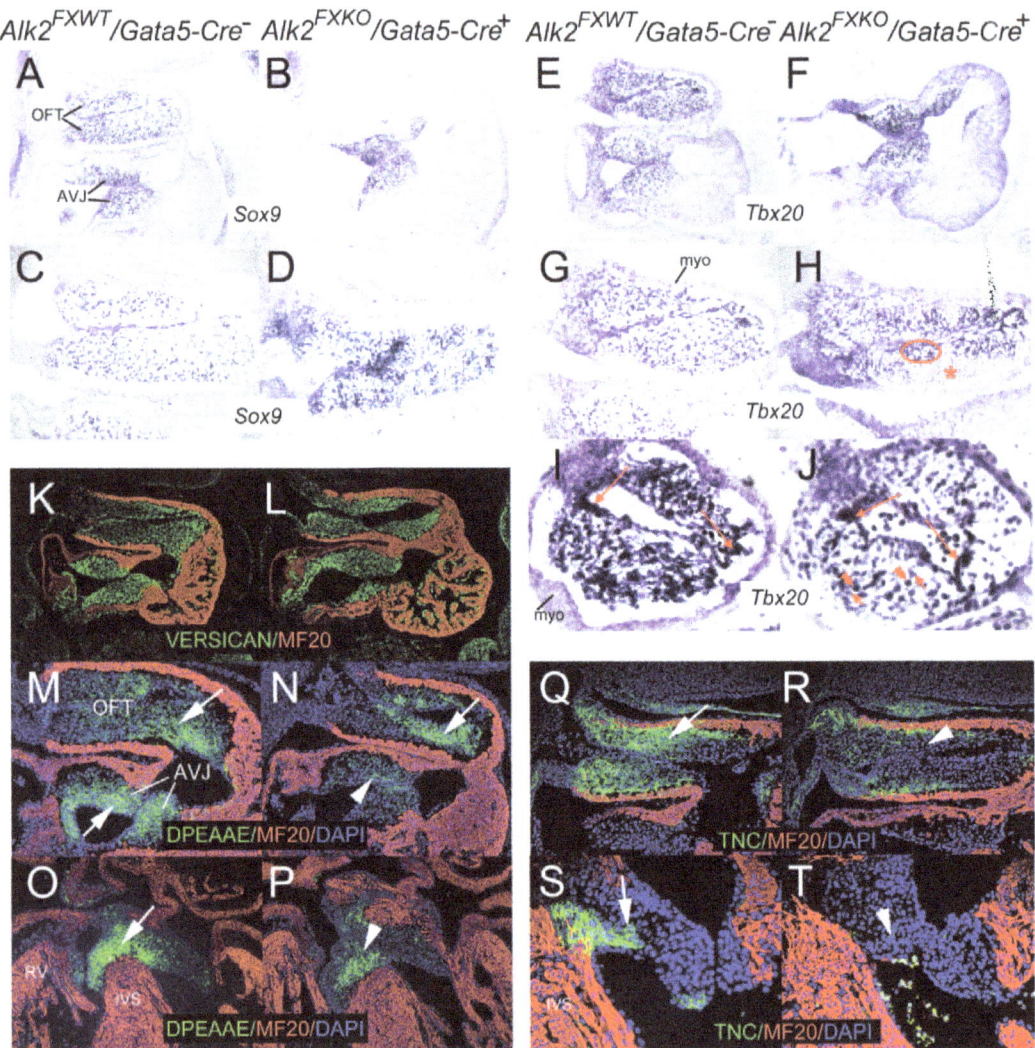

$Alk2^{FXWT}/Gata5\text{-}Cre^-$ $Alk2^{FXKO}/Gata5\text{-}Cre^+$ $Alk2^{FXWT}/Gata5\text{-}Cre^-$ $Alk2^{FXKO}/Gata5\text{-}Cre^+$

Figure 6. *Sox9* and *Tbx20* **expression and less cleaved versican and tenascin-C in endocardial cushions and valve leaflets in controls and** *Alk2/Gata5-Cre* **mutants.** In situ hybridization for *Sox9* (A–D) and *Tbx20* (E–J) on sagittal (A–H) and transverse (I, J) sections of E11 control and *Alk2/Gata5-Cre* mutant hearts. Prominent expression of both genes in atrioventricular (AVJ) and outflow tract (OFT) cushions in both control and mutant samples. Stronger staining detectable in certain regions of endocardium (*Tbx20*: red arrows in I, J) in equivalent areas of both control and mutant. Although staining for both *Sox9* and *Tbx20* in cushion mesenchyme also varied between adjacent cells (illustrated in J: short arrow lower vs double arrowhead higher), mutant but not control had groups of adjacent groups cells of lower (such as red asterisk in H) and higher (red ellipse) *Tbx20* signal. Immunostaining for total versican on sagittal E11 control (K) and *Alk2/Gata5-Cre* mutant (L) sections (green: versican; red: MF20). M–P, immunostaining for cleaved versican using anti-DPEAAE antibody on control (M,O) and *Alk2/Gata5-Cre* (N,P) sections. M–N, sagittal sections at E11; O–P, transverse sections at E14; green: cleaved versican; red: MF20. Staining in control AVJ mesenchyme (arrow in M,O) more extensive than mutant (arrowhead in N,P), though both similar in OFT. Immunostaining for tenascin-C on control (Q,S) and *Alk2/Gata5-Cre* mutant (R,T) sections; Q,R, sagittal sections at E11; S,T, transverse sections at E14. Green, tenascin-C (TNC); red, MF20. Staining in control mesenchyme (arrow) more extensive than mutant (arrowhead). AVJ, atrioventricular cushions; OFT, outflow tract cushions; IVS, ventricular septum; myo, OFT myocardium; RV, right ventricle.

Discussion

Abnormal *Alk2* function has been implicated in human cardiac disease [29,30]. However, our current knowledge about the role of *Alk2* in cardiac development is limited to endocardial EMT and neural crest cell migration [26,39,40], and it is not known which Alk2-mediated processes fail in human patients that show disease-causing mutations in the *Alk2* gene. Since EMT fails in *Alk2/Tie2-Cre* mutants, efficient analysis of a later role for Alk2 in endocardium or its derivatives in post-EMT septum and valve development in isolation is not possible using this model. Similarly, in *Alk2/Wnt1-Cre* mutants, recombination in neural crest cells occurs very early and affects not only the initial distribution of these cells in the OFT but

also causes malformations in adjacent structures that could affect valve morphogenesis indirectly [39]. To overcome these limitations, we used the *Gata5-Cre* transgenic mouse line. This was originally designed as an epicardium-specific driver but this and our earlier studies have shown that *Alk2* does not play a detectable essential role in the epicardium (Figure S1) or working myocardium [26]. Recombination in endocardium commences after the main phase of Alk2-dependent EMT, and, in contrast with AV events, no defects in OFT septation or arterial valve development were detected in *Alk2/Tie2-Cre* mutants [26]. In the present study we show that *Gata5-Cre* induces efficient recombination in all cushion mesenchyme soon after EMT or migration. Using this driver line, we found that, following abrogation of *Alk2* in the endocardial cushion

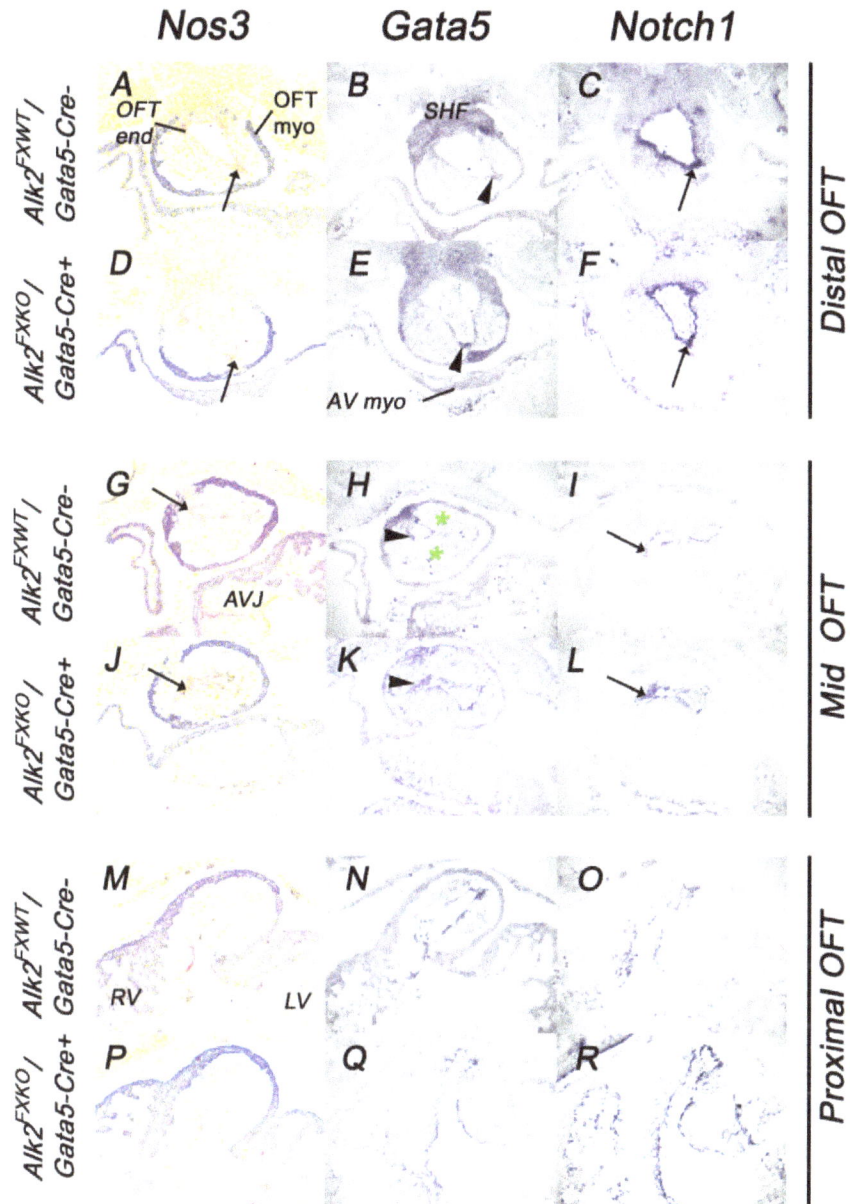

Figure 7. Regional patterns of BAV-associated gene expression do not differ between control and *Alk2/Gata5-Cre* mutant outflow tracts. Sections transverse to distal (A–F), mid (G–L) and proximal (M–R) outflow tracts of control (A–C; G I, M O) and mutant (D–F; J–L; P–R) embryos showing expression patterns of Nos3 (Immunostaining: Nos3, pink; myocardium, blue-purple; nuclei, yellow; images color-inverted so that signal in single layer of endocardium is visible), (A, D, G, J, M, P); *Gata5* (ISH: B, E, H, K, N, Q) and *Notch1* (ISH: C, F, I, L, O, R). Staining for Nos3 and *Notch1* present in virtually all endocardial cells in the OFT; *Gata5* (e.g., arrow heads) detected above background in endocardium lateral to rather than over the two main cushions (septal, parietal: *) where *Notch1* and Nos3 also more strongly expressed (arrows). Non-coronary leaflet develops from the intercalated cushion on the left in these images, right coronary from the adjacent part of the parietal cushion (* in the more anterior position). *Gata5* also detected in second heart field (SHF) cells/most distal OFT wall. OFT, myo: outflow tract myocardium; OFT end, OFT endocardium; AV myo, atrioventricular myocardium; AVJ, atrioventricular cushion; RV, right ventricle; LV, left ventricle.

mesenchyme, cushion growth was attenuated, and VSD and functional BAVs developed.

In a recent detailed analysis of BAV development [11], two morphologically and etiologically different rodent models were studied: the mouse model lacking *Nos3*, where BAVs results from right and non-coronary (R-N) leaflet precursor fusion present at or before OFT septation occurs, and a well-established hamster model where right-left coronary (R-L) leaflet fusions are associated with abnormal OFT septation morphology. The R-N and R-L BAV phenotypes are the two more common in humans, and have

different clinical implications. In pediatric patients, R-N BAVs are more likely to progress rapidly to aortic insufficiency and stenosis, while those with R-L BAVs develop more rapid aortic wall regeneration [3]. Our analysis of the *Alk2/Gata5-Cre* mutant aortic valve during its embryonic morphogenesis shows no evidence of BAV formed by R-L leaflet fusion, but a spectrum of defects including fusion of R-N leaflet precursors, and functional bicuspid valve composed of separate right and left leaflets each adjacent to a coronary orifice, and only a very small, poorly formed leaflet in the non-coronary position. Genetic mutants surviving to adulthood

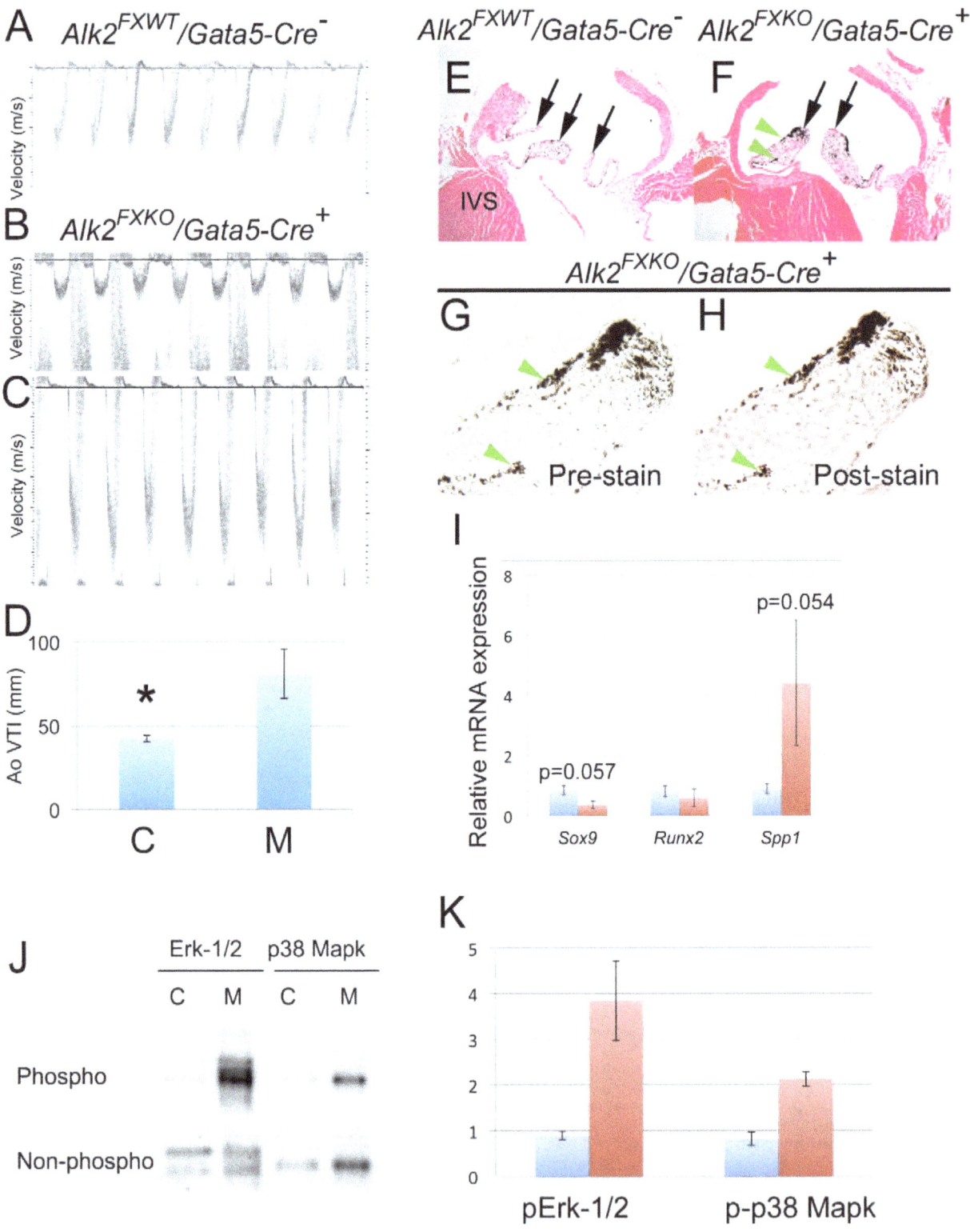

Figure 8. Aortic stenosis and insufficiency in *Alk2/Gata5-Cre* mutants. Echocardiography of a control (A), an *Alk2/Gata5-Cre* mutant with aortic stenosis and insufficiency (B) and an *Alk2/Gata5-Cre* mutant with aortic stenosis (C). A bar graph (D) depicts the two-fold difference in aortic velocity index between controls (C) and stenotic mutants (M) (n = 6). Aortic valve leaflets (arrows) of stenotic *Alk2/Gata5-Cre* mutant thickened and hypercellular (F) when compared to those of age- and sex-matched control (E) (Von Kossa-stained sections with nuclear red counterstain). Dark patches are endogenous melanin, not evidence of calcification: Alizarin Red staining on sister section to (F) (pre-staining, G; post staining H) shows dark patches (e.g., green arrowheads) match precisely and no bright red positive stain for calcium. I, Relative real-time RT-PCR quantification of *Sox9*, *Runx2* and *Spp1 (osteopontin)* in isolated valve leaflets of controls and *Alk2/Gata5-Cre* mutants with aortic stenosis and insufficiency (n = 2). J, Up-regulation of phospho-Erk1/2 and phospho–p38 in samples with aortic stenosis and insufficiency (n = 2). Bar graph (K) depicts relative quantification of phospho-Erk1/2 and phospho-p38 between controls and *Alk2/Gata5-Cre* mutants shown in J (n = 2). Error bars, SEM; *p<0.05.

were more likely to develop stenosis and insufficiency than controls. In investigating the mechanism underlying these phenotypes, we looked for a relationship with the *Nos3* (and related *Gata5*) R-N fusion models. We could find no difference in expression of *Nos3* or *Gata5* immediately prior to the stage at which morphological abnormalities were apparent in these models, suggesting that Alk2 lies downstream or a different pathway is involved. Although the category of BAV resulting from altered expression of Notch1 signaling has not been reported, we also established that expression of *Notch1* itself was not altered prior to cushion maturation. Notch signaling is also implicated in preventing calcification, which is frequently associated with thickened or mechanically compromised valves with stenosis in humans, but no evidence of calcification was found in our adult mutant mice with stenosis suggesting that either Notch signaling is not compromised, or other aspects of the abnormal phenotype of the valve cells were simultaneously protective. Some pro-osteogenic differences (lower *Sox9* and higher *Spp1* expression and higher Erk1/2 phosphorylation in mutant valve leaflets) were detected, but not others: *Runx2* expression and Bmp Smad phosphorylation were not elevated. Calcification in mouse valves with compromised Notch1 signaling results only after a further perturbation (high cholesterol diet) [41] and involves inflammatory cells in which abnormal Notch signaling is also implicated as responsible for their contributing to the calcified phenotype as well as valve interstitial cells. We found no evidence of higher expression of two markers of inflammation in stenotic adult *Alk2/Gata5-Cre* mutant aortic valves, suggesting that inflammation was not causal to the stenosis. Together with absence of calcification, reduced Notch signaling as a result of *Alk2* deficiency in the valves of adult *Gata5-Cre/Alk2* mutants valves is also unlikely.

Further to establishing the mechanism underlying the BAV phenotype present by E14, we examined other aspects of cell behavior in the precursor tissues. *Alk2/Gata5-Cre* mutant cushions contained plenty of mesenchymal cells, and cushion organization closely resembled that in controls soon after recombination. However, we detected a 40% reduction in mesenchymal cell proliferation rate at E11 and E12, greater than the 20–25% reported for *Gata5*-deficient cushion mesenchyme [7], and reduced phosphorylation of Bmp Smads in OFT tissues at E12. Transcription factors Sox9 and Tbx20 have been implicated in promoting proliferation over differentiation in cushion mesenchyme and we have found some evidence that our mutant cushions contain patches of mesenchyme with reduced *Tbx20* expression. Some altered expression of cleaved versican and tenascin-C were also found, but there was no simple correlation with later morphological differences between control and mutants. Levels of cleaved versican were reduced in AV cushions but an increase in cellularity was not observed. Subtle abnormalities in *Alk2/Gata5-Cre* right atrioventricular but not left atrioventricular AV valve leaflets were detected at E18 but the tenascin-C expression adjacent to both valves was altered in mutants. AV and OFT septation, which might be expected to be compromised by a reduction in mesenchyme cell number, still occurred, and the incidence of VSDs was reduced by more than 50% between E14 and E18, suggesting that abnormalities created by Alk2 signaling deficiency might be rescued or ameliorated over time.

Aortic leaflets of *Alk2/Gata5-Cre* mutants did not appear of abnormal thickness or cellularity at a late embryonic stage. Leaflets from mutant adult valves with stenosis were abnormally thickened, in common with diseased human valves (data not shown), but we did not detect evidence of higher cell proliferation than that in control valve tissues after diagnosis, so the timing and mechanisms underlying this process remain to be determined, and may be

secondary to the morphology rather than the altered Alk2 function. Even in aortic valves with three leaflets, there is a correlation between developing valve disease and the deviation of leaflet size away from equality in humans. The abnormal mechanical stresses on valve leaflets in these settings could lead to abnormal organization and repair of valve components [18], even without the direct effects of an abnormal valve cell genotype being taken into account.

Detailed studies by others [7,11] have started to provide information about the morphological events underlying the development of BAV in rodents during embryonic development. Our work here on the *Alk2/Gata5-Cre* model also reveals a novel morphological feature not reported by others. Rather than only two leaflet cushions, or a simple R-N, or fusing intermediate phenotype, being present by E14, and at E17, our evidence demonstrates that in most cases a small third cushion in the non-coronary position was still present in mutant aortic valves, although the other two leaflets appose one another across the lumen and are performing the valvar function at this time. The presence of such a structure may further compromise function after birth if it maintains its relative size by impeding apposition of the other valve leaflets. It remains to be determined why this structure and not the pulmonary equivalent, is altered. Both are formed from intercalated cushions in the OFT, and, as our detailed ISH analysis here shows for the first time, expression of BAV-implicated genes *Nos3*, *Gata5*, *Hey1* and *Notch1* was highest in the OFT endocardium in 'lateral' positions that include where the intercalated cushions develop immediately before morphological abnormalities are first detectable in these models. All OFT cushions contain mesenchymal cells formed by EMT, but, unlike the larger (parietal and septal) cushions, intercalated cushion mesenchyme includes a molecularly distinct population that may be of pharyngeal mesoderm origin (Robert Anderson, personal communication (Sizarov et al 2012 in press)), as well as far fewer neural crest cells [11]. However, as the intercalated cushions lie on opposite sides of the OFT lumen, they are also adjacent to myocardial populations that differ in their molecular identity [42], and, as the aortic and pulmonary valve precursors are differently positioned within the OFT relative to other structures, they may experience different flow conditions even before septation [43]. Experimentally altered flow patterns can result in abnormal cushion formation in earlier embryos [44] and in valve leaflets [45] and secondary shear stress or flow-related mechanisms might contribute to the phenotypes identified in animal models of BAV. *Nos3* expression is regulated by flow [46,47], which affects endothelial motility and EMT [48]. Moreover, Fernandez et al [21] suggest a mechanism whereby *Nos3* deficiency results in abnormalities in endocardial generation of mesenchyme (EMT), which leads to a failure to form separate precursor cushions for the right and non-coronary leaflets. Notch1 signaling is also implicated in EMT and this might contribute to its role in BAV in humans. It is important to note that in none of the descriptions of animal BAV models [7,49](this paper) is there definitive evidence of fusion between separate, fully formed, excavated leaflets, and that therefore the term 'fused' or 'fusion' used when defining BAV morphology should not be presumed to imply such a process. Instead the BAVs in both *Nos3* (and perhaps *Gata5*) –deficient R-N mice and R-L hamster phenotypes originate as a lack of failure to develop separate leaflets through the failure to develop normal separate leaflet cushions at a much earlier stage. Nevertheless, further remodeling of mature valve leaflets through flow-mediated or other mechanisms, and early death, might be expected to contribute to the variable penetrance of BAV and other phenotypes in postnatal animals in this and other models ($Nos3^{-/-}$: 5/12 BAV in adults [6]; Gata5-/- 25% BAV in adults,

3% in controls [7]; Nkx2-5+/−: 0%, 2%, 11% depending on background, up to 8 times that of controls [5]). Inadequate function of the more abnormal aortic valves at birth, and reduced cardiac efficiency where ventricular septation had not occurred are obvious candidates to account for the 55% death rate amongst early postnatal *Alk2/Gata5-Cre* mutants and thus reduce the penetrance of BAV greatly from its late embryonic rate.

The absence of OFT septal defects and the reduction in penetrance of VSD during prenatal development ventricular septation are consistent with roles for *Alk2* in septal and valvar maturation that are partially redundant or subject to genetic modifiers that affect the severity of the phenotype, or involve processes in which there is a degree of plasticity in timing. Whether always three leaflet, or the result of postnatal 'recovery' from a prenatal functional BAV phenotype, the incidence of stenosis argues that three leaflet aortic valves in *Alk2* mutants still remain susceptible to stenosis and insufficiency.

Materials and Methods

Mice

Mice carrying the conditional *Alk2-flox* allele ($Alk2^{FX}$) and *Gata5-Cre* transgenic mice were used and genotyped as previously described [31,39]. *Tbx18-Cre* mice were kindly provided by Dr. S Evans [50] and were genotyped for the presence of *Cre* by PCR (oligo sequences; Cre-F, 5'-cgtttctgagcatacctgga-3'; Cre-R, 5'-atttctcccaccgtcagtacg-3'). Timed matings between male mice that were heterozygous for the *Alk2* knockout allele ($Alk2^{WTKO}$) carrying a heterozygous *Gata5-Cre* (or *Tbx18-Cre*) transgene, and female mice homozygous for the *Alk2-flox* allele ($Alk2^{FXFX}$) were used to obtain $Alk2^{FXKO}$/*Gata5-Cre*$^+$ tissue-specific mutant embryos (herein called *Alk2/Gata5-Cre*). As controls, we used $Alk2^{FXWT}$/*Gata5-Cre*$^-$ littermates, which have two functional *Alk2* alleles.

Ethics Statement

This study was carried out in strict accordance with the recommendations in the Guide for the Care and Use of Laboratory Animals of the National Institutes of Health. The experiments described in this study were specifically approved by the University Committee on Use and Care of Animals of the University of Michigan-Ann Arbor (Protocol Number: #09944).

R26R lineage tracing

For lineage tracing experiments, timed matings were set up between $Alk2^{WTKO}$/*Gata5-Cre*$^+$ males and $Alk2^{FXFX}$/$R26R^{lacz/lacz}$ females as previously described [51]. The embryos were harvested (E10-E11) and stained for the presence *of β-galactosidase* activity as described [52].

Histology, immunohistochemistry, apoptosis and BrdU incorporation assays

Embryos were fixed in 4% paraformaldehyde for 12–18 hours at 4°C, dehydrated and embedded in Leica Histowax according to standard procedures. After embedding, sections were cut at 5–7 µm. Histological analysis was performed on sections stained with hematoxylin and eosin according to standard procedures. For immunohistochemistry, citrate antigen retrieval was performed where necessary (and before anti-BrdU antibody use, where combined staining was performed). Primary antibodies (listed below) were detected using either Alexafluor-594 or Alexafluor-488 secondary antibodies (Invitrogen) on sections mounted in Vectashield containing DAPI or propidium iodide nuclear counterstains (Vector Labs Inc). Primary antibodies to the following used were: periostin (Abcam ab14041), versican

(Chemicon AB1033), cleaved versican (DPEAAE) (Thermoscientific PA1-86354), MF20 (DSHB), Nos3 (eNos) (Thermoscientific RB9279-P) and WT1(Santa Cruz Biotechnology sc-192). Apoptotic cells were detected using the 'Dead End' TUNEL assay kit (Promega) following manufacturer's instructions. For cell proliferation analyses i.p. injections of cell proliferation labeling reagent (RPN201, Amersham/GE Healthcare) were performed. BrdU-labelled cells were detected on sectioned wax-embedded tissues using anti-BrdU antibody (RPN202, Amersham/GE Healthcare) according to manufacturer's instructions. Fluorescent images were viewed on an Olympus BX51 microscope and documented using an Olympus DP71 camera. Adobe Photoshop CS4 was used to invert the image colors to enable the results to be visible. Each assay was repeated at least once; see figure texts for details.

In situ hybridization (ISH)

For RNA in situ hybridization, embryos were fixed in 4% buffered paraformaldehyde for 12–18 hours, dehydrated and either stored in 95% ethanol at −20°C until needed or processed for embedding in Leica Histowax or BlueRibbon embedding medium. In situ hybridization was performed [53] on 10 µm sections using non radio-active DIG-labeled RNA probes made according to manufacturer's instructions (Roche Applied Science). Each analysis was performed on 2–3 independent samples per genotype. Probes for *Sox9*, *Tbx20*, *Notch1* and *Hey2* were made from templates kindly provided by Nobby Kamiya [54], Richard Harvey [55] and Irma Thesleff [56], respectively. Probes for *Alk2* (nts 814–1414 and nts1281–2024 of NM_001110204) *Gata5* (nts 1460–2061 of NM_008093) and *Hey1* (nts 205–1105 of NM_010423) were made from cloned templates containing PCR-amplified sequences from total mouse cDNA. Results were viewed on an Olympus BX51 or Leica MZ95 microscope and documented using an Olympus DP71 camera and software.

Real-time Quantitative PCR

Total RNAs were isolated from individual aortic valves (trimmed to include mainly leaflets) placed in RLT buffer (Qiagen) and DTT using the RNeasy microkit (Qiagen), and used immediately to synthesize cDNA using Omniscript reverse-transcriptase (Qiagen) and random priming according to manufacturer's instructions. cDNA aliquots (one tenth each total cDNA prep) were then pre-amplified for 10 cycles using Taqman PreAmp Mastermix (Applied Biosystems) and the same batch of diluted mix of primers used for subsequent quantitative PCR assays, and the resulting products diluted, all according to manufacturer's instructions. β-actin (*Actb*) primers were included in the pre-amplification mix. Real-time qPCR analyses were performed using Universal ProbeLibrary-based assays (Roche Applied Science) with gene-specific primer sequences generated by the manufacturer's online site (https://www.roche-applied-science.com/sis/rtpcr/upl/index.jsp?id=UP030000). Each 30 µl reaction included 2 µl of sample as prepared above, 1 µl each forward and reverse primer (stock 20 µM), 0.5 µl Probe and 15 µl Taqman Universal PCR Master Mix (Applied Biosystems). 45-cycle assays were performed using the ABI 7300 PCR and Detection System (Applied Biosystems) and analysed using 7500 System v1.2.2 software. *βactin* was used to standardize relative quantities. Results with C_ts outside 15–30 cycles were excluded. cDNAs from aortic valve tissue from three different control and mutant mice were analyzed simultaneously.

Immunoblotting

For Western blots, tissues were lysed in 2× Laemmli sample buffer [57], heated at 80°C for 10 minutes, and quantified by

Quant-It protein assay reagents (Invitrogen). Samples (3 μg protein per lane) were loaded onto NuPaGE 4–12% Bis-Tris gels (Invitrogen) and run at 200 V for 50 minutes. Proteins were transferred onto nitrocellulose filters using an iBlot dry blotting system (Invitrogen). For immunodetection, filters were blocked with 5% milk for 1 hour and incubated with primary antibodies for 12–16 hours at +4°C in 2%milk. Primary antibodies to the following antigens were used (all Cell Signaling Technology unless otherwise stated) phospho-Smad 1,5,8 (9511), phospho-Erk1/2 (4376), Erk1/2 (4695), phospho-p38Mapk (4511), p38Mapk (Santa Cruz Biotechnology sc-728), β-actin (Sigma A1978). The filters were washed in TBST, incubated for 30 mins with HRP-labeled secondary antibodies washed again in TBST and incubated for 5 minutes in Immobilon HRP Substrate (Millipore). Detection and quantification was accomplished by using the BioSpectrum AC imaging system (UVP).

Echocardiography

Induction of anesthesia was performed in an enclosed container filled with 4% isoflurane. After induction, the mice were placed on a warming pad to maintain body temperature. 1–1.5% isoflurane was supplied via a nose cone to maintain a surgical plane of anesthesia. The hair was removed from the upper abdominal and thoracic area with depilatory cream. ECG was monitored via non-invasive resting ECG electrodes. Transthoracic echocardiography was performed in the supine or left lateral position. Two-dimensional, M-mode, Doppler and tissue Doppler echocardiographic images were recorded using a Visual Sonics' Vevo 770 high resolution in vivo micro-imaging system. LV ejection fraction was measured from the two-dimensional long axis view. Systolic and diastolic dimensions and wall thickness were measured by M-mode in the parasternal short axis view at the level of the papillary muscles. Fractional shortening and ejection fraction were also calculated from the M-mode parasternal short axis view. Diastolic function was assessed by conventional pulsed-wave spectral Doppler analysis of mitral valve inflow patterns (early [E] and late [A] filling waves). Doppler tissue imaging (DTI) was used to measure the early (Ea) diastolic tissue velocities of the septal and lateral annuluses of the mitral valve in the apical 4-chamber view. Echo was performed on 3 month-old (3 male, 3 female), 7.5 month-old (4 male, 4 female) and 13 month or older (4 male, 4 female) Alk2/Gata5-Cre mutants, along with male and female control animals of the same ages.

Histological detection of calcification

Von Kossa staining with nuclear red counterstaining was performed on rehydrated 7 μm formalin-fixed tissue sections using the Diagnostic Biosystems kit (Pleasanton CA) according to manufacturer's instructions. Alzarin Red staining was performed on sister sections with freshly prepared alizarin red using a standard protocol. Resulting sections were viewed on an Olympus BX51 microscope and documented using an Olympus DP71 camera and software.

Statistical analysis

Statistical analysis was done by Mann-Whitney U test. P values<0.05 were considered significant. Error bars represent SEM in all bar graphs.

Supporting Information

Figure S1   No detectable cardiac defects in epicardium-specific Alk2 mutants. Coronary vasculature smooth muscle and cardiac fibroblast cells are both epicardium-derived. R26R-driven βgal staining (blue) shows that abrogation of Alk2 function in epicardial cells using the Tbx18-Cre driver line did not cause detectable defects in the smooth muscle cell layer surrounding coronary arteries (E18: white arrows in A, B) or in generation and migration of epicardially derived WT1-positive cells (white arrowheads) into the ventricular walls (C, D) (E13: immunostaining for WT1, green; for MF20, red). A and C, controls; B and D, Alk2/Gata5-Cre mutants.

Figure S2   No difference in regional patterns of Notch1 target genes Hey1 and Hey2 between control and Alk2/Gata5-Cre mutant outflow tracts. ISH performed on sections transverse to distal (A–D), mid (E–H) and proximal (I–L) outflow tract of control (A, B, E, F, I, J) and mutant (C, D, G, H, K, L) embryos showing expression patterns (blue) of Hey1 (A, C, E, G, I, K) and Hey2 (ISH: B, D, F, H, J, L). Hey1 expression in OFT endocardium (arrow head) restricted to cells lateral to but not over the two main OFT cushions (parietal, septal *). ISH staining for Hey1 on sagittal sections (distal to the left) of control (I') and mutant (K') also not above background in mesenchymal cells of the proximal OFT cushions (Prox OFT). Hey2 detected in most OFT endocardial cells but stronger in areas lateral to the main OFT cushions (arrows). Non-coronary leaflet will develop from the intercalated cushion on the left side in these images. Hey1 also detected in atrial appendage myocardium (A Myo) and epicardium (green arrow). Hey2 also detected in ventricular wall myocardium (V Myo).

Figure S3   Expression findings in valve leaflets of Alk2/Gata5-Cre mutants with aortic stenosis and insufficiency. A, Scatter plot demonstrates inverse relationship between Spp1 and Sox9 expression in aortic valve leaflets of stenotic Alk2/Gata5-Cre mutants measured by real-time RT-PCR. B, Bar graph illustrates no difference in relative expression of inflammation markers Alox5 and Cd68, and of proliferation marker Pcna, in stenotic mutant (red) and normal control (blue) aortic valve leaflets measured by real-time RT-PCR quantification (n = 3). Error bars, SEM.

Acknowledgments

We thank Nobby Kamiya, Richard Harvey, Deepak Srivastava and Irma Thesleff for probe templates, Kimber Converso-Baran and Mark Russell for Echo analyses, Sylvia Evans for Tbx18-Cre mice and Robert H. Anderson for very helpful suggestions for morphological analysis.

Author Contributions

Conceived and designed the experiments: PST SS VK. Performed the experiments: PST SS VK. Analyzed the data: PST VK. Contributed reagents/materials/analysis tools: PR-L. Wrote the paper: PST VK.

References

1. Siu SC, Silversides CK (2010) Bicuspid aortic valve disease. J Am Coll Cardiol 55: 2789–2800.

2. Yener N, Oktar GL, Erer D, Yardimci MM, Yener A (2002) Bicuspid aortic valve. Ann Thorac Cardiovasc Surg 8: 264–267.

3. Braverman AC, Guven H, Beardslee MA, Makan M, Kates AM, et al. (2005) The bicuspid aortic valve. Curr Probl Cardiol 30: 470–522.

4. Garg V, Muth AN, Ransom JF, Schluterman MK, Barnes R, et al. (2005) Mutations in NOTCH1 cause aortic valve disease. Nature 437: 270–274.

5. Biben C, Weber R, Kesteven S, Stanley E, McDonald L, et al. (2000) Cardiac septal and valvular dysmorphogenesis in mice heterozygous for mutations in the homeobox gene Nkx2-5. Circ Res 87: 888–895.

6. Lee TC, Zhao YD, Courtman DW, Stewart DJ (2000) Abnormal aortic valve development in mice lacking endothelial nitric oxide synthase. Circulation 101: 2345–2348.

7. Laforest B, Andelfinger G, Nemer M (2011) Loss of Gata5 in mice leads to bicuspid aortic valve. J Clin Invest 121: 2876–2887.

8. Krug EL, Runyan RB, Markwald RR (1985) Protein extracts from early embryonic hearts initiate cardiac endothelial cytodifferentiation. Dev Biol 112: 414–426.

9. Person AD, Klewer SE, Runyan RB (2005) Cell biology of cardiac cushion development. IntRevCytol 243: 287–335.

10. Markwald RR, Krook JM, Kitten GT, Runyan RB (1981) Endocardial cushion tissue development: structural analyses on the attachment of extracellular matrix to migrating mesenchymal cell surfaces. Scan Electron Microsc. pp 261–274.

11. Jiang X, Rowitch DH, Soriano P, McMahon AP, Sucov HM (2000) Fate of the mammalian cardiac neural crest. Development 127: 1607–1616.

12. Ya J, Schilham MW, Clevers H, Moorman AF, Lamers WH (1997) Animal models of congenital defects in the ventriculoarterial connection of the heart. J Mol Med (Berl) 75: 551–566.

13. Tomanek RJ (2005) Formation of the coronary vasculature during development. Angiogenesis 8: 273–284.

14. Hurle JM, Colvee E, Blanco AM (1980) Development of mouse semilunar valves. Anat Embryol (Berl) 160: 83–91.

15. Sacks MS, Yoganathan AP (2007) Heart valve function: a biomechanical perspective. Philos Trans R Soc Lond B Biol Sci 362: 1369–1391.

16. Hinton RB, Yutzey KE (2011) Heart valve structure and function in development and disease. Annu Rev Physiol 73: 29–46.

17. David Merryman W (2010) Mechano-potential etiologies of aortic valve disease. J Biomech 43: 87–92.

18. Vollebergh FE, Becker AE (1977) Minor congenital variations of cusp size in tricuspid aortic valves. Possible link with isolated aortic stenosis. Br Heart J 39: 1006–1011.

19. Stewart BF, Siscovick D, Lind BK, Gardin JM, Gottdiener JS, et al. (1997) Clinical factors associated with calcific aortic valve disease. Cardiovascular Health Study. J Am Coll Cardiol 29: 630–634.

20. Sievers HH, Schmidtke C (2007) A classification system for the bicuspid aortic valve from 304 surgical specimens. J Thorac Cardiovasc Surg 133: 1226–1233.

21. Fernandez B, Duran AC, Fernandez-Gallego T, Fernandez MC, Such M, et al. (2009) Bicuspid aortic valves with different spatial orientations of the leaflets are distinct etiological entities. J Am Coll Cardiol 54: 2312–2318.

22. Fernandes SM, Sanders SP, Khairy P, Jenkins KJ, Gauvreau K, et al. (2004) Morphology of bicuspid aortic valve in children and adolescents. J Am Coll Cardiol 44: 1648–1651.

23. Schaefer BM, Lewin MB, Stout KK, Byers PH, Otto CM (2007) Usefulness of bicuspid aortic valve phenotype to predict elastic properties of the ascending aorta. Am J Cardiol 99: 686–690.

24. Sugi Y, Yamamura H, Okagawa H, Markwald RR (2004) Bone morphogenetic protein-2 can mediate myocardial regulation of atrioventricular cushion mesenchymal cell formation in mice. DevBiol 269: 505–518.

25. Ma L, Lu MF, Schwartz RJ, Martin JF (2005) Bmp2 is essential for cardiac cushion epithelial-mesenchymal transition and myocardial patterning. Development 132: 5601–5611.

26. Wang J, Sridurongrit S, Dudas M, Thomas P, Nagy A, et al. (2005) Atrioventricular cushion transformation is mediated by ALK2 in the developing mouse heart. DevBiol 286: 299–310.

27. Song L, Fassler R, Mishina Y, Jiao K, Baldwin HS (2007) Essential functions of Alk3 during AV cushion morphogenesis in mouse embryonic hearts. DevBiol 301: 276–286.

28. Rivera-Feliciano J, Tabin CJ (2006) Bmp2 instructs cardiac progenitors to form the heart-valve-inducing field. DevBiol 295: 580–588.

29. Smith KA, Joziasse IC, Chocron S, van Dinther M, Guryev V, et al. (2009) Dominant-negative ALK2 allele associates with congenital heart defects. Circulation 119: 3062–3069.

30. Joziasse IC, Smith KA, Chocron S, van Dinther M, Guryev V, et al. (2011) ALK2 mutation in a patient with Down's syndrome and a congenital heart defect. Eur J Hum Genet 19: 389–393.

31. Merki E, Zamora M, Raya A, Kawakami Y, Wang J, et al. (2005) Epicardial retinoid X receptor alpha is required for myocardial growth and coronary artery formation. ProcNatlAcadSciUSA 102: 18455–18460.

32. Dudas M, Sridurongrit S, Nagy A, Okazaki K, Kaartinen V (2004) Craniofacial defects in mice lacking BMP type I receptor Alk2 in neural crest cells. MechDev 121: 173–182.

33. Angelini A, Ho SY, Anderson RH, Devine WA, Zuberbuhler JR, et al. (1989) The morphology of the normal aortic valve as compared with the aortic valve having two leaflets. J Thorac Cardiovasc Surg 98: 362–367.

34. Dupuis LE, McCulloch DR, McGarity JD, Bahan A, Wessels A, et al. (2011) Altered versican cleavage in ADAMTS5 deficient mice; a novel etiology of myxomatous valve disease. Dev Biol 357: 152–164.

35. Hurle JM, Garcia-Martinez V, Ros MA (1990) Immunofluorescent localization of tenascin during the morphogenesis of the outflow tract of the chick embryo heart. Anat Embryol (Berl) 181: 149–155.

36. Nagy E, Andersson DC, Caidahl K, Eriksson MJ, Eriksson P, et al. (2011) Upregulation of the 5-lipoxygenase pathway in human aortic valves correlates with severity of stenosis and leads to leukotriene-induced effects on valvular myofibroblasts. Circulation 123: 1316–1325.

37. Peacock JD, Huk DJ, Ediriweera HN, Lincoln J (2011) Sox9 transcriptionally represses spp1 to prevent matrix mineralization in maturing heart valves and chondrocytes. PLoS One 6: e26769.

38. Gu X, Masters KS (2009) Role of the MAPK/ERK pathway in valvular interstitial cell calcification. Am J Physiol Heart Circ Physiol 296: H1748–1757.

39. Kaartinen V, Dudas M, Nagy A, Sridurongrit S, Lu MM, et al. (2004) Cardiac outflow tract defects in mice lacking ALK2 in neural crest cells. Development 131: 3481–3490.

40. Desgrosellier JS, Mundell NA, McDonnell MA, Moses HL, Barnett JV (2005) Activin receptor-like kinase 2 and Smad6 regulate epithelial-mesenchymal transformation during cardiac valve formation. DevBiol 280: 201–210.

41. Nus M, MacGrogan D, Martinez-Poveda B, Benito Y, Casanova JC, et al. (2011) Diet-induced aortic valve disease in mice haploinsufficient for the Notch pathway effector RBPJK/CSL. Arterioscler Thromb Vasc Biol 31: 1580–1588.

42. Bajolle F, Zaffran S, Meilhac SM, Dandonneau M, Chang T, et al. (2008) Myocardium at the base of the aorta and pulmonary trunk is prefigured in the outflow tract of the heart and in subdomains of the second heart field. Dev Biol 313: 25–34.

43. Ya J, van den Hoff MJ, de Boer PA, Tesink-Taekema S, Franco D, et al. (1998) Normal development of the outflow tract in the rat. Circ Res 82: 464–472.

44. Manner J, Seidl W, Steding G (1993) Correlation between the embryonic head flexures and cardiac development. An experimental study in chick embryos. Anat Embryol (Berl) 188: 269–285.

45. Colvee E, Hurle JM (1983) Malformations of the semilunar valves produced in chick embryos by mechanical interference with cardiogenesis. An experimental approach to the role of hemodynamics in valvular development. Anat Embryol (Berl) 168: 59–71.

46. Nadaud S, Philippe M, Arnal JF, Michel JB, Soubrier F (1996) Sustained increase in aortic endothelial nitric oxide synthase expression in vivo in a model of chronic high blood flow. Circ Res 79: 857–863.

47. Gan LM, Selin-Sjogren L, Doroudi R, Jern S (2000) Temporal regulation of endothelial ET-1 and eNOS expression in intact human conduit vessels exposed to different intraluminal pressure levels at physiological shear stress. Cardiovasc Res 48: 168–177.

48. Egorova AD, Khedoe PP, Goumans MJ, Yoder BK, Nauli SM, et al. (2011) Lack of primary cilia primes shear-induced endothelial-to-mesenchymal transition. Circ Res 108: 1093–1101.

49. Fernandes SM, Khairy P, Sanders SP, Colan SD (2007) Bicuspid aortic valve morphology and interventions in the young. J Am Coll Cardiol 49: 2211–2214.

50. Cai CL, Martin JC, Sun Y, Cui L, Wang L, et al. (2008) A myocardial lineage derives from Tbx18 epicardial cells. Nature 454: 104–108.

51. Soriano P (1999) Generalized lacZ expression with the ROSA26 Cre reporter strain. NatGenet 21: 70–71.

52. Hogan B, Beddington R, Costantini F, Lacy E (1994) Manipulating the mouse embryo. A laboratory manual. New York: Cold Spring Harbor Laboratory Press.

53. Moorman AF, Houweling AC, de Boer PA, Christoffels VM (2001) Sensitive nonradioactive detection of mRNA in tissue sections: novel application of the whole-mount in situ hybridization protocol. JHistochemCytochem 49: 1–8.

54. Tamamura Y, Otani T, Kanatani N, Koyama E, Kitagaki J, et al. (2005) Developmental regulation of Wnt/beta-catenin signals is required for growth plate assembly, cartilage integrity, and endochondral ossification. J Biol Chem 280: 19185–19195.

55. Stennard FA, Costa MW, Lai D, Biben C, Furtado MB, et al. (2005) Murine T-box transcription factor Tbx20 acts as a repressor during heart development, and is essential for adult heart integrity, function and adaptation. Development 132: 2451–2462.

56. Mitsiadis TA, Lardelli M, Lendahl U, Thesleff I (1995) Expression of Notch 1, 2 and 3 is regulated by epithelial-mesenchymal interactions and retinoic acid in the developing mouse tooth and associated with determination of ameloblast cell fate. J Cell Biol 130: 407–418.

57. Harlow E, Lane D (1988) Antibodies. A Laboratory Manual. New York: CSH Press.

12

Ultra High-Resolution Gene Centric Genomic Structural Analysis of a Non-Syndromic Congenital Heart Defect, Tetralogy of Fallot

Douglas C. Bittel[1]*, Xin-Gang Zhou[2], Nataliya Kibiryeva[1], Stephanie Fiedler[3], James E. O'Brien Jr.[1], Jennifer Marshall[1], Shihui Yu[4], Hong-Yu Liu[2]*

1 The Ward Family Heart Center, Children's Mercy Hospitals and Clinics and University of Missouri-Kansas City School of Medicine, Kansas City, Missouri, United States of America, **2** Section of Cardiovascular Surgery, The First Affiliated Hospital of Harbin Medical University, Harbin, China, **3** Department of Pathology, Children's Mercy Hospitals and Clinics and University of Missouri-Kansas City School of Medicine, Kansas City, Missouri, United States of America, **4** Department of Laboratory Medicine and Pathology, Seattle Children's Hospital and Department of Laboratory Medicine, University of Washington School of Medicine, Seattle, Washington, United States of America

Abstract

Tetralogy of Fallot (TOF) is one of the most common severe congenital heart malformations. Great progress has been made in identifying key genes that regulate heart development, yet approximately 70% of TOF cases are sporadic and nonsyndromic with no known genetic cause. We created an ultra high-resolution gene centric comparative genomic hybridization (gcCGH) microarray based on 591 genes with a validated association with cardiovascular development or function. We used our gcCGH array to analyze the genomic structure of 34 infants with sporadic TOF without a deletion on chromosome 22q11.2 (n $_{male}$ = 20; n $_{female}$ = 14; age range of 2 to 10 months). Using our custom-made gcCGH microarray platform, we identified a total of 613 copy number variations (CNVs) ranging in size from 78 base pairs to 19.5 Mb. We identified 16 subjects with 33 CNVs that contained 13 different genes which are known to be directly associated with heart development. Additionally, there were 79 genes from the broader list of genes that were partially or completely contained in a CNV. All 34 individuals examined had at least one CNV involving these 79 genes. Furthermore, we had available whole genome exon arrays from right ventricular tissue in 13 of our subjects. We analyzed these for correlations between copy number and gene expression level. Surprisingly, we could detect only one clear association between CNVs and expression (GSTT1) for any of the 591 focal genes on the gcCGH array. The expression levels of GSTT1 were correlated with copy number in all cases examined (r = 0.95, p = 0.001). We identified a large number of small CNVs in genes with varying associations with heart development. Our results illustrate the complexity of human genome structural variation and underscore the need for multifactorial assessment of potential genetic/genomic factors that contribute to congenital heart defects.

Editor: Barbara Bardoni, CNRS UMR7275, France

Funding: Endowment came from the Fraternal Order of Eagles, Kansas. The funders had no role in study design, data collection and analysis, decision to publish, or preparation of the manuscript.

Competing Interests: The authors have declared that no competing interests exist.

* E-mail: dbittel@cmh.edu (DCB); hyliu1963@163.com (HYL)

Introduction

Tetralogy of Fallot (TOF) consists of a ventricular septal defect, obstruction of the right ventricular outflow tract, override of the ventricular septum by the aortic root, and right ventricular hypertrophy [1]. As the most prevalent form of cyanotic heart disease, it occurs in about five to seven per 10,000 live births, and accounts for 5–7% of all congenital heart defects (CHD). The occurrence of CHD in the offspring of mothers with TOF is approximately 3.1%, supporting a genetic contribution to the developmental defect [2–4]. With the tremendous advancements in surgical and medical management, the morbidity and mortality of those born with TOF in the last 20 years is significantly improved. However, long-term sequelae, including ventricular dysfunction, arrhythmia, and life-long disability, are still challenges in this patient population [1,5]. As with most congenital heart defects, the etiology of TOF is poorly understood. Improved

understanding of possible causes will permit insight into the pathobiological basis of TOF, and allow for improved definition of disease risk. It may also empower health care practitioners with improved diagnosis, prognosis, and therapy.

Based on studies of recurrence and transmission risks, it is hypothesized that the etiology of all CHD (including TOF) is most likely multifactorial in origin [2,6]. The sporadic nature of most non-syndromic CHD probably involves a multitude of susceptibility genes with low-penetrance mutations (common variants), or intermediate-penetrance mutations (rare variants), superimposed on unfavorable environmental factors. Conceptually, an individual's genetic configuration interacts with environmental and epigenetic factors to reach a threshold of "noise" in the cell to cell communication exceeding the ability of feedback regulatory mechanisms to compensate, resulting in a congenital heart defect [7]. Although widely accepted, this hypothesis remains difficult to prove, and only a few studies describing accumulation and/or interaction effects in CHD have been reported [8].

The influence of genetic factors is evident by the association of TOF with chromosomal abnormalities such as microdeletion of chromosome 22q11.2, and trisomy 21, 18, or 13 [5]; however, these patients usually have multiple non-cardiac abnormalities concurrently with TOF. Multiple genetic studies have shown many signaling pathways, including WNT, NOTCH, BMP (bone morphogenetic protein), and FGF (fibroblast growth factor), play critical regulatory roles in the secondary heart field and contribute to the formation of the outflow tract and right ventricle [9]. Distinct changes in gene expression in these signaling pathways have been found in human heart tissues from individuals with TOF [10]. Haploinsufficiency of cardiac transcription factor genes that regulate these pathways (NKX2.5, TBX1, TBX5 and GATA4) or the transmembrane receptors, NOTCH1 and NOTCH2 and their ligand JAG1, can cause TOF and other heart defects [8]. In addition, recent genome wide association studies (GWAS) of single nucleotide polymorphisms in subjects with TOF revealed a significant associations between SNPs located on chromosomes 12q24.11–13 and 13q32 [11], and 15q26.3 and 18q21.2 [12]. Additionally, somatic mutations that reduce the expression of GATA6 have been associated with TOF [13].

Most non-syndromic CHDs, which account for 80% of all CHDs, occur sporadically, and families with clear monogenic inheritance of non-syndromic CHD are rare. This makes the identification of human disease genes involved in non-syndromic CHD by a classical positional genetics approach difficult [8]. There has been great interest in using aCGH to identify copy number variants (CNVs) that may contribute to CHD [14–22]. GWAS studies and aCGH have identified some new candidate risk factors for CHD, but there remains a significant amount of heritability that remains unexplained.

Genome-wide microarray-based comparative genomic hybridization (aCGH) or SNP microarray analysis is now recommended as a first-tier test for patients with intellectual disabilities, autism, and/or congenital anomalies [23,24]. Considering that next generation sequencing (NGS) methods are not yet reliable enough to detect genomic CNVs; aCGH still represents the gold standard for identifying pathogenic chromosomal abnormalities as small as several hundred base pairs, and up to several megabases. We report our analysis of genomic DNA from 34 infants with sporadic non-syndromic TOF using a novel ultra high-resolution custom gene-centric comparative genomic hybridization (gcCGH) microarray. This array was used to identify CNVs involving genes known to be important for vertebrate heart development and/or function.

Materials and Methods

Ethics Statement

The Children's Mercy Hospitals and Clinics institutional review board approved this research protocol. The parents of all subjects provided written consent for participation after reading the consent document and having their questions answered.

Sample Collection

Genomic DNA was extracted from the peripheral blood of 34 infants with sporadic TOF (n $_{male}$ = 20; n $_{female}$ = 14; age range of 2 to 10 months). None of these infants had a 22q11.2 deletion, and most had no other clinical features (Clinical summary, Table S1). Gene expression analysis was done on right ventricular (RV) tissue that was discarded during reconstructive surgery, de-identified, flash frozen and stored in liquid nitrogen until processing. All tissue samples removed during surgery were excised by the performing surgeon for clinical indications utilizing standard of care procedures. The normally developing comparison RV tissues (cryo-preserved pulmonary homografts, described in detail in [25]) were thawed per protocol in sterile conditions. The attending surgeon (JEO) dissected the normally developing graft tissue to ensure the graft tissues were from the equivalent location as the tissue obtained from surgery.

Construction of a Gene Centric Comparative Genomic Hybridization (gcCGH) Microarray

We used the Ingenuity Pathways Analysis (IPA, Redwood City, CA) database to derive a list of genes which contained the word "cardiac" or "heart" in their description (2237 IPA genes). In addition, we derived a refined subset of genes with validated roles in cardiovascular development or function (594 validated genes) using the three online databases: Cardiovascular Gene Ontology Annotation Initiative (http://www.ebi.ac.uk/GOA/CVI/prioritized_gene_list.html); CHD Wiki (http://homes.esat.kuleuven.be/~bioiuser/chdwiki/index.php/Main_Page); and HuGE Navigator (version 2.0) (http://www.hugenavigator.net/HuGENavigator/startPagePhenoPedia.do). Finally, in order to focus on genes that are more likely to impact cardiac development, we used IPA to derive a list of 229 genes that comprise five networks with experimentally confirmed roles in regulating vertebrate heart development: WNT; Notch; Sonic Hedgehog; cardiomyocyte differentiation via BMP receptors; and factors promoting cardiogenesis in vertebrates (development of these lists of genes is described in greater detail in [25] and the complete list is in Table S2).

The ultra high-resolution gene centric microarray was designed by Oxford Gene technology (OGT, Begbroke, Oxfordshire, UK). The genes from the five heart development networks and the 594 genes in our validated list were saturated with probes throughout the length of the gene, provided the sequence met length, GC content and Tm requirements for the array. The remaining genes from the IPA search had less dense probe assignment, and the remaining genome was covered at approximately 1 probe per 9.4 Kb.

Array Hybridization

All gcCGH tests were performed, analyzed and validated based on the protocols described previously [26,27]. In brief, all DNA samples were assessed for genomic DNA concentration and purity. Agarose gel electrophoresis was used to assess the quality of the genomic DNA samples. The test DNA (3 μg) and reference DNA (3 μg, pooled normal human male or female DNAs were used as reference DNA; purchased from Promega, Madison, WI) were digested with AluI and RsaI (Promega), and then labeled using the Agilent Genomic DNA Labeling Kit PLUS (Agilent Technologies, Santa Clara, CA). The individually labeled test and reference samples were then purified using Microcon YM-30 filters (Millipore, Billerica, MA). Following purification, the appropriately labeled test DNA and reference DNA were mixed together and hybridized to the custom gcCGH array. The hybridization was followed by four washing steps, and slides were scanned on an Agilent Microarray Scanner G2565BA with 5-μm resolution. Captured images were assessed with Feature Extraction Software, version 9.5 (Agilent), and the data were then imported into Agilent CGH Analytics 3.2.5 software for statistical analysis.

aCGH Analysis

The analysis and visualization of aCGH-244 K data was performed using the Aberration Detection Method 2 (ADM2) within Agilent CGH Analytics 3.2.5 software as used in our clinical laboratory evaluations, and as described in detail previously [26]. Briefly, the ADM2 quality-weighted interval score algorithm identifies aberrant intervals in samples that have consistently high or low log ratios based on their statistical score. The score represents the deviation of the weighted average of the normalized log ratios from its expected value of zero calculated with Derivative Log2 Ratio Standard Deviation algorithm. Our threshold settings for the CGH analytics software to make a positive call were 6.0 for sensitivity, 0.25 for minimum absolute average log ratio per region, 10,000 for maximum number of aberrant regions, and 3 consecutive probes with the same polarity were required for the minimum number of probes per region.

Exon-level Expression Microarrays

We previously analyzed the gene expression patterns in 13 of the subjects included in this genomic assessment. Detailed descriptions of subjects used for expression analysis and array preparation can be found in our previous publication [25]. Briefly, RNA was extracted from ~10 mg of frozen right ventricular tissue using a mirVana microRNA isolation kit (Applied Biosystems/ Ambion, Austin, TX) according to the manufactures instructions.

The exon-level expression arrays were Affymetrix HuEx-1_0-st-v2 (Affymetrix, Santa Clara, CA), and the experimental data were deposited in the Gene Expression Omnibus (GEO accession # GSE35776). These file are embargoed until June 2014, however, the files will be made available upon request prior to release from embargo. All arrays were run at the Kansas University Medical Center-Microarray Facility (KUMC-MF) according to the manufacturer's protocols. The KUMC-MF is supported by the Kansas University-School of Medicine, KUMC Biotechnology Support Facility, the Smith Intellectual and Developmental Disabilities Research Center (HD02528), and the Kansas IDeA Network of Biomedical Research Excellence (RR016475). All analyses were performed using statistical software: Partek Genomics Suite software version 6.6 (Partek Inc, St. Louis). Raw data (CEL. files) were uploaded into Partek Genomics Suite for normalization and statistical analysis. Robust Multichip Analysis (RMA) was used for background correction followed by quantile normalization with baseline transformation to the median of the control samples. Only probes with intensity values above 20% of background value, in at least one of the conditions, were included for additional analysis. The Ingenuity Pathways Analysis (IPA) version 9.0 was used to explore networks, canonical pathways and predefined functional categories. A Fisher's exact test was used to calculate a p-value determining the probability that the association between the genes in the dataset and the pathway was explained by chance alone. All biological functions and/or diseases in IPA's database were considered for the analysis without bias. Significance was defined as a p-value ≤ 0.05.

Real-Time Quantitative Polymerase Chain Reaction (q-PCR) and Quantitative Reverse Transcription-PCR (qRT-PCR)

CNV status was validated by q-PCR performed on a subset of genes/regions with copy number changes using specific primers (genes and primers are listed in Table S3 in Tables S3 and S4) and SYBR green as previously described [10,28]. Gene expression was verified by qRT-PCR performed on a subset of genes using gene specific primers (primers are listed in Table S3) and SYBR green

as previously described [10,28]. For each sample, real-time q-PCR or qRT-PCR was performed in triplicate on an ABI 7000 sequence detection instrument. The point at which the intensity level crossed the PCR cycle threshold (C_T) was used to compare individual reactions. We used *RNU24* and *GAPDH* to normalize our q-PCR or qRT-PCR results as done previously [10,25,27].

UCSC Visualization

CNV and expression data were uploaded into the UCSC Genomics Bioinformatics browser website (http://genome.ucsc.edu/) in bed graph format according to the website instructions to allow for graphic inspection of the data. Expression level was based on comparison to tissue from normally developing individuals as described previously [10,25].

Results and Discussion

Heart formation and function are precisely controlled by networks of transcription factors that link upstream signaling systems with the protein-coding genes required for cardiac myogenesis, morphogenesis and contractility. Single gene defects have been identified which cause CHDs, but they are rare. Thus, most of the heritability of congenital heart defects remains to be identified. Several reports examining CNVs associated with CHDs to date have added several additional potential candidate genes/ regions that may contribute to dysregulated heart development, but the resolution of these reports was limited to CNVs greater than about 100 kb. Therefore, we created an ultra high-density custom microarray focused on the genes known to be associated with cardiovascular development and function. We placed genes in three levels of importance based on potential impact on heart development using current annotation regarding potential developmental significance for the heart.

Our primary objective was to search for CNVs that were unlikely to be detected by previous assessments using standard aCGH or GWAS. We found many small CNVs that have the potential to impact the function of genes in our high priority list of genes, as well as the much larger number in the second and third tier genes. CNVs were detected for every chromosome within our cohort of children with TOF. Using the criteria described in the Methods section to identify CNVs, a total of 613 CNVs ranging from 74 base pairs to 19.5 Mb were detected. These included 402 deletions with an average size of 511 kb, and 211 duplications with an average size of 142 kb. We detected four CNVs larger than 5 Mb in size, and 216 that were less than 10 Kb. Summary information about the distribution and size of CNVs is listed in Table 1, and the specific distribution of these CNVs on individual chromosomes is listed in Table S4 in Tables S3 and S4. The entire list of CNVs is presented in Table S5 (the original aCGH files are available upon request from the first corresponding author).

Among the CNVs detected in these 34 subjects, there were 16 subjects with 33 different CNVs involving 13 genes that are known to be critical for regulating development of the right ventricle making them good candidate genes for contributing to TOF (the genes were identified using the GO terms *right ventricle morphogenesis* or *outflow track morphogenesis*; Table 2). Two of these genes are known to be pathogenic, *JAG1* [18,29] and *NOTCH1* [29], on chromosomes 9 and 20 respectively. Additionally, there were 79 genes from the list of 591 validated genes (genes that were experimentally determined to have a role in vertebrate heart development or function extracted from IPA) that were partially or completely contained in a CNV. Interestingly, all 34 individuals examined had at least one CNV involving these 79 genes. See Table S5 for a complete list of all CNVs detected.

Table 1. Summary of CNVs Detected in 34 Subjects using ultra-High Resolution CGH.

	Duplicated CNVs	Deleted CNVs	Total CNVs
Overall			
No. of CNVs	211	402	613
Range of CNVs (bp)	79–1,482,399	74–19,485,749	74–19,485,749
CNVs per individual	6.2	11.8	18.0
Total size (bp)	30,013,063	205,345,525	235,358,588
Average size per CNV (bp)	142,377	511,828	384,573
Average size per individual (bp)	1,158,165	1,423,255	2,581,420
No. of CNVs≥5 Mb (bp)	0	4	4

Comparison to CNVs in Individuals without Heart Defects

Our custom gene centered array was not available for analysis of subjects without heart defects. Therefore, in order to study whether the CNVs we identified were present in individuals without heart defects, we downloaded the datasets from Mills et al, and Jiang et al [30,31]. These datasets were used for assessments of small CNVs in 24 individuals from the Hapmap project [30], and 32 individuals with autism [31] using genome sequencing tools. The subjects in these two reports had no reported evidence of heart defects. We eliminated SNPs and small indels less than 100 bp from our comparison. We manually searched the datasets for CNVs involving the 13 genes from pathways regulating heart development. We searched for small CNVs anywhere in the gene, or 10 kb upstream or downstream, in order to include regions where the CNV would be most likely to affect gene expression or function. These comparison dataset searches were limited to CNVs less than 10 kb (Table 2).

The dataset from Jiang et al [31] contained far more CNVs than the Mills et al [30] dataset. This is undoubtedly due to technical differences in the way the CNVs were identified, but may also reflect the higher burden of CNVs in general, in individuals with developmental disorders. Only one CNV involving our 13 critical genes did not have counterparts in the two comparison datasets: *HEY1*, (Table 2). HEY1 is a member of the Notch pathway, and is a transcription factor involved in determining cell fate and boundary formation. There were 4 deletions and 3 duplications involving *Hey1* in our cohort. *Hey1* knockout mice had no apparent phenotype, but the combined knockout of *Hey1* and *Hey2* caused embryonic lethality due to inadequate vascular remodeling [32]. Thus, *Hey1/Hey2* are critical for cardiovascular development. Therefore, alteration of the dosage of *HEY1* in these infants may have contributed to the inadequate communication between the first and second heart field and thus resulted in TOF and merits further investigation.

Previously Identified Candidate Regions

One patient had a deletion encompassing *JAG1*, and a second deletion encompassing *NOTCH1*. A second patient had a deletion encompassing *NOTCH1* (Table 2). The JAGGED genes (*JAG1* and *JAG2*) encode NOTCH ligands. *NOTCH1* is one of four NOTCH family receptors. NOTCH is an ancient cell-signaling system that regulates cell fate via local cell-cell interactions, and can initiate diverse and tissue-specific downstream effects such as cell fate specification, progenitor cell maintenance, cell proliferation, apoptosis and boundary formation [33]. *JAG1* mutations have been found in patients with Alagille syndrome which can include TOF, and also in patients with non-syndromic right-sided heart

defects such as pulmonary stenosis and TOF [29,34–36]. Likewise, *NOTCH1* mutations have been shown to cause bicuspid aortic valve (BAV), as well as TOF [8]. These large deletions would be detected by standard aCGH, and are probable contributors to the TOF of these two infants.

The interest in identifying risk factors for CHD has resulted in recent large GWAS studies reporting significant associations between SNPs located on chromosomes 12q24.11–13 and 13q32 [11], and 15q26.3 and 18q21.2 [12]. We did not see any of our CNVs within or near these regions, with the exception of 15q26.3. We observed one subject with a 126 kb duplication in this region (see Table S5). However, it was detected by our background probes, and only impacted 3 open reading frame sequences; not within a target gene. This is an interesting coincidence, but is of uncertain significance. Additionally, a recent case report of somatic mutations that reduce the expression of *GATA6* have been associated with TOF [13]. We observed two deletions involving part of *GATA6*, and this strengthens the link between *GATA6* and TOF.

Inheritance

The CNVs containing *JAG1*, *TBX2*, *GATA6* or *NOTCH1* were particularly interesting because of their known association with heart defects. Therefore, we tested these to determine whether they were de novo or inherited. Each CNV had at least one case that was inherited, and all but the CNV containing *JAG1* had a case that was de novo in origin (Table 2). Regardless of the origin of the CNV, CNVs involving some or all of a gene could make subtle differences in expression or function that could have contributed to TOF, and certainly warrant further investigation.

CNVs in High Frequency in the TOF Cohort

Three CNVs containing genes associated with cardiovascular development or function, but not known to directly regulate heart development, occurred in high frequency in our cohort of infants with TOF: *CHL1*, *NKX2-1* and *GSTT1*. In addition to the above mentioned datasets, we used the Database of Genomic Variants (DGV, http://projects.tcag.ca/variation/) to search for additional reports of CNVs involving these three genes in normal individuals. These data are summarized in Table 2. Our cohort contained 19 CNVs (19 of 34; 56%) involving much of the promoter and the first 2 exons of *CHL1*, and all 19 CNVs were deletions. Two reports in the DGV indicated frequencies of 1 duplication in 30 subjects [37], and 2 duplications in 450 subjects [38]. In our cohort there were 13 deletions involving part of *NKX2-1* (13/34; 38%). The DGV contained one report with 2 deletions in 450 control subjects examined [38]. Finally, our cohort had 25 CNVs

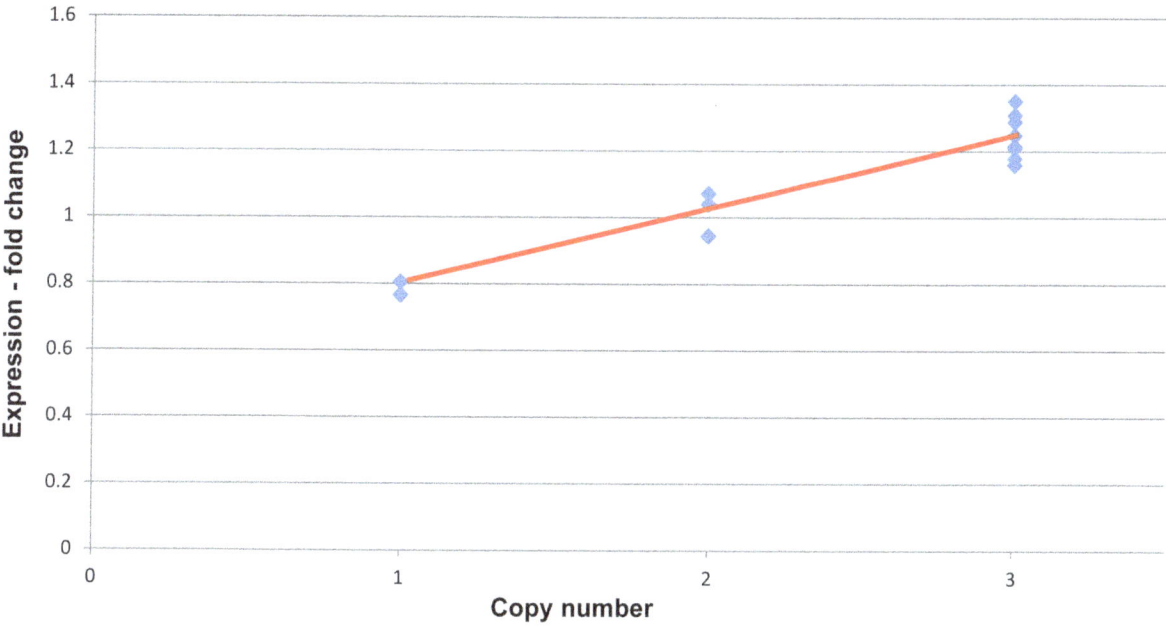

Figure 1. Correlation between copy number and gene expression of *GSTT1*. *GSTT1* expression in tissue from the right ventricle of infants with TOF relative to controls. Pearson correlation coefficient; r = 0.95, p = 0.001.

involving *GSTT1* (3 deletions and 22 duplications, 26/34; 76%). The frequencies reported in the DGV were 21 deletions in 30 subjects [37], and 630 CNVs (301 deletions and 329 duplications) in 1184 subjects [39]. The frequency of CNVs for these three genes in our cohort were all significantly higher than those seen in the DGV (chi square test of proportions, p<0.001) with the exception of the CNVs involving *GSTT1* compared to the observed frequency reported by Perry et al [37] (our TOF cohort, 26/34 = 76%; Perry et al. 21/30 = 70%), which, although there was a higher frequency in our cohort, it was not statistically significant.

Although CNVs involving these genes are relatively common in normal individuals, they occurred at a significantly higher frequency in our cohort of subjects with TOF. These three genes have no known direct influence on heart development. However, within the context of accumulating "noise" in the communication between the first and second heart field, alterations in the behavior of these genes might contribute to the dysregulation that leads to TOF.

Correlation between CNVs and Gene Expression

We had genome wide expression exon arrays available for 13 of our subjects who also underwent gcCGH analysis. The expression analysis was done using RNA extracted from right ventricular tissue removed at the time of surgical correction of the defect [10,25]. We examined the data from these two platforms to look for correlations between CNVs and gene expression in the RV. We used gene expression data at the probe (exon) level, as well as the whole gene level, to test for CNV/expression correlation. We limited our correlational assessment to CNVs associated with the genes in the list of 591 validated genes. Each of the 13 subjects with expression analysis had at least one CNV involving one or more genes on the list. In these 13 subjects, there were a total of 79 CNVs meeting the inclusion criteria. There were 41 different genes with a CNV encompassing part or all of the genes, never the less, most of the genes within the CNVs occurred too infrequently

to allow conclusions to be made about the correlation between the CNV and expression in the ventricular tissue.

GSTT1 was the only gene with a clear correlation between copy number and gene expression in the RV (Pearson's correlation coefficient, r = 0.95, p = 0.001; 7 duplications, 2 deletions from the 13 subjects examined with expression arrays). Figure 1 shows the relationship between *GSTT1* copy number and gene expression in the RV tissue of infants with TOF (compared to RV control tissue). We uploaded the CGH data and the probe intensity data to the UCSC browser to visualize the relationship between the CNVs and probe level expression (Figure S1). The TOF subjects without CNVs involving *GSTT1* did not have significant changes in *GSTT1* expression when compared to the tissue from normally developing controls. Those with deletions had significantly less *GSTT1* expression, and those with duplications had significantly more expression of *GSTT1* in the right ventricular tissue, compared to normally developing subjects. This included all the probes within the affected region (Figure S1). *GSTT1* is the first step in glutathione detoxification, and null genotypes of glutathione transferases have recently been associated with risk of CHD, particularly when parents were exposed to environmental toxins [40]. But since our cohort with TOF had individuals with under- and over-expression of *GSTT1* relative to control subjects, it seems rather unlikely that CNVs involving *GSTT1* represent a strong risk factor for TOF.

In addition, we used qRT-PCR to examine the expression of 5 genes of particular relevance for heart development, *TBX2* (3 duplications, 1 deletion), *GATA6* (2 deletions), *NOTCH1* (2 deletions), *NOTCH2* (2 deletions) and *JAG1* (1 deletion) in RV tissue from subjects with CNVs involving these genes compared to the pooled RNA from our control samples (data not shown). We did not have exon expression microarrays on any of these subjects, but extracted RNA from archived RV in order to examine expression. Expression of *NOTCH1*, *GATA6* and *JAG1* did not significantly differ from the expression of the control samples regardless of CNV status. Interestingly, the expression of *TBX2* and *NOTCH2* were reduced in the RV tissue of all TOF subjects for whom we examined expression data relative to the control samples from normally developing infants. This no doubt reflects other regulatory mechanisms that are independent of copy number.

It should be emphasized that our expression data was limited in scope to a small sample, and expression at 6 months of age may not reflect expression during early gestation when the heart fields were misaligned. In addition, subtle changes in expression that are not within the resolution of our tools could be important for precise regulation of early heart development.

Conclusions

Our study was designed to examine structural variation at very high resolution in genes with potential significance for heart development or function. We identified a large number of relatively small CNVs, not previously reported. With the possible exception of the CNVs involving *JAG1* and *NOTCH1*, our small sample size precludes any conclusion about the broader impact of these CNVs. However, it seems likely that some of these CNVs, together with other genetic and epigenetic variants, and probably environmental factors, may have contributed to the developmental deficiency that caused TOF. Delineating the impact of multiple small contributions to developmental irregularity remains a challenge. However, new high-resolution technologies are aiding in the identification of potentially important genetic elements that may eventually provide a molecular genetic explanation for complex developmental disorders like tetralogy of Fallot.

Supporting Information

Figure S1 Representative examples of copy number variants involving GSTT1 and expression of GSTT1 in cardiac tissues from infants with TOF relative to controls as graphically displayed in the UCSC Genome Browser.

Table S1 Patient Characteristics.

Table S2 List of genes used to create the gene centric array.

Tables S3 and S4 Includes Table S3 and S4. Table S3. Primers used for CNVs containing genes of primary importance for heart development. Table S4. Summary of chromosomal distribution of CNVs.

Table S5 Complete list of CNVs.

Acknowledgments

We thank Drs. Stephen Scherer and Ryan Yuen for providing their dataset [31].

Author Contributions

Conceived and designed the experiments: DCB SY. Performed the experiments: DCB NK SF. Analyzed the data: DCB XGZ NK JEO JM SY HYL. Contributed reagents/materials/analysis tools: DCB SY SF HYL. Wrote the paper: DCB XGZ SY.

References

1. Apitz C, Webb GD, Redington AN (2009) Tetralogy of Fallot. Lancet 374: 1462–1471.
2. Burn J, Brennan P, Little J, Holloway S, Coffey R, et al. (1998) Recurrence risks in offspring of adults with major heart defects: results from first cohort of British collaborative study. Lancet 351: 311–316.
3. Veldtman GR, Connolly HM, Grogan M, Ammash NM, Warnes CA (2004) Outcomes of pregnancy in women with tetralogy of Fallot. J Am Coll Cardiol 44: 174–180.
4. Zellers TM, Driscoll DJ, Michels VV (1990) Prevalence of significant congenital heart defects in children of parents with Fallot's tetralogy. Am J Cardiol 65: 523–526.
5. Bailliard F, Anderson RH (2009) Tetralogy of Fallot. Orphanet J Rare Dis 4: 2.
6. Roessler E, Ouspenskaia MV, Karkera JD, Velez JI, Kantipong A, et al. (2008) Reduced NODAL signaling strength via mutation of several pathway members including FOXH1 is linked to human heart defects and holoprosencephaly. Am J Hum Genet 83: 18–29.
7. Pierpont ME, Basson CT, Benson DW, Jr., Gelb BD, Giglia TM, et al. (2007) Genetic basis for congenital heart defects: current knowledge: a scientific statement from the American Heart Association Congenital Cardiac Defects Committee, Council on Cardiovascular Disease in the Young: endorsed by the American Academy of Pediatrics. Circulation 115: 3015–3038.
8. Wessels MW, Willems PJ (2010) Genetic factors in non-syndromic congenital heart malformations. Clin Genet 78: 103–123.
9. Rochais F, Mesbah K, Kelly RG (2009) Signaling pathways controlling second heart field development. Circ Res 104: 933–942.
10. Bittel DC, Butler MG, Kibiryeva N, Marshall JA, Chen J, et al. (2011) Gene expression in cardiac tissues from infants with idiopathic conotruncal defects. BMC Med Genomics 4: 1.
11. Cordell HJ, Topf A, Mamasoula C, Postma AV, Bentham J, et al. (2013) Genome-wide association study identifies loci on 12q24 and 13q32 associated with tetralogy of Fallot. Hum Mol Genet 22: 1473–1481.
12. Flaquer A, Baumbach C, Pinero E, Garcia Algas F, de la Fuente Sanchez MA, et al. (2013) Genome-wide linkage analysis of congenital heart defects using MOD score analysis identifies two novel loci. BMC Genet 14: 44.
13. Huang RT, Xue S, Xu YJ, Yang YQ (2013) Somatic mutations in the GATA6 gene underlie sporadic tetralogy of Fallot. Int J Mol Med 31: 51–58.
14. Breckpot J, Thienpont B, Arens Y, Tranchevent LC, Vermeesch JR, et al. (2011) Challenges of interpreting copy number variation in syndromic and non-syndromic congenital heart defects. Cytogenet Genome Res 135: 251–259.
15. Breckpot J, Thienpont B, Peeters H, de Ravel T, Singer A, et al. (2011) Array comparative genomic hybridization as a diagnostic tool for syndromic heart defects. J Pediatr 156: 810–817, 817 e811–817 e814.
16. Erdogan F, Larsen LA, Zhang L, Tumer Z, Tommerup N, et al. (2008) High frequency of submicroscopic genomic aberrations detected by tiling path array comparative genome hybridisation in patients with isolated congenital heart disease. J Med Genet 45: 704–709.
17. Goldmuntz E, Paluru P, Glessner J, Hakonarson H, Biegel JA, et al. (2012) Microdeletions and microduplications in patients with congenital heart disease and multiple congenital anomalies. Congenit Heart Dis 6: 592–602.
18. Greenway SC, Pereira AC, Lin JC, DePalma SR, Israel SJ, et al. (2009) De novo copy number variants identify new genes and loci in isolated sporadic tetralogy of Fallot. Nat Genet 41: 931–935.
19. Hitz MP, Lemieux-Perreault LP, Marshall C, Feroz-Zada Y, Davies R, et al. (2012) Rare copy number variants contribute to congenital left-sided heart disease. PLoS Genet 8: e1002903.
20. Silversides CK, Lionel AC, Costain G, Merico D, Migita O, et al. (2012) Rare copy number variations in adults with tetralogy of Fallot implicate novel risk gene pathways. PLoS Genet 8: e1002843.
21. Soemedi R, Wilson IJ, Bentham J, Darlay R, Topf A, et al. (2012) Contribution of global rare copy-number variants to the risk of sporadic congenital heart disease. Am J Hum Genet 91: 489–501.
22. Tomita-Mitchell A, Mahnke DK, Struble CA, Tuffnell ME, Stamm KD, et al. (2012) Human gene copy number spectra analysis in congenital heart malformations. Physiol Genomics 44: 518–541.
23. Manning M, Hudgins L, Professional P, Guidelines C (2010) Array-based technology and recommendations for utilization in medical genetics practice for detection of chromosomal abnormalities. Genet Med 12: 742–745.
24. Miller DT, Adam MP, Aradhya S, Biesecker LG, Brothman AR, et al. (2010) Consensus statement: chromosomal microarray is a first-tier clinical diagnostic test for individuals with developmental disabilities or congenital anomalies. Am J Hum Genet 86: 749–764.
25. O'Brien JE, Jr., Kibiryeva N, Zhou XG, Marshall JA, Lofland GK, et al. (2012) Noncoding RNA expression in myocardium from infants with tetralogy of Fallot. Circ Cardiovasc Genet 5: 279–286.

26. Yu S, Bittel DC, Kibiryeva N, Zwick DL, Cooley LD (2009) Validation of the Agilent 244 K oligonucleotide array-based comparative genomic hybridization platform for clinical cytogenetic diagnosis. Am J Clin Pathol 132: 349–360.

27. Yu S, Kielt M, Stegner AL, Kibiryeva N, Bittel DC, et al. (2009) Quantitative real-time polymerase chain reaction for the verification of genomic imbalances detected by microarray-based comparative genomic hybridization. Genet Test Mol Biomarkers 13: 751–760.

28. Bittel DC, Kibiryeva N, Sell SM, Strong TV, Butler MG (2007) Whole genome microarray analysis of gene expression in Prader-Willi syndrome. Am J Med Genet A 143: 430–442.

29. Bauer RC, Laney AO, Smith R, Gerfen J, Morrissette JJ, et al. (2010) Jagged1 (JAG1) mutations in patients with tetralogy of Fallot or pulmonic stenosis. Hum Mutat 31: 594–601.

30. Mills RE, Luttig CT, Larkins CE, Beauchamp A, Tsui C, et al. (2006) An initial map of insertion and deletion (INDEL) variation in the human genome. Genome Res 16: 1182–1190.

31. Jiang YH, Yuen RK, Jin X, Wang M, Chen N, et al. (2013) Detection of clinically relevant genetic variants in autism spectrum disorder by whole-genome sequencing. Am J Hum Genet 93: 249–263.

32. Fischer A, Schumacher N, Maier M, Sendtner M, Gessler M (2004) The Notch target genes Hey1 and Hey2 are required for embryonic vascular development. Genes Dev 18: 901–911.

33. de la Pompa JL (2009) Notch signaling in cardiac development and disease. Pediatr Cardiol 30: 643–650.

34. Colliton RP, Bason L, Lu FM, Piccoli DA, Krantz ID, et al. (2001) Mutation analysis of Jagged1 (JAG1) in Alagille syndrome patients. Hum Mutat 17: 151–152.

35. Krantz ID, Colliton RP, Genin A, Rand EB, Li L, et al. (1998) Spectrum and frequency of jagged1 (JAG1) mutations in Alagille syndrome patients and their families. Am J Hum Genet 62: 1361–1369.

36. Li L, Krantz ID, Deng Y, Genin A, Banta AB, et al. (1997) Alagille syndrome is caused by mutations in human Jagged1, which encodes a ligand for Notch1. Nat Genet 16: 243–251.

37. Perry GH, Ben-Dor A, Tsalenko A, Sampas N, Rodriguez-Revenga L, et al. (2008) The fine-scale and complex architecture of human copy-number variation. Am J Hum Genet 82: 685–695.

38. Conrad DF, Pinto D, Redon R, Feuk L, Gokcumen O, et al. (2010) Origins and functional impact of copy number variation in the human genome. Nature 464: 704–712.

39. International HapMap C, Altshuler DM, Gibbs RA, Peltonen L, Altshuler DM, et al. (2010) Integrating common and rare genetic variation in diverse human populations. Nature 467: 52–58.

40. Cresci M, Foffa I, Ait-Ali L, Pulignani S, Gianicolo EA, et al. (2011) Maternal and paternal environmental risk factors, metabolizing GSTM1 and GSTT1 polymorphisms, and congenital heart disease. Am J Cardiol 108: 1625–1631.

13

The Ambiguous Role of *NKX2-5* Mutations in Thyroid Dysgenesis

Klaartje van Engelen[1,2,3]*, **Mathilda T. M. Mommersteeg**[4¤], **Marieke J. H. Baars**[2], **Jan Lam**[5], **Aho Ilgun**[4], **A. S. Paul van Trotsenburg**[6], **Anne M. J. B. Smets**[7], **Vincent M. Christoffels**[4], **Barbara J. M. Mulder**[1,3], **Alex V. Postma**[4]

1 Department of Cardiology, Academic Medical Center, Amsterdam, The Netherlands, 2 Department of Clinical Genetics, Academic Medical Center, Amsterdam, The Netherlands, 3 Interuniversity Cardiology Institute of The Netherlands (ICIN), Utrecht, The Netherlands, 4 Heart Failure Research Centre, Department of Anatomy and Embryology, Academic Medical Center, Amsterdam, The Netherlands, 5 Department of Pediatric Cardiology, Academic Medical Center, Amsterdam, The Netherlands, 6 Department of Pediatric Endocrinology, Academic Medical Center, Amsterdam, The Netherlands, 7 Department of Radiology, Academic Medical Center, Amsterdam, The Netherlands

Abstract

NKX2-5 is a homeodomain-containing transcription factor implied in both heart and thyroid development. Numerous mutations in *NKX2-5* have been reported in individuals with congenital heart disease (CHD), but recently a select few have been associated with thyroid dysgenesis, among which the p.A119S variation. We sequenced *NKX2-5* in 303 sporadic CHD patients and 38 families with at least two individuals with CHD. The p.A119S variation was identified in two unrelated patients: one was found in the proband of a family with four affected individuals with CHD and the other in a sporadic CHD patient. Clinical evaluation of heart and thyroid showed that the mutation did not segregate with CHD in the familial case, nor did any of the seven mutation carriers have thyroid abnormalities. We tested the functional consequences of the p.A119S variation in a cellular context by performing transactivation assays with promoters relevant for both heart and thyroid development in rat heart derived H10 cells and HELA cells. There was no difference between wildtype NKX2-5 and p.A119S NKX2-5 in activation of the investigated promoters in both cell lines. Additionally, we reviewed the current literature on the topic, showing that there is no clear evidence for a major pathogenic role of *NKX2-5* mutations in thyroid dysgenesis. In conclusion, our study demonstrates that p.A119S does not cause CHD or TD and that it is a rare variation that behaves equal to wildtype NKX2-5. Furthermore, given the wealth of published evidence, we suggest that *NKX2-5* mutations do not play a major pathogenic role in thyroid dysgenesis, and that genetic testing of *NKX2-5* in TD is not warranted.

Editor: Marian Ludgate, Cardiff University, United Kingdom

Funding: This study was funded by the Academic Medical Center (government funding). The funders had no role in study design, data collection and analysis, decision to publish, or preparation of the manuscript.

Competing Interests: The authors have declared that no competing interests exist.

* E-mail: k.vanengelen@amc.uva.nl

¤ Current address: Department of Cell & Developmental Biology, University College London, London, United Kingdom

Introduction

Persistent congenital hypothyroidism of thyroidal origin is a relatively common disorder, occurring in about 1/2500 live births [1]. In 85% of cases it is caused by thyroid dysgenesis (TD), consisting of agenesis, hypoplasia or ectopia of the thyroid gland [2]. TD is a heterogeneous disorder that occurs mostly sporadically, though 2% of cases are reported as familial [3]. The pathogenesis of TD is largely unknown; possible roles for environmental, genetic and epigenetic factors have been suggested, and in a minority of humans with TD mutations in *NKX2-1* [4], *FOXE1* [5], *PAX8* [6] and *TSHR* [7] have been identified. Additionally, in a recent study mutations in *NKX2-5* were reported hypothyroidism [8].
in a small proportion of patients with persistent congenital

NKX2-5 encodes a homeodomain-containing transcription factor that is expressed during thyroid development (for review see [9]), but it is mainly known to play a crucial role in heart development [10]. *NKX2-5* mutations have been found in a subset of patients with congenital heart disease (CHD), mostly septal defects [11,12]. As CHD is overrepresented among children with TD and vice versa, a developmental association between the cardiac and thyroid systems has been suggested [13–15].

We screened families and individual patients with CHD for mutations in *NKX2-5*. In this paper we focus on the p.A119S variation, which we found in two probands. Dentice *et al.* reported this as a causative mutation in a child with ectopic thyroid gland, with functional studies showing a dominant negative effect of the mutation [8]. We evaluated the heart and the thyroid gland in our two families with a total of seven p.A119S carriers and we performed follow-up functional studies. Additionally, we discuss existing literature on the connection between *NKX2-5* mutations and TD.

Methods

Ethics Statement

This study was approved by the Medical Ethical Committee of the Academic Medical Center in Amsterdam. Written informed consent was obtained from all participants.

Patients and Clinical Evaluation

DNA from 303 patients with primum atrial septal defect (ASDI, n = 271) or secundum atrial septal defect (ASDII, n = 32) was extracted from CONCOR, a nationwide registry and DNA bank for adult patients with CHD, described in detail elsewhere [16]. Additionally, probands of 38 families with multiple (at least two) affected patients with several forms of CHD, identified at the departments of clinical genetics or cardiology of the AMC, were included. In this study, we focused on patients who were found to carry the p.A119S NKX2-5 variation. Probands with this variation, as well as their available family members, were clinically evaluated. Medical records were analyzed and all individuals underwent physical examination with attention to syndromic features. Cardiologic examination consisted of a 12-lead electrocardiogram (ECG) and two-dimensional echocardiography, which were assessed by a cardiologist who was blinded for the mutational status. Thyroid ultrasound and thyroid function analysis were used to investigate the thyroid gland. TSH and free T4 were measured by time-resolved fluoroimmunoassay (Delfia, hTSH Delfia Ulta resp. FT4 Delfia, Perkin Elmer, Turku, Finland), detection limits: 0.01 mU/L for TSH and 2 pmol/L for free T4, total assay variation: 4–5% for TSH and 6–7% for free T4. Thyreoglobulin and anti-TPO were measured by chemiluminescence immunoassay (LUMI-test Tg resp. anti-TPO, BRAHMS, Berlin, Germany), detection limits: 1 pmol/L for Tg and 30 kU/L for anti-TPO, total assay variation: 7–13% for Tg and 8–12% for anti-TPO. The results of the ultrasound were analyzed by a radiologist who was blinded for mutational status as well as cardiologic status.

Mutation Analysis

Genomic DNA of CHD patients as well as relatives of patients carrying the A119S variation was extracted from peripheral blood according to standard procedures. Coding regions and intron–exon boundaries of NKX2-5 (NM_004387.3) were analyzed using direct sequence analysis on an ABI3730xl capillary sequencer using Big-Dye Terminator v3.1 (Applied Biosystems). Data were analyzed using Codoncode analysis software (v3.1, CodonCode Corporation). In the proband with the p.A119S variation who had aortic coarctation and bicuspid aortic valve, sequence analysis of the NOTCH1 gene was also performed.

Plasmid Constructs and Transfections

Human clones for NKX2-5 and TBX5 were obtained from the IMAGE consortium [17]. The human clones were in the following vectors: pCMVSport6-hNKX2-5 and pcDNA3.1-hTBX5. Promoter construct for ANF-luc is as described before [18], the promoters for Dio2, Tg and TPO were cloned from their appropriate species, as described before [8], and subcloned into pGL3 basic expression vectors (Promega). Expression and promoter constructs were all sequence verified. pCMVSport6-hNKX2-5 mutants (p.A119S, p.N188K) were constructed using site-directed mutagenesis (Strategene). Transfections were performed using polyethylenimine (25 kDa, linear, Brunschwick).

EMSA, Probe Annealing

Radioactive Electrophoretic Mobility Shift Assay (EMSA) was performed using the following wildtype sequence as probes: 5′-

TCTGCTCTTCTCACACCT**TTGAAGTGGGG**GCCTCTT and its complementary oligo (5′-GCCTCAAGAGGC**CCC-CACTTCAA**AGGTGTG), as described before [18], The specific conditions were as follows: bandshift buffer (BB) (10 mM Tris pH 7.9, 10% glycerol, 50 mM NaCl, 0.5 mM EDTA); non-specific competitor Spermidine 3-HCl (Sigma, S2501) at a concentration of 1 μg/μl;prepared according manufacturers instruction. First 5.0 μg crude nuclear cell extracts were pre-incubated for 5 min at +15 to +25°C in a reaction containing 14 μl BB, 1 μl of the non-specific competitor spermidine, 1 μg BSA, 1 mM DTT and supplemented with H20 up to 20 μl. Input was corrected for Nkx2.5 expression and total amount protein was kept constant at 5.0 μg by addition of empty vector nuclear extracts. Then 2 μl of labelled Nkx-specific probe (30000 c.p.m) was added. Complexes were allowed to form for 20–25 min at +15 to +25°C. The samples were loaded on 6%-TBE polyacrylamide gel which was prerunned at RT for 30 min at 25 V. Complexes were separated at 4 V/cm at RT for 60 min. Gels were dried unfixed on Whatman 3 MM and exposed for autoradiography.

Luciferase Assay

Neonatal rat heart myocytes, immortalized with a temperature-sensitive SV40 antigen (H10 cells [19], were grown in standard 12-wells plates in DMEM supplemented with 10% FCS (Gibco-BRL) and glutamine. HeLa cells were grown according to standard culturing conditions [20]. 700 ng Nppa/TPO/Dio2/Tg-luciferase constructs were co-transfected with 1 ng of cmv-renilla vector, as normalization control (Promega), together with appropriate combinations of expression constructs (pCMVSport6-hNKX2-5, pcDNA3.1-hTBX5) up to 900 ng. Measurements were performed on a Glomax 20/20 luminometer. Triplo transfection experiments were repeated at least three times for each condition, data were corrected for intersession variation as described [21]. Statistical analysis was performed using two-tailed t-test, P<0.05 was considered significant.

Nuclear Localization

Cos7 cells [22] were seeded in standard 12-wells plates and transfected with 500 ng WT or p.A119S NKX2.5. 24 h post-transfection, cells were fixed in 2% paraformaldehyde, permeabilized using 0.3% Triton X-100, and incubated with rabbit anti-Nkx2-5 (Santra cruz) and DAPI (Sigma).

Results

Mutational Analysis

We identified a total of three missense NKX2-5 variations in our cohort of 341 CHD patients: a p.C270Y variant in a patient with ASDI and cleft mitral valve, and twice the p.A119S variant in separate probands (see below). We will only discuss the results of the p.A119S variant, as the other variation is outside the scope of this study.

The nucleotide change from G to T at codon 119 in NKX2-5 was identified in two patients. This results in the substitution of an alanine for a serine leading to p.A119S. This variation was present once in a proband from one of the 38 families tested and once in a proband from 303 sporadic patients with ASD. The p.A119S variation was not found in 200 local controls. Data from the NHLBI exome sequencing project shows that it is a very rare variation with a minor allele frequency of 0.001% (7/6470 individuals, rs1378526) [23]. Alignment of the aminoacids of proteins of different species shows that this position is conserved up to rat Nkx2-5 (Figure 1A). However, chicken Nkx2-5 protein actually has a serine at this position, though the surrounding

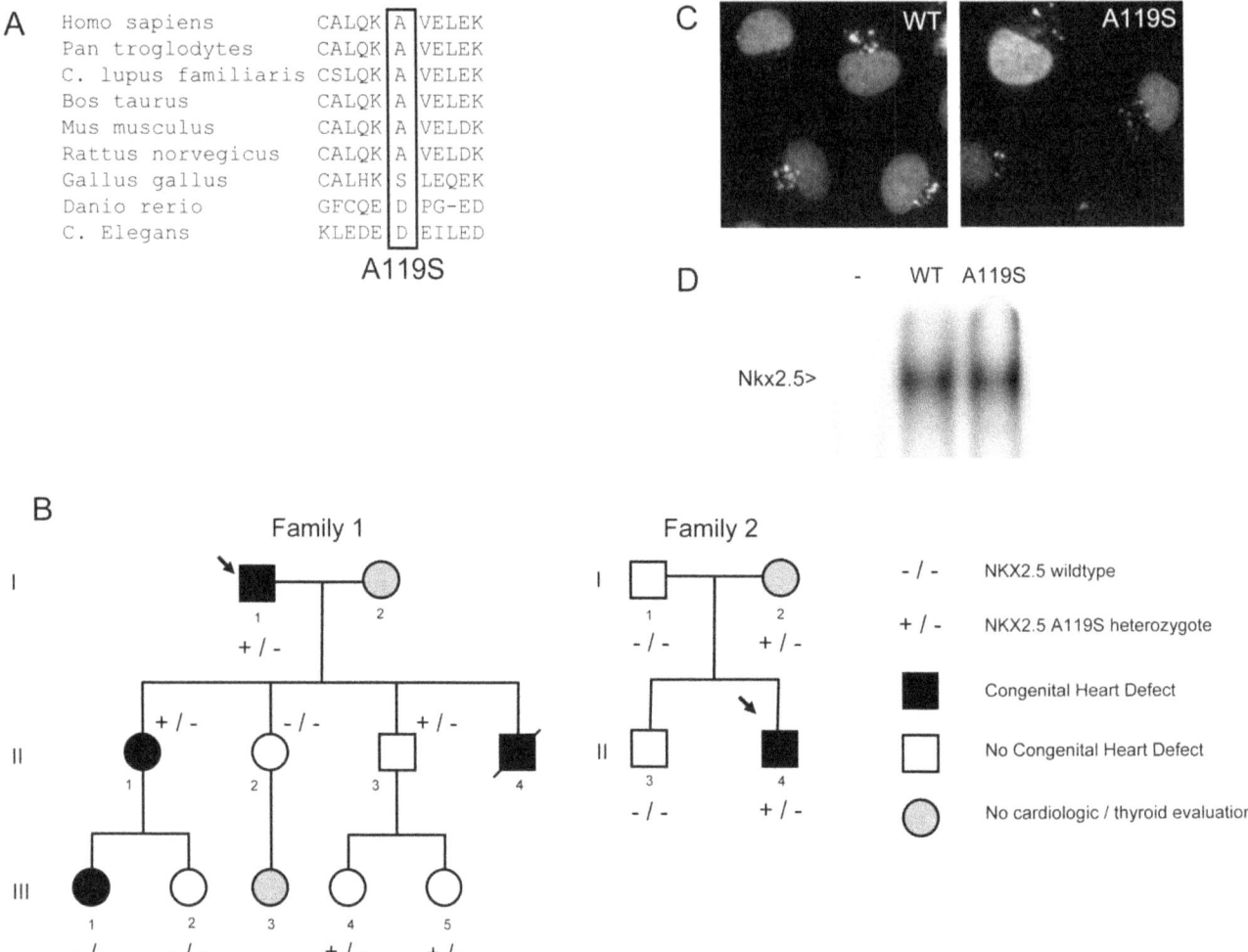

Figure 1. Family pedigrees, aminoacid alignments, nuclear localization of NKX2-5 protein and electro mobility shift assay. A. Pedigrees of the two families with the p.A119S NKX2-5 mutation. Individuals with congenital heart defects are indicated with a filled black symbol, while individuals with normal echocardiography are indicated with a white symbol. Grey symbols represent individuals that have not been evaluated clinically. A slash denotes a deceased individual; the proband is indicated by an arrow. None of the evaluated family members showed thyroid abnormalities. Heterozygous carriers of p.A119S are represented by +/− and non-carriers by −/−. B. Multiple alignments of aminoacids of the region surrounding p.A119 for various species. C. Nuclear localization of either wildtype or p.A119S NKX2-5 protein in COS7 cells. Nuclei are stained in green, red represents either the wildtype or mutant protein, orange indicates nuclei that are positive for wildtype or mutant protein. D. Electro mobility shift assay in cos7 cells, using the published nkx2.5 binding site [26]. Wildtype nkx2.5 protein and p.A119S Nkx2.5 protein bind equally well, − is untransfected control.

aminoacids differ. The pedigrees of the families with the p.A119S variation are shown in Figure 1B. Table 1 summarizes the clinical features of both families. Analysis of NOTCH1 in the proband of family 1, who had aortic coarctation and bicuspid aortic valve, did not show a pathogenic mutation.

Family Phenotypes

Family 1. The p.A119S variation was found in the proband (I-1), who had an aortic coarctation and bicuspid aortic valve diagnosed at age 45 years. The coarctation was surgically corrected at age 45 years and an artificial aortic valve was implanted at age 73 years because of severe calcification and stenosis. The probands' youngest son (II-4) died 20 days after birth, post-mortem pathology revealing aortic coarctation. The oldest daughter of the proband (II-1) was born with a ventricular septal defect (VSD) that closed spontaneously during childhood. Her oldest daughter (III-1) also had a VSD which was surgically

closed when she was 7 months old. Echocardiography was normal in the other family members. Normal location, volume and structure of the thyroid gland were shown by ultrasound in all investigated family members. Thyroid function was also normal in all individuals. The p.A119S variation did not segregate with the cardiac defects within the family, as III-1 is affected but she does not have the mutation and several family members without any evidence of CHD carried the mutation (II-3, III-4, III-5).

Family 2. The p.A119S variation was also found in a sporadic patient with ASDI with cleft mitral valve as well as small ASDII, for which a surgical correction took place at the age of 5 years. Thyroid ultrasound showed normal location and volume of the gland, but a small nodule was present in the left lobe. Additionally, anti-TPO antibodies were positive (620 kU/l) with normal thyroid function tests. These abnormalities are frequent in the general population [24,25], and we

Table 1. Clinical details of the family members.

Patients	Sex/age at evaluation (years)	A119S	Heart		Thyroid								Remarks
			CHD	ECG	Position in neck	Aspect	Volume left lobe (ml)	Volume right lobe (ml)	TSH (mE/L)	Free T4 (pmol/L)	Thyreoglobulin (pmol/L)	Anti-TPO antibodies	
Family 1													
I-1	M/81	+	CoA, BAV	Atrial fibrillation	Normal	Homogenous	9.5	9.0	2.20	14.5	4	Neg	
II-1	F/51	+	VSD	Normal	Normal	Homogenous	4.6	3.3	3.60	12.7	9	Neg	
II-2	F/49	−	None	Low voltages	Normal	Homogenous	3.7	3.9	1.60	12.3	5	Neg	
II-3	M/48	+	None	Normal	Normal	Homogenous	5.0	7.5	2.10	14.4	6	ND	
II-4	M/10 days	ND	CoA	ND	ND	ND	ND	ND	ND	ND	ND	ND	Deceased at age 10 days
III-1	F/24	−	VSD	Rigth axis deviation	Normal	Homogenous	2,9	3	1.70	13.6	9	Neg	
III-2	F/21	−	None	Normal	Normal	Homogenous	4.6	4.8	1.50	13.4	6	Neg	
III-4	F/20	+	None	Normal	Normal	Homogenous	3.0	6.0	1.40	15.3	6	Neg	
III-5	F/12	+	None	Normal	Normal	Homogenous	2.6	3.5	ND	ND	ND	ND	
Family 2													
I-1	M/60	−	None	ND	Normal	Homogenous	4.4	5.9	1.80	16.2	4	Neg	
I-2	F/62	+	None reported	ND	ND	ND	ND	ND	ND	ND	ND	ND	
II-1	M/35	−	None	ND	Normal	Homogenous	6.7	8.9	1.50	14.2	6	Neg	
II-2	M/31	+	ASDI, ASDII	RBBB	Normal	Homogenous	5.6	5.0	1.40	17.0	2	Pos (620 kU/l)	Homogenous solid nodule in left thyroid lobe, diameter 6 mm

ND, not determined; neg, negative; pos, positive; CHD, congenital heart disease; CoA, aortic coarctation; BAV, bicuspid aortic valve; VSD, ventricular septal defect; ASDI, ostium primum atrial septal defect; ASDII, ostium secundum atrial septal defect; RBBB, right bundle branch block.Anti-TPO antibodies 'negative' means value <50 kU/l.

therefore do not consider them to fall outside the range of expected findings. The probands' mother was found to carry the p.A119S variation and the father and brother did not. The mother was not available for clinical evaluation, though she did not have a history of cardiac or thyroid disorders. The probands' father had a myocardial infarction at age 55. He did not have CHD. Echocardiography in the probands' brother did not show CHD either. Thyroid evaluation of the probands' father and brother was also normal.

Normal Sub Cellular Distribution of the NKX2-5 p.A119S Protein

To be able to regulate transcription and exert its function, the NKX2-5 protein needs to be present in the nucleus. The localization of the p.A119S NKX2-5 protein was assessed by transfecting it into rat heart-derived cells (H10) and COS7 cells. The localization of mutant and WT proteins was visualized with an antibody against Nkx2-5. Figure 1C shows that both the wildtype and p.A119S NKX2-5 protein localize exclusively inside the nucleus, indicating that the process of nuclear import is not affected by the variation.

No Functional Defect in DNA Binding of p.A119S Nkx2.5

The transcription factor Nkx2.5 activates its target genes by binding to the DNA. To test whether the DNA binding capacity of p.A119S Nkx2.5 was altered, we used an electrophoretic mobility shift assay (EMSA) [18]. A fragment of the *Nppa* promoter was used, a well characterized promoter relevant in heart development, containing a functional Nkx2.5 binding element [26]. As shown in figure 1D, both wildtype and p.A119S Nkx2.5 protein bind equally well, indicating that there is no difference in DNA binding capacity between p.A119S and wildtype Nkx2.5 protein.

No Difference in Promoter Activations of Wildtype NKX2-5 or p.A119S NKX2-5

To test the functional consequences of the p.A119S variation in a relevant cellular context, we used reporter assays in which the proximal *NPPA* promoter (-270 to $+1$) [26], and the *Dio2*, *Tg* and *TPO* [8] promoters involved in thyroid gland function, were fused to a luciferase reporter. These promoters all contain functional binding sites for NKX2-5. We also tested NKX2-5 in combination with the TBX5 transcription factor as TBX5 synergizes with NKX2-5 in the activation of the *NPPA* promoter [26]. These transactivation assays were performed in both H10 cells and HELA cells, as used in the original publication of Dentice *et al.* on the possible connection between p.A119S and TD [8]. As a negative control we also used the p.N188K NKX2-5 mutant, reported as causative in a family with five affected presenting with atrial septal defects, Ebsteins anomaly and abnormal AV conduction [27]. No thyroid abnormalities were reported for this mutation. p.N188K introduces a mutation in the homedomain of Nkx2.5, an element conserved in all members of the Nkx protein family and known to directly contact adenine in the major groove of DNA. The p.N188K mutation leads to a complete loss-of-function in DNA binding [28] and can therefore serve as a negative control.

In the H10 cells, the wildtype NKX2-5 and the p.A119S protein both significantly activated the *NPPA* promoter driven reporter. When transfected together with TBX5 both wildtype NKX2-5 and p.A119S NKX2-5 also activated the reporter construct synergistically (Figure 2A). There was no difference between wildtype NKX2-5 and p.A119S NKX2-5 in the activation of the *NPPA* promoter construct for any condition tested. Likewise, we

observed no difference in activation of the *Dio2*, *Tg* or *TPO* promoter constructs between wildtype and p.A119S in H10 cells. We repeated all experiments in HELA cells, and found stronger activation of all constructs in comparison to the H10 cells. However, once again, we observed no difference in activation of any promoter tested between wildtype NKX2-5 and p.A119S NKX2-5 (Figure 2B).

Discussion

In our population of 303 patients with ASD and 38 probands from families with CHD, we found the NKX2-5 p.A119S variation in two patients. The variation did not segregate with CHD in the familial case, nor were any signs of TD present in the seven mutation carriers. Furthermore, functional studies showed no difference between wildtype and p.A119S protein in activation of four different promoters in either H10 cells or HELA cells. Taken together, our results strongly suggest that the p.A119S variation behaves similar to wild type NKX2-5 and that it has no discernible pathogenic role in either CHD or TD.

NKX2-5 belongs to the NK-2 family of homeodomain-containing transcription factors, which are conserved from flies to humans [10]. Its role as a transcription regulator during early embryonic heart developmental has been known for many years, and mutations in NKX2-5 are found in patients with CHD [10–12]. NKX2-5 has also been shown to be required for thyroid development in animal studies [8,29]. The link between thyroid development and NKX2-5 was highlighted by a recent publication of Dentice *et al.* [8], who reported three variations in NKX2.5 in four of the 241 patients with persistent congenital hypothyroidism studied, amongst them the p.A119S variation. They performed functional studies and showed a reduced DNA binding capacity and reduced transactivation properties with a dominant negative effect for p.A119S in comparison to wildtype Nkx2-5. The p.A119S mutation identified by Dentice *et al.* occurred in a girl with an ectopic thyroid gland. Her mother, who also carried the mutation, had auto-immune hypothyroidism but no evidence of TD and both were without evidence of CHD. Our molecular testing of the p.A119S variation in both rat heart derived (H10) cells and HELA cells showed no difference in transactivation of any of the four promoters tested (*NPPA*, *Tg*, *Dio2*, *TPO*), which is in contrast to the results obtained by Dentice *et al.* Nevertheless, the results of our functional studies are in agreement with our clinical data as the mutation did not segregate with CHD in our familial case and none of our seven mutation carriers had thyroid disease. Moreover, the A119S variation is present in the general population at a low rate (0.001%) and classified as a SNP [23]. In general, we conclude that we cannot uphold the results obtained by Dentice *et al.*, and it is unclear why the molecular results between the two studies are different, as the same proteins, promoters and cell lines were used. One difference is the fact that we did include a negative control (p.N188K) to show that our assay is robust and no confounding variables acted on the experiment.

Given the above, an important question is to what extent NKX2-5 mutations are involved in the pathogenesis of TD. In addition to p.A119S, three other NKX2-5 variations have been reported in literature thus far to be associated with TD: p.R25C, p.S265R and p.R161P [8,30]. The p.R25C variation has been identified in several patients with CHD, none of whom were reported to have TD [31]. Moreover, this variation is present in 1% of the general population as a SNP (rs2893667) [23], making it unlikely that it plays any pathogenic role in TD. In contrast, both the p.S265R and the p.R161P variation have not been reported in

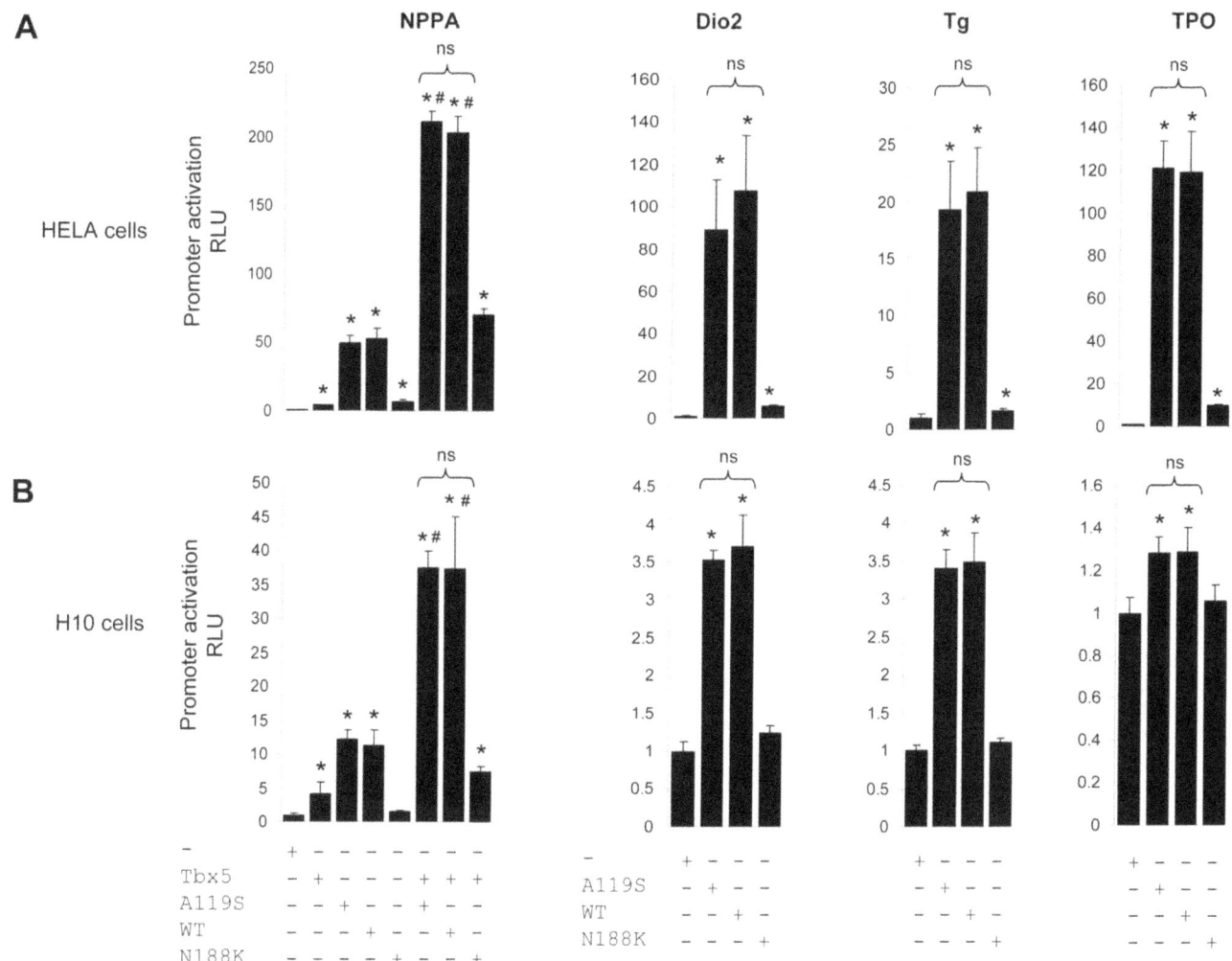

Figure 2. Relative activation of the Nppa, Dio2, Tg and TPO promoters in combination with wildtype NKX2-5, p.A119S NKX2-5, p.N188K NKX2-5 or TBX5. A. In H10 cells. B. In HELA cells. Significant differences between vector and condition tested are marked with *, P<0.05. # denotes a significant difference between conditions tested with and without TBX5, P<0.05. Error bars represent standard deviation (SD). Each condition has been tested at least in three independent triplicate experiments.

the general population. The p.S265R variation was reported in a girl with TD who also carried a mutation in the PAX8 promoter region [30] and the mutant protein was shown to have a reduced function. However, as the girls' healthy brother, father and grandmother also carried the NKX2-5 variation and the PAX8 mutation may have accounted for TD in the girl, there is no direct evidence that the p.S265R variation causes TD. The p.R161P NKX2-5 variation was found in a TD patient; however her father also carried the mutation but had no TD or CHD. Taken together, none of the four currently published NKX2-5 variations have been demonstrated to segregate with a phenotype of TD within a family. Although incomplete penetrance cannot be totally excluded, there is no strong genetic evidence of a clear pathogenic effect of the mutations.

To gain further insight into the role of NKX2-5 mutations in TD, a cohort of TD patients can be investigated for mutations in NKX2-5. However, the NKX2-5 gene has been analyzed in over 460 congenital hypothyroidism patients to date, but no additional mutations were identified (Table 2) [14,15,32–35]. Interestingly, 51 of these patients also had CHD [14,33]. Furthermore, none of

the more than 150 CHD patients with a demonstrated NKX2-5 mutation [12] were reported to have thyroid problems.

Although there is a lack of evidence for a strong pathogenic effect of NKX2-5 mutations in human TD, Nkx2-5 has been shown to be involved in thyroid development. Evidence for this comes from studies using wildtype Nkx2-5 mice, showing Nkx2-5 expression in the thyroid primordium up to E11.5 [8]. Moreover, Nkx2-5 knockout mice demonstrate thyroid bud hypoplasia [8,28]. Although these studies suggest that absence of Nkx2-5 could lead to (a form of) TD, one should keep in mind that these observations are based on Nkx2-5 null mice, which die around E9-10 [36]. In contrast, heterozygous knockout mice are viable and are not reported to have TD [37]. This suggests that the loss of one Nkx2-5 allele is tolerated, perhaps by compensation during development by paralogue genes such as NKX2-1, which activates the same promoter regions as NKX2-5.

Altogether, given the wealth of published evidence, we believe that NKX2-5 mutations do not play a major pathogenic role in TD. A role of NKX2-5 as a genetic modifier cannot entirely be excluded though. To our opinion, there is currently not enough evidence to warrant routine genetic testing for NKX2-5 mutations

Table 2. Studies analyzing *NKX2-5* in patients with persistent congenital hypothyroidism.

Author	Type of patients	N of patients	N of mutation carriers (%)	Remarks
Dentice et al., 2006 [8]	Persistent CH (athyreosis 53; thyroid ectopy 98; thyroid hypoplasia 15; 75 CH without goiter)	241	4 (1,7)	Two mutations (p.A119S and p.R25C), present in 3/4 patients, have been reported as a SNP [23].
Al Taji et al., 2007 [33]	Persistent primary non-auto-immune, non-goitre hypothyroidism AND CHD	15	0 (0)	
Ramos et al., 2009 [15]	Thyroid hypoplasia or athyreosis	35	0 (0)	
Cangul et al., 2009 [32]	Primary non-auto-immune, non-goitre hypothyroidism, from consanguineous families	9	0 (0)	In an additional 130 patients from consanguineous families linkage to the NKX2.5 locus was assumed to be excluded because heterozygosity for the gene was detected (no mutational analysis performed).
Narumi et al., 2010 [35]	Permanent primary CH diagnosed by neonatal screening (thyroid ectopy 37; thyroid aplasia 6; thyroid hypoplasia 8; other 51)	102	0 (0)	
Passeri et al., 2011 [14]	CHD and non-autoimmune CH (normal thyroid volume 35; hemiagenesis 1)	36	0 (0)	
Hermanns et al., 2011 [30]	nm	nm	1	Case report: the p.S265R variation was identified in a girl with thyroid dysgenesis who also carried a mutation in the PAX8 promoter region.
Brust et al., 2012 [34]	Thyroid dysgenesis (thyroid ectopy 13; hypoplasia 11; athyreosis 3)	27	0 (0)	

CHD, Congenital Heart Disease; CH, Congenital Hypothyroidism; nm, not mentioned.

in TD patients, and vice versa, to evaluate the thyroid in individuals carrying an NKX2-5 mutation.

In conclusion, the results of our study demonstrate that p.A119S does not cause CHD or TD and that it is a rare variation that behaves equal to wildtype NKX2-5. Furthermore, given the lack of clear evidence of pathogenicity of the reported NKX2-5 mutations, the high amounts of patients with TD without an NKX2-5 mutation and the absence of TD in NKX2-5 mutation carriers, we suggest that NKX2-5 mutations do not play a major pathogenic role in thyroid dysgenesis and that genetic testing for NKX2-5 in TD is not warranted. A role of NKX2-5 as a genetic modifier cannot entirely be excluded.

Acknowledgments

We are grateful to the patients and family members for their kind participation. We also thank E. Endert (Laboratory for Endocrinology, Academic Medical Center) for the performance of thyroid function analyses.

Author Contributions

Conceived and designed the experiments: KvE MJHB BJMM AVP. Performed the experiments: KvE MTMM JL AI AMJBS. Analyzed the data: KvE AVP. Contributed reagents/materials/analysis tools: ASPvT AVP. Wrote the paper: KvE MJHB VMC AVP.

References

1. Kempers MJ, Lanting CI, van Heijst AF, van Trotsenburg AS, Wiedijk BM, et al. (2006) Neonatal screening for congenital hypothyroidism based on thyroxine, thyrotropin, and thyroxine-binding globulin measurement: potentials and pitfalls. J Clin Endocrinol Metab 91: 3370–3376.
2. van Vliet G (2003) Development of the thyroid gland: lessons from congenitally hypothyroid mice and men. Clin Genet 63: 445–455.
3. Castanet M, Polak M, Bonaiti-Pellie C, Lyonnet S, Czernichow P, et al. (2001) Nineteen years of national screening for congenital hypothyroidism: familial cases with thyroid dysgenesis suggest the involvement of genetic factors. J Clin Endocrinol Metab 86: 2009–2014.
4. Krude H, Schutz B, Biebermann H, von MA, Schnabel D, et al. (2002) Choreoathetosis, hypothyroidism, and pulmonary alterations due to human NKX2-1 haploinsufficiency. J Clin Invest 109: 475–480.
5. Clifton-Bligh RJ, Wentworth JM, Heinz P, Crisp MS, John R, et al. (1998) Mutation of the gene encoding human TTF-2 associated with thyroid agenesis, cleft palate and choanal atresia. Nat Genet 19: 399–401.
6. Macchia PE, Lapi P, Krude H, Pirro MT, Missero C, et al. (1998) PAX8 mutations associated with congenital hypothyroidism caused by thyroid dysgenesis. Nat Genet 19: 83–86.
7. Sunthornthepvarakui T, Gottschalk ME, Hayashi Y, Refetoff S (1995) Brief report: resistance to thyrotropin caused by mutations in the thyrotropin-receptor gene. N Engl J Med 332: 155–160.
8. Dentice M, Cordeddu V, Rosica A, Ferrara AM, Santarpia L, et al. (2006) Missense mutation in the transcription factor NKX2-5: a novel molecular event in the pathogenesis of thyroid dysgenesis. J Clin Endocrinol Metab 91: 1428–1433.

9. Fagman H, Nilsson M (2011) Morphogenetics of early thyroid development. J Mol Endocrinol 46: R33–R42.
10. Bartlett H, Veenstra GJ, Weeks DL (2010) Examining the cardiac NK-2 genes in early heart development. Pediatr Cardiol 31: 335–341.
11. Schott JJ, Benson DW, Basson CT, Pease W, Silberbach GM, et al. (1998) Congenital heart disease caused by mutations in the transcription factor NKX2-5. Science 281: 108–111.
12. Reamon-Buettner SM, Borlak J (2010) NKX2-5: an update on this hypermutable homeodomain protein and its role in human congenital heart disease (CHD). Hum Mutat 31: 1185–1194.
13. Olivieri A, Stazi MA, Mastroiacovo P, Fazzini C, Medda E, et al. (2002) A population-based study on the frequency of additional congenital malformations in infants with congenital hypothyroidism: data from the Italian Registry for Congenital Hypothyroidism (1991–1998). J Clin Endocrinol Metab 87: 557–562.
14. Passeri E, Frigerio M, De FT, Valaperta R, Capelli P, et al. (2011) Increased Risk for Non-Autoimmune Hypothyroidism in Young Patients with Congenital Heart Defects. J Clin Endocrinol Metab : E1115–E1119.
15. Ramos HE, Nesi-Franca S, Boldarine VT, Pereira RM, Chiamolera MI, et al. (2009) Clinical and molecular analysis of thyroid hypoplasia: a population-based approach in southern Brazil. Thyroid 19: 61–68.
16. van der Velde ET, Vriend JW, Mannens MM, Uiterwaal CS, Brand R, et al. (2005) CONCOR, an initiative towards a national registry and DNA-bank of patients with congenital heart disease in the Netherlands: rationale, design, and first results. Eur J Epidemiol 20: 549–557.

17. Lennon G, Auffray C, Polymeropoulos M, Soares MB (1996) The I.M.A.G.E. Consortium: an integrated molecular analysis of genomes and their expression. Genomics 33: 151–152.

18. Postma AV, van de Meerakker JB, Mathijssen IB, Barnett P, Christoffels VM, et al. (2008) A gain-of-function TBX5 mutation is associated with atypical Holt-Oram syndrome and paroxysmal atrial fibrillation. Circ Res 102: 1433–1442.

19. Jahn L, Sadoshima J, Greene A, Parker C, Morgan KG, et al. (1996) Conditional differentiation of heart- and smooth muscle-derived cells transformed by a temperature-sensitive mutant of SV40 T antigen. J Cell Sci 109 (Pt 2): 397–407.

20. Gey GO, Coffman WD, Kubicek MT (1952) Tissue culture studies of the proliferative capacity of cervical carcinoma and normal epithelium. Cancer Res 12: 264–265.

21. Ruijter JM, Thygesen HH, Schoneveld OJ, Das AT, Berkhout B, et al. (2006) Factor correction as a tool to eliminate between-session variation in replicate experiments: application to molecular biology and retrovirology. Retrovirology 3: 2.

22. Gluzman Y (1981) SV40-transformed simian cells support the replication of early SV40 mutants. Cell 23: 175–182.

23. Tennessen JA, Bigham AW, O'Connor TD, Fu W, Kenny EE, et al. (2012) Evolution and Functional Impact of Rare Coding Variation from Deep Sequencing of Human Exomes. Science 337: 64–69.

24. Dean DS, Gharib H (2008) Epidemiology of thyroid nodules. Best Pract Res Clin Endocrinol Metab 22: 901–911.

25. Spencer CA, Hollowell JG, Kazarosyan M, Braverman LE (2007) National Health and Nutrition Examination Survey III thyroid-stimulating hormone (TSH)-thyroperoxidase antibody relationships demonstrate that TSH upper reference limits may be skewed by occult thyroid dysfunction. J Clin Endocrinol Metab 92: 4236–4240.

26. Habets PE, Moorman AF, Clout DE, van Roon MA, Lingbeek M, et al. (2002) Cooperative action of Tbx2 and Nkx2.5 inhibits ANF expression in the atrioventricular canal: implications for cardiac chamber formation. Genes Dev 16: 1234–1246.

27. Benson DW, Silberbach GM, Kavanaugh-McHugh A, Cottrill C, Zhang Y, et al. (1999) Mutations in the cardiac transcription factor NKX2.5 affect diverse cardiac developmental pathways. J Clin Invest 104: 1567–1573.

28. Kasahara H, Lee B, Schott JJ, Benson DW, Seidman JG, et al. (2000) Loss of function and inhibitory effects of human CSX/NKX2.5 homeoprotein mutations associated with congenital heart disease. J Clin Invest 106: 299–308.

29. Lints TJ, Parsons LM, Hartley L, Lyons I, Harvey RP (1993) Nkx-2.5: a novel murine homeobox gene expressed in early heart progenitor cells and their myogenic descendants. Development 119: 419–431.

30. Hermanns P, Grasberger H, Refetoff S, Pohlenz J (2011) Mutations in the NKX2.5 Gene and the PAX8 Promoter in a Girl with Thyroid Dysgenesis. J Clin Endocrinol Metab 96: E977–E981.

31. Beffagna G, Cecchetto A, Dal BL, Lorenzon A, Angelini A, et al. (2012) R25C mutation in the NKX2.5 gene in Italian patients affected with non-syndromic and syndromic congenital heart disease. J Cardiovasc Med (Hagerstown).

32. Cangul H, Morgan NV, Forman JR, Saglam H, Aycan Z, et al. (2010) Novel TSHR mutations in consanguineous families with congenital nongoitrous hypothyroidism. Clin Endocrinol (Oxf) 73: 671–677.

33. Al Taji E, Biebermann H, Limanova Z, Hnikova O, Zikmund J, et al. (2007) Screening for mutations in transcription factors in a Czech cohort of 170 patients with congenital and early-onset hypothyroidism: identification of a novel PAX8 mutation in dominantly inherited early-onset non-autoimmune hypothyroidism. Eur J Endocrinol 156: 521–529.

34. Brust ES, Beltrao CB, Chammas MC, Watanabe T, Sapienza MT, et al. (2012) Absence of mutations in PAX8, NKX2.5, and TSH receptor genes in patients with thyroid dysgenesis. Arq Bras Endocrinol Metabol 56: 173–177.

35. Narumi S, Muroya K, Asakura Y, Adachi M, Hasegawa T (2010) Transcription factor mutations and congenital hypothyroidism: systematic genetic screening of a population-based cohort of Japanese patients. J Clin Endocrinol Metab 95: 1981–1985.

36. Lyons I, Parsons LM, Hartley L, Li R, Andrews JE, et al. (1995) Myogenic and morphogenetic defects in the heart tubes of murine embryos lacking the homeo box gene Nkx2–5. Genes Dev 9: 1654–1666.

37. Biben C, Weber R, Kesteven S, Stanley E, McDonald L, et al. (2000) Cardiac septal and valvular dysmorphogenesis in mice heterozygous for mutations in the homeobox gene Nkx2–5. Circ Res 87: 888–895.

14

Contribution of Rare Copy Number Variants to Isolated Human Malformations

Clara Serra-Juhé[1,2], Benjamín Rodríguez-Santiago[3], Ivon Cuscó[1,2], Teresa Vendrell[4], Núria Camats[5], Núria Torán[5], Luis A. Pérez-Jurado[1,2]*

1 Unitat de Genètica, Universitat Pompeu Fabra, Barcelona, Spain, **2** Centro de Investigación Biomédica en Red de Enfermedades Raras (CIBERER), Barcelona, Spain, **3** Quantitative Genomic Medicine Laboratories (qGenomics), Barcelona, Spain, **4** Programa de Medicina Molecular i Genètica, Hospital Universitari Vall d'Hebron, Barcelona, Spain, **5** Servei d'Anatomia Patològica, Hospital Universitari Vall d'Hebron, Barcelona, Spain

Abstract

Background: Congenital malformations are present in approximately 2–3% of liveborn babies and 20% of stillborn fetuses. The mechanisms underlying the majority of sporadic and isolated congenital malformations are poorly understood, although it is hypothesized that the accumulation of rare genetic, genomic and epigenetic variants converge to deregulate developmental networks.

Methodology/Principal Findings: We selected samples from 95 fetuses with congenital malformations not ascribed to a specific syndrome (68 with isolated malformations, 27 with multiple malformations). Karyotyping and Multiplex Ligation-dependent Probe Amplification (MLPA) discarded recurrent genomic and cytogenetic rearrangements. DNA extracted from the affected tissue (46%) or from lung or liver (54%) was analyzed by molecular karyotyping. Validations and inheritance were obtained by MLPA. We identified 22 rare copy number variants (CNV) [>100 kb, either absent (n = 7) or very uncommon (n = 15, <1/2,000) in the control population] in 20/95 fetuses with congenital malformations (21%), including 11 deletions and 11 duplications. One of the 9 tested rearrangements was *de novo* while the remaining were inherited from a healthy parent. The highest frequency was observed in fetuses with heart hypoplasia (8/17, 62.5%), with two events previously related with the phenotype. Double events hitting candidate genes were detected in two samples with brain malformations. Globally, the burden of deletions was significantly higher in fetuses with malformations compared to controls.

Conclusions/Significance: Our data reveal a significant contribution of rare deletion-type CNV, mostly inherited but also *de novo*, to human congenital malformations, especially heart hypoplasia, and reinforce the hypothesis of a multifactorial etiology in most cases.

Editor: Francesc Palau, Instituto de Ciencia de Materiales de Madrid - Instituto de Biomedicina de Valencia, Spain

Funding: This work was supported by grants from the Spanish Ministry of Health (PI042063), the CIBERER (Centro de Investigación Biomédica en Red de Enfermedades Raras)(U735-3) and the VI Framework Programme of the European Union (LSHG-CT-2006-037627). CS-J and BR-S were supported by predoctoral (FIS FI08/00365) and posdoctoral fellowships (FIS CD06/00019) of the Fondo de Investigación Sanitaria, respectively. The funders had no role in study design, data collection and analysis, decision to publish, or preparation of the manuscript.

Competing Interests: Benjami´n Rodri´guez-Santiago and Luis A. Pe´rez-Jurado are currently employee and scientific advisor, respectively, of qGenomics SL.

* E-mail: luis.perez@upf.edu

Introduction

A potentially lethal or disabling major malformation occurs in 2–3% of liveborn infants and 20% of stillborn fetuses [1]. Congenital malformations have become the main cause of infant mortality during the first years of life [2] and are associated with long term morbidity [3,4]. In particular, congenital heart defects (CHD) represent a high percentage of clinically significant birth defects. The incidence of CHD is approximately 8 per 1,000 livebirths making CHD the most common malformation [5,6].

Congenital malformations often occur in the setting of multiple congenital anomalies, including dysmorphic facial features, developmental aberrations of different organs, or growth abnormalities [7,8]. In these cases with a more complex syndrome, chromosomal aberrations are a frequent cause of disease, although point mutations in developmental or metabolic genes have also been described in specific syndromes [9,10]. Standard karyotyping can detect numerical and structural anomalies larger than 5–10 Mb and other techniques, such as fluorescent in situ hybridization (FISH) [11] or MLPA [12–14], allow the identification of submicroscopic chromosomal imbalances. In the last decade, the development of molecular karyotyping by array comparative genomic hybridization (aCGH) or single-nucleotide-polymorphism (SNP) microarrays, globally termed chromosomal microarray analysis (CMA), has allowed the detection of as much as 15–24% of causative segmental aneusomies in patients with multiple congenital anomalies and/or intellectual disability [15,16]. Retrospective studies in fetuses with multiple malformations have obtained a detection rate of causative chromosomal imbalances from 8 to 15% by using CMA [17–19], and the clinical utility of a targeted CMA has been demonstrated in standard invasive prenatal diagnosis [20,21]. CHD are among the malformations in which genomic rearrangements have been shown to play a major role. For instance, microdeletions at 22q11.2 [22,23] and microduplications at 1q21.1 [24,25] are a common cause of conotruncal heart defects.

In an important proportion of cases, only one malformation is detected without the presentation of other minor or major defects. Although some isolated congenital malformations can be caused by environmental risk factors, such as maternal diseases or exposure to teratogenic agents during pregnancy [4], there is strong evidence that genetics plays a major role, as epidemiological studies have shown an increased risk of this type of anomalies in siblings and offspring of individuals with sporadic congenital malformations, as well as increased paternal age and high concordance in monozygotic twins [26–28]. A small percentage can be attributed to point mutations in development related genes [29,30], although this type of genetic alterations have been insufficiently tested until recently. Submicroscopic deletions and duplications may play a significant role in the etiology of this condition, either as direct cause or as possible genetic risk factor for isolated congenital anomaly [31]. Nevertheless, the mechanisms underlying the majority of non-chromosomal or sporadic congenital malformations are poorly understood.

Finding the cause of congenital malformations is necessary to better understand the pathophysiological basis of these developmental anomalies and define disease risks, both critical elements to ensure proper genetic counseling and disease prevention. Genetic counseling has become more relevant in this area considering not only the recurrence risk of healthy parents after having an index case, but also that more individuals with congenital malformations are living into adulthood due to advances in medical and surgical care and may have the opportunity to reproduce [7].

We have searched for cryptic genomic rearrangements in fetuses with isolated congenital malformations and fetuses with more than one congenital anomaly. Our data illustrate a significant contribution of rare deletion-type CNV, mostly inherited but also *de novo*, to human congenital malformations. These genomic rearrangements could represent the single genetic etiology of the disease, perhaps as part of a more complex syndrome without other recognizable manifestations at this stage of development, or genetic susceptibility factors contributing to the mutational load in multifactorial disorders.

Methods

Ethics Statement

All studies were performed as part of an expanded diagnostic protocol approved by the Medical Ethical Committee of the Vall d'Hebron Hospital, after receiving written informed consent from the family.

Samples/Patients

Fetuses were selected from medically terminated pregnancies between 17 and 22 weeks of gestation owing to one or more malformations with bad prognosis detected during pregnancy. Samples were collected from frozen tissues stored in the Tissue Bank of Vall d'Hebron Hospital. A complete fetopathological examination had been performed and the samples were classified in two different groups: 1) 68 samples with an isolated congenital malformation, including 33 with isolated CHD, 26 with isolated central nervous system (CNS) malformation and 9 with isolated renal malformation; 2) 27 fetuses with more than a unique malformation. Prenatal GTG banding chromosome analysis was

Table 1. Overview of malformations in the 95 analyzed fetuses.

MALFORMATION	SAMPLES
Congenital heart disease	
Conotruncal defect	13
Heart hypoplasia	17
Other	3
Central nervous system malformation	
Neural tube defect	16
Holoprosencephaly	3
Hydrocephalus	3
Ventriculomegaly	3
Agenesis of the corpus callosum	1
Renal malformations	
Agenesis	5
Dysplasia	3
Nephronophthisis	1
Multiple malformations	27

normal for all 95 fetuses. An overview of the clinical features of the fetuses included in the study is summarized in table 1 (detailed in Tables S1, S2, S3, S4).

Parental blood samples were collected in cases in which an alteration was identified.

DNA extraction from tissue and blood samples

In fetuses with an isolated congenital malformation, the affected tissue (heart, brain or kidney) was obtained when available (n = 44); liver or lung tissue was used for the remaining samples with insufficient target tissue (n = 24). For fetuses with multiple congenital anomalies (n = 27), liver or lung tissue was used. Parental DNA was isolated from total blood. DNA was extracted using the Gentra Puregene Blood kit (Qiagen) according to manufacturer's instructions.

Multiplex Ligation-dependent Probe Amplification (MLPA)

Genomic rearrangements in subtelomeric regions (P036 and/or P070, MRC Holland) as well as recurrent microdeletion or microduplication syndromes (custom made, Table S5) were also discarded prior to selection by using two MLPA panels.

An MLPA assay was also designed to validate the genomic alterations detected by CMA and to study the inheritance in those cases with available parental samples. A total of 100 ng of genomic DNA from each sample was subject to MLPA using specific synthetic probes [Table S6] designed to target the specific CNV detected by different types of array. All MLPA reactions were analyzed on an ABI PRISM 3100 Genetic analyzer according to manufacturers' instructions. Each MLPA signal was normalized and compared to the corresponding peak height obtained in control samples [32,33].

Molecular karyotyping by CMA

The entire cohort was studied by using BAC (Bacterial Artificial Chromosome) aCGH. DNA samples (1 μg) were labeled by random priming with Cy3-dCTP and Cy5-dCTP and hybridized against a reference pool of the same gender. Samples were hybridized onto a BAC aCGH containing 5,600 clones with a backbone mean coverage of ~1 Mb and increased density in hotspot regions for genomic rearrangements (subtelomeres, pericentromeres and regions flanked by segmental duplications). Analyses of BAC-aCGH data were performed as previously described [32].

A total of 25 samples were also studied by using an oligonucleotide Agilent H244K aCGH. Samples were processed and hybridized according to manufacturer's recommendations (Agilent Protocol v6.0, ref. G4410-90010). This technique allowed us to validate and better map the breakpoints of the alterations detected by BAC aCGH, as well as to increase the resolution of the study in samples in which no alteration had been detected using BAC aCGH. Only CNVs with genes, longer than 100 kb and with a frequency in control samples lower than 1/2,000 were considered. The frequency of each CNV in the control population was determined using 1 M Illumina SNP array data from a control database of 8,329 samples already reported [34], along with data from 1,991 Spanish adult samples from the Spanish Bladder Cancer/EPICURO study including 1034 patients with urothelial cell carcinoma of the bladder and 957 hospital-based generally healthy controls with a mean age of 63.7 years [35].

DNA from 70 samples was studied by using the 370K Illumina SNP array. This technique permitted us to increase the resolution in samples in which no alteration had been identified using BAC aCGH. Moreover, using SNP array uniparental disomy and regions with high level of homozygosity were studied. Copy number changes were identified using the PennCNV software with stringent filtering, as previously described [35]. Only CNVs with genes, longer than 100 kb and with a frequency in control samples lower than 1/2,000 were considered. A search for possible mosaic copy number and copy neutral changes was also performed using the MAD algorithm [36].

Genetic counseling

Genetic counseling was offered to all couples when an alteration was identified in order to explain the findings and the need for further testing including parental samples. After the study of the parents' samples, follow-up counseling was provided along with a written report explaining the alteration, the putative relation with the phenotype and the implications to the family.

Bioinformatic and statistical analyses

The frequency of each CNV in the population was determined using 1 M Illumina SNP array data from a control database of 8,329 samples already reported [34], along with data from 1,991 Spanish adult samples studied in our laboratory with the same arrays [35].

In addition, already available data from a randomly selected cohort of 168 generally healthy Spanish adult control individuals (Spanish Bladder Cancer/EPICURO study genotyped with Illumina 1 M SNP array [35]) was used in order to compare the different frequencies of rare rearrangements between controls and fetuses with congenital malformations (global CNV burden and CNV combinations). In order to avoid or minimize a possible bias due to the different detection yield of the array platforms used, we only considered alterations larger than 100 kb that should be detected with any of the platform arrays. For the comparative analyses, only CNVs with genes, a minimum length of 100 kb and a frequency in control samples lower than 1/2,000 were considered. Alterations totally overlapping with segmental duplications were also excluded to minimize biases due to the different probe coverage among microarray platforms.

Gene content and enrichment analyses

The gene content (genes included or disrupted) of the rare CNVs identified in the cohort of fetuses was analyzed using a computational resource, Consensus Path DB [37], to obtain an overview of the pathways that could be altered. Pathways were considered overrepresented when their p-value was above 0.05.

Results

Prenatal GTG banding chromosome analysis was normal for all 95 fetuses. Known microdeletion/microduplication syndromes and subtelomeric genomic rearrangements were also discarded by MLPA in all cases. All samples were first studied using BAC aCGH and then by oligonucleotide or SNP array (Fig. 1).

Globally, CMA detected 22 CNVs fulfilling the established criteria (>100 kb, gene containing and present in <1/2000 controls) in 20 samples (21.05%), 11 deletions and 11 duplications (100.6–2,324 kb in length), with 2 samples harboring two rearrangements. MLPA probes were designed to define the inherited or *de novo* nature of the CNVs in all 9 cases from whom parental samples were available. In 8 cases the alterations were inherited, while the rearrangement was *de novo* in a single case. The detected alterations are listed in table 2, including information about the genomic coordinates, size, microarrays used for detection and validation, inheritance and genes included in the region. Among the 22 alterations identified, 7 (4 duplications and 3 deletions) have never been found in the 10,320 adults used as controls. Two aberrations, both of them identified in fetuses with CHD, overlap with previously reported alterations associated with developmental anomalies and are likely the underlying genetic cause [38–40]: 1) A 363 kb *de novo* deletion in 16q24.1, encompassing five genes (*FOXF1, FOXC2, MTHFSD, FLJ30679* and *FOXL1*), was detected in a fetus with left heart hypoplasia (case 2); 2) the recurrent 2.2 Mb 15q13.3 deletion was identified in a fetus with right heart hypoplasia as well as in the healthy mother (case 1). The remaining 20 rearrangements have not been described in patients with disease.

Although not included in the listed 22 aberrations because its reported frequency in controls is 0.14% (>1/1,000), we also detected the recurrent 1.6 Mb 16p13.11 duplication in two samples, one case of CNS malformation (neural tube defect and Arnold-Chiari malformation) and another with multiple malformations (anal imperforation, right heart hypoplasia and esophagus atresia). The reciprocal deletion of this region has been clearly associated with increased risk for congenital malformations and developmental difficulties but published data for the duplication are not clearly conclusive [41].

In order to define whether the global burden of rare CNVs in the fetuses with congenital malformations was or not significantly increased, we compared it with a cohort of 168 control subjects analyzed with the Illumina 1 M SNP array. For consistency, only CNVs larger than 100 kb, containing genes, not totally overlapping with segmental duplications, and found at a frequency <1/2,000 were considered (listed in Table S7). Rare CNVs fulfilling criteria were identified in 17.86% of the control samples including 2 samples with 2 alterations. These rare CNVs in controls were predominantly duplications (78.12% vs 21.88% deletions). Thus, the global CNV burden in malformed fetuses was only slightly increased with respect to that in normal controls (21.05% vs 17.86%).

The proportion of samples with rearrangements was different between the different groups of malformations, being higher in fetuses with CHD (10/33 samples, 30.30%) and even higher if only heart hypoplasia was considered (8/17, 47.06%). The

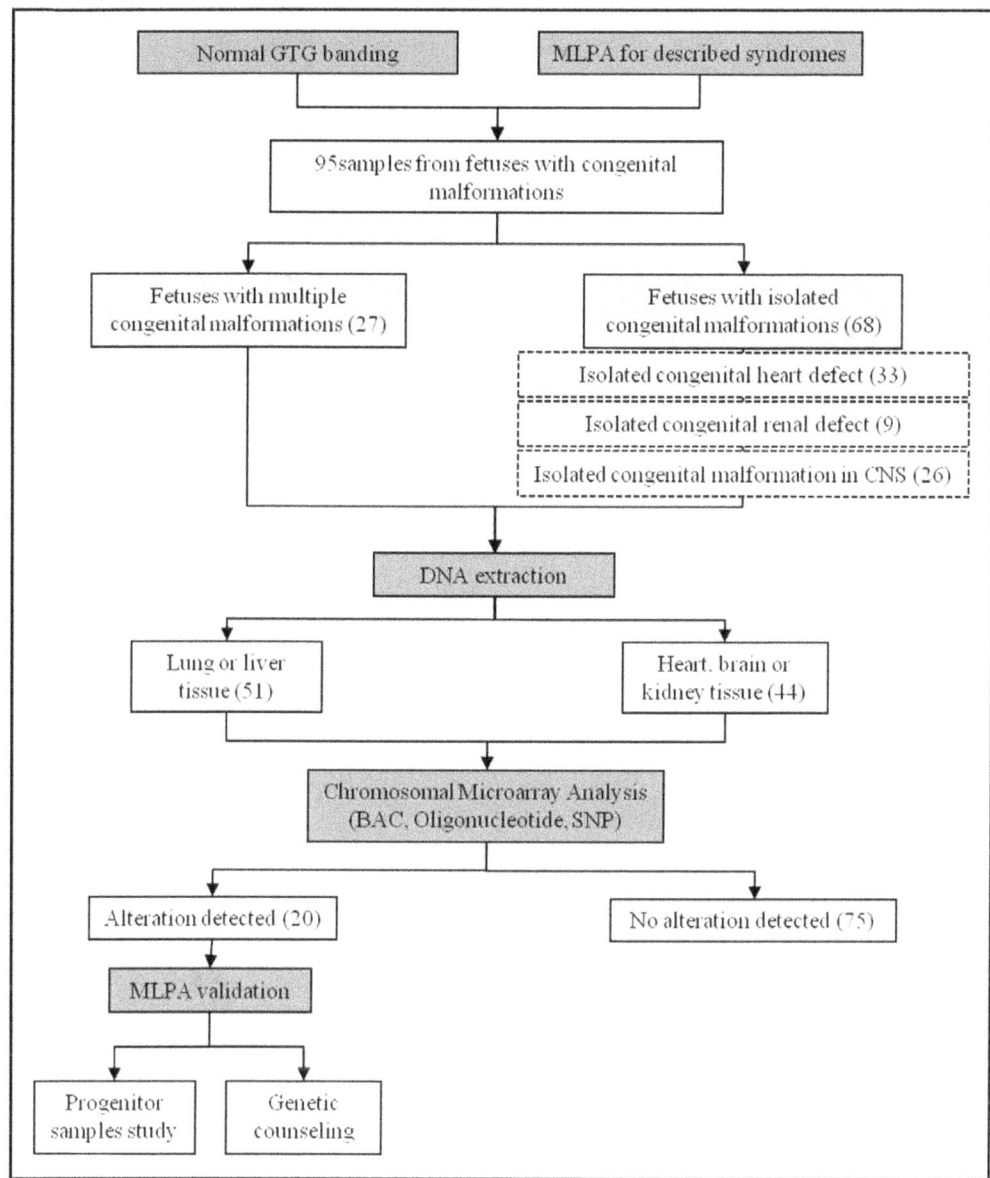

Figure 1. Strategy followed to study samples of fetuses with congenital malformations. MLPA: multiplex ligation-dependent probe amplification; CNS: central nervous system; BAC: bacterial artificial chromosome; SNP: single nucleotide polymorphism.

difference in aberration frequency between groups was statistically significant comparing fetuses with heart hypoplasia and controls (p = 0.009). The difference in the frequency of deletion-type CNV between cases and controls was also statistically significant (50% vs 21.88%, p = 0.03) and more evident comparing only fetuses with heart hypoplasia and controls (p = 0.001). These differences were due to the increased number of deletions, but not duplications, in cases with congenital malformations (Table 3). The frequency of individuals with more than one CNV hit fulfilling the established criteria was not different between cases and controls, around 2% (Table 3).

Regarding the overrepresentation analysis, phosphatidylinositol phosphate metabolism was the only pathway significantly overrepresented in cases with respect to controls. Three genes directly involved in this pathway, *PIK3C2G*, *GPLD1* and *INPP5A*, are included in the CNVs identified in two fetuses. Interestingly, two

of these genes are located in two deletions found in the same sample, a fetus with holoprosencephaly. One deletion encompassing three genes, *ALDH5A1*, *GPLD1* and *MRS2*, was inherited from the mother, while the other one including only one gene, *PIK3C2G*, was inherited from the father (Fig. 2). An additional sample with two events was a fetus with hydrocephalus found to have two duplication CNVs, on chromosome bands 1p33 (including the genes *FAAH*, *DMBX1* and *KNCN*) and 10q11.22 (containing the genes *SYT15*, *GPRIN2* and *PPYR1*), but parental samples were not available in this case.

No large stretches of homozygosity suggestive of parental consanguinity or uniparental disomy (UPD) were identified in any sample (70/95 fetuses studied with SNP arrays). In addition, despite the use of DNA from the affected tissue in 46% of cases, no events of copy number or copy neutral changes suggestive of somatic mutations were detected.

Table 2. Summary of copy number variations detected in 95 fetuses with congenital malformations.

Case #	Malformation	Gain/Loss	Region	Length (kb)	Start	End	Array used	Inheritance	Genes in the region	Control frequency (10,320)
6	CHD	Gain	5q35.2	297.3	175798945	176096236	SNP	-	ARL10, CLTB, EIF4E1B, FAF2, GPRIN1, HIGD2A, NOP16, PCDH24, RNF44, SNCB, TSPAN17	0
2	CHD	Loss	16q24.1	363.5	86382121	86745576	SNP	De novo	FOXF1, FOXC2, MTHFSD, FLJ30679, FOXL1	0
4	CHD	Loss	16q23.3	120.3	83869776	83990089	SNP	Paternal	MLYCD, OSGIN1	1
23	CHD	Loss	6p25.1	139.4	5249765	5389206	Oligonucleotide	-	LYRM4, FARS2	1
24	CHD	Gain	2p25.3	108.5	3579585	3688127	SNP	-	COLEC11, RNASEH1, RPS7	1
29	CHD	Gain	3p26.3	246.5	2869944	3116438	SNP	Paternal	CNTN4, IL5RA	1
1	CHD	Loss	15q13.3	2207	30755144	32962148	BAC and Oligo	Maternal	FAN1, MTMR10, TRPM1, LOC283710, KLF13, OTUD7A, CHRNA7	1
3	CHD	Loss	13q21.2	288.1	60410392	60698463	BAC and SNP	Maternal	DIAPH3	2
15	CHD	Gain	10q26.3	181.4	134572478	134753880	Oligonucleotide	-	INPP5A, NKX6-2, TTC40	2
13	CHD	Gain	9p21.1	369.2	28659143	29028380	SNP	-	LINGO2	4
48	CNS	Loss	17p12	1383.3	14090300	15473646	Oligonucleotide	-	COX10, CDRT15, HS3ST3B1, PMP22, TEKT3, CDRT4, FAM18B2	0
57	CNS	Loss	6p22.2	112.9	24401654	24514569	SNP	Maternal	ALDH5A1, GPLD1, MRS2	0
50	CNS	Loss	12p12.3	311.6	18337494	18649057	SNP	Paternal	PIK3C2G	4
	CNS	Gain	1p33	139.2	46814268	46953453	Oligonucleotide	-	FAAH, DMBX1, KNCN	0
	CNS	Gain	10q11.22	197.3	46951237	47148490	Oligonucleotide	-	SYT15, GPRIN2, PPYR1	4
59	CNS	Gain	5p13.2	150.3	37411054	37561355	BAC and Oligo	-	WDR70	4
53	CNS	Loss	18q22.1	2324.0	63733025	66057032	SNP	Maternal	CDH19, DSEL, LOC643542	4
65	Renal	Loss	4q12	883	52798624	53681594	SNP	Maternal	DANCR, LRRC66, SGCB, SNORA26, SPATA18, USP46	1
72	Multiple	Gain	10p14	128.4	11815455	11943885	SNP	-	C10orf47, LOC219731	0
82	Multiple	Gain	5q35.3	752.9	179833485	180586413	SNP	-	BTNL3, BTNL8, BTNL9, CNOT6, FLT4, LOC729678, MGAT1, OR2V2, OR2Y1, SCGB3A1, ZFP62	0
85	Multiple	Loss	7p14.1	130.1	40264889	40394987	SNP	-	C7orf10	1
84	Multiple	Gain	1p34.1	100.6	46252717	46353332	SNP	-	MAST2	5

Control frequency refers to the frequency of the same type of rearrangement found in the fetus, deletion or duplication. Hg19 assembly. CHD: congenital heart defect; CNS: central nervous system; SNP: single nucleotide polymorphism; BAC: bacterial artificial chromosome.

Table 3. Comparisons of rare copy number changes >100 kb detected in the fetuses with congenital malformations and controls.

GROUP	ALTERATIONS	DELETIONS	DUPLICATIONS	DOUBLE HIT	SAMPLES
Controls (168)	32	7 (4.2%/21.88%)	25 (14.9%/78.12%)	2 (1.19%)	30 (17.86%)
Fetuses (95)	22	11 (11.6%/50%)	11 (11.6%/50%)	2 (2.11%)	20 (21.05%)
CHD (33)	10	5 (15.2%/50%)	5 (15.2%/50%)	0 (0%)	10 (30.30%)
*Heart hypoplasia (17)	8	5 (29.4%/62.5%)	3 (17.6%/37.5%)	0 (0%)	8 (47.06%)
CNS malformations (26)	7	4 (15.4%/57.14%)	3 (11.5%/42.86%)	2 (7.69%)	5 (19.23%)
Renal malformations (9)	1	1 (11.1%/100%)	0 (0%/0%)	0 (0%)	1 (11.11%)
Multiple malformations (27)	4	1 (3.7%/25%)	3 (11.1%/75%)	0 (0%)	4 (14.81%)

In brackets the proportion of samples with the CNV and the proportion of the specific type of rearrangement. *A subcategory of CHD only considering heart hypoplasia has been added to the table due to remark the different frequency of CNVs with respect to the other CHD. CHD: congenital heart defect; CNS: central nervous system.

Discussion

Chromosomal aberrations have been reported as a frequent cause of congenital malformations, especially when they are associated with growth or developmental delay, malformations affecting a second organ or dysmorphic features [6,16,18,42]. Many of the chromosomal unbalances associated with such syndromes are large and encompass multiple genes. A detection rate of 10% of chromosomal abnormalities, including one marker chromosome, one rearrangement of 9 Mb and another rearrangement of 13 Mb, has been reported studying by aCGH a population of 50 fetuses with at least three malformations or a severe brain anomaly [42]. A yield of 16.3%, considering known syndromes, was found in a cohort of 49 fetuses with birth defects [18]. The role of submicroscopic deletions and duplications in isolated congenital malformations has been documented for CHD with the identification of 18 putatively pathogenic CNVs (17.1%) in 105 samples from infants with isolated CHD [31], including recurrent rearrangements in 22q11.2 (responsible of DiGeorge syndrome), 17p11 (causative of Smith-Magenis syndrome) and 1q21.1, a large alteration of 14 Mb and an aberration with no genes.

In our series, chromosomal alterations detected by karyotyping and cryptic alterations in subtelomeric regions or known microdeletion/microduplication syndromes were previously excluded. Rare CNVs larger than 100 kb were detected in 21% of fetuses with prenatally detected malformations, with a yield of 30.3% in fetuses with CHD. The CNV burden was slightly but significantly higher in malformed fetuses compared with controls (21.05% vs 17.86%). Deletions were also more prevalent in cases than controls (50% vs 21.88%). As expected, large CNVs and mostly deletions are more likely to affect gene expression with relevant effect on developmental pathways. The difference in the detection rate in comparison with other studies might be explained by the different selection criteria and resolution of the array platforms used.

We detected abnormalities previously reported as causative of CHD in two cases. A 363 kb *de novo* deletion in 16q24.1 encompassing the *FOX* gene cluster was detected in a fetus with left heart hypoplasia. Overlapping deletions have been previously reported in patients with alveolar capillary dysplasia, misalignment of pulmonary veins and distinct malformations including congenital heart defect, specifically hypoplastic left heart [38]. Deletion of *FOXF1* is thought to be responsible for alveolar capillary dysplasia while *FOXC2* is related to the lymphoedema-distichiasis syndrome. Larger deletions, as in our case, may cause a more complex

syndrome which includes CHD likely due to additive effects of haploinsufficiency for contiguous genes [38].

We also identified the recurrent 2.2 Mb 15q13.3 deletion in a fetus with right heart hypoplasia, inherited from the healthy mother. Interestingly, the brother of the mother also had a cardiac malformation on anamnesis but he rejected to be studied. Deletions and duplications at 15q13.3 have been related to different developmental anomalies, such as dysmorphic features, intellectual disability, seizures, schizophrenia, and in 17% of patients congenital heart defects [39]. Based on previous studies in animal models, *KLF13*, encoding the Kruppel-like factor 13, is the best candidate gene for the cardiac defects associated with the 15q13.3 deletion. *KLF13* knockdown in Xenopus embryos caused atrial septal defects and hypotrabeculation similar to those observed in humans or mice with hypomorphic *GATA4* alleles [40]. Rearrangements in this region show incomplete penetrance and variable expressivity, with various cases in which the deletion or duplication is inherited from a healthy progenitor, as in our case [39]. Given this incomplete penetrance of clinical manifestations and the relatively low proportion of patients affected by cardiac disease, it is assumed that factors other than the 15q13.3 deletion should also be involved in the appearance of the clinical traits. In this case, no additional genomic alterations were detected.

Among the additional rare rearrangements identified in fetuses with malformations, all tested were inherited from an apparently healthy progenitor, which is consistent with previous data [31,39]. The rarity and gene content of some of these rearrangements suggest their possible pathogenic implication in congenital malformations. Nevertheless, like in some recurrent microdeletion syndromes, the existence of healthy carriers among progenitors and the adult population indicates that the rearrangements are not the only cause of the disease. Considering the epidemiologic evidence for multifactorial etiology of major malformations, these rearrangements could represent just one of the several factors involved. In this regard, a case with holoprosencephaly showed two deletions, one inherited from the mother and the other from the father, both harboring genes of the same pathway (phosphatidylinositol metabolism). Two duplication-type CNV events were also found in a fetus with hydrocephalus, although parental samples were not available to determine their inheritance pattern. However, candidate genes for brain malformation were also located in both CNVs: *DMBX1* codes for a diencephalon-mesencephalon homeobox implicated in brain development and *GPRIN2* encodes a G-protein regulated inducer of neurite overgrowth involved in formation and extension of neurite-like processes [43,44]. Given the very low frequency of these alterations in controls, the functional relationship of altered genes

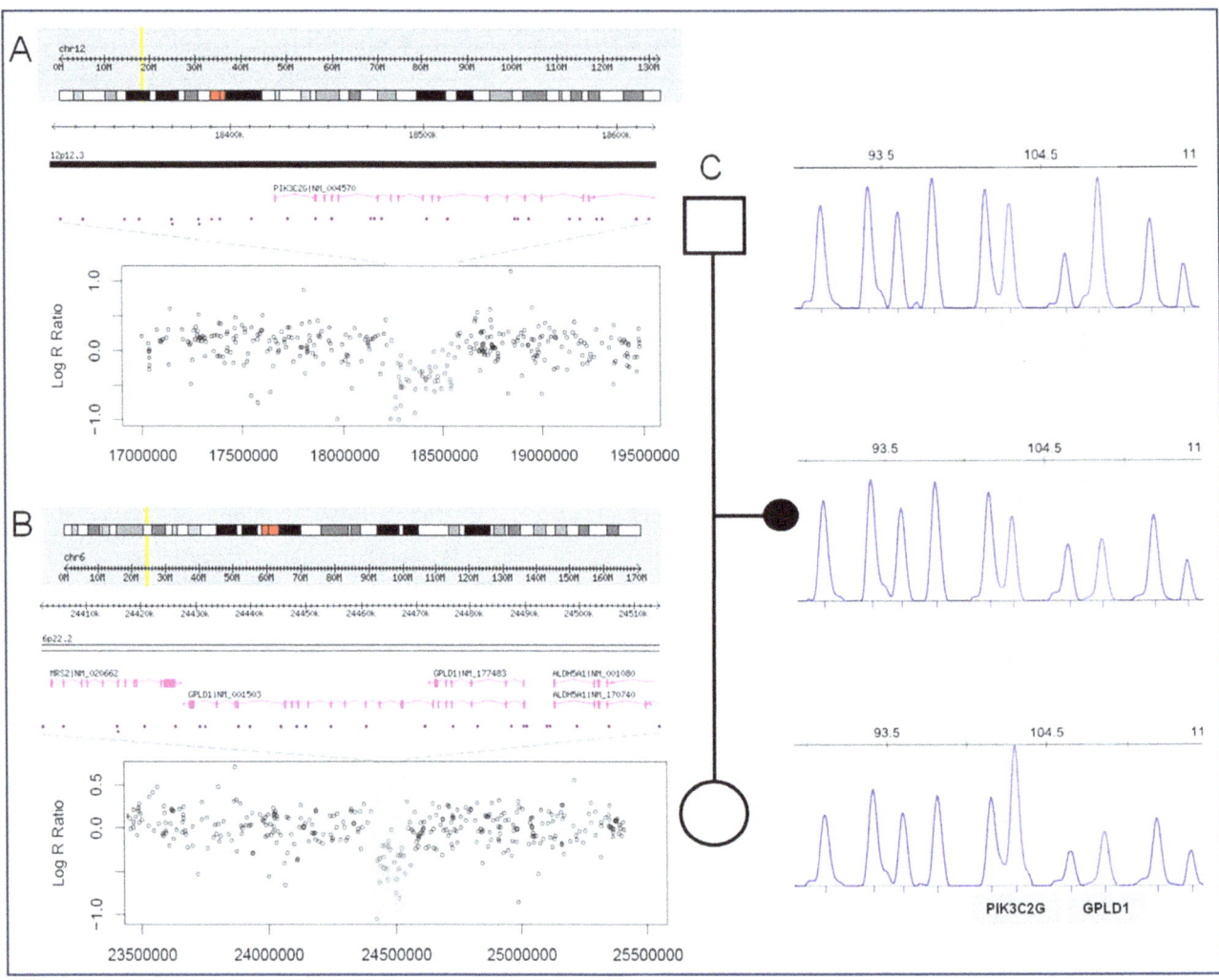

Figure 2. Detection, validation and inheritance of the two chromosomal deletions in case 57. A and B: Ideogram showing the location of the rearrangement and the corresponding regional plot of the Log R Ratio values of the SNP array (deleted and flanking regions). C: MLPA pattern in the familial trio showing the inheritance of both deletions. Hg19 assembly. MLPA: multiplex ligation-dependent probe amplification; SNP: single nucleotide polymorphism.

and their inheritance from different progenitors at least in the first case, it is logical to propose that the double hit may have contribute to the fetal malformations by additive effect of the CNVs on altering developmental regulation. A two-hit model with several recurrent and non-recurrent CNVs has been already reported for neurobehavioral and relatively severe phenotypes [45].

In addition, we also detected the 16p13.11 1.6 Mb duplication in two cases with different phenotypes. This duplication has been found in 0.14% normal adult controls (12/8,329 controls) and in 0.27% patients with developmental delay and/or malformations (42/15,767) [34]. Given the higher frequency of this duplication in our series (2%) as well as in reported patients with developmental anomalies [41], the data highly suggest that this CNV is indeed a susceptibility variant for developmental disorders including congenital malformations. The different phenotypes related to the microduplication might also be related to the concurrence of this contiguous gene alteration with other undefined genetic or environmental second hit. Depending on the other concurrent factors that may contribute to reach the gene dysfunction threshold in a specific tissue or developmental time, the phenotype

would correspond to different diseases or malformations. Although additional CNVs were not found with increased frequency in cases with respect to controls in our cohort, including the two cases with 16p13.11, secondary events of other type, such as point mutations or epimutations cannot be ruled out.

On the other hand, UPD and shared homozygosity regions were discarded by SNP array and mosaic alterations were also not identified. Although the number of samples studied is low, UPD does not seem to be a common cause of isolated congenital defects. Since DNA from the affected tissue was analyzed in 46 samples, we can also conclude that mosaicism for large rearrangements in the abnormally developed tissue is not frequent in isolated congenital malformations.

In addition to the most common aneuploidies and genomic disorders also detected by karyotyping and targeted assays, CMA significantly increases the detection yield of cryptic segmental aneuploidies in fetuses with congenital malformations. The highest yield for rare CNVs was found in samples with hypoplasia of the left/right heart, doubling the frequency of any other group of malformations and suggesting a higher genetic component for this type of malformation, which is consistent with its higher heritability [46,47]. A higher frequency of rearrangements in patients with left heart hypoplasia comparing with controls has been recently reported, even though the difference was only statistically significant for aberrations smaller than 60 kb [48]. However, from a clinical perspective, CMA can detect the single causative alteration in a relatively low percentage of cases with isolated congenital malformations, about 2% once the most common aneuploidies and recurrent rearrangements are discarded. Therefore, although many rare CNVs detectable by CMA, like those reported here, presumably contribute to the disorder, they should be considered as variants of unknown significance until more information is available to better predict phenotype based on genotype.

Accumulation of multiple rare genomic and epigenetic variants converging to deregulate developmental genes leading to mutational loading of developmental networks may cause congenital malformations [49]. Rare copy number variants, point mutations and/or epigenetic variations, either inherited or *de novo*, can impact gene function or alter dosage and contribute to mutational load. Changes affecting multiple genes and networks related to development may induce developmental anomalies. This concept implies that if threshold levels of flux are exceeded, compensatory mechanisms may fail, leading to an inadequate development. This hypothesis has been tested in mouse model and some results suggest that the accumulation of alterations in regulatory development networks results in an inadequate development [50]. Although it is reasonable to expect homologous genes to behave similarly in humans, more evidence supporting this hypothesis is needed. Further studies, including whole genome sequencing and epigenomic analyses as well as expression profiles of genes related to development should be done in order to improve the knowledge of the etiology and the diagnostic tools for isolated congenital malformations.

Supporting Information

Table S1 List of heart malformations present in the cohort of 33 studied fetuses with isolated congenital heart defect. RHH: right heart hypoplasia; IVC: interventricular communication; LHH: left heart hypoplasia; VSD: ventricular septal defect; D-TGA: dextro-transposition of the great arteries; L-TGA: levo-transposition of the great arteries; AVSD: atrioventricular septal defect. IAC: interatrial communication.

Table S2 Overview of the central nervous system malformations in 26 of the analyzed fetuses. CNS: central nervous system.

Table S3 Type of renal malformations observed in 9 of the studied fetuses.

Table S4 Overview of the affected organs and systems in fetuses with multiple malformations. CHD: congenital heart defect; CNS: central nervous system; IUGR: intrauterine growth restriction. VATER: Vertebrae, Anus, Trachea, Esophagus, and Renal. OEIS: omphalocele, exstrophy, imperforate anus, spinal defects.

Table S5 MLPA probes used to discard well-known genetic alterations related to MCA/MR. Hg19 assembly.

Table S6 MLPA probes used to validate the alterations detected by CMA and to study parental samples. Hg19 assembly.

Table S7 Summary of rare copy number variations >100 kb detected in samples of 168 control subjects. Hg19 assembly.

Acknowledgments

We would like to thank Verena Terrado and Raquel Flores for technical assistance, as well as Gabriela Palacios and the anonymous reviewer of the manuscript for critical comments and suggestions. We also would like to thank all participant families for their consent and support.

Author Contributions

Conceived and designed the experiments: CS-J TV LAP-J. Performed the experiments: CS-J. Analyzed the data: CS-J BR-S IC LAP-J. Contributed reagents/materials/analysis tools: BR-S NT NC. Wrote the paper: CS-J LAP-J. Selection of the samples: CS-J TV NC NT LAP-J. Revising the article critically for important intellectual content: CS-J BR-S IC TV NC NT LAP-J. Final approval of the version to be submitted: CS-J BR-S IC TV NC NT LAP-J..

References

1. Kalter H, Warkany J (1983) Medical progress. Congenital malformations: etiologic factors and their role in prevention (first of two parts). N Engl J Med 308(8):424–31.

2. Kalter H, Warkany J (1983) Congenital malformations (second of two parts). N Engl J Med 308(9):491–7.

3. De Galan-Roosen AE, Kuijpers JC, Meershoek AP, van Velzen D (1998) Contribution of congenital malformations to perinatal mortality. A 10 years prospective regional study in The Netherlands. Eur J Obstet Gynecol Reprod Biol 80(1):55–61.

4. Botto LD, Correa A (2003) Decreasing the burden of congenital heart disease: an epidemiologic evaluation of risk factors and survival. Prog Pediatr Cardiol 18:111–21.

5. Mitchell SC, Sellmann AH, Westphal MC, Park J (1971) Etiologic correlates in a study of congenital heart disease in 56,109 births. Am J Cardiol 28(6):653–7.

6. Richards AA, Santos LJ, Nichols HA, Crider BP, Elder FF, et al. (2008) Cryptic chromosomal abnormalities identified in children with congenital heart disease. Pediatr Res 64(4):358–63.

7. Pierpont ME, Basson CT, Benson DW, Jr., Gelb BD, et al. (2007) Genetic basis for congenital heart defects: current knowledge: a scientific statement from the American Heart Association Congenital Cardiac Defects Committee, Council on Cardiovascular Disease in the Young: endorsed by the American Academy of Pediatrics. Circulation 115(23):3015–38.

8. Thienpont B, Mertens L, de Ravel T, Eyskens B, Boshoff D, et al. (2007) Submicroscopic chromosomal imbalances detected by array-CGH are a frequent cause of congenital heart defects in selected patients. Eur Heart J 28(22):2778–84.

9. Ogata T, Yoshida R (2005) PTPN11 mutations and genotype-phenotype correlations in Noonan and LEOPARD syndromes. Pediatr Endocrinol Rev 2(4):669–74.

10. Ng SB, Bigham AW, Buckingham KJ, Hannibal MC, McMillin MJ, et al. (2010) Exome sequencing identifies MLL2 mutations as a cause of Kabuki syndrome. Nat Genet 42(9):790–3.

11. Popp S, Schulze B, Granzow M, Keller M, Holtgreve-Grez H, et al. (2002) Study of 30 patients with unexplained developmental delay and dysmorphic features or congenital abnormalities using conventional cytogenetics and multiplex FISH telomere (M-TEL) integrity assay. Hum Genet 111(1):31–9.

12. Rooms L, Reyniers E, van Luijk R, Scheers S, Wauters J, et al. (2004) Subtelomeric deletions detected in patients with idiopathic mental retardation using multiplex ligation-dependent probe amplification (MLPA). Hum Mutat 23(1):17–21.

13. Bendavid C, Dubourg C, Pasquier L, Gicquel I, Le Gallou S, et al. (2007) MLPA screening reveals novel subtelomeric rearrangements in holoprosencephaly. Hum Mutat 28(12):1189–97.

14. Koolen DA, Nillesen WM, Versteeg MH, Merkx GF, Knoers NV, et al. (2004) Screening for subtelomeric rearrangements in 210 patients with unexplained mental retardation using multiplex ligation dependent probe amplification (MLPA). J Med Genet 41(12):892–9.

15. Vissers LE, de Vries BB, Osoegawa K, Janssen IM, Feuth T, et al. (2003) Array-based comparative genomic hybridization for the genome wide detection of submicroscopic chromosomal abnormalities. Am J Hum Genet 73(6):1261–70.

16. Shaw-Smith C, Redon R, Rickman L, Rio M, Willatt L, et al. (2004) Microarray based comparative genomic hybridisation (array-CGH) detects submicroscopic

chromosomal deletions and duplications in patients with learning disability/ mental retardation and dysmorphic features. J Med Genet 41(4):241–8.

17. Schaeffer AJ, Chung J, Heretis K, Wong A, Ledbetter DH, et al. (2004) Comparative genomic hybridization-array analysis enhances the detection of aneuploidies and submicroscopic imbalances in spontaneous miscarriages. Am J Hum Genet 74(6):1168–74.

18. Le Caignec C, Boceno M, Saugier-Veber P, Jacquemont S, Joubert M, et al. (2005) Detection of genomic imbalances by array based comparative genomic hybridisation in fetuses with multiple malformations. J Med Genet 42(2):121–8.

19. Vialard F, Molina Gomes D, Leroy B, Quarello E, Escalona A, et al. (2009) Array comparative genomic hybridization in prenatal diagnosis: another experience. Fetal Diagn Ther 25(2):277–84.

20. Tyreman M, Abbott KM, Willatt LR, Nash R, Lees C, et al. (2009) High resolution array analysis: diagnosing pregnancies with abnormal ultrasound findings. J Med Genet 46(8):531–41.

21. Armengol L, Nevado J, Serra-Juhé C, Plaja A, Mediano C, et al. (2011) Clinical utility of chromosomal microarray analysis in invasive prenatal diagnosis. Hum Genet 131(3):513–523.

22. Momma K (2010) Cardiovascular anomalies associated with chromosome 22q11.2 deletion syndrome. Am J Cardiol 105(11):1617–24.

23. Webber SA, Hatchwell E, Barber JC, Daubeney PE, Crolla JA, et al. (1996) Importance of microdeletions of chromosomal region 22q11 as a cause of selected malformations of the ventricular outflow tracts and aortic arch: a three-year prospective study. J Pediatr 129(1):26–32.

24. Brunetti-Pierri N, Berg JS, Scaglia F, Belmont J, Bacino CA, et al. (2008) Recurrent reciprocal 1q21.1 deletions and duplications associated with microcephaly or macrocephaly and developmental and behavioral abnormalities. Nat Genet 40(12):1466–71.

25. Greenway SC, Pereira AC, Lin JC, DePalma SR, Israel SJ, et al. (2009) De novo copy number variants identify new genes and loci in isolated sporadic tetralogy of Fallot. Nat Genet 41(8):931–5.

26. Pietrzyk JJ (1997) A search for environmental and genetic background for neural tube defects: twenty-five years of experience. Cent Eur J Public Health. 5(2):86–9.

27. Nora JJ, Nora AH (1976) Recurrence risks in children having one parent with a congenital heart disease. Circulation 53:701–2.

28. Hardin J, Carmichael SL, Selvin S, Lammer EJ, Shaw GM (2009) Increased prevalence of cardiovascular defects among 56,709 California twin pairs. Am J Med Genet A. 149A(5):877–86.

29. Butler TL, Esposito G, Blue GM, Cole AD, Costa MW, et al. (2010) GATA4 mutations in 357 unrelated patients with congenital heart malformation. Genet Test Mol Biomarkers 14(6):797–802.

30. Sperling S, Grimm CH, Dunkel I, Mebus S, Sperling HP, et al. (2005) Identification and functional analysis of CITED2 mutations in patients with congenital heart defects. Hum Mutat 26(6):575–82.

31. Erdogan F, Larsen LA, Zhang L, Tümer Z, Tommerup N, et al. (2008) High frequency of submicroscopic genomic aberrations detected by tiling path array comparative genome hybridisation in patients with isolated congenital heart disease. J Med Genet 45(11):704–9.

32. Cusco I, del Campo M, Vilardell M, González E, Gener B, et al. (2008) Array-CGH in patients with Kabuki-like phenotype: identification of two patients with complex rearrangements including 2q37 deletions and no other recurrent aberration. BMC Med Genet 9:27.

33. Rodriguez-Santiago B, Brunet A, Sobrino B, Serra-Juhé C, Flores R, et al. (2010) Association of common copy number variants at the glutathione S-transferase genes and rare novel genomic changes with schizophrenia. Mol Psychiatry 15(10):1023–33.

34. Cooper GM, Coe1 BP, Girirajan S, Rosenfeld JA, Vu TH, et al (2011) A copy number variation morbidity map of developmental delay. Nat Genet 43(9):838–46.

35. Rodriguez-Santiago B, Malats N, Rothman N, Armengol L, Garcia-Closas M, et al. (2010) Mosaic uniparental disomies and aneuploidies as large structural variants of the human genome. Am J Hum Genet 87(1):129–38.

36. González JR, Rodríguez-Santiago B, Cáceres A, Pique-Regi R, Rothman N, et al. (2011) A fast and accurate method to detect allelic genomic imbalances underlying mosaic rearrangements using SNP array data. BMC Bioinformatics 12:166.

37. Kamburov A, Wierling C, Lehrach H, Herwig R (2009) ConsensusPathDB–a database for integrating human functional interaction networks. Nucleic Acids Res 37:623–628.

38. Stankiewicz P, Sen P, Bhatt SS, Storer M, Xia Z, et al. (2009) Genomic and genic deletions of the FOX gene cluster on 16q24.1 and inactivating mutations of FOXF1 cause alveolar capillary dysplasia and other malformations. Am J Hum Genet 84(6):780–91.

39. van Bon BW, Mefford HC, Menten B, Koolen DA, Sharp AJ, et al. (2009) Further delineation of the 15q13 microdeletion and duplication syndromes: a clinical spectrum varying from non-pathogenic to a severe outcome. J Med Genet 46(8):511–23.

40. Lavallee G, Andelfinger G, Nadeau M, Lefebvre C, Nemer G, et al. (2006) The Kruppel-like transcription factor KLF13 is a novel regulator of heart development. Embo J 25(21):5201–13.

41. Nagamani SC, Erez A, Bader P, Lalani SR, Scott DA, et al. (2011) Phenotypic manifestations of copy number variation in chromosome 16p13.11. Eur J Hum Genet 19(3):280–6.

42. Valduga M, Philippe C, Bach Segura P, Thiebaugeorges O, Miton A, et al. (2010) A retrospective study by oligonucleotide array-CGH analysis in 50 fetuses with multiple malformations. Prenat Diagn 30(4):333–41.

43. Ohtoshi A, Behringer RR (2004) Neonatal lethality, dwarfism, and abnormal brain development in Dmbx1 mutant mice. Molec Cell Biol 24(17):7548–58.

44. Chen LT, Gliman AG, Kozasa T (1999) A candidate target for G protein action in brain. J Biol Chem 274(38):26931–8.

45. Girirajan S, Rosenfeld JA, Cooper GM, Antonacci F, Siswara P, et al. (2010) A recurrent 16p12.1 microdeletion supports a two-hit model for severe developmental delay. Nat Genet 42(3):203–9.

46. Hinton RB Jr, Martin LJ, Tabangin ME, Mazwi ML, Cripe LH, et al. (2007) Hypoplastic left heart syndrome is heritable. J Am Coll Cardiol 50(16):1590–5.

47. Iascone M, Ciccone R, Galletti L, Marchetti D, Seddio F, et al. (2011) Identification of de novo mutations and rare variants in hypoplastic left heart syndrome. Clin Genet.

48. Ashleigh R, Payne AR, Chang SW, Koenig SN, Zinn AR, et al. (2012) Submicroscopic Chromosomal Copy Number Variations Identified in Children With Hypoplastic Left Heart Syndrome. Pediatr Cardiol.

49. Bentham J, Bhattacharya S (2008) Genetic mechanisms controlling cardiovascular development. Ann N Y Acad Sci 1123:10–9.

50. Bittel DC, Butler MG, Kibiryeva N, Marshall JA, Chen J, et al. (2011) Gene expression in cardiac tissues from infants with idiopathic conotruncal defects. BMC Med Genomics 4(1):1.

15

Real-Time 3-Dimensional Echocardiographic Assessment of Ventricular Volume, Mass, and Function in Human Fetuses

Minjuan Zheng[1,2,9], **Micheal Schaal**[1,9], **Yan Chen**[3,9], **Xiaokui Li**[1], **Weihui Shentu**[1], **Pengyuan Zhang**[1], **Muhammad Ashraf**[1], **Shuping Ge**[4]*, **David J. Sahn**[1]*

1 Pediatric Cardiology, Oregon Health and Science University, Portland, Oregon, United States of America, 2 Department of Ultrasound, Xijing Hospital/Fourth Military Medical University, Xi'an, China, 3 Department of Oncology, Xijing Hospital/Fourth Military Medical University, Xi'an, China, 4 Section of Cardiology, St. Christopher's Hospital for Children/Drexel University College of Medicine, Philadelphia, Pennsylvania, United States of America

Abstract

Objectives: We sought to determine the feasibility and reproducibility of real-time 3-dimensional echocardiography (RT3DE) for evaluation of cardiac volume, mass, and function and to characterize maturational changes of these measurements in human fetuses.

Methods: Eighty pregnant women in the 2nd and 3rd trimesters (59 with normal fetuses and 21 with fetuses with congenital heart disease [CHD]) were enrolled. We acquired RT3DE images using a matrix-array transducer. RT3DE measurements of volume, mass, stroke volume (SV), combined cardiac output (CCO), and ejection fraction (EF) were obtained. Images were scored and analyzed by two blinded independent observers. Inter- and intraobserver variabilities and correlations between fetal cardiac indices and gestational age were determined.

Results: Fifty-two of 59 normal data sets (88%) and 9 of 21 CHD data sets (43%) were feasible for analysis. In normal fetuses, the right ventricle (RV) is larger than the left ventricle (LV) ($P<0.05$), but no difference exists between the LV and RV in mass, SV, CO, and CO/CCO. The EFs for the LV and RV were diminished; the RVSV/LVSV was reduced in CHD fetuses compared with normal fetuses ($P<0.05$). Fetal ventricular volumes, mass, SV, and CCO fit best into exponential curves with gestational age, but LVEF, RVEF, and RVSV/LVSV remain relatively constant.

Conclusions: RT3DE is feasible and reproducible for assessment of LV and RV volume, mass, and function, especially in normal fetuses. Gestational growth of these measures, except for EF, is exponential in normal and CHD fetuses. CHD fetuses exhibit diminished LV and RV EFs.

Editor: Erik L. Ritman, Mayo Clinic College of Medicine, United States of America

Funding: This work was supported by Oregon Health and Science University (http://www.ohsu.edu/xd/). The funder had no role in study design, data collection and analysis, decision to publish, or preparation of the manuscript.

Competing Interests: The authors have declared that no competing interests exist.

* E-mail: shuping.ge@tenethealth.com (SG); sahnd@ohsu.edu (DJS)

9 These authors contributed equally to this work.

Introduction

Ventricular volumetrics are crucial measures for evaluating fetal cardiovascular maturational growth, especially for fetuses with cardiac and extracardiac defects. Accurate and reliable methods for assessing ventricular volumes, mass, stroke volume (SV), cardiac output (CO), and ejection fraction (EF) will provide information to guide medical and surgical management of fetuses with structural and functional abnormalities. Conventional quantitative assessments of these indices in fetuses using 2-dimensional echocardiography (2DE) and pulse-wave Doppler have intrinsic technical limitations in terms of accuracy and have not gained wide acceptance [1]. A spatiotemporal image correlation (STIC) technique and virtual organ computer-aided analysis (VOCAL) have recently been used to assess fetal cardiac volume [2–6].

Although the results of these studies have validated the feasibility and accuracy of this technique, it is an indirect motion-gated offline scanning mode rather than a real-time 3-D echocardiography (RT3DE) technique [7].

Technological development in matrix-array and RT3DE allows acquisition of full-volume data sets within seconds in children and adults [8]. To date, although data reported that RT3DE based on matrix probe allows examination of fetal structures from multiple perspectives in real time, which is helpful to confirm normal cardiac structure and detect congenital anomalies [9–13], measurements of fetal ventricular volumes, mass, SV, combined cardiac output (CCO), and EF have not been systematically evaluated using matrix-array RT3DE. In addition, the changing roles of the right and left ventricles during fetal growth and development warrant further investigation using a more reliable method. Therefore, our aims were to (1) evaluate the feasibility and reproducibility of RT3DE for measuring ventricular indices in fetuses with normal and abnormal cardiac structures; and (2) evaluate the roles and performance of the left ventricle (LV) and right ventricle (RV) during the second and third trimesters.

Methods

Study Subjects

A total of 80 consecutive pregnant women using the perinatal services of the Oregon Health & Science University were enrolled in this study. Written informed consent form was provided by each participant before study. Consent procedure and research protocol were approved by the institutional review board of Oregon Health & Science University. Participants included women with normal fetuses (n = 59; age 18–42 years; fetal gestational age 16.7–34.6 weeks, mean 24.6±5.6 weeks) and women with fetuses with CHD (n = 21; age 20–35 years; gestational age 21.1–35.1 weeks, mean 27.5±4.8 weeks).

In the group with normal fetuses, the indications for ultrasound were confirmation of gestational age and fetal growth, advanced maternal age, abnormal screening test results, previous obstetric complications, family history of congenital heart anomalies, and suspicion of cardiac or extracardiac anomalies. All of the pregnancies met the following criteria: no maternal or fetal complications and normal results on a fetal echocardiogram. The indications for ultrasound in the group with fetuses with CHD are shown in Table 1. Routine obstetric ultrasound scans were followed by 3DE scans. According to the protocol, RT3DE acquisition time was limited to 15 minutes. Women with multiple fetuses were excluded. Postnatal confirmation of CHD was obtained by neonatal echocardiography, cardiac catheterization, or autopsy.

Image Acquisition

The RT3DE data sets were obtained using a 2- to 4-MHz matrix array X4 transducer and 3DE ultrasound system (HP SONOS 7500, Philips Medical Systems, Andover, MA). The resolution of this system is approximately 0.7×0.7×0.5 mm to 1.2×1.2×0.8 mm as measured by voxel size. 3D data were

acquired by Sahn DJ, and Li X and analyzed by Zheng M, Schaal M. When typical four-chamber views were shown, with least fetal movement and with abdomen upwords, it was the best position for fetal heart 3D data acquisition. The image or region of interest was optimized for gain, compression, scanning depth, image width, angles, transmission focus, and line density. We used an external signal generator that was timed to be in synchrony with the observed fetal heart beats on the real time 2D echocardiography, which was used as a trigger for the 3D acquisition. Acquisitions were performed during fetal quiescence with multiple complete cardiac cycles. Each acquisition speed varied from approximately 5 s to 7 s. An average of 5 to 7 loops were obtained and later transferred to a workstation for offline analysis.

RT3DE Data Analysis

Image quality assessment. All the RT3DE data were assessed by scores. The image quality of each data set was assigned to the following score criterion: 1': unacceptable-image quality was not measurable; 2': poor-image was judged as measurable but was suboptimal with artifacts; 3': acceptable-image was clear, measurable and diagnostic; 4': good-image was good, easily measurable and artifact was rarely present; 5': excellent-image was extremely clear with all sharp borders for confident diagnosis and measurement.

LV analysis. LV 3D data were analyzed by a 4-plane algorithm (4D LV-Analysis software package, Research-Arena, TomTec, Munich, Germany) (Figure 1). First, the data set was oriented, adjusted, and displayed in four views, including three long-axis views (apical 4-, 3-, and 2-chamber views) and an orthogonal short-axis view. Second, an end diastolic (ED) frame was chosen as the largest chamber size and an end systolic (ES) frame, as the smallest chamber size. Third, initial manual tracing of the endocardial and epicardial contours was performed using the 4-, 3- and 2-chamber views during end diastole and end systole and adjustment was made with reference to the short-axis view and cine loops. Finally, semiautomatic endocardial and epicardial tracing was undertaken on both end diastole and end systole, and 4-dimensional LV indices were calculated. A minimum of 3 loops were traced to derive the average for each data set.

Table 1. Characteristics of the congenital heart defects examined by RT3DE.

Disease	Gestational Age(weeks)	No. of fetus	RT3DE information Quality	
			Not measurable*	Useful†
Hypoplastic left heart syndrome	31~35	4	4	0
Tetralogy of Fallot(TOF)	30~35	2	1	1
Situs inversus,dextrocardia,complete transposition of the great vessels(TGA)	21~24	2	2	0
Secundum atrial septum defect(ASD)	23~32	4	1	3
Ventricular septum defect(VSD)	24~30	4	0	4
Double outlet right ventricle, TGA	20~23	2	2	0
Tachycardia,VSD,atrial septal aneurysm	21	1	0	1
Pulmonary atresia with a hypoplastic right ventricle	24	1	1	0
Truncus arteriosus	21	1	1	0
Total cases		21	12	9

*information derived from RT3DE was unclear for diagnosis.
†information derived from RT3DE was useful and obligatory for the diagnosis.

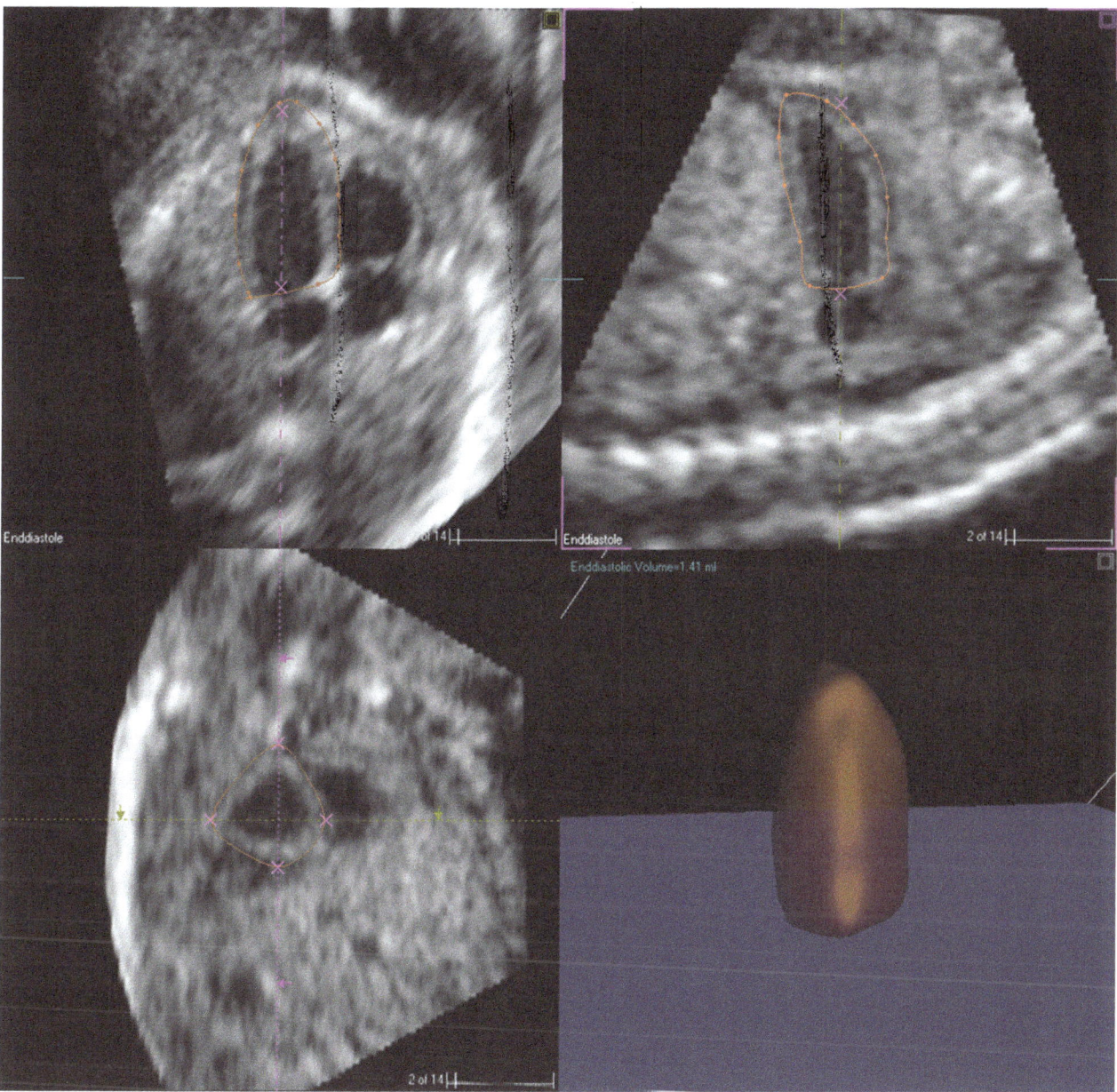

Figure 1. RT3DE image analysis for LV volumes and mass based on 3 orthogonal planes. Upper left, 4-chamber view with easily identifiable morphological markers. Upper right,2-chamber view planes, Lower left, short-axis view of both ventricles, lower right, calculated LV volume and shape display.

RV analysis. RV 3D data were analyzed in a similar fashion using a 4D RV-Function software package (Research-Arena, TomTec, Munich, Germany). By contrast, the landmarks were set using the center of the tricuspid valve, mitral valve, RV, and LV. The 3D data were oriented, adjusted, and displayed in sagittal, 4-chamber, and coronal views (Figure 2). Again, initial manual tracing of the endocardial and epicardial contours was performed using these images. Finally, semiautomatic endocardial and epicardial tracing was undertaken on end diastole and end systole, and 4-dimensional RV indices were calculated.

LV and RV calculations. Stroke volume (SV) was calculated as $SV = EDV - ESV$. Ejection fraction (EF) was calculated as $EF = (EDV - ESV)/EDV$. Cardiac output (CO) was calculated as $CO = SV \times$ heart rate (HR). Combined cardiac output (CCO) was calculated as $CCO = LV\ CO + RV\ CO$. Myocardial mass was calculated as myocardial volume × myocardial density (1.05 g/mL) [14], where myocardial volume was the difference between epicardial and endocardial shells of the LV or RV. Papillary muscle and trabeculae were included in the endocardial rim, but the apical RV moderator band was excluded and considered as cavity volume.

Intra- and Interobserver Variability of RT3DE Measurements

A total of 30 3DE data sets were selected randomly. Tracings and measurements were performed by two blinded experienced observers to determine intra- and interobserver variability. To ascertain intraobserver variability, one observer, who was blinded

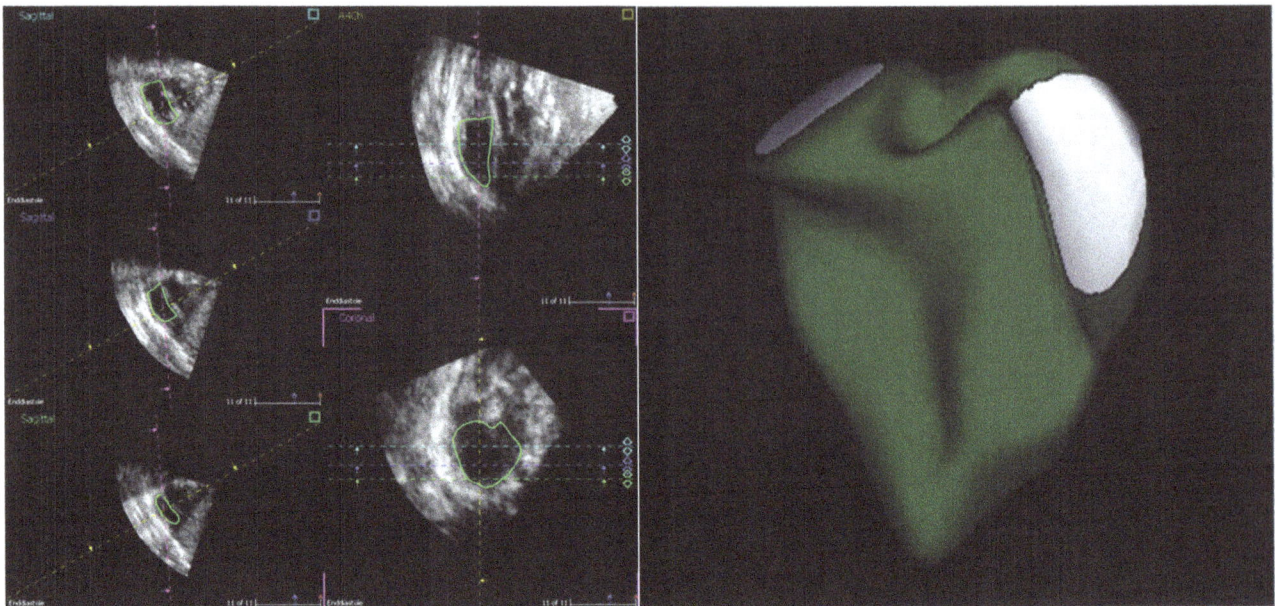

Figure 2. RV volume analysis by RT3DE image package. Left, the 3D data displayed in sagittal, 4-chamber, and coronal views, right, displayed RV volume and shape.

to the first analysis and measurements, repeated the RT3DE data analysis at a 4-week interval. To determine interobserver variability, a second observer analyzed and measured the RT3DE data independently, blinded to the results of the first observer. Intra- and interobserver variability was expressed as a percentile of the differences (difference between the measurements/mean of the measurements ×100%).

Statistical Analysis

Continuous variables were shown as the mean ± the standard deviation. Interobserver agreement of image scores was assessed using kappa statistics, with a kappa value greater than 0.8 and 0.61 to 0.80 representing good and substantial agreement, respectively [15]. The Pearson chi-square test was used to check for independence between image scores and gestational age. The Bland–Altman analysis was used to examine agreement within or between observers. Correlation and regression analyses were used to determine the relationships between gestational age and ventricular indices derived by RT3DE. The significance of the biases was tested using a 2-tailed t test. Levene's test was used to assess the equality of variance. Statistical significance was defined as $P<0.05$. Statistical analyses were done using the SPSS statistical software package (version 13.0; SPSS Inc, Chicago, IL) and Microsoft Excel 2007 (Microsoft Corporation, Redmond, WA).

Results

Feasibility and Reproducibility of RT3DE Fetal Measurements

As shown in Table 2, the feasibility of RT3DE measurements of 80 fetuses (59 normal and 21 CHD) were assessed by an image quality scores system. Of the 59 normal fetuses, 88% (52/59) were suitable for 3DE analysis (n = 52; age 18–42 years; gestational age 16.7–34.6 weeks, mean 23.7±4.2). For fetuses with CHD, 43% (9/21) of the data sets were acceptable for 3D analysis. The characteristics of the CHD fetuses are summarized in Table 1

(n = 9; age 27–35; gestational age 21–35 weeks, mean 27.1±4.9). No adverse event occurred.

When image quality was assessed, a chi-square test of image scores and gestational age showed $\chi^2 = 12.86$, $P = 0.12$. The kappa statistics indicated interobserver agreement for 3D image quality scores (κ value = 0.76; $P<0.001$). The inter- and intraobserver variabilities for RT3DE measurements were 1.3±3.9% and 0.7±6.1% for volumes, and 1.0±3.6% and 2.5±5.4% for ventricular mass.

RT3DE Assessment of Fetal Ventricular Volume, Mass, and Function

RV and LV cardiac indices were obtained from each adequate image set. The time necessary for analyzing both LV and RV volumes and mass after image acquisition was from 7 to 26 minutes (average 12.9±7.8 minutes). The mean values of EDV,

Table 2. RT3DE image quality scores.

Gestational Age (weeks)	Image Quality Scores					
	1'	2'	3'	4'	5'	total
≥16~<21	5(6.25%)	2(2.5%)	9(11.3%)	4(5.0%)	0	20
≥21~<29	8(10.0%)	4(5.0%)	12(15.0%)	7(8.75%)	14(17.5%)	45
≥29~<40	6(7.5%)	2(2.5%)	3(3.75%)	3(3.75%)	1(1.25%)	15
Total	19	61				80

The 3D image quality was assessed as follows:
1': *unacceptable*-image quality was not measurable;
2': *poor*-image was judged as measurable but was suboptimal with artifacts;
3': *acceptable*-image was clear, measurable and diagnostic;
4': *good*-image was good, easily measurable and artifact was rarely present;
5': *excellent*-image was extremely clear with all sharp borders for confident diagnosis and measurement.

Table 3. Mean Ventricular Volumes, Mass by RT3DE in Normal and CHD Fetuses.

	Age	GA	HR	LVEDV,ml	LVESV,ml	RVEDV,ml	RVESV,ml	LVmass,gm	RVmass,gm
Normal (n = 52)	28.6±5.6	23.7±4.2	136.7±5.4	1.88±1.56*	0.90±0.78*	2.04±1.50	1.05±0.80	1.77±1.45	1.79±1.19
CHD (n = 9)	30.0±2.6	27.1±4.9	132.3±8.0	1.89±0.95	0.80±0.49	1.89±0.93	0.80±0.43	1.63±1.07	1.54±0.97

*P<0.05: compared with right ventricle; P>0.05: compared normal group with CHD group in all indices.
GA: gestational age, HR: heart rate.

ESV, and mass obtained with RT3DE are shown in Table 3. There was no significant difference in EDV, ESV, and mass between the normal and CHD groups (*P*>0.05). However, RVEDV and RVESV were significantly larger than LVEDV and LVESV in normal fetuses, respectively (*P*<0.05).

When ventricular volumes, masses, SV, and CCO in both normal and CHD groups were correlated with gestational age (Figures 3, 4, 5), the best fits were curvilinear, that is, exponential with gestational age. Although we found no statistically significant difference between the normal and CHD groups, the two groups exhibited different regressions.

Right and left ventricular SV, CO, CCO, and EF for the normal and CHD groups are shown in Table 4. No difference was seen in SV and CO between the LV and RV in both normal and CHD groups, nor was any difference noted in the LVCO/CCO and RVCO/CCO. Furthermore, although the results trended toward increased RV and LV SV, CO, and CCO in the group with CHD, the difference was statistically insignificant. However, we noted a significant decrease in RVEF, LVEF, and RV/LV SV in the CHD group compared with the normal group (Table 4). In addition, the RVSV/LVSV ratio, LVEF, and RVEF seemed declined with gestational age in the normal group, but only

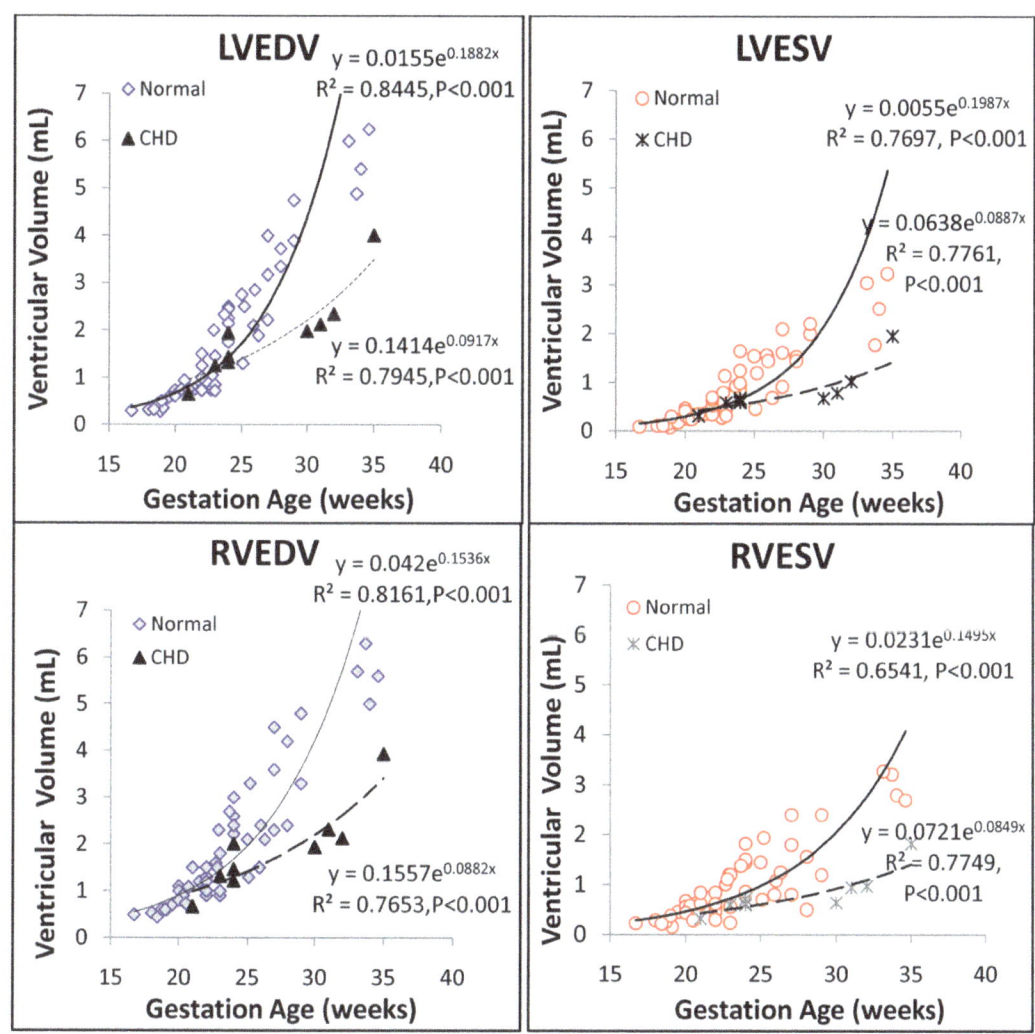

Figure 3. Gestational growth of LV and RV volumes in normal and CHD fetuses.

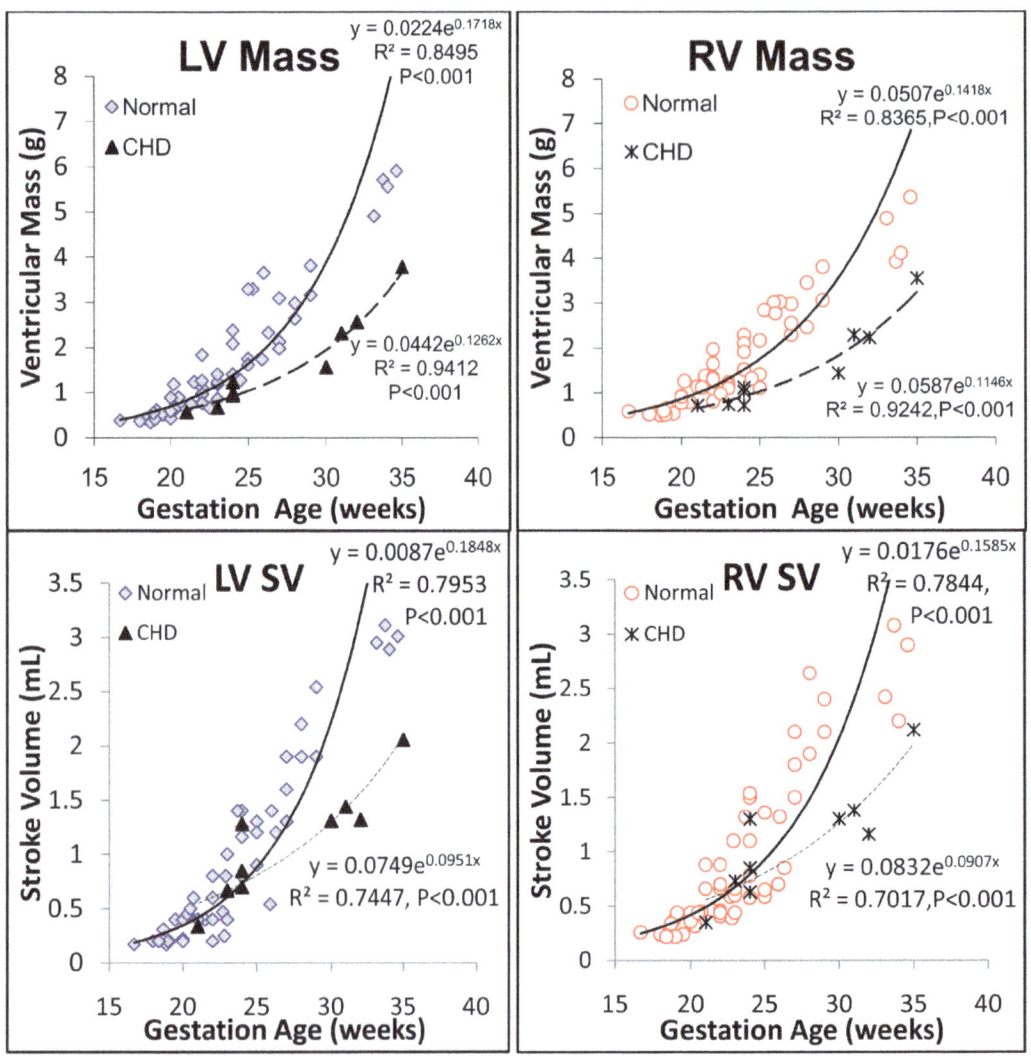

Figure 4. Growth of LV and RV mass and stroke volume with gestational age in normal and CHD fetuses.

RVSV/LVSV ratio and RVEF showed a significant negative correlation (Figure 5).

Discussion

Real-time 3-Dimensional Fetal Echocardiography

Previous assessment of fetal ventricular volume growth and functional maturation has largely been based on invasive means in instrumented animals and M-mode or 2D studies in humans [16,17]. Whereas these measurements have been validated in adult, children, and fetuses, evidence is growing that these measurements have limited accuracy and reproducibility compared with current real-time 3D echocardiography in both adults and children. M-mode echocardiography is highly dependent on the incident ultrasound beam and geometric assumptions of the ventricles. It has limited accuracy and repeatability [18]. As many as 40% of normal fetuses can have falsely increased cardiac dimensions on random 2D measurements compared with phase-specific M-mode dimensions [19]. It has also been shown that 2D-based methods provide reasonable estimates of ventricular indices for the LV but are problematic for the RV [20,21]. In an adult study, the 2D-based echocardiographic calculations overestimated

RV volumes by as much as 30% to 35% [14]. These potential measurement errors may be more problematic when the small size of the ventricles and the small absolute functional changes are evaluated in human fetuses with normal and congenital heart defects.

Three-dimensional echocardiography has become available for prenatal diagnosis of heart defects. Quantitative 3D echocardiography has also been used to determine ventricular volume, mass, and function in both children and adults [22–24]. Most 3DE fetal studies have used the spatiotemporal image correlation (STIC) technique [2–7]. The STIC technique is based on motion-gated offline reconstruction of consecutive subvolumes during a cardiac cycle. The automated volume acquisition is made possible because the array in the transducer performs a slow single sweep, recording a single 3D data set consisting of many 2D frames, one behind the other, then combining frames from the identical phase in the cycle from consecutive slices. When the cardiac abnormality involves dyssynchrony between ventricles, this method may lead to inaccurate estimation of maximum and minimum volume, such as EDV and ESV.

In contrast, 3DE with xMatrix transducer technology can facilitate real-time 3D visualization of the fetal heart. In this

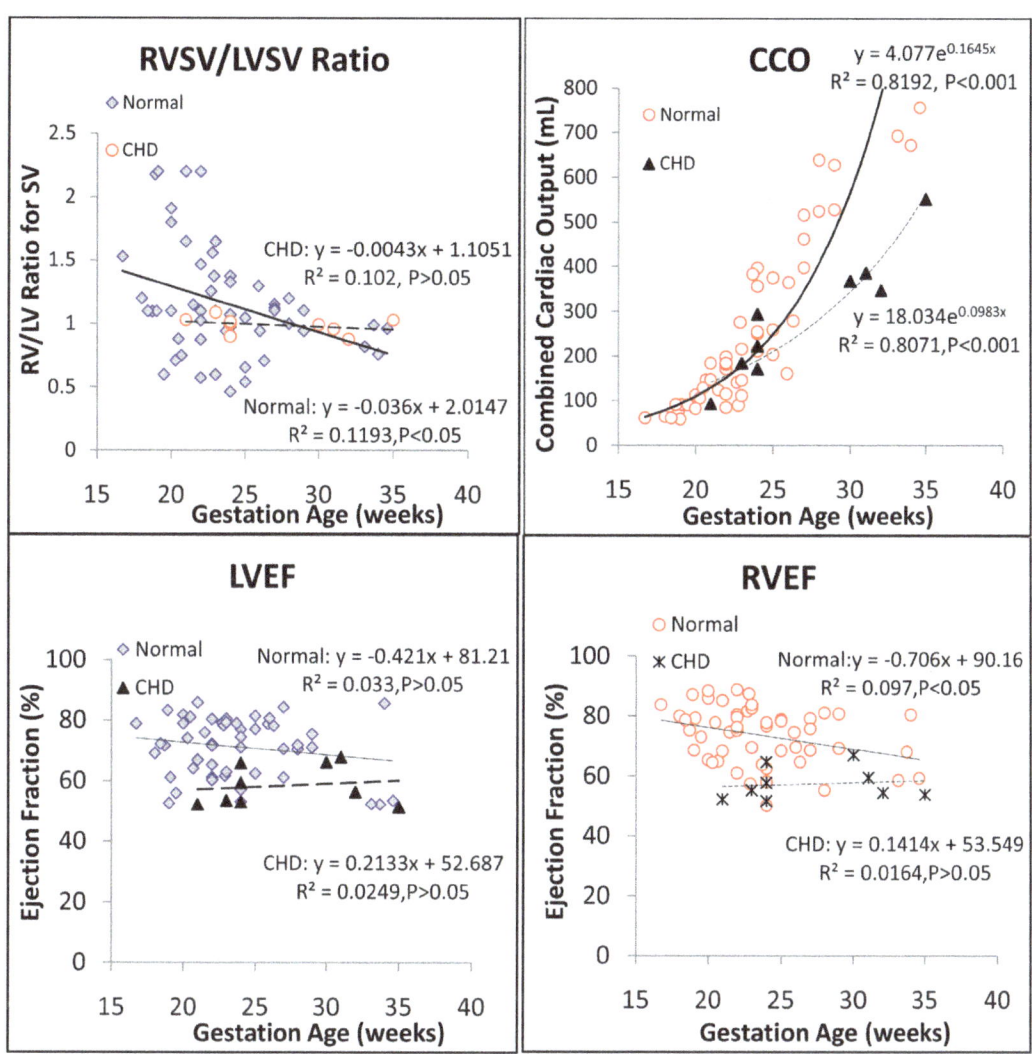

Figure 5. Gestational growth and maturation of RV to LV SV ratio, LV and RV EFs, and CCO.

approach, the transducer is usually built with 3000 active elements to capture data to generate real-time 3D images instead of reconstructing 2D images with STIC technology.

Feasibility and Reproducibility

Based on the feasibility data obtained in this study, 3D data from 88% normal and 43% CHD fetuses were adequate for analysis. The correlation between the 3D image scores and gestational age showed that the image quality did not change significantly after 16 weeks of gestation, suggestive of the multifactorial contribution to the 3D image quality, probably related to fetal position, maternal acoustic window, and amniotic

fluid quantity and clarity, in addition to gestational age. In our study, feasibility was low for 3D data set for CHD fetuses (9/21, 43%). In this cohort, the success rate of fetal RT3DE was related to whether we can get ideal four chamber view. In the 9 measurable cases, 8 cases were with simple CHD and had nearly normal size ventricles (3 ASD, 5 VSD, Table 1). In other 12 cases not suitable for 3D analysis, mostly were complex CHD, including 7 cases with significantly hypoplastic ventricles or large septal defects (4 Hypoplastic left heart syndrome, 1 TOF, 1Pulmonary atresia with a hypoplastic right ventricle, 1Truncus arteriosus), or malpositioned-ventricles and/or with significantly altered ventricular geometry (4 TGA, 2 of them were situs inversus and

Table 4. Ventricular SV, CO, CCO and EF by RT3DE in Normal and CHD Fetuses.

	LVSV,ml	RVSV,ml	LVCO,ml	RVCO,ml	CCO,ml	LVCO/CCO	RVCO/CCO	LVEF,%	RVEF,%	RV/LV SV
Normal(n = 52)	0.98±0.82	0.99±0.77	131.2±107.3	133.1±100.7	264.3±205.1	0.48±0.09	0.52±0.09	71.3±9.8*	73.5±9.5*	1.16±0.44*
CHD (n = 9)	1.10±0.51	1.09±0.52	146.7±70.0	144.3±69.8	291.1±139.4	0.50±0.01	0.50±0.02	58.5±6.6	57.4±5.4	0.99±0.07

*P<0.05, compared with CHD group. P>0.05, compared left ventricle with right ventricle in all indices.

dextrocardia), which were not suitable for LV and RV analysis algorism and software. The kappa statistics indicated good interobserver agreement for 3D image quality scores (κ value = 0.76; $P<0.001$). In addition, Bland–Altman analyses showed good inter- and intraobserver reproducibility for ventricular volumes and mass.

Ventricular Volume, Mass, and Function

A number of studies have pursued the use of reconstructive 3D echocardiography and STIC to quantify fetal heart volumes, mass, and function [2–6,25]. Simioni et al established nomograms for fetal SV, CO and EF by STIC modality, finding SV and CO increased exponentially with gestation and EF remained fairly stable through gestation (around 63%) [26]. Our finding is accordant with theirs with exponentially increased SV, CO, and relative stable EF (Figure 4 and 5). The ranges of these variables were wider, which may due to wider gestation age ranges (16.7 to 34.6 weeks compared with 20 to 34 weeks). Messing et al also estimated fetal ventricular mass using STIC with VOCAL inversion mode [27]. LV and RV mass values derived from this method was larger than our data (especially RV mass). Besides systematic variation between STIC VOCAL and RT3DE, this difference may also caused by their larger sample size (106 fetus including normal and abnormal), and with larger ranged of ventricular sizes (including cardiomyopathy cases with enlarged chambers). Like RT3DE, STIC volumes can also be calculated automatically. Rizzo G et al reported good agreement between VOCAL and sonographic automatic volume calculation (sonoAVC) for fetal ventricular volume measurements (intraclass correlation coefficients 0.978 and 0.985 for LV and RV), and the time necessary to measure the SV was significantly shorter with sonoAVC (2.8 versus 11.7 minutes) than with VOCAL [28].

Using real-time 3D echocardiography, we demonstrated an exponential growth pattern for ventricular volumes and mass. When we compared data from the normal group with those from the CHD group, although we noted a trend toward smaller chamber size, mass, SV, CO, and CCO, we found no significant difference in EDV, ESV, mass, SV, CO, or CCO. However, we did find a significant difference in EF and the RV to LV ratio for SV. These findings may be due to the small number of fetuses with CHD relative to the number of normal fetuses. However, it is also plausible that EF and the lesser role RV played as compared with LV were more sensitive to fetal functional compromise and adaptation secondary to CHD.

Fetal Cardiac Output and Distribution

Much of our current understanding about fetal cardiac output and distribution is derived from studies in fetal sheep. In these studies, fetal CO and distribution were measured using the radionuclide-labeled microsphere method or electromagnetic flow transducers applied around the ascending aorta and the pulmonary trunk [29,30]. Results from these methods indicated that, in the fetal lamb, the RV ejected approximately two-thirds and the LV ejected one-third of the combined ventricular output. Results from previous human fetal studies using Doppler echocardiographic measurements of the CCO indicated that, although the RV was dominant in the human fetus, the human RV to LV ratio was smaller (1.2–1.5) than that in the fetal lamb (1.8) [30–32]. According to our RT3DE data, the RV-to-LV ratio for SV in the normal group was 1.16±0.44, which was different from that for the CHD group (0.99±0.07), yielding values closer to those obtained using Doppler echocardiography than were found in the sheep studies.

In fetal circulation, the LV output is directed into the ascending aorta to supply the upper body, including the brain, whereas the RV output supports the lower body and placenta through the ductus arteriosus. Therefore, the large brain mass of humans compared with that of sheep may explain the higher LV output and the lower ratio between the RV and LV output.

For the gestational EF changes and the RV/LV ratio of SV as linear regression fits, a trend toward a decrease in EF and RV/LV SV with gestational age was observed (Figure 4); again, we found no statistical significance, except for RV/LV SV and RVEF for normal fetuses, which was only a modest correlation ($R^2 = 0.12$, $P<0.05$, $R^2 = 0.10$, $P<0.05$, respectively) (Figure 5).

Study Difficulties and Limitations

The study has several limitations: We do not have a gold standard, either ex vivo or in vivo, for validation of RT3DE technology; nor do we have experimental data to corroborate the findings from 3D echocardiography, such as direct comparison with 3D volume and mass by fetal cardiac MRI. Most of the available validation studies derived from adults and children show the superior accuracy and reproducibility of 3D versus 2D or M-mode echocardiography for measurement of volumes, mass, and function. As with 2D studies, the 3D method cannot be used to study fetal hearts before 15 gestational weeks because the volumes may be under the lower limit of image resolution. At a fetal gestational age greater than 37 weeks, one may encounter difficulties stemming from fetal position and calcification of the thoracic cavity. In addition, this study is a prospective study from a single institution. The sample size was limited, especially for the group with CHD, and a subgroup analysis based on the type of CHD was not possible. Another limitation that we did not perform a direct comparisons between RT3DE with STIC technology for assessment of cardiac volumes, since the 2 different techniques would require 2 imaging modalities with 2 separate 3D data acquisition and analysis systems.

Despite these limitations, the results are of interest from a developmental perspective and add new and possibly more quantitative measures for fetal cardiac growth and maturational changes in normal and CHD fetuses.

Conclusions

RT3DE is feasible and reproducible for assessment of LV and RV volume, mass, and function after 15 weeks of gestation, especially in normal fetuses. Increases during gestation of these measures, except for EF, are exponential in both normal and CHD fetuses. Although RV is the dominant ventricle, the ratio of the RV and LV contribution to the combined CO is lower in humans than in experimental animals. LV and RV EFs are compromised in CHD fetuses compared with normal fetuses and may serve as sensitive measures for evaluation of fetal cardiac function.

Acknowledgments

The authors thank Pamela Fried of Drexel University College of Medicine Academic Publishing Services for editorial help.

Author Contributions

Conceived and designed the experiments: SG DJS. Performed the experiments: MZ MS XL DJS. Analyzed the data: MS YC. Contributed reagents/materials/analysis tools: WS PZ MA. Wrote the paper: MZ.

References

1. DeKoninck P, Steenhaut P, Van Mieghem T, Mhallem M, Richter J, et al. (2012) Comparison of Doppler-based and three-dimensional methods for fetal cardiac output measurement. Fetal Diagn Ther32: 72–78.
2. Messing B, Cohen SM, Valsky DV, Rosenak D, Hochner-Celnikier D, et al. (2007) Fetal cardiac ventricle volumetry in the second half of gestation assessed by 4D ultrasound using STIC combined with inversion mode. Ultrasound Obstet Gynecol 30: 142–151.
3. Simioni C, Araujo Júnior E, Martins WP, Rolo LC, da Rocha LA, et al. (2012) Fetal cardiac output and ejection fraction by spatio-temporal image correlation (STIC): comparison between male and female fetuses. Rev Bras Cir Cardiovasc 27: 275–282.
4. Barreto EQ, Milani HJ, Haratz KK, Araujo Júnior E, Nardozza LM, et al. (2012) Reference intervals for fetal heart volume from 3-dimensional sonography using the extended imaging virtual organ computer-aided analysis method at gestational ages of 20 to 34 weeks. J Ultrasound Med 31: 673–678.
5. Rizzo G, Capponi A, Cavicchioni O, Vendola M, Arduini D (2007) Fetal cardiac stroke volume determination by four-dimensional ultrasound with spatio-temporal image correlation compared with two-dimensional and Doppler ultrasonography. Prenat Diagn 27: 1147–1150.
6. Molina FS, Faro C, Sotiriadis A, Dagklis T, Nicolaides KH (2008) Heart stroke volume and cardiac output by four-dimensional ultrasound in normal fetuses. Ultrasound Obstet Gynecol 32: 181–187.
7. Yagel S, Cohen SM, Shapiro I, Valsky DV (2007) 3D and 4D ultrasound in fetal cardiac scanning: a new look at the fetal heart. Ultrasound Obstet Gynecol 29: 81–95.
8. Soriano BD, Hoch M, Ithuralde A, Geva T, Powell AJ, et al. (2008) Matrix-array 3-dimensional echocardiographic assessment of volumes, mass, and ejection fraction in young pediatric patients with a functional single ventricle: a comparison study with cardiac magnetic resonance. Circulation 117: 1842–1848.
9. Sklansky MS, DeVore GR, Wong PC (2004) Real-time 3-dimensional fetal echocardiography with an instantaneous volume-rendered display: early description and pictorial essay. J Ultrasound Med23: 283–9.
10. Gonçalves LF, Nien JK, Espinoza J, Kusanovic JP, Lee W, et al. (2006). What does 2-dimensional imaging add to 3- and 4-dimensional obstetric ultrasonography? J Ultrasound Med 25: 691–699.
11. Gonçalves LF, Espinoza J, Kusanovic JP, Lee W, Nien JK, et al. (2006) Applications of 2-dimensional matrix array for 3- and 4-dimensional examination of the fetus: a pictorial essay. J Ultrasound Med 25: 745–755.
12. Hung J, Lang R, Flachskampf F, Shernan SK, McCulloch ML,et al. (2007) 3D echocardiography: a review of the current status and future directions. J Am Soc Echocardiogr 20: 213–233.
13. Acar P, Dulac Y, Taktak A, Abadir S (2005) Real-time three-dimensional fetal echocardiography using matrix probe. Prenat Diagn 25: 370–375.
14. Myerson SG, Montgomery HE, World MJ, Pennell DJ (2002) Left ventricular mass: reliability of M-mode and 2-dimensional echocardiographic formulas. Hypertension 40: 673–678.
15. Landis JR, Koch GG (1977) The measurement of observer agreement for categorical data. Biometrics 33: 159–174.
16. Schmidt KG, Silverman NH, Van Hare GF, Hawkins JA, Cloez JL, et al. (1990) Two-dimensional echocardiographic determination of ventricular volumes in the fetal heart. Validation studies in fetal lambs. Circulation 81: 325–333.
17. Schmidt KG, Silverman NH, Hoffman JI (1995) Determination of ventricular volume in human fetal hearts by two-dimensional echocardiography. Am J Cardiol 76: 1313–1316.
18. Simpson JM, Cook A (2002) Repeatability of echocardiographic measurements in the human fetus. Ultrasound Obstet Gynecol 20: 332–339.
19. DeVore GR, Platt LD (1985) The random measurement of transverse diameter of the fetal heart: a potential source of error. J Ultrasound Med 4: 335–341.
20. Graham TP Jr, Jarmakani JM, Atwood GF, Canent RV Jr (1973) Right ventricular volume determinations in children. Normal values and observations with volume or pressure overload. Circulation 47: 144–153.
21. Chang FM, Hsu KF, Ko HC, Yao BL, Chang CH, et al. (1997) Fetal heart volume assessment by three-dimensional ultrasound. Ultrasound Obstet Gynecol 9: 42–48.
22. Sapin PM, Gopal AS, Clarke GB, Smith MD, King DL (1996) Three-dimensional echocardiography compared to two-dimensional echocardiography for measurement of left ventricular mass anatomic validation in an open chest canine model. Am J Hypertens 9: 467–474.
23. Lu X, Nadvoretskiy V, Bu L, Stolpen A, Ayres N, et al. (2008) Accuracy and reproducibility of real-time 3-dimensional echocardiography for assessment of right ventricular volumes and ejection fraction in children. J Am Soc Echocardiogr 21: 84–89.
24. Lu X, Xie M, Tomberlin D, Klas B, Nadvoretskiy V, et al. (2008) How accurately, reproducibly and efficiently can we measure left ventricular indexes in children using m-mode, 2D and 3D echocardiography? Am Heart J155: 946–953.
25. Bhat AH, Corbett V, Carpenter N, Liu N, Liu R, et al. (2004) Fetal ventricular mass determination on three-dimensional echocardiography: studies in normal fetuses and validation experiments. Circulation 110: 1054–1060.
26. Simioni C, Nardozza LM, Araujo Júnior E, Rolo LC, Zamith M, et al. (2011) Heart stroke volume, cardiac output, and ejection fraction in 265 normal fetus in the second half of gestation assessed by 4D ultrasound using spatio-temporal image correlation. J Matern Fetal Neonatal Med 24: 1159–1167.
27. Messing B, Cohen SM, Valsky DV, Shen O, Rosenak D, et al. (2011) Fetal heart ventricular mass obtained by STIC acquisition combined with inversion mode and VOCAL. Ultrasound Obstet Gynecol 38: 191–197.
28. Rizzo G, Capponi A, Pietrolucci ME, Arduini D (2010) Role of sonographic automatic volume calculation in measuring fetal cardiac ventricular volumes using 4-dimensional sonography: comparison with virtual organ computer-aided analysis. J Ultrasound Med 29: 261–270.
29. Siimes AS, Creasy RK, Heymann MA, Rudolph AM (1978) Cardiac output and its distribution and organ blood flow in the fetal lamb during ritodrine administration. Am J Obstet Gynecol 132: 42–48.
30. Rudolph AM, Heymann MA (1976) Cardiac output in the fetal lamb: the effects of spontaneous and induced changes of heart rate on right and left ventricular output. Am J Obstet Gynecol 124: 183–192.
31. De Smedt MC, Visser GH, Meijboom EJ (1987) Fetal cardiac output estimated by Doppler echocardiography during mid- and late gestation. Am J Cardiol 60: 338–342.
32. Mielke G, Benda N (2001) Cardiac output and central distribution of blood flow in the human fetus. Circulation 103: 1662–1668.

16

Functional Significance of SRJ Domain Mutations in *CITED2*

Chiann-mun Chen[1,2❂]**, Jamie Bentham**[1,2❂]**, Catherine Cosgrove**[1,2]**, Jose Braganca**[1,2]**, Ana Cuenda**[4]**, Simon D. Bamforth**[1,2,3]**, Jürgen E. Schneider**[1,2]**, Hugh Watkins**[1,2]**, Bernard Keavney**[3]**, Benjamin Davies**[2]**, Shoumo Bhattacharya**[1,2]*

1 Department of Cardiovascular Medicine, Wellcome Trust Centre for Human Genetics, University of Oxford, Oxford, United Kingdom, **2** Wellcome Trust Centre for Human Genetics, University of Oxford, Oxford, United Kingdom, **3** Institute of Genetic Medicine, Newcastle University, Newcastle, United Kingdom, **4** Centro Nacional de Biotecnología, CSIC, Madrid, Spain

Abstract

CITED2 is a transcriptional co-activator with 3 conserved domains shared with other CITED family members and a unique Serine-Glycine Rich Junction (SRJ) that is highly conserved in placental mammals. Loss of *Cited2* in mice results in cardiac and aortic arch malformations, adrenal agenesis, neural tube and placental defects, and partially penetrant defects in left-right patterning. By screening 1126 sporadic congenital heart disease (CHD) cases and 1227 controls, we identified 19 variants, including 5 unique non-synonymous sequence variations (N62S, R92G, T166N, G180-A187del and A187T) in patients. Many of the CHD-specific variants identified in this and previous studies cluster in the SRJ domain. Transient transfection experiments show that T166N mutation impairs TFAP2 co-activation function and ES cell proliferation. We find that CITED2 is phosphorylated by MAPK1 *in vitro* at T166, and that MAPK1 activation enhances the coactivation function of CITED2 but not of CITED2-T166N. In order to investigate the functional significance *in vivo*, we generated a T166N mutation of mouse *Cited2*. We also used PhiC31 integrase-mediated cassette exchange to generate a *Cited2* knock-in allele replacing the mouse *Cited2* coding sequence with human *CITED2* and with a mutant form deleting the entire SRJ domain. Mouse embryos expressing only CITED2-T166N or CITED2-SRJ-deleted alleles surprisingly show no morphological abnormalities, and mice are viable and fertile. These results indicate that the SRJ domain is dispensable for these functions of CITED2 in mice and that mutations clustering in the SRJ region are unlikely to be the sole cause of the malformations observed in patients with sporadic CHD. Our results also suggest that coding sequence mutations observed in case-control studies need validation using *in vivo* models and that predictions based on structural conservation and *in vitro* functional assays, or even *in vivo* global loss of function models, may be insufficient.

Editor: Fabio Martelli, IRCCS-Policlinico San Donato, Italy

Funding: This work was supported by grants from the Wellcome Trust (083228/Z/07/Z to S.B. and 090532/Z/09/Z to the Wellcome Trust Centre for Human Genetics; www.wellcome.ac.uk), and grants from the British Heart Foundation (CH/09/003 and PG/07/045/22690; www.bhf.org.uk). The funders had no role in study design, data collection and analysis, decision to publish, or preparation of the manuscript.

Competing Interests: The authors have declared that no competing interests exist.

* E-mail: sbhattac@well.ox.ac.uk

❂ These authors contributed equally to this work.

Introduction

Congenital heart disease (CHD) is one of the major causes of childhood morbidity and mortality in the West. The incidence of CHD in live-born infants ranges from 0.4 to 1.2% [1,2], and increases in first-degree relatives to 2–5% [2], suggesting a role for genetic or environmental variations which may contribute to disease risk. Chromosomal and Mendelian syndromes account for approximately 20% (11.9% and 7.4% respectively) of CHD cases [3,4]. The genetic architecture underlying the remaining 80% of "sporadic" CHD remains elusive and cannot be addressed by standard family based linkage studies. However, genetic variants have been shown to be associated with sporadic, non-Mendelian/non-chromosomal CHD as non-synonymous disease-associated mutations have previously been found in case-control studies [5].

CITED2 is a CREBBP/EP300-interacting protein that is present in all vertebrates. It is highly conserved in placental mammals, with 95% identity between human and mouse. It has three regions (CR1-3) that are conserved in other CITED family members, and also an unusual Serine-glycine Rich Junction (SRJ, residues 161–199), which is unique to CITED2 [6–10]. The function of CR2 (residues 215–270) is to bind the CH1 domain of CREBBP and EP300 transcriptional co-activators, and *in vitro* studies indicate that it is necessary for all known biological activities of CITED2 [10–13]. CITED2 competitively inhibits hypoxia-activated gene transcription by blocking the interaction between CREBBP/EP300 and HIF-1A [10]. CITED2 also functions as a transcriptional co-activator, by recruiting CREBBP/EP300 to chromatin via the DNA-binding transcription factor AP2 (TFAP2) [11,14,15]. The functions of CR1, CR3 and the SRJ domain are not known. The SRJ domain has been hypothesized to be a mutational hotspot as variants clustering in this region have previously been reported in patients with CHD [16,17].

Cited2 is essential for normal mouse development. Mice lacking *Cited2* die *in utero* with cardiac and aortic arch malformations, adrenal gland agenesis, small cranial and dorsal root ganglia, exencephaly, and neural crest and left-right patterning defects [11,15,18–22]. The cardiac malformations in mice lacking *Cited2* are diverse and include atrial and ventricular septal defects, double outlet right ventricle, common arterial trunk, tetralogy of Fallot, transposition of the great arteries, and interrupted and aberrant aortic arches.

In this study, we have investigated the involvement of *CITED2* in CHD by direct sequencing of a cohort of CHD patients and controls and confirmed the clustering of non-synonymous mutations to the SRJ domain. *In vitro* experiments indicated that a specific residue in the SRJ domain (T166) was a functional target of MAPK1, and was necessary for TFAP2 co-activation. We used gene-targeting technologies in the mouse to functionally assess the contribution of T166 and the SRJ domain, as a whole, to disease. Mouse embryos expressing only CITED2-T166N or CITED2 SRJ-deleted alleles surprisingly showed no structural abnormalities by magnetic resonance imaging, and mice were viable and fertile. These results suggest that the SRJ domain is dispensable for CITED2 function in mice. Thus, point mutations and deletions clustering in the SRJ region are unlikely to be the sole cause of the malformations observed in patients with sporadic CHD, and may require additional factors to cause disease.

Results

Rare variants are infrequently found in *CITED2* in CHD and cluster in the SRJ domain

We sequenced the entire *CITED2* open reading frame in 1126 CHD cases and 1227 ethnically matched controls (Table 1 and Table S1). Nineteen sequence variants were identified. Of the non-synonymous variants found, five (T166N, R92G, N62S, A187T and G180-A187del) were unique to cases, while two (P36R, Q40H) were present only in controls. Three non-synonymous variants (H39del, H160L, G194-G195del) were present in both cases and controls. Three of the five non-synonymous variants found only in cases were inherited from unaffected parents (N62S, T166N and G180-A187del). Although there was an excess of non-synonymous variants that were unique to cases, this was not statistically significant using a 2-tailed Fisher's exact test. H39del was found in 10 cases and 1 control; however, we were unable to confirm this ratio in a replicate cohort (9/566 in cases vs. 43/2394 in controls, p = n.s., Text S1).

Three of the five non-synonymous variants identified uniquely in cases in this study, three of six in the study by Sperling et al. [16] and four of four in the study by Yang et al. [17], lie within the SRJ region of *CITED2* (Fig. 1A). The SRJ domain is highly conserved in placental mammals. It is, however, substantially abbreviated in marsupials and is absent in other vertebrates (Fig. 1B). Using the RONN program [23], we find that the SRJ domain is predicted to have a highly disordered secondary structure. However, none of the SRJ domain mutations listed above affected the disorder plot to any significant extent (Fig. S1). A number of functions have been indicated for intrinsically disordered regions, including molecular recognition, ligand binding, protein, DNA and RNA interactions, and as flexible linkers between domains [24].

CITED2 T166N mutation ablates TFAP2 coactivation function in vitro

Using the program NetPhos, we found that T166 is predicted to be a phosphorylation site for proline directed kinases [25,26]. The T166N mutation is predicted to abolish this putative phosphor-

Table 1. Synonymous and non-synonymous mutations identified through direct sequencing of 1126 cases with CHD and 1227 controls.

Variation	Protein	Cases	Controls	Diagnosis
Non-Synonymous, Unique				
c.559G>A	p.Ala187Thr	1	0	PS
c.497C>A	p.Thr166Asn	1	0	TGA
c.274A>G	p.Arg92Gly	1	0	ASD
c.185A>G	p.Asn62Ser	1	0	TOF
c.538-561del	p.Gly180_Ala187del	1	0	AVSD
c.107C>G	p.Pro36Arg	0	1	Control
c.120G>C	p.Gln40His	0	1	Control
Synonymous, Unique				
c.762T>C	p.Asp254Asp	1	0	Ebstein,VSD
c.612C>T	p.Ser204Ser	1	0	TGA
c.471C>T	p.Asn157Asn	1	0	ASD
c.381C>T	p.His127His	1	0	TOF
c.276G>A	p.Arg92Arg	1	0	VSD
c.117C>T	p.His39His	0	1	Control
c.120G>A	p.Gln40Gln	0	1	Control
Both				
c.115-117delCAC	p.His39del	10	1	
c.479A>T	p.His160Leu	11	9	
c.582C>T	p.Gly194Gly	7	13	
c.21C>A	p.Ala7Ala	306	336	
c.580-585delGGCGGC	p.Gly194_Gly195del	6	10	

5 unique non-synonymous variants are observed in the cases and 2 in the control group. Abbreviations: PS, pulmonic stenosis; TGA, transposition of great arteries; ASD, atrial septal defect; TOF, Tetralogy of Fallot; AVSD, atrioventricular septal defect; VSD, ventricular septal defect.

ylation site. To assess the functional significance of the T166N variant we examined its ability to co-activate a TFAP2 isoform. We performed transient transfection assays in Hep3B cells using a TFAP2 luciferase reporter containing three copies of the human metallothionein IIa TFAP2-binding site [11,14]. As reported previously [11,14], transfection of CITED2 alone did not affect reporter activity, and co-transfection of TFAP2C and CITED2, enhanced reporter activity 2 fold over that achieved with TFAP2C alone. In comparison, CITED2-T166N was severely defective for TFAP2C co-activation (Fig. 2).

Another molecular function of CITED2 is to represses HIF1 transactivation by interfering with the interaction between the carboxy-terminus of HIF1A, and EP300/CREBBP [10,27,28]. We tested the ability of CITED2 to repress the trans-activation of a fusion protein that contains the yeast GAL4 DNA-binding domain fused to the carboxy-terminus transactivation domain of HIF1A (residues 723–826, GAL4-HIF1A [10]). This is a weak transactivator under normoxic conditions but is strongly activated by either hypoxia or the iron chelator desferrioxamine (DFO) [10]. We found that T166N was identical to wild-type CITED2 in repressing GAL4-HIF1A transactivation. We also found that CITED2-T166N is expressed at wild-type levels, binds EP300 and TFAP2 efficiently *in vitro*, and is localised to the nucleus thus

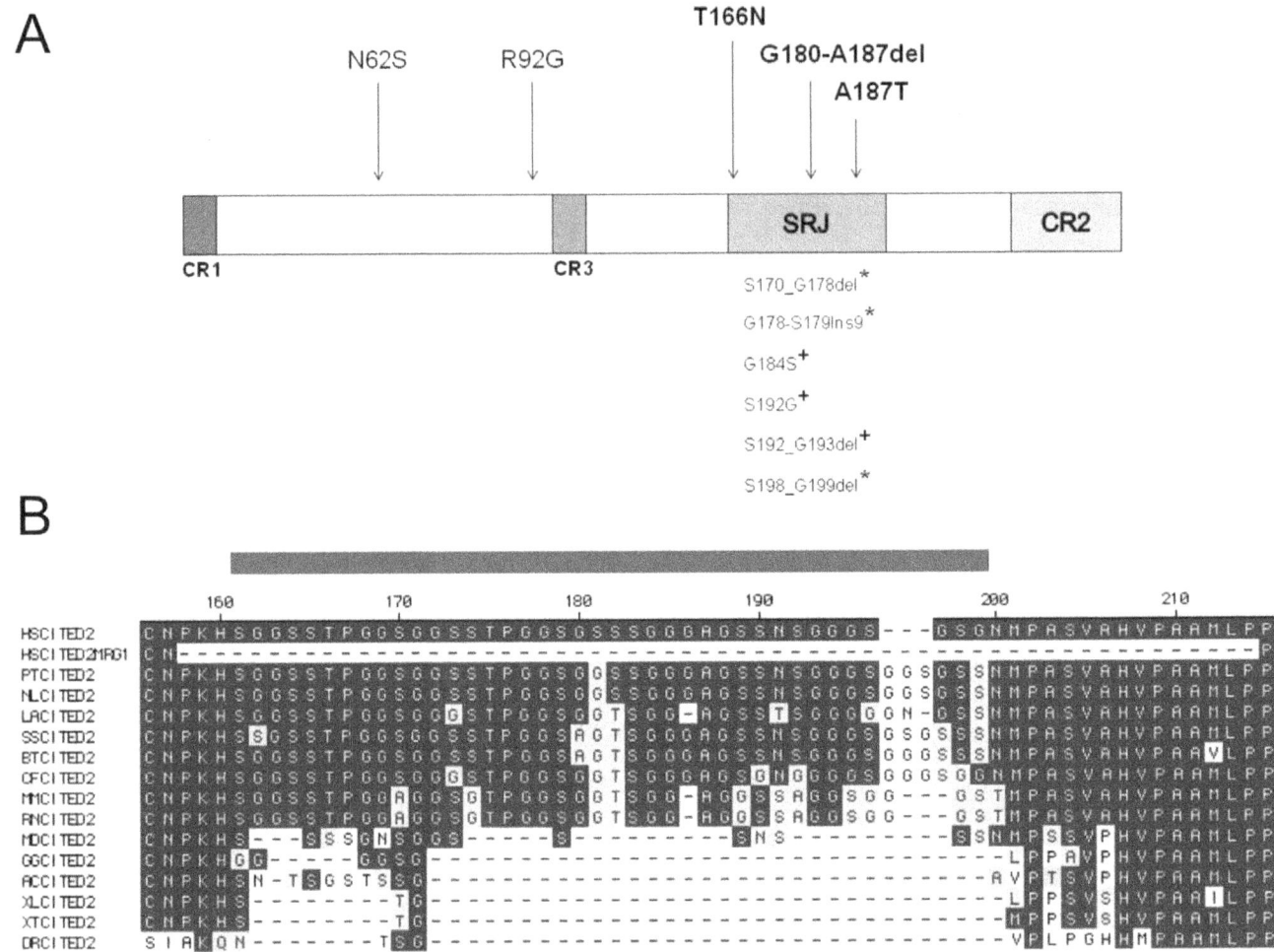

Figure 1. Structure of CITED2. (A) Schematic diagram of human CITED2 showing conserved regions (CR) 1–3 and the serine-glycine rich junction (SRJ). Also indicated are the locations of CITED2 variants. All unique non-synonymous variants found in this study are shown above the figure with variants found in the SRJ highlighted. Unique non-synonymous variants found by Sperling et al., 2005 (*) and Yang et al., 2010 (+) are shown below. SRJ comprises AA 161 to 199. (B) The CITED2 peptide sequence is shown for *Homo sapiens* (Human, HSCITED2, AF129290), CITED2-MRG1 (Human, HSCITED2 MRG1 isoform lacking the entire SRJ), *Pan troglodytes* (Chimapanzee, PTCITED2), *Nomascus leucogenys* (Gibbon, NLCITED2), *Loxodonta africana* (Elephant, LACITED2), *Sus scrofa* (Pig, SSCITED2), *Bos taurus*, (Cow, BTCITED2), *Canis familiaris* (Dog, CFCITED2), *Mus musculus* (Mouse, MMCITED2), *Rattus norvegicus* (Rat, RNCITED2), *Monodelphis domestica* (Opossum, MDCITED2), *Gallus gallus* (Chicken, GGCITED2), *Anolis carolinensis* (Anole lizard, ACCITED2), *Xenopus laevis* (African clawed frog, XLCITED2), *Xenopus tropicalis* (Western clawed frog, XTCITED2), and *Danio rerio* (Zebrafish, DRCITED2). Sequence alignments taken from the latest genome builds from EBI Ensembl. SRJ domain spans region marked with grey bar above corresponding to AA161 to 199 in the human protein sequence.

excluding these factors as possible mechanisms for impaired function (Fig. S2).

CITED2 is phosphorylated by MAPK1 at S85, T166 and T175

We examined the phosphorylation of CITED2 by MAPK1 (ERK2, Fig. 3). Recombinant human CITED2 was phosphorylated *in vitro* by active MAPK1. The phosphorylated CITED2 was then digested with trypsin and the resulting peptides were chromatographed on a Vydac C18 column. Three major peaks of ^{32}P radioactivity, termed A1 to A3, were observed. Both peaks A1 and A2 contained a peptide corresponding to residues 71–92 of CITED2 phosphorylated at Ser85. Interestingly, CITED2-Ser85 is not followed by a proline residue. Although all MAP Kinases phosphorylate preferentially Ser or Thr followed by Pro, non-canonical phosphorylation sites, such as the one found in CITED2, have previously been shown [29–32]. No mass

spectrometry data was obtainable for the A3 group of peaks but phosphoaminoacid analysis indicated that only phosphoThreonine was present (data not shown). In addition, Edman degradation showed the presence of ^{32}P at residues 7 and 16. Only one tryptic peptide occurs in CITED2 that is consistent with tryptic cleavage at Lys/Arg followed by Threonine residues at positions 7 and 16 and it consists of residues 160–239, (k)hsggsstpggsggsstpggsgsssgggagssnsgggsgsgnmpasvahvpaamlppn-vidtdfidedeevlmslviemgldr. Varying oxidation states of the 4 Methionine residues in this sequence could account for its complexity on the HPLC elution profile. Taken together, it suggests that peak A3 is a mixture of peaks of ^{32}P radioactivity containing a diphosphopeptide corresponding to residues 160–239 phosphorylated at Thr166 and Thr175 (three minor peaks of radioactivity were also observed eluting at 25–40 min, but the identity of the phosphorylated residue(s) eluting in them could not be determined). Phosphorylation of the mutant CITED2-T166N

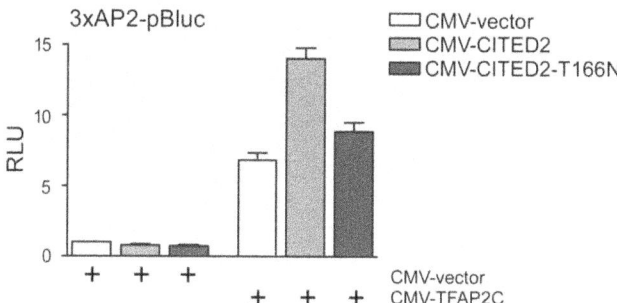

Figure 2. CITED2 mutation and its functional consequences. Hep3B cells were transiently transfected with the 3xAP2-luciferase reporter and the indicated plasmids and with CMV-lacZ. Results (mean±SEM, three independent experiments) are presented as relative luciferase units (RLU), corrected for β-galactosidase activity. The control transfection value (at the extreme left) in each case (with CMV-vector) is set at 1.

by MAPK1 was also analyzed by chromatography on a Vydac C18 column after tryptic digestion. The same three major (called A4 to A6 in the Fig. 3) and minor peptides phosphorylated on wild type CITED2 were phosphorylated in CITED2-T166N, however, the radioactivity of peak A3 was significantly reduced in the mutant and some other minor peaks appeared (85–95 min on the elution profile). Peaks A4 and A5 contained the peptide (residues 71–92) of CITED2 phosphorylated at Ser85. Peak A6 contained a peptide with ^{32}P radioactivity released at cycle 16 and containing phospho-Thr (phosphoaminoacid analysis and Edman degradation, data not shown). On the basis of its similar HPLC elution profile to peak A3 of wild type CITED2, this is most likely the peptide containing residues 160–239 phosphorylated at Thr175. The diphosphopeptide with phosphoThr166 was not found due to the T166N mutation.

CITED2 coactivation is enhanced by activation of MAPK1 and requires T166

The above results suggested that CITED2 phosphorylation by MAPK1 at T166 may be required for its coactivation function. To test this, we performed coactivation studies in Hep3B cells. Here, we co-transfected a TFAP2 reporter plasmid, and plasmids encoding CITED2, CITED2T166N, MAPK1, and variants of the MAPK1-activating kinase, MAPKK1S221A (a constitutively inactive mutant) or MAPKK1-S217ES221E (a constitutively active mutant). No significant effect of MAPK1 and MAPKK1 plasmids was observed on activity of the reporter in the absence of TFAP2 (not shown) (Fig. 4). However a major effect (3-fold over CITED2 alone) was observed on TFAP2C coactivation by CITED2 in the presence of MAPK1+MAPKK1-S217ES221E. In comparison to TFAP2C without CITED2, this represents a ~6 fold activation of the reporter (Fig. 4). Co-expression of MAPK1 or MAPKK1 did not affect the expression of CITED2 (Fig. S3). CITED2-T166N did not respond to MAPK1 activation. These results indicate that activated MAPK1 enhances co-activation function of CITED2 (Fig. 4). The effect is specific to TFAP2C in these experiments, and also requires the T166 residue. Taken together these results support the idea that T166 is the target of a proline-directed kinase, and its phosphorylation enhances CITED2 coactivation function.

T166 is essential for maintaining ES proliferation in the absence of Leukemia Inhibitory Factor (LIF)

We next sought to determine if T166 is necessary for the ability of CITED2 to maintain mouse embryonic stem (ES) cell proliferation. ES cells can proliferate indefinitely in culture, and are pluripotent [33]. In mouse ES cells this requires the growth factors LIF and BMP [34] and is correlated with the expression of alkaline phosphatase [35]. Gain-of-function experiments have shown that *Nanog* and *Cited2* can bypass the requirement for LIF in mouse ES cells [35–37]. We used a previously described episomal expression system in ES cells for these experiments [36]. We transfected plasmids bearing *Nanog*, *CITED2*, *CITED2-T166N*, and empty vector controls in E14/T ES cells. Following puromycin selection, cells were plated in the absence of LIF, and numbers estimated using crystal violet staining at daily intervals thereafter. These experiments showed that both *Nanog* and *CITED2* maintained the proliferation of ES cells in the absence of LIF, whereas empty vector did not. *CITED2-T166N* had a markedly reduced ability to maintain ES cell proliferation in the absence of LIF suggesting that T166 is essential for maintaining ES proliferation in the absence of LIF (Fig. 5).

Generation of mice harboring the non-synonymous T166N variant within the *Cited2* SRJ domain

In order to investigate the functional significance of the T166N variant *in vivo*, the orthologous amino acid change was introduced into the mouse *Cited2* locus using homologous recombination in ES cells (Fig. 6A). *Cited2* $^{+/T166N}$ embryos (n = 9) and *Cited2* $^{T166N/T166N}$ embryos (n = 2) at 15.5 days post coitum (dpc) analyzed by magnetic resonance imaging (MRI) were found to be anatomically normal, showing no dominant effect. In addition, they were viable and fertile. One possibility in the human situation is that the wild-type allele may not sufficiently compensate for lack of activity of the mutant allele. To determine if a single allele of *Cited2* ^{T166N} would support normal embryonic development, we studied *Cited2* $^{-/T166N}$ mouse embryos. *Cited2* $^{-/T166N}$ mice were generated by crossing *Cited2* $^{+/T166N}$ to *Cited2* $^{+/-}$. 31 out of 31 *Cited2* $^{-/T166N}$ mouse embryos at 15.5 days post coitum (dpc) analyzed by magnetic resonance imaging (MRI) were found to be anatomically normal. They revealed none of the structural developmental anomalies associated with the loss of *Cited2* and had normal sized adrenal glands (Fig. 7C, H and M, Fig. S4). Furthermore, *Cited2* $^{-/T166N}$ mice were born at the expected Mendelian ratios (6/20, Table 2A, $X^2(3) = 0.4$; p = n.s.) and were viable and fertile.

Development of a system to efficiently introduce human *CITED2* variants into mouse *Cited2*

In order to introduce human *CITED2* variants into the mouse *Cited2* gene at high efficiency, we adapted a Recombinase Mediated Cassette Exchange (RMCE) system that uses PhiC31 integrase [38,39]. Using homologous recombination, the *Cited2* gene was targeted in C57BL/6N mouse ES cells so that exon 2 (which contains the entire open reading frame, ORF) became flanked with *attP* sites, resulting in the generation of ES cell line, *Cited2* ^{attP} (Fig. 6B). Using this ES cell line, the *Cited2* ORF can be manipulated and exchanged with sequences introduced using the exchange plasmids harboring analogously positioned *attB* sites. Co-transfection with PhiC31 integrase results in their stable integration at high efficiency within the *Cited2* gene (data not shown).

Generation of mice lacking the CITED2 SRJ domain

As variants found in patients tend to cluster in the SRJ domain, and having found that a non-synonymous mutation within the SRJ

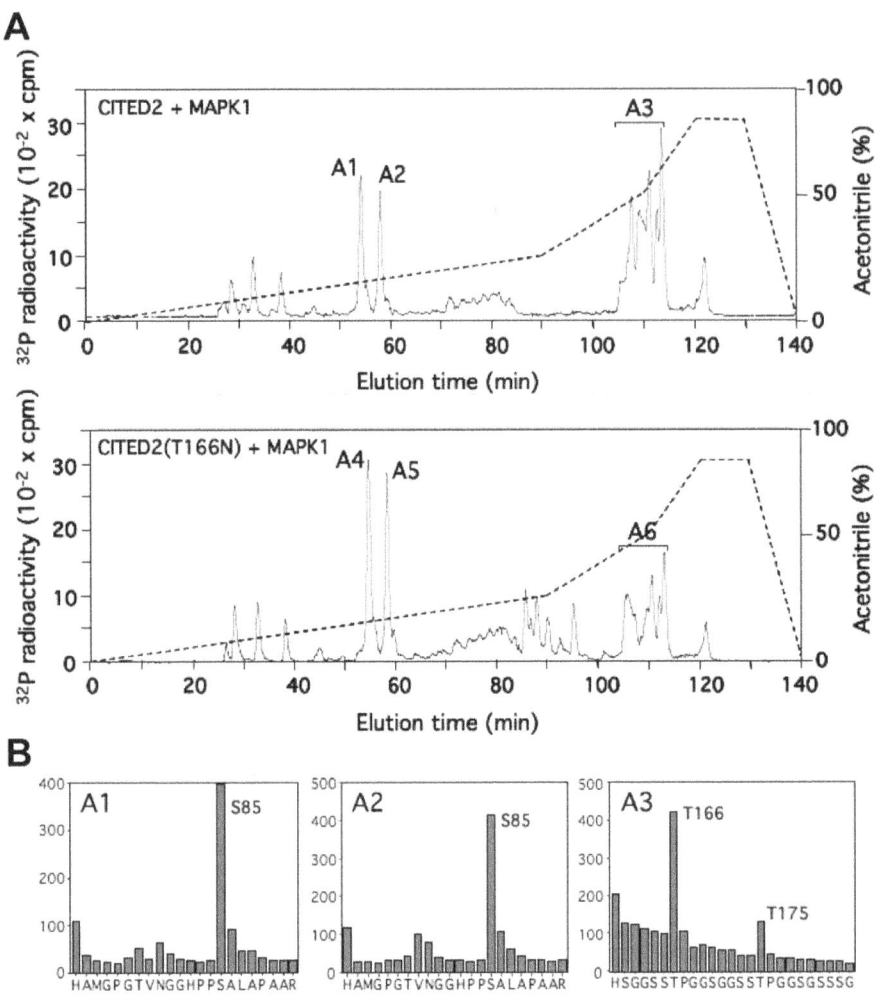

Figure 3. Identification of residues in CITED2 wild type or CITED2T166N phosphorylated by ERK2 (MAPK1). (A) GST-CITED2 wild type or mutant GST-CITED2T166N were incubated with Mg [^{32}P]ATP in the presence of ERK2 and subjected to SDS-PAGE. The phosphorylated CITED2 was excised from the gel, digested with trypsin and the peptide separated by chromatography on a Vydac C18 column. The column was developed with an acetonitrile gradient (broken line) and ^{32}P-radioactivity is shown (full line). The phosphopeptides A1 to A6 are indicated. (B) The major peaks (A1 to A6) of ^{32}P-radioactivity were analysed by MALDI-TOF, MALDI TOF-TOF, Edman degradation and phosphoamino acid analysis as described in Materials and Methods and the data for A1–A3 is shown. The sequence inferred from this data is shown underneath each figure.

domain was compatible with normal embryonic development, we sought to understand the function of the SRJ domain as a whole by assessing the effect of replacing the mouse *Cited2* ORF with that of the human *CITED2* MRG1 isoform [6,7]. This isoform lacks residues 158–214 (i.e. the SRJ region plus 18 flanking amino acids) and is a rare variant of CITED2 (ENSP00000376126, Fig. 1B) which likely arises from non-canonical splice sites within exon 2 [10]. In order to achieve this, the endogenous mouse *Cited2* ORF in *Cited2*^{attP} ES cells was replaced using RMCE with the *CITED2*^{MRG1} ORF (referred to as *Cited2*^{MRG1}) and its corresponding control, full-length human *CITED2* ORF (referred to as *Cited2*^{HUM}, Fig. 6C).

The SRJ domain of CITED2 is dispensable for function

Cited2$^{-/MRG1}$ embryos, generated by crossing *Cited2*$^{+/MRG1}$ to *Cited2*$^{+/-}$ mice, were devoid of wild type *Cited2* and expressed only a single copy of the CITED2-MRG1 isoform. This was confirmed by western blotting and by Reverse Transcription Polymerase Chain Reaction (RT-PCR) followed by sequencing of the PCR products (Fig. 8A and B). 74 of 75 *Cited2*$^{-/MRG1}$ embryos harvested at 15.5 dpc and analyzed using MRI showed no overt cardiac or other

anatomical developmental anomalies associated with loss of *Cited2*, and they all showed normal sized adrenal glands (Fig. 7D, I and N and Fig. S4). One embryo presented with ectopia cordis, small ventricular septal defect, oedema and other structural anomalies (Fig. S5). *Cited2*$^{-/MRG1}$ and *Cited2*$^{MRG1/MRG1}$ mice were found to be viable and fertile. Furthermore, *Cited2*$^{-/MRG1}$ mice were found at the expected Mendelian ratio at weaning (12/41, Table 2B, X^2 (3): 0.46, p = n.s.). The same analysis was carried out for the control, full length *Cited2*^{HUM} allele. No anatomical anomalies were found in *Cited2*$^{-/HUM}$ embryos (0/20). *Cited2*$^{HUM/HUM}$ mice were also viable and fertile as were *Cited2*$^{-/HUM}$ (data not shown).

Discussion

Our resequencing study reported here and those reported elsewhere [16,17] indicate that non-synonymous mutations of *CITED2* can be observed in patients with congenital heart disease, and that these mutations tend to cluster in the SRJ domain. Cell-based assays investigating some of these variants have indicated that they can affect HIF1A-repression and/or TFAP2-coactivation

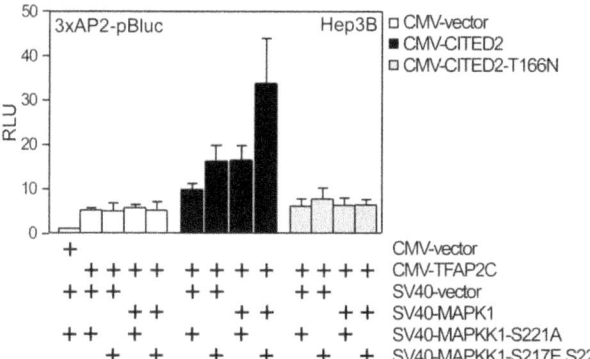

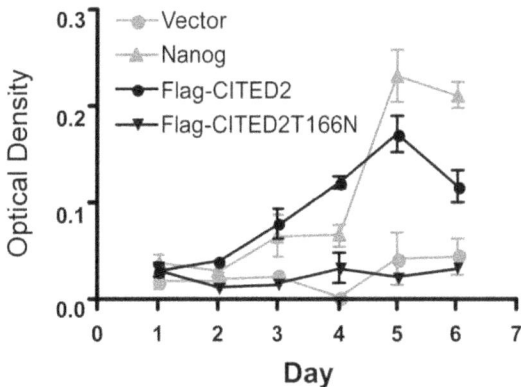

Figure 4. MAPK signalling to CITED2 enhances its co-activation function. Hep3B cells were transiently transfected with the 3xAP2-luciferase reporter, with CMV-lacZ, CITED2-expressing plasmid or the control vector and plasmids expressing MAPK1 or the control vector and with plasmids expressing a defective MAPKK1 (SV40-MAPKK1-S221A) or a constitutively active MAPKK1 (SV40-MAPKK1-S217ES221E). Results are presented as relative luciferase units corrected for lacZ activity. The control transfection value (at the extreme left) in each case (with CMV-vector) is set at 1.

Figure 5. ES cell proliferation rescue by wild-type CITED2 and CITED2-T166N in the absence of leukemia inhibitory factor (LIF). E14/T ES cells transfected by electroporation with the indicated plasmids were selected in puromycin. Surviving cells were plated in quadruplicate into 12-well plates in medium containing puromycin, but in the absence of LIF. The cells were fixed at the indicated time points using 10% formalin. The relative number of ES cells was determined by staining with 0.1% crystal violet, extracting cell-associated dye using 10% acetic acid, and measuring absorbance at A590. Results are presented as mean±SEM. Results represent a single experiment. Similar results were obtained from three independent experiments.

functions of CITED2 [16]. The SRJ domain, although highly conserved in placental mammals, is substantially abbreviated in marsupials (e.g. the opossum *Monodelphys domesticus*) and in monotremes (e.g. the platypus *Ornithorhynchus anatinus*), and is absent in other vertebrates (Fig. 1B). Thus, the region may have appeared relatively recently in evolutionary terms and may conceivably be of relevance to differences in cardiac development and structure between placental mammals and other vertebrates [40–43].

Structurally, the SRJ region is predicted to be disordered and potentially functions as a flexible linker [24]. The T166 residue within this domain is predicted to be a target of proline directed kinases [25,26], and our studies indicated that the T166 residue can be phosphorylated by MAPK1, and that activation of MAPK1 promoted co-activation function. Moreover cell-based studies indicated that the T166N mutation had a deleterious effect on TFAP2 co-activation function, and on the ability of CITED2 to promote ES cell proliferation in the absence of LIF.

Surprisingly, our *in vivo* study of mice carrying the T166N variant and the deletion of the SRJ domain indicate that in mice, under normal laboratory conditions, neither the complete deletion of the SRJ domain nor the introduction of a variant which could potentially lead to the loss of a phosphorylation site of CITED2 are detrimental to its function. In a single *Cited2* $^{-/MRG1}$ embryo out of 75 that we studied, we observed an ectopia cordis phenotype. Since ectopia cordis is not a phenotype which has previously been associated with the loss of *Cited2* [11,15,17,21,22,44–47], and this embryo has normal adrenal glands (absence of which is a hallmark of *Cited2* deficiency), it is most unlikely that it is a consequence of the loss of the SRJ domain. Animals of this genotype are also viable and fertile. However, *in vitro* data indicate that the T166N mutation can have functional significance, and previous studies have indicated that other SRJ mutations also affect its function [16]. It is possible that the partial impairment of CITED2 function revealed by *in vitro* experiments is insufficient to affect development.

Taken together, the results obtained from mouse studies indicate that the SRJ domain is dispensable during mouse cardiac development and for viability and fertility. On the other hand, three independent human studies show that non-synonymous

mutations, predominantly clustering in the SRJ domain, are mainly observed in patients with CHD and not in controls suggesting that this region is important for normal cardiac development. How can we explain these divergent observations? One possibility is that the SRJ is indeed dispensable for mammalian heart development, and that the observations from patients may be misleading. Supporting this idea, there is considerable lack of conservation in this domain between placental and non-placental mammals. Furthermore, the mutations in the SRJ do not significantly affect the disordered nature of the domain, indicating that it may be able to accommodate mutations without adversely affecting the overall structure and function of the protein. Moreover, in no case has it been shown that the mutation has either arisen *de novo* or been transmitted from an affected parent. Another possibility that partially reconciles the mouse and human observations is that variants found clustered in the SRJ in CHD patients may not, by themselves, be causative of disease and may require additional factors, such as second site genetic modifiers or environmental stress, for a phenotypic manifestation. Supporting this idea, we have previously shown that a maternal high-fat diet can alter the penetrance of left-right patterning defects and cleft palate in *Cited2* deficient mouse embryos [48]. In addition, we have also shown that *Cited2* can genetically interact with other developmental genes: loss of *Lmo4* can affect the *Cited2* phenotype [49]. A third possibility to be considered is human and mouse discordance where the mouse model fails to phenocopy the human disease. For instance, mutations in EVC and DHCR7 result in heart defects in humans (Ellis van Creveld Syndrome, OMIM 225500, Smith-Lemli-Opitz syndrome OMIM 270400) but not in the mouse [33,50,51].

To summarise, using a case-control approach we found, like others, that non-synonymous variants cluster in the SRJ region of CITED2 in CHD patients but not in controls. A point mutation (T166N) in this region greatly affects CITED2 co-activation function and LIF-independent growth of ES cells and is likely phosphorylated by MAPK1. We found that mice harboring, either the T166N point mutation or a deletion of the entire SRJ domain and 18 adjacent amino acids, undergo normal cardiac develop-

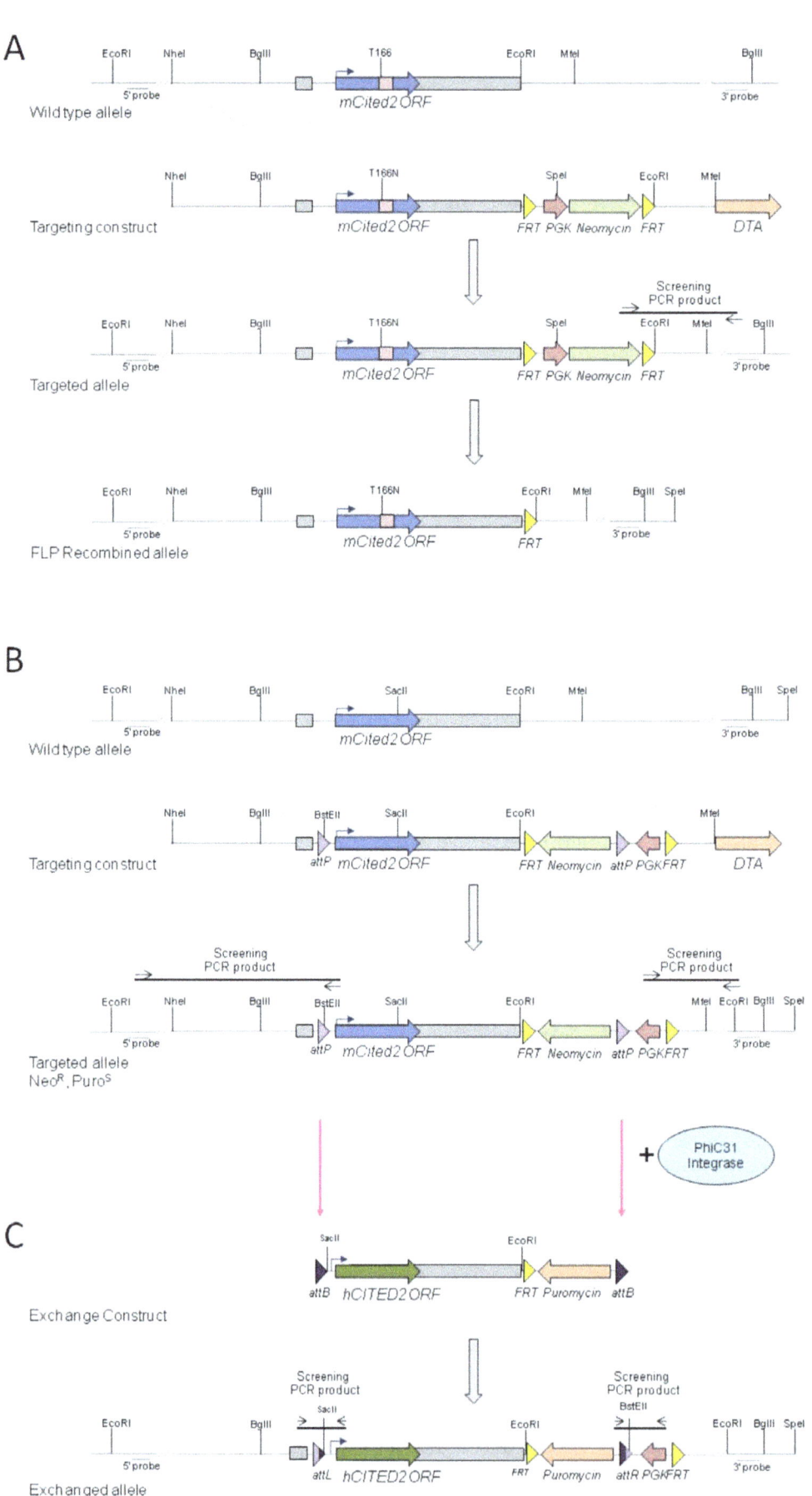

Figure 6. Generation of *Cited2* alleles. (A) Targeting strategy for the generation of *Cited2* ^{T166N} allele by homologous recombination. The T to N change was introduced by site directed mutagenesis into the orthologous residue in the mouse sequence. The structure of the wildtype *Cited2* allele, targeting vector, targeted allele, and its structure after FLP mediated recombination are shown. The open reading frame (ORF, blue arrow) is entirely contained within exon 2 (exons indicated by grey rectangles). The targeting vector has an *frt-PGK-NeoR-frt* selection cassette downstream of exon 2, followed by a DTA (diphtheria toxin) cassette. (B) Targeting strategy for the generation of the *Cited2*^{attP} ES cell line. A 5′ *attP* site was introduced into the first intron, upstream of the ATG and a 3′ *attP* site downstream of the stop codon and exon 2 as part of the neomycin selection cassette, in between the PGK promoter and the neomycin coding region. A DTA cassette was also introduced downstream of the 3′ homology arm for negative selection. (C) The human CITED2^{MRG1} isoform (not shown) and the human full length CITED2 were targeted into the *Cited2* locus via PhiC31 integrase mediated cassette exchange. The exchange event occurs between the *attP* and *attB* sites giving rise to *attL* and *attR* sites. Successful exchange replaces the mouse *Cited2* ORF with that of either the MRG1 isoform of *CITED2* or the full length human *CITED2* and brings the puromycin resistance gene under control of the PGK promoter.

ment and are viable and fertile. Thus, under normal conditions in mice, T166 and the SRJ domain are dispensable for these functions. We suggest that point mutations and deletions clustering in the SRJ region may require additional genetic or environmental factors to cause disease. Our results suggest that coding sequence mutations observed in case-control studies need validation using *in vivo* models and that predictions based on structural conservation and *in vitro* functional assays, or even *in vivo* global loss of function models, may be insufficient. This has implications for the interpretation of data arising from exon resequencing programs currently being pursued in cardiac and other developmental diseases.

Materials and Methods

Cases and controls

Patients (all of North West European White Caucasian ancestry) were ascertained through referring clinicians as part of the Genetic Origins of Congenital Heart Disease Study (GO-CHD) at several UK paediatric and adult congenital heart disease centres and were evaluated by physical examination and echocardiography. Samples were also obtained through collaboration with the University of Newcastle. Patients with CHD where the genetic mechanism was known were excluded (Down syndrome and DiGeorge syndrome amongst others). Ethnicity was determined by questionnaire and based on all four grandparents using the 2001 UK census of the population categories. Blood or saliva was collected from each affected individual and their parents, where available, and DNA was extracted using standard techniques. Written informed consent for inclusion in molecular genetic studies was obtained in each case. Approval for this study was obtained from a national ethics committee (MREC for Wales, REF 05/MRE09/89). 1227 unselected control samples were obtained from North West European White Caucasian individuals from the 1958 UK birth cohort (1041) and from the Wellcome Trust Case Control Consortium UK blood donor collection (186).

DNA sequencing

Oligonucleotides were designed from flanking intronic and exonic sequence of the CITED2 gene (Accession No. AF129290) to produce two ~500 bp PCR products. The following PCR primer pairs were used. To amplify the N terminal product: forward primer: 5′ TGTGGCGCGGGTCTCATTATC, reverse primer: 5′ CTGGTTTGTCCCGTTCATCTG; to amplify the C terminal product: forward primer 5′ TCACCCCTACCCCCA-CAACC, reverse primer 5′ TTCACGCCGAAGAAGTTGGG. Both strands of each product were sequenced on an automated ABI3730 sequencer using BigDye terminator cycle sequencing reagents (Applied Biosystems, CA, USA). Chromatographs were analyzed using PHREDPHRAP, Sequencher (v4.8, Gene Codes Corp., MI, USA) and GAP4 in house software (Wellcome Trust

Sanger Institute, Cambridge, UK). Parental samples were analyzed where available to determine inheritance.

Transient transfection and pull-down experiments

Plasmids, transfection conditions for transient transfection experiments, and luciferase assays have been previously described [10,14]. Site directed mutagenesis was performed using the QuikChange™ Site-Directed Mutagenesis Kit (Stratagene) as per manufacturer's instructions, and oligonucleotides 5′-GCGGCGGCAGCAG-CAACCCGGGCGGCTCGGGCGGC and 5′-GCCGCCCGA-GCCGCCCGGGTTGCTGCTGCCGCCGC were used to create the T166N mutation which was confirmed by sequencing. GST pulldown experiments and desferrioxamine treatments were performed as previously described [10]. MAPK1 expression plasmid was a gift from Ralf Janknecht [52]. MAPKK1, MAPKK1S221A and MAPKK1-S217ES221E plasmids were gifts from Chris Marshall [53].

Identification of phosphorylation sites in CITED2

Phosphorylation of CITED2 by active GST-ERK2 was carried out as described [54]. Wild type human GST-CITED2 (~2 mM) or mutant GST-CITED2-T166N were incubated for 60 min at 30°C with activated human GST-ERK2 (2 U/ml), 10 mM magnesium acetate and 1 mM [γ³²P]ATP (Amersham Bioscience) in 50 mM Tris-HCl, pH 7.5, 0.1 mM EGTA, 0.1 mM sodium orthovanadate and 0.1% (v/v) 2-mercaptoethanol. The procedure for mapping the phosphorylation sites is detailed elsewhere [55]. The ³²P-labelled protein was reduced with DTT and incubated with 0.5% (v/v) iodoacetamide to alkylate cysteine residues and subjected to SDS-PAGE. The band corresponding to ³²P-labeled GST-CITED2 was excised, digested with trypsin and chromatographed on a Vydac C18 column (218TP5215, 2 mm i.d. ×15 cm) equilibrated in 0.1% (v/v) trifluoroacetic acid (TFA). The column was developed with a gradient of acetonitrile in 0.1% (v/v) TFA from 0–30% acetonitrile (0–90 min), 30–50% acetonitrile (90–110 min) and 50–100% acetonitrile (110–120 min). The flow rate was 0.2 ml/min, fractions of 0.1 ml were collected and the ³²P radioactivity determined by Cerenkov counting. Briefly, sites of phosphorylation within the peptides were determined by a combination of MALDI-TOF and MALDI TOF-TOF (matrix assisted laser-desorption ionization-time-of-flight/time-of-flight) mass spectrometry on an Applied Biosystems 4700 TOF/TOF Proteomics Analyser (utilising 5 mg/ml alpha cyano-cinnamic acid in 10 mM ammonium phosphate 50% acetonitrile as the matrix), and solid-phase Edman sequencing of peptides coupled to a Sequelon-arylamine membrane (on an Applied Biosystems 494C protein sequencer). The release of ³²P radioactivity after each cycle of Edman degradation was counted. Phosphoaminoacid analysis was performed as described [54].

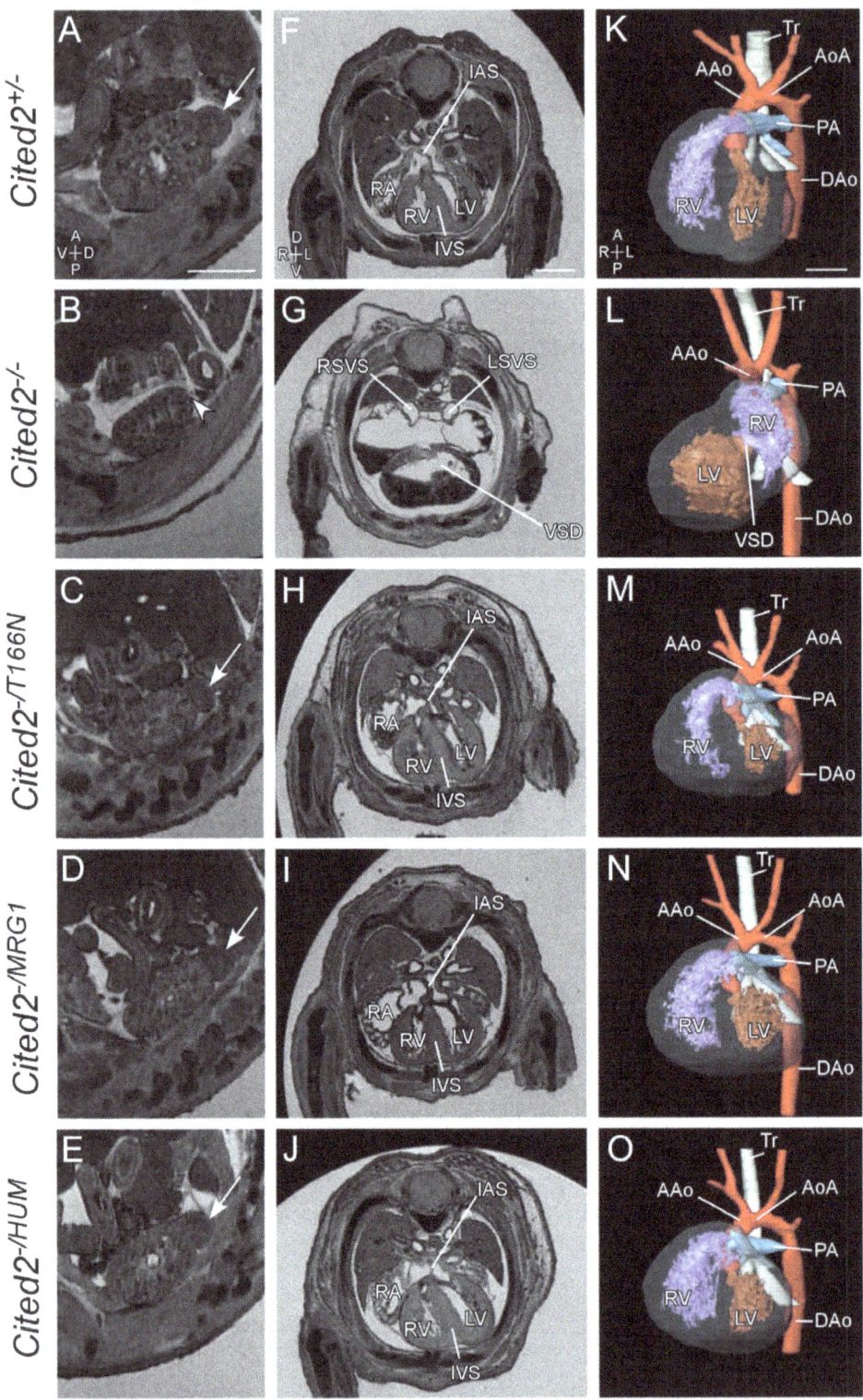

Figure 7. Phenotypic analysis of mouse embryos expressing CITED2 variants. MRI analysis of embryos 15.5 days post coitum (dpc). Genotypes are indicated as shown. Sagittal sections through the left kidney (A–E) are shown to indicate the left adrenal gland where present (arrows), and absent (arrowhead). Transverse sections through the thorax (F–J) and 3D reconstructions (K–O) are shown to demonstrate cardiac anatomy. Loss of *Cited2* leads to adrenal agenesis (B, arrowhead), right atrial isomerism, ventricular septal defect (VSD) and common atrium (G), and abnormal ventricular topology (L). Embryos expressing only the T166N variant, the MRG1 isoform, or full length human CITED2 have normal adrenal glands and hearts. RA, Right Atria; RV, Right Ventricle; LV, Left Ventricle; IVS, Interventricular Septum; IAS, Intra-atrial Septum; AAo, Aorta; AoA, Aortic Arch; Tr, Trachea; DAo, Dorsal Aorta; LSVS and RSVS, Left and Right Systemic Venous Sinus. Axis: A, Anterior; P, Posterior; V, Ventral; D, Dorsal; L, Left; R, Right. Scale bars: 0.5 mm.

Table 2. Mice expressing a single copy of the Cited2 ^{T166N} (A) or Cited2 ^{MRG1} (B) allele are found at the expected Mendelian ratios at weaning.

	Expected	Observed
Cited2 $^{+/-}$ ♂ X Cited2 $^{+/T166N}$ ♀		
Cited2 $^{+/T166N}$	5	5
Cited2 $^{-/T166N}$	5	6
Cited2 $^{+/+}$	5	5
Cited2 $^{+/-}$	5	4
Cited2 $^{+/-}$ ♂ X Cited2 $^{+/MRG1}$ ♀		
Cited2 $^{+/MRG1}$	10.25	10
Cited2 $^{-/MRG1}$	10.25	12
Cited2 $^{+/+}$	10.25	10
Cited2 $^{+/-}$	10.25	9

Mice were genotyped at 3 weeks of age. All genotypes are present at the expected Mendelian ratios.

ES cell pluripotency

E14/T cells [56] (gift from Austin Smith) were transfected with pPyCAGIP-CITED2 or CITED2-T166N episomal expression vectors, pPyCAGIP-Nanog vector (positive control) and empty vector [36]. Cells were selected with puromycin, and then tested for maintenance of cell proliferation in the absence of LIF. Cell proliferation was assayed using crystal violet staining as described [13].

Generation of Cited2 ^{T166N} mice

The T166N mutation was introduced into the endogenous Cited2 gene by gene targeting in murine 129Sv embryonic stem (ES) cells (Fig. 6A). The targeting vector was constructed using Cited2 genomic sequences isolated from a λFIXII-129SvJ genomic library (Stratagene). The C-A change which converts Threonine 166 to Arginine was introduced via site directed mutagenesis which also introduced an adjacent, silent PasI restriction site 7 bp downstream. Further cloning and primer information is available upon request. The frt-PGK-NeoR-frt selection cassette was inserted 1.581 kb downstream of the stop codon. A DTA cassette was also introduced downstream of the 3′ homology arm for negative selection. The targeting vector was linearized with NheI and electroporated into ES cells at GenOway (France). ES cells were selected in 350 ug/ul G418. Correct targeting of the Cited2 gene at the 3′arm was detected by long range PCR spanning the homology region and at the 5′arm by Southern blotting (data not shown). Correctly targeted ES cell clones were injected into C57BL/6J blastocysts and chimeras crossed to C57BL/6J females. Following successful germline transmission, targeting was confirmed to be correct by Southern blotting (Fig. 8C). Heterozygous mice were crossed to FLPeR [57] mice in a C57BL/6J background to remove the frt-PGK-NeoR-frt selection cassette. The resulting FLP recombined Cited2 $^{+/T166N}$ mice were backcrossed to C57BL/6J for at least 2 further generations prior to the start of experiments and maintained by backcrossing to C57BL/6J mice. All studies involving animals were performed in accordance with UK Home Office Animals (Scientific Procedures) Act 1986 and approved by the University of Oxford's Local Ethical Review Process.

Generation of the Cited2 ^{attP} ES cell line

The Cited2 ^{attP} ES cell line was generated via homologous recombination in C57BL/6N ES cells (Fig. 6B). A targeting construct was assembled by introducing two PhiC31 integrase attP sites into the Cited2 locus of genomic DNA isolated from BAC RP23-450-B12 DNA. The 5′ attP site was introduced into the first intron, upstream of the ATG and the 3′ attP site 1.551 kb downstream of the stop codon as part of the Neomycin selection cassette, in between the PGK promoter and the Neomycin coding region. A DTA cassette was also introduced downstream of the 3′ homology arm for negative selection. Further details on the cloning are available upon request. The NotI linearized vector was electroporated into mouse JM8.F6 ES cells, a C57BL/6N ES cell line [58], followed by selection in G418 (175 µg/ml). Neomycin resistant colonies were analyzed by long range PCR spanning both the 3′ and 5′ homology arms for correct targeting of the Cited2 gene and integration of the 5′ attP site. Primer pairs used for long range PCR were the following: for the 5′ homology arm: forward primer 5′ CCAGGATGGGAAACCCTGACT and reverse primer 5′ CTCAGTTGGGGGCGTAGTTCG, and for the 3′ homology arm: forward primer 5′ CCCTACCCGGTA-GAAGTTCCT and reverse primer 5′ AGATATCACGTAG-GATCTGCT. The generated ES cells were validated as being suitable for subsequence manipulation by injection into albino C57BL/6J (C57BL/6J-Tyr $^{c-2J}$/J) blastocysts. Successful germline transmission was confirmed by the aforementioned long range PCR. Mice carrying the Cited2 ^{attP} allele were bred to homozygosity and in trans to a Cited2 null allele (Cited2 ^{tm1Bha}) [11] to ensure that the tagged Cited2 allele did not disrupt CITED2 function and to validate the ES cell resource for future manipulation.

Generation of Cited2 ^{MRG1} and Cited2 ^{HUM} alleles by Recombinase Mediated Cassette Exchange (RMCE)

Cited2 ^{MRG1} and Cited2 ^{HUM} targeted ES cell lines were generated via RMCE using the previously targeted Cited2 ^{attP} ES cells (Fig. 6C). Exchange vectors were designed to only replace the mouse Cited2 ORF with either human full length CITED2 or CITED2 ^{MRG1} ORF, whilst retaining the intact mouse 5′ and 3′ UTRs. The vectors were assembled by introducing one attB PhiC31 integrase recognition site upstream of either human full length CITED2 or MRG1 at the same location in the first intron where the attP recognition site had previously been inserted. The second attB site was introduced upstream of the promoterless puromycin expression cassette. Successful RMCE was thus designed to reconstitute a functional puromycin resistance cassette.

1×10^6 Cited2 ^{attP} ES cells were co-electroporated with 5 µg of either the full length human CITED2 or the CITED2 ^{MRG1} exchange plasmid and 5 µg of pPhiC31o [59] using the Neon transfection system (Invitrogen) (3×1400 V, 10 ms) and plated on puromycin resistant fibroblast feeder layers. After approximately 7 days of selection in 600 ng/ml puromycin, 24 resistant colonies were isolated per construct, expanded and screened by PCR for the correct cassette exchange events at the 5′ and 3′ ends using specific primers which amplify across the the resulting attL and attR sites (to amplify across the attL: forward primer 5′ CAG-CAGGTCCGCCGAGGTAGC and reverse primer 5′ AACC-GAGACCGGTTCAACAGC, and to amplify across the attR: forward primer 5′ CACGCTTCAAAAGCGCACGTCTG and reverse primer 5′ CGCGTGAGGAAGAGTTCTTGCA). The generation of the attL site was confirmed by digesting the PCR product with SacII. Correct exchange was further confirmed by long range PCR (For 5′ homology arm: 5′ CCAGGATGG-GAAACCCTGACT and 5′ CAGCAGGTCCGCCGAGG-TAGC, and for the 3′ homology arm: 5′ CAGAAATCGCAAA-

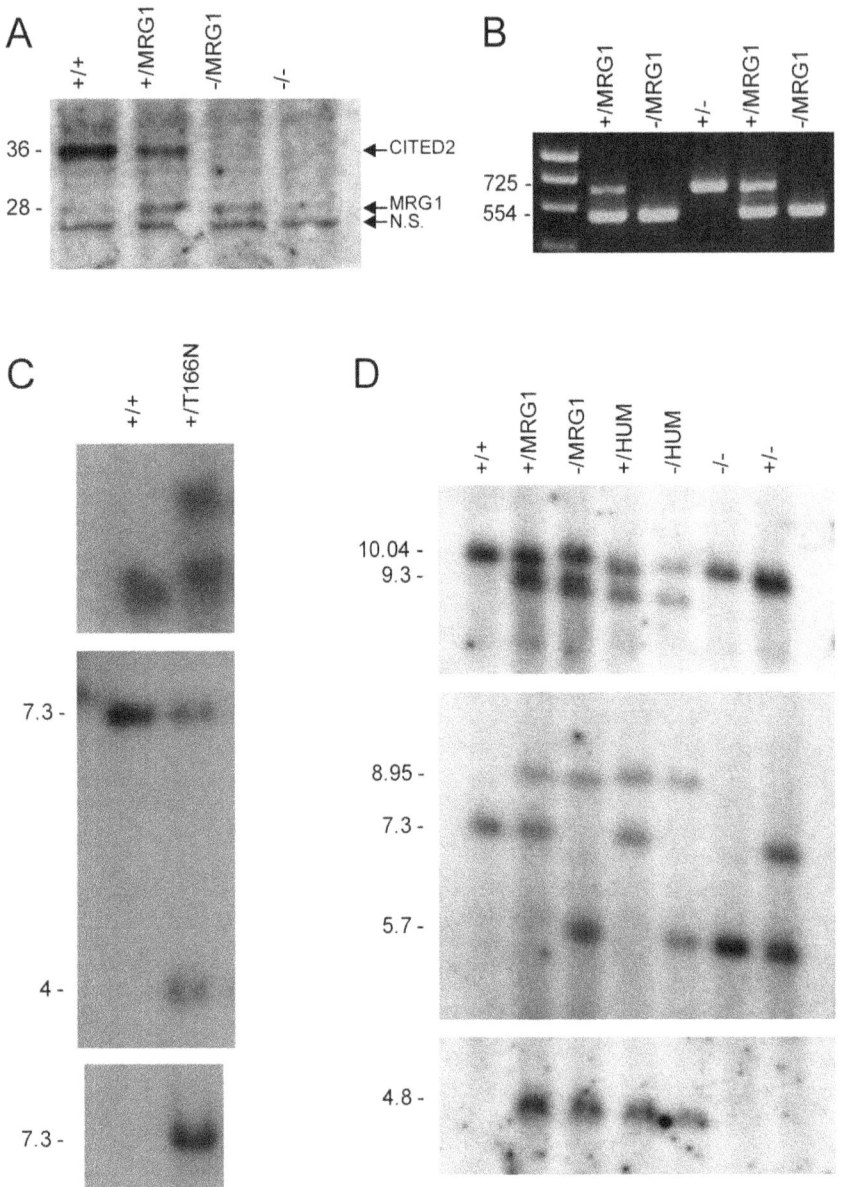

Figure 8. Molecular characterization of the *Cited2 T166N*, *Cited2 MRG1* and *Cited2 HUM* alleles. (A) Western blot of total protein lysates from mouse embryonic fibroblasts (MEFs), probed with anti-CITED2 antibody. CITED2 and CITED2-MRG1 are indicated, as is a non-specific band (N.S.) that migrates at 25 kDa. (B) RT-PCR showing RNA products expressed by embryos of various genotypes. PCR primers were designed to differentiate between the endogenous mouse *Cited2* transcript and the *Cited2 MRG1* transcript by their size difference. Wild type mouse *Cited2*, containing the SRJ domain produces the larger 725 bp band. (C) Southern blots of *Cited2 T166N* allele. Top, Southern blot of *EcoRI* digested genomic DNA probed with a 5′-probe. Middle, Southern blot of *BglII* digested genomic DNA, probed with a 3′-probe. Probe positions are indicated in Fig. 3. Bottom, Southern blot of *SpeI* digested genomic DNA hybridized with an internal (Neomycin) probe, to confirm single copy integration. (D) Southern blots of *Cited2 MRG1* and *Cited2 HUM* alleles. Top, Southern blot of *EcoRI/SacII* digested genomic DNA, probed with a 5′-probe. Middle, Southern blot of *BglII* digested genomic DNA, probed with a 3′-probe. The position of the probes is indicated in Fig. 3. Bottom, Southern blot of *EcoRI* digested genomic DNA hybridized with an internal (Puromycin) probe to confirm single copy integration.

GACGGAAG and 5′ AGATATCACGTAGGATCTGCT) followed by sequencing of the PCR products.

ES cells from correctly exchanged colonies were injected into albino C57BL/6J blastocysts. The resulting chimeras were mated with albino C57BL/6J females. Successful germline transmission yielded black pups and was confirmed by long range PCR and Southern blotting for correct targeting and exchange at both 5′ and 3′ ends. F1 pups were also screened by Southern blotting to ensure that no ectopic integration of the exchange cassette had

occurred (Fig. 8D). Southern blotting was performed using standard protocols. Mouse colonies were maintained by backcrossing to C57BL/6J mice.

Cell Culture

Mouse ES cells were cultured in Knockout DMEM (Dulbecco's Modified Eagle Medium, Invitrogen) supplemented with 2 mM L-Glutamine (PAA), 1× non-essential amino acids (PAA), 0.1 mM β-mercaptoethanol (Sigma), 1000 U/ml ESGRO (Millipore) and

10% fetal bovine serum (Invitrogen). Hep3B cells (ATCC No. HB-8064) were grown in Minimum Essential Medium (MEM) supplemented with 2 mM L-glutamine, 1% penicillin-streptomycin, and 10% FBS. All cells were cultured at 37°C in a humidified atmosphere containing 5% CO_2.

Generation and analysis of embryos

Cited2 $^{+/T166N}$, *Cited2* $^{+/MRG1}$ and *Cited2* $^{+/HUM}$ were crossed to mice heterozygous for the *Cited2* ^{tm1Bha} null allele (*Cited2* $^{+/-}$). Embryos were dissected at 15.5 dpc and harvested and processed for Magnetic Resonance Imaging (MRI) as previously described [11]. MRI was performed on a horizontal 9.4 T/21 cm VNMRS Direct Drive™ MR system (Varian Inc., Palo Alto, CA, USA) as described previously [60]. Genotype deviation from expected Mendelian ratios was analysed using the X^2 test. The calculated probability of a type 1 error was calculated using the CHIDIST function in Excel (Microsoft Office 2007, Microsoft, Redmond, WA, USA).

Western Blotting

Mouse embryonic fibroblasts (MEFs) isolated using standard protocols from decapitated and eviscerated 13.5 dpc embryos were lysed in lysis buffer (50 mM Tris, 150 mM NaCl, 0.5% Tx100) containing protease inhibitors (cOmplete, EDTA-free Protease Inhibitor Cocktail, Roche) at 4°C for 20 minutes, followed by centrifugation and removal of the non-soluble pellet. Protein concentrations were quantified using the Bicinchoninic acid (BCA) protein assay kit (Pierce). 60 ug of whole cell lysate were loaded into each well of a NuPage NOVEX 4–12% Bis-Tris gel (Invitrogen) and blotted onto a nitrocellulose membrane using standard protocols. Western blots using Hep3B cells were processed in a similar manner. Mouse monoclonal antibody against CITED2 (JA22) was used at 1:500 (Abcam).

RT-PCR

Total RNA was isolated from the caudal half of 13.5 dpc embryos using the RNeasy Tissue Kit (Qiagen) and first strand cDNA was synthesized using Quantitect Reverse Transcription Kit (Qiagen) as per manufacturer's instructions using 1 ug of total RNA. 1/20th of the reverse transcription product was used per PCR reaction. PCR products were gel purified and sequenced to confirm identity. The following PCR primers were used: forward primer 5′ CAGAAATCGCAAAGACGGAAG and reverse primer 5′ CTCGTCGATGAAATCAGTGTC.

Supporting Information

Figure S1   Disorder plot of mouse wild type CITED2 and variants. RONN (http://www.strubi.ox.ac.uk/RONN) was used to predict protein disorder. The highest peak, representing the highest probability of disorder, resides over residues corresponding to the SRJ (161–199) (red box). The CR2 domain (green box) has the lowest probability of disorder, consistent with it harboring all known biological functions of CITED2. CR1 (blue box) and CR3 (purple box) are also marked in the graph for the wild type protein. The location of the molecular lesions in each variant is indicated with a black arrow. The location of the SRJ and flanking residues which have been removed in the MRG1 isoform is marked with the red arrow.

Figure S2   CITED2 T166N mutation does not impair CITED2's ability to repress HIF1 transactivation. (A) Hep3B cells were transiently cotransfected with GAL4-HIF1A

(40 ng), 3xGAL4-luciferase reporter (100 ng), CMV-lacZ (100 ng), and increasing amounts (4 and 40 ng) of CITED2 or mutant plasmids. GAL4-HIF1A transactivation was stimulated by adding desferrioxamine (DFO, 100 μM) as indicated. Results are presented as in (Fig. 2). (B) Western blots were performed using whole cell extracts prepared from Hep3B cells transfected with the indicated CITED2 plasmids. CITED2 was detected using a monoclonal anti-CITED2 antibody (top panels). Loading was monitored by probing the membrane with a monoclonal anti-β-tubulin antibody (bottom panels). (C, D) *Top panels:* Autoradiograms of gels showing the binding of 35S-labelled CITED2 and CITED2-p.T166N to GST (lanes 3, 4, 9, 10), GST-TFAP2A (lanes 5 and 6) and GST-p300CH1 (lanes 11–12). *Bottom panels:* Coomassie blue stain of the gels showing relative amounts of GST, GST-TFAP2A and GST-EP300CH1 proteins. (E) Hep3B cells were transfected with CITED2 plasmids expressing the indicated CITED2 proteins. These were detected forty-eight hours after transfection by indirect immunofluorescence, using a monoclonal anti-CITED2 antibody and a secondary rabbit anti-mouse antibody coupled to FITC (green). Nuclei were counterstained with DAPI (blue). The merged image is shown in the panels on the extreme right.

Figure S3   Co-expression of MAPK1 or MAPKK1 did not affect the expression of CITED2. Western blot were performed using whole cell extracts prepared from Hep3B cells co-transfected with the plasmid expressing CITED2, a plasmid expressing MAPK1 and with plasmids expressing a kinase inactive MAPKK1 (SV40-MAPKK1-S221A) or a constitutively active MAPKK1 (SV40-MAPKK1-S217ES221).

Figure S4   Adrenal gland size measurements. The volume of adrenal glands of 15.5 dpc embryos were measured by segmentation analysis using Amira 5.3 (Visage, Berlin). All measurements were corrected for embryo weight. Values represent measurements obtained from 6 embryos from each genotype. Error bars represent SEM.

Figure S5   E15.5 *Cited2* $^{-/MRG1}$ **embryo with ectopia cordis.** Single embryo out of 75 of the same genotype to present with any structural developmental anomaly. (A) External side view, (B) frontal view and (C) MRI image of sagittal section through embryo showing the ectopic heart (arrowhead) rostral to the umbilical hernia (arrow); the left forelimb has been removed. (D) Sagittal section through left adrenal gland (Ad). (E) Transverse section through the heart showing the heart outside the chest cavity and (F) 3D reconstruction of the heart and major vessels showing normal topology of the right and left ventricles (RV, LV) and a small ventricular septal defect (VSD). RA, Right Atria; LA, Left Atria; IVS, intraventricular septum; Tr, Trachea; AoA, Aortic Arch; DAo, Dorsal Aorta. Scale bars: 0.5 mm.

Text S1

Table S1   Diagnostic characteristics for all 1126 cases sequenced. Many patients have multiple diagnoses and for these the patient is recorded in the diagnostic category for the lesion most likely to need clinical intervention. Abbreviations: Transposition of the great arteries (TGA; cc – congenitally corrected), secundum atrial septal defect (ASD), Tetralogy of Fallot (TOF), atrioventricular septal defect (AVSD), ventricular septal defect (VSD), pulmonary atresia with intact ventricular septum (PA/IVS), pulmonary atresia with ventricular septal defect (PA-VSD), coarctation of aorta (CoA), aortic stenosis (AS), hypoplastic left heart syndrome (HLHS), mitral valve abnormalities (MV abn), patent ductus arteriosus (PDA), double outlet right ventricle (DORV), pulmonary stenosis (PS), common arterial trunk (CAT), aorto-pulmonary (AP) window, tricuspid atresia (TA), double inlet left ventricle (DILV), discordant ventriculo-arterial connections (discordant VA) and partial and total anomalous venous drainage (PAPVD and TAPVD respectively).

Acknowledgments

We would like to thank Carol Broadbent, Michal Bilski, Daniel Andrew, David Campbell, Akshay Ahuja, Michelle Hammett, Daniel Biggs and Christopher Dean Preece for expert technical assistance, Kamel El Omari for advice on protein structure and the use of the RONN program, and Shankar Srinivas for critical reading of the manuscript. We would also like to thank Arjamand Shauq, Edmond Ladusans, Michael Gatzoulis, Sonya V. Babu-Narayan, Satish Adwani, John Deanfield, Philip Roberts, Sachin Khambadkone, Willem Ouwehand, Alison Coffey and Edward Blair for patient samples, Austin Smith for T14/T cells, Ralf Janknecht and Chris Marshall for plasmids.

Author Contributions

Conceived and designed the experiments: CMC J. Bentham J. Braganca AC SDB HW BK BD SB. Performed the experiments: CMC J. Bentham CC J. Braganca AC SDB. Analyzed the data: CMC J. Bentham CC J. Braganca AC. Contributed reagents/materials/analysis tools: JES BD. Wrote the paper: CMC BD SB.

References

1. Hoffman JIE (2002) Incidence, mortality and natural history. In: Anderson RH, Baker EJ, Macartney FJ, Rigby ML, Shinebourne EA et al., editors. Paediatric Cardiology. London: Churchill Livingstone. pp. 111–139.

2. Burn J, Goodship J (2002) Congenital heart disease. In: Rimoin DL, Connor JM, Pyeritz RE, Korf BR, editors. Principles and Practice of Medical Genetics. London: Churchill Livingstone.

3. Ferencz C, Boughman JA, Neill CA, Brenner JI, Perry LW (1989) Congenital cardiovascular malformations: questions on inheritance. Baltimore-Washington Infant Study Group. J Am Coll Cardiol 14: 756–763.

4. Ferencz C, Boughman JA (1993) Congenital heart disease in adolescents and adults. Teratology, genetics, and recurrence risks. Cardiol Clin 11: 557–567.

5. Bentham J, Bhattacharya S (2008) Genetic mechanisms controlling cardiovascular development. Ann N Y Acad Sci 1123: 10–19.

6. Shioda T, Fenner MH, Isselbacher KJ (1996) msg1, a novel melanocyte-specific gene, encodes a nuclear protein and is associated with pigmentation. Proceedings of the National Academy of Sciences 93: 12298–12303.

7. Shioda T, Fenner MH, Isselbacher KJ (1997) MSG1 and its related protein MRG1 share a transcription activating domain. Gene 204: 235–241.

8. Dunwoodie SL, Rodriguez TA, Beddington RSP (1998) Msg1 and Mrg1, founding members of a gene family, show distinct patterns of gene expression during mouse embryogenesis. Mech Dev 72: 27–40.

9. Sun HB, Zhu YX, Yin T, Sledge G, Yang YC (1998) MRG1, the product of a melanocyte-specific gene related gene, is a cytokine-inducible transcription factor with transformation activity. Proc Natl Acad Sci U S A 95: 13555–13560.

10. Bhattacharya S, Michels CL, Leung MK, Arany ZP, Kung AL, et al. (1999) Functional role of p35srj, a novel p300/CBP binding protein, during transactivation by HIF 1. Genes Dev 13: 64–75.

11. Bamforth SD, Braganca J, Eloranta JJ, Murdoch JN, Marques FI, et al. (2001) Cardiac malformations, adrenal agenesis, neural crest defects and exencephaly in mice lacking Cited2, a new Tfap2 co-activator. Nat Genet 29: 469–474.

12. Braganca J, Swingler T, Marques FI, Jones T, Eloranta JJ, et al. (2002) Human CREB-binding Protein/p300-interacting Transactivator with ED-rich Tail (CITED) 4, a New Member of the CITED Family, Functions as a Co-activator for Transcription Factor AP-2. J Biol Chem 277: 8559–8565.

13. Kranc KR, Bamforth SD, Braganca J, Norbury C, Van Lohuizen M, et al. (2003) Transcriptional Coactivator Cited2 Induces Bmi1 and Mel18 and Controls Fibroblast Proliferation via Ink4a/ARF. Mol Cell Biol 23: 7658–7666.

14. Braganca J, Eloranta JJ, Bamforth SD, Ibbitt JC, Hurst HC, et al. (2003) Physical and Functional Interactions among AP-2 Transcription Factors, p300/CREB-binding Protein, and CITED2. J Biol Chem 278: 16021–16029.

15. Bamforth SD, Braganca J, Farthing CR, Schneider JE, Broadbent C, et al. (2004) Cited2 controls left-right patterning and heart development through a Nodal-Pitx2c pathway. Nat Genet 36: 1189–1196.

16. Sperling S, Grimm CH, Dunkel I, Mebus S, Sperling HP, et al. (2005) Identification and functional analysis of CITED2 mutations in patients with congenital heart defects. Hum Mutat 26: 575–582.

17. Yang XF, Wu XY, Li M, Li YG, Dai JT, et al. (2010) [Mutation analysis of Cited2 in patients with congenital heart disease]. Zhonghua Er Ke Za Zhi 48: 293–296.

18. Barbera JP, Rodriguez TA, Greene ND, Weninger WJ, Simeone A, et al. (2002) Folic acid prevents exencephaly in Cited2 deficient mice. Hum Mol Genet 11: 283–293.

19. Yin Z, Haynie J, Yang X, Han B, Kiatchoosakun S, et al. (2002) The essential role of Cited2, a negative regulator for HIF-1{alpha}, in heart development and neurulation. Proc Natl Acad Sci U S A 99: 10488–10493.

20. Weninger WJ, Lopes Floro K, Bennett MB, Withington SL, Preis JI, et al. (2005) Cited2 is required both for heart morphogenesis and establishment of the left-right axis in mouse development. Development 132: 1337–1348.

21. Withington SL, Scott AN, Saunders DN, Lopes Floro K, Preis JI, et al. (2006) Loss of Cited2 affects trophoblast formation and vascularization of the mouse placenta. Dev Biol 294: 67–82.

22. Lopes Floro K, Artap ST, Preis JI, Fatkin D, Chapman G, et al. (2011) Loss of Cited2 causes congenital heart disease by perturbing left-right patterning of the body axis. Hum Mol Genet 20: 1097–1110.

23. Yang ZR, Thomson R, McNeil P, Esnouf RM (2005) RONN: the bio-basis function neural network technique applied to the detection of natively disordered regions in proteins. Bioinformatics 21: 3369–3376.

24. Dunker AK, Brown CJ, Lawson JD, Iakoucheva LM, Obradovic Z (2002) Intrinsic disorder and protein function. Biochemistry 41: 6573–6582.

25. Blom N, Gammeltoft S, Brunak S (1999) Sequence and structure-based prediction of eukaryotic protein phosphorylation sites. J Mol Biol 294: 1351–1362.

26. Roux PP, Blenis J (2004) ERK and p38 MAPK-activated protein kinases: a family of protein kinases with diverse biological functions. Microbiol Mol Biol Rev 68: 320–344.

27. Freedman SJ, Sun ZY, Kung AL, France DS, Wagner G, et al. (2003) Structural basis for negative regulation of hypoxia-inducible factor-1alpha by CITED2. Nat Struct Biol 10: 504–512.

28. De Guzman RN, Martinez-Yamout MA, Dyson HJ, Wright PE (2004) Interaction of the TAZ1 domain of the CREB-binding protein with the activation domain of CITED2: regulation by competition between intrinsically unstructured ligands for non-identical binding sites. J Biol Chem 279: 3042–3049.

29. Cheung PC, Campbell DG, Nebreda AR, Cohen P (2003) Feedback control of the protein kinase TAK1 by SAPK2a/p38alpha. Embo J 22: 5793–5805.

30. Mody N, Campbell DG, Morrice N, Peggie M, Cohen P (2003) An analysis of the phosphorylation and activation of extracellular-signal-regulated protein kinase 5 (ERK5) by mitogen-activated protein kinase kinase 5 (MKK5) in vitro. Biochem J 372: 567–575.

31. Kuma Y, Campbell DG, Cuenda A (2004) Identification of glycogen synthase as a new substrate for stress-activated protein kinase 2b/p38beta. Biochem J 379: 133–139.

32. Feijoo C, Campbell DG, Jakes R, Goedert M, Cuenda A (2005) Evidence that phosphorylation of the microtubule-associated protein Tau by SAPK4/p38delta at Thr50 promotes microtubule assembly. J Cell Sci 118: 397–408.

33. Fitzky BU, Moebius FF, Asaoka H, Waage-Baudet H, Xu L, et al. (2001) 7-Dehydrocholesterol-dependent proteolysis of HMG-CoA reductase suppresses sterol biosynthesis in a mouse model of Smith-Lemli-Opitz/RSH syndrome. J Clin Invest 108: 905–915.

34. Ying QL, Nichols J, Chambers I, Smith A (2003) BMP induction of Id proteins suppresses differentiation and sustains embryonic stem cell self-renewal in collaboration with STAT3. Cell 115: 281–292.

35. Pritsker M, Ford NR, Jenq HT, Lemischka IR (2006) Genomewide gain-of-function genetic screen identifies functionally active genes in mouse embryonic stem cells. Proc Natl Acad Sci U S A 103: 6946–6951.

36. Chambers I, Colby D, Robertson M, Nichols J, Lee S, et al. (2003) Functional expression cloning of Nanog, a pluripotency sustaining factor in embryonic stem cells. Cell 113: 643–655.

37. Mitsui K, Tokuzawa Y, Itoh H, Segawa K, Murakami M, et al. (2003) The homeoprotein Nanog is required for maintenance of pluripotency in mouse epiblast and ES cells. Cell 113: 631–642.

38. Hitz C, Wurst W, Kuhn R (2007) Conditional brain-specific knockdown of MAPK using Cre/loxP regulated RNA interference. Nucleic Acids Res 35: e90.

39. Chen CM, Krohn J, Bhattacharya S, Davies B (2011) A comparison of exogenous promoter activity at the ROSA26 locus using a PhiC31 integrase mediated cassette exchange approach in mouse ES cells. PLoS ONE 6: e23376.

40. Anderson RH, Webb S, Brown NA, Lamers W, Moorman A (2003) Development of the heart: (3) formation of the ventricular outflow tracts, arterial valves, and intrapericardial arterial trunks. Heart 89: 1110–1118.

41. Qayyum SR, Webb S, Anderson RH, Verbeek FJ, Brown NA, et al. (2001) Septation and valvar formation in the outflow tract of the embryonic chick heart. Anat Rec 264: 273–283.

42. Runciman SI, Gannon BJ, Baudinette RV (1995) Central cardiovascular shunts in the perinatal marsupial. Anat Rec 243: 71–83.

43. Karel F. Liem WB, Warren Walker, Lance Grande (2001) Functional Anatomy of the Vertebrates: An Evolutionary Perspective. Fort Worth: Harcourt College Publishers.

44. Weninger WJ, Floro KL, Bennett MB, Withington SL, Preis JI, et al. (2005) Cited2 is required both for heart morphogenesis and establishment of the left-right axis in mouse development. Development 132: 1337–1348.

45. Chen Y, Doughman YQ, Gu S, Jarrell A, Aota S, et al. (2008) Cited2 is required for the proper formation of the hyaloid vasculature and for lens morphogenesis. Development 135: 2939–2948.

46. Chen Y, Haviernik P, Bunting KD, Yang YC (2007) Cited2 is required for normal hematopoiesis in the murine fetal liver. Blood 110: 2889–2898.

47. Kranc KR, Schepers H, Rodrigues NP, Bamforth S, Villadsen E, et al. (2009) Cited2 is an essential regulator of adult hematopoietic stem cells. Cell Stem Cell 5: 659–665.

48. Bentham J, Michell AC, Lockstone H, Andrew D, Schneider JE, et al. (2010) Maternal high-fat diet interacts with embryonic Cited2 genotype to reduce Pitx2c expression and enhance penetrance of left-right patterning defects. Hum Mol Genet 19: 3394–3401.

49. Michell AC, Braganca J, Broadbent C, Joyce B, Franklyn A, et al. (2010) A novel role for transcription factor Lmo4 in thymus development through genetic interaction with Cited2. Dev Dyn 239: 1988–1994.

50. Ruiz-Perez VL, Blair HJ, Rodriguez-Andres ME, Blanco MJ, Wilson A, et al. (2007) Evc is a positive mediator of Ihh-regulated bone growth that localises at the base of chondrocyte cilia. Development 134: 2903–2912.

51. Wassif CA, Zhu P, Kratz L, Krakowiak PA, Battaile KP, et al. (2001) Biochemical, phenotypic and neurophysiological characterization of a genetic mouse model of RSH/Smith–Lemli–Opitz syndrome. Hum Mol Genet 10: 555–564.

52. Janknecht R, Nordheim A (1996) Regulation of the c-fos promoter by the ternary complex factor Sap-1a and its coactivator CBP. Oncogene 12: 1961–1969.

53. Cowley S, Paterson H, Kemp P, Marshall CJ (1994) Activation of MAP kinase kinase is necessary and sufficient for PC12 differentiation and for transformation of NIH 3T3 cells. Cell 77: 841–852.

54. Cuenda A, Cohen P, Buee-Scherrer V, Goedert M (1997) Activation of stress-activated protein kinase-3 (SAPK3) by cytokines and cellular stresses is mediated via SAPKK3 (MKK6); comparison of the specificities of SAPK3 and SAPK2 (RK/p38). EMBO J 16: 295–305.

55. Campbell DG, Morrice NA (2002) Identification of protein phosphorylation sites by a combination of mass spectrometry and solid phase Edman sequencing. J Biomol Tech 13: 119–130.

56. Nichols J, Evans EP, Smith AG (1990) Establishment of germ-line-competent embryonic stem (ES) cells using differentiation inhibiting activity. Development 110: 1341–1348.

57. Farley FW, Soriano P, Steffen LS, Dymecki SM (2000) Widespread recombinase expression using FLPeR (Flipper) mice. genesis 28: 106–110.

58. Pettitt SJ, Liang Q, Rairdan XY, Moran JL, Prosser HM, et al. (2009) Agouti C57BL/6N embryonic stem cells for mouse genetic resources. Nat Meth 6: 493–495.

59. Raymond CS, Soriano P (2007) High-Efficiency FLP and ΦC31 Site-Specific Recombination in Mammalian Cells. PLoS ONE 2: e162.

60. Schneider JE, Bamforth SD, Farthing CR, Clarke K, Neubauer S, et al. (2003) Rapid identification and 3D reconstruction of complex cardiac malformations in transgenic mouse embryos using fast gradient echo sequence magnetic resonance imaging. J Mol Cell Cardiol 35: 217–222.

17

Mice Carrying a Hypomorphic Evi1 Allele are Embryonic Viable but Exhibit Severe Congenital Heart Defects

Emilie A. Bard-Chapeau[1], Dorota Szumska[2], Bindya Jacob[3], Belinda Q. L. Chua[1], Gouri C. Chatterjee[4], Yi Zhang[5], Jerrold M. Ward[1], Fatma Urun[6], Emi Kinameri[6], Stéphane D. Vincent[7], Sayadi Ahmed[1], Shoumo Bhattacharya[2], Motomi Osato[3], Archibald S. Perkins[5], Adrian W. Moore[6], Nancy A. Jenkins[1¤], Neal G. Copeland[1*¤]

1 Institute of Molecular and Cell Biology, Singapore, Singapore, 2 Welcome Trust Centre for Human Genetics, Oxford, United Kingdom, 3 Cancer Science Institute, Singapore, Singapore, 4 MYSM School of Medicine, Yale University School of Medicine, New Haven, Connecticut, United States of America, 5 Department of Pathology and Laboratory Medicine, University of Rochester Medical Center, Rochester, New York, United States of America, 6 RIKEN Brain Science Institute, 2-1 Hirosawa, Wako-shi, Saitama, Japan, 7 Department of Development and Stem Cells, Institut de Génétique et de Biologie Moléculaire et Cellulaire, CNRS UMR 7104, Inserm U964, Université de Strasbourg, Illkirch, France

Abstract

The ecotropic viral integration site 1 (Evi1) oncogenic transcription factor is one of a number of alternative transcripts encoded by the Mds1 and Evi1 complex locus (Mecom). Overexpression of Evi1 has been observed in a number of myeloid disorders and is associated with poor patient survival. It is also amplified and/or overexpressed in many epithelial cancers including nasopharyngeal carcinoma, ovarian carcinoma, ependymomas, and lung and colorectal cancers. Two murine knockout models have also demonstrated Evi1's critical role in the maintenance of hematopoietic stem cell renewal with its absence resulting in the death of mutant embryos due to hematopoietic failure. Here we characterize a novel mouse model (designated Evi1^{fl3}) in which Evi1 exon 3, which carries the ATG start, is flanked by loxP sites. Unexpectedly, we found that germline deletion of exon3 produces a hypomorphic allele due to the use of an alternative ATG start site located in exon 4, resulting in a minor Evi1 N-terminal truncation and a block in expression of the Mds1-Evi1 fusion transcript. Evi1$^{\delta ex3/\delta ex3}$ mutant embryos showed only a mild non-lethal hematopoietic phenotype and bone marrow failure was only observed in adult Vav-iCre/+, Evi1$^{fl3/fl3}$ mice in which exon 3 was specifically deleted in the hematopoietic system. Evi1$^{\delta ex3/\delta ex3}$ knockout pups are born in normal numbers but die during the perinatal period from congenital heart defects. Database searches identified 143 genes with similar mutant heart phenotypes as those observed in Evi1$^{\delta ex3/\delta ex3}$ mutant pups. Interestingly, 42 of these congenital heart defect genes contain known Evi1-binding sites, and expression of 18 of these genes are also effected by Evi1 siRNA knockdown. These results show a potential functional involvement of Evi1 target genes in heart development and indicate that Evi1 is part of a transcriptional program that regulates cardiac development in addition to the development of blood.

Editor: Hiromi Yanagisawa, UT-Southwestern Med Ctr, United States of America

Funding: This work was supported by the Biomedical Research Council (BMRC), Agency for Science, Technology and Research (A*STAR), Singapore; a Japan Society for Promotion of Sciences (JSPS) Grants-in-Aid Young Scientists (B), and a RIKEN Brain Science Institute (BSI) core grant to A.W.M.; and the Cancer Prevention Research Institute of Texas (CPRIT) (N.G.C. and N.A.J.). N.G.C. and N.A.J. are both CPRIT Scholars in Cancer Research. The funders had no role in study design, data collection and analysis, decision to publish, or preparation of the manuscript.

Competing Interests: The authors have declared that no competing interests exist.

* E-mail: ncopeland@tmhs.org

¤ Current address: Methodist Hospital Research Institute, Houston, Texas, United States of America

Introduction

The complexity of an organism is defined not only by the number of its genes, but also how expression of these genes is controlled. This also includes several post-transcriptional events that control protein production, including alternative splicing, translational repression, microRNA-induced mRNA degradation, and the regulated generation of distinct gene products through the alternative use of translational initiation sites. These various mechanisms provide a tremendous diversity of protein sequence, structure and function [1,2]. Much improvement has been made in defining the molecular basis of these regulations. However, it remains a major challenge to integrate this knowledge into a complete understanding of the resulting physiological functions, in normal and pathological conditions.

The MDS1 and EVI1 complex locus (MECOM) contains several transcription start sites and alternative splice options. It produces multiple transcripts coding for nuclear transcription factors. One of its major gene products is ecotropic viral integration site 1 (EVI1), an oncogenic zinc finger transcription factor (TF) whose overexpression in myeloid disorders such as acute and chronic myeloid leukemia (AML and CML), and myelodysplastic syndrome (MDS) has been extensively studied and correlated with poor patient survival [3–5]. Amplification and/or overexpression of EVI1 have also been observed in multiple epithelial cancers, including nasopharyngeal carcinoma, ovarian

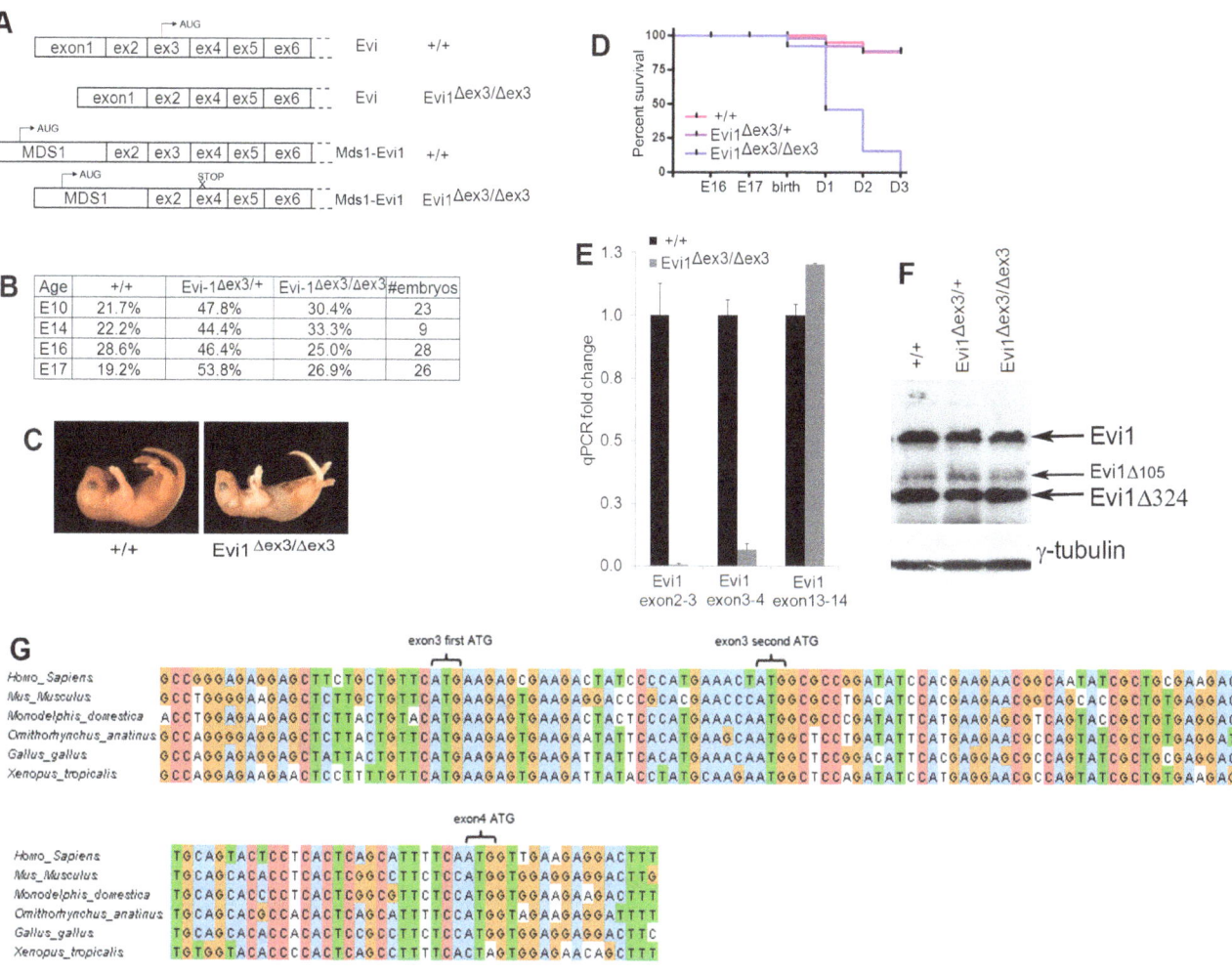

Figure 1. Deletion of Evi1 exon3 generates a hypomorphic allele. (A) Sequenced products obtained after 5'RACE from wild type or Evi1[δex3/][δex3] mutant embryos. (B) Table showing the fraction of embryos of each genotype detected at different stages of embryonic development. The Mendelian ratios were not affected by the Evi1 exon3 deletion. (C) Pictures of 28 hr-old littermates highlight the poor health of dying Evi1[δex3/δex3] pups. (D) Kaplan-Meyer curves for wild type, Evi1[δex3/+] and Evi1[δex3/δex3] progeny indicate lethality of all Evi1[δex3/δex3] pups by three days after birth (n = 5 to 16 per genotype). Log rank test, Chi square p value <0.0001. (E) RT-qPCR from cDNA of E14.5 embryos. The primers used amplified the regions between Evi1 exons 2 and 3, 3 and 4 or 13 and 14. Mean of three different samples per condition. The standard deviation is shown. (F) Expression of Evi1 and γ-tubulin protein products in E14.5 wild type or E17.5 Evi1[δex3/+] and Evi1[δex3/δex3] mutant embryos (100 μg protein/lane). (G) Nucleotide sequence of Evi1 cDNA in the exon 3 and 4 genomic region. Two ATG sites are present in exon 3 and one in exon 4. All ATGs are conserved in higher vertebrates.

carcinoma, ependymomas, and lung and colorectal cancers [6–11]. In addition, EVI1 controls several aspects of embryonic development including hematopoiesis where it has been shown to be important for hematopoietic stem cell (HSC) renewal [12] and angiogenesis [13]. The most oncogenic human MECOM isoform, EVI1, encodes a 1051 amino acid protein containing two zinc finger domains, a central transcriptional repression domain and an acidic C-terminal region [5,14,15]. The seven zinc finger domains located in the N-terminus are known to bind to a GATA-like consensus motif [13,16–19], while the three zinc finger domains in the C-terminus bind to an ETS-like motif [16,20]. Additional alternative splicing of MECOM in human and mouse produces, amongst others, two major isoforms, EVI1δ324 and MDS1-EVI1 [5,14,15,21]. MDS1-EVI1 is a larger MECOM variant. Although MDS1 was originally described as a distinct gene, it is now recognized to be an alternative transcription start site and part of the MECOM locus. MDS1-EVI1 contains a 188 amino acid extension at its N-terminus, adding the so-called PR domain,

which is a derivative of the SET domain [5,14,15,22]. Several lines of evidence suggest that the form of EVI1 lacking the PR domain and MDS1-EVI1 display opposite functions. The shorter isoform (EVI1) acts as an aggressive oncogene while expression of the longer isoform (MDS1-EVI1) is linked to good prognosis in cancer [23–25]. MDS1-EVI1 was also recently described as a regulator of long term HSC repopulating activity [21]. Another important MECOM isoform, called EVI1δ324, resembles EVI1 but lacks zinc fingers motifs 6 and 7, which prevents its binding to GATA-like sites. Additional alternative splicing lead to the deletion of 9aa in the repressor domain of EVI1, MDS1-EVI1, or EVI1δ324 [14,26–28], thus producing additional isoforms.

The exact physiological roles of these various MECOM products remain to be characterized. Two mouse knockout models have been previously reported that target MECOM. The first one was produced by deletion of Evi1 exon 7 [13,29] while the second represents a conditional deletion of exon 4 [12]. For both alleles, homozygous Evi1[-/-] mice resulted in the deletion of both Evi1 and

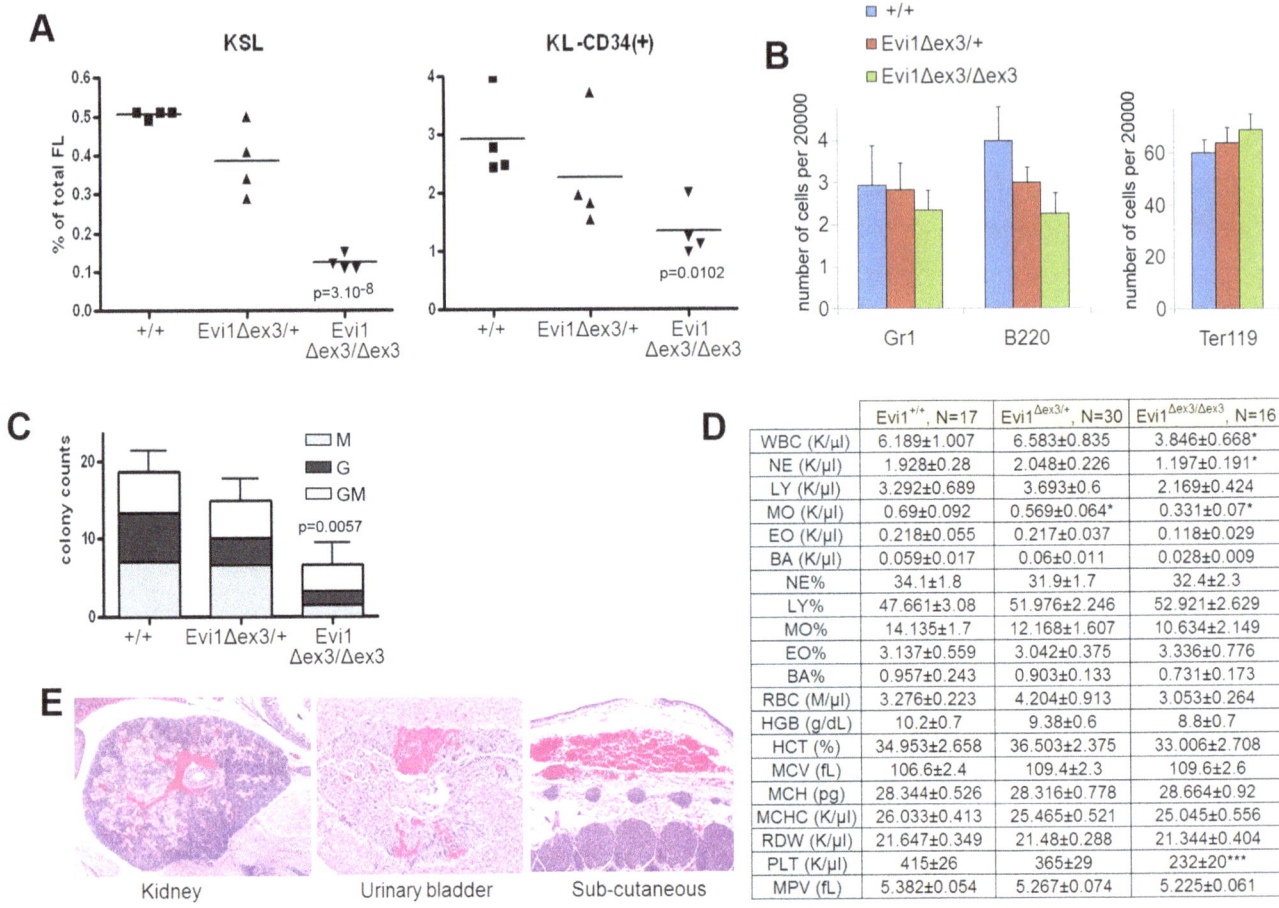

Figure 2. Disruption of hematopoiesis in Evi1$^{\delta ex3/\delta ex3}$ newborn mice. (A,B) Flow cytometric profiles of wild type, Evi1$^{\delta ex3/+}$ and Evi1$^{\delta ex3/\delta ex3}$ littermate fetal livers at E14.5. (A) HSC and progenitor cell subpopulations were detected by a combination of markers (KSL: c-Kit$^+$, S: Sca-1$^+$, L: lineage$^-$, or KL-CD34$^+$). We found a significant reduction of cells in the Evi1-deleted samples; p values are from an unpaired t-test between +/+ and Evi1$^{\delta ex3/\delta ex3}$ fetal livers. (B) Bar graph shows the number of granulocytes (Gr1), B-lymphocytes (B220) and erythroid cells (Tert119) in fetal livers of various different genotypes. (C) Colony forming counts from cells of 3 fetal livers of each genotype at E14.5 We observed a significant reduction in colony formation between +/+ and Evi1$^{\delta ex3/\delta ex3}$ fetal livers, p = 0.0057 (unpaired t-test). No BFU-E or CFU-Mix colonies were identified. (D) Hemogram results for 4 hr- to 24 hr-old wild type (N = 17), Evi1$^{\delta ex3/+}$, (N = 30) and Evi1$^{\delta ex3/\delta ex3}$ (N = 16) littermate pups. Mean ± SEM is indicated. *p<0.05, **p<0.01, ***p<0.001, unpaired t-test. Leukocyte counts in peripheral blood and white blood cell differentials reveal a mild leucopenia in Evi1$^{\delta ex3/\delta ex3}$ newborn mice. Platelet (PLT) counts and mean platelet volume (MPV) results show a mild hypoproliferative thrombocytopenia in Evi1$^{\delta ex3/\delta ex3}$ pups. Normal erythrocyte counts, hemoglobin quantification and hematocrit assessment in the peripheral blood of Evi1$^{\delta ex3/\delta ex3}$ animals. Mean corpuscular volume (MCV), mean corpuscular hemoglobin (MCH), mean corpuscular hemoglobin concentration (MCHC) and red cell distribution widths (RDW) are shown. (E) Hematoxylin and eosin staining of 5 μm sections of 24 hr- to 48 hr-old Evi1$^{\delta ex3/\delta ex3}$ pups. Mild hemorrhages were seen in 31% of the mice (4 out of 13 pups).

Mds1-Evi1 transcripts. Both phenotypes showed embryonic lethality and impairment of hematopoiesis due to the loss of HSC renewal ability.

In this study, we analyzed a new conditional mutant allele of Mecom that was produced by flanking Evi1 exon 3, also Mds1-Evi1 exon 4, with loxP sites. The removal of Evi1 exon 3 is predicted to generate a frame shift mutation that would block the translation of Mds1-Evi1 protein. As Evi1 and Evi1δ324 both have translational initiation site located in exon3, it was also predicted that their protein expression would be blocked. However, Evi1 and Evi1δ324 proteins are produced in Evi1$^{\delta ex3/\delta ex3}$ tissues, likely due to an alternative translation start site located in exon 4. Thus, only the Mds1-Evi1 isoform is fully disrupted in Evi1$^{\delta ex3/\delta ex3}$ mice. Evi1$^{\delta ex3/\delta ex3}$ animals do not die in utero and display a different phenotype compared to exon 4 and 7 knockout mice. The analysis of this new hypomorphic exon 3 Evi1 allele has uncovered novel physiological functions for MECOM in the formation of the circulatory system and provided a better understanding of the function of the various MECOM transcripts.

Experimental Procedures

Animals

The Institute of Molecular and Cell Biology Animal Care and Use Committee approved all animal protocols used in this study. The Evi1 exon 3 floxed allele, $Evi1^{fl3}$ [21], was maintained in a pure C57BL/6 background. After crossing to a β-actin-Cre deleter strain to generate the $Evi1^{\delta ex3}$ null allele, $Evi1^{\delta ex3}$ bearing mice were a mixture of strains 129/Sv and C57BL/6. They were made congenic on a C57BL/6 background over the course of the study, with no observed change in the experimental results. Mice were genotyped by PCR using primers F1 (5'- GGAGTGT-TAAGCTTGAATTCC-3'), F2 (5'-GAAGAGCTCTTGCTG-TTCATG-3'), and R7 (5'- CAGCTTAGACCTCAGCTAAC-

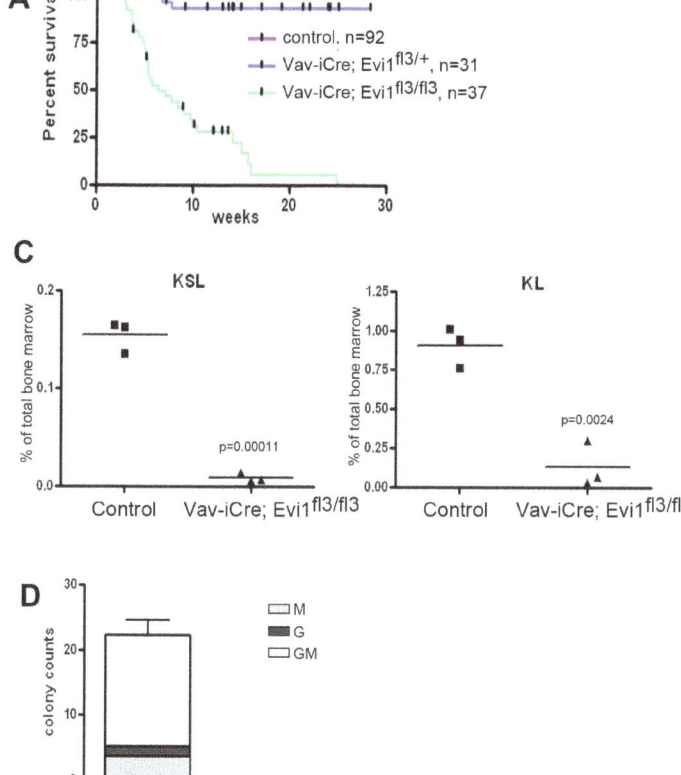

B	littermate control, N=5	Cre/+;Evi1 ^{fl3/fl3}, N=5
WBC (K/µl)	7.23±0.44	5±0.69*
NE (K/µl)	1.47±0.23	0.53±0.12**
LY (K/µl)	4.95±0.66	4.14±0.73
MO (K/µl)	0.342±0.033	0.202±0.036*
EO (K/µl)	0.362±0.171	0.106±0.007
BA (K/µl)	0.106±0.05	0.016±2.416
NE%	20.73±3.53	11.42±2.31*
LY%	67.9±6.5	81.2±4
MO%	4.79±0.46	4.76±2.22
EO%	5.06±2.28	2.35±0.59
BA%	1.49±0.66	0.27±0.11
RBC (M/µl)	8.77±0.49	1.54±0.33***
HGB (g/dL)	11.62±0.67	3.06±0.63***
HCT (%)	41.8±3.38	9.92±2.56***
MCV (fL)	47.4±1.6	63.6±5.2**
MCH (pg)	13.3±0.6	20.4±1.5**
MCHC (K/µl)	28.2±1.8	32.4±2.5
RDW (K/µl)	24.9±1.4	33±2.8
PLT (K/µl)	724±147.2	65.8±15.8**
MPV (fL)	4.8±0.33	6.38±0.37*

Figure 3. Profound depletion of hematopoietic cells in adult mice carrying an Evi1 exon3 deletion. (A) Kaplan-Meyer survival curves indicate significant lethality in Vav-iCre; Evi1 ^{fl3/fl3} mice, with a median survival of 7.7 weeks (Log rank test, Chi square p value <0.0001). (B) Hemograms for 6 to 9 week-old Vav-iCre; Evi1 ^{fl3/fl3} mice. These adult mice displayed leucopenia, severe anemia and thrombocytopenia. Mean ± SEM is indicated. *p<0.05, **p<0.01, ***p<0.001, unpaired t-test. (C) Flow cytometric profiles of bone marrow cells from Vav-iCre/+;Evi1 ^{fl3/fl3} and littermate control mice (Evi1 ^{fl3/+} or Evi1 ^{fl3/fl3}). HSC and progenitor cell subpopulations were detected by a combination of markers (KSL: c-Kit⁺, S: Sca-1⁺, L: lineage[−]). We found a significant reduction of cells in Evi1-deleted samples, p = 0.00011 and p = 0.0024, for KSL and KL, respectively (unpaired t-test). (D) Colony forming counts for cells from bone marrow of Vav-iCre;Evi1 ^{fl3/fl3} and littermate control mice (Evi1 ^{fl3/+} or Evi1 ^{fl3/fl3}). N=3 for each group, p = 0.0019 (unpaired t-test). No BFU-E and CFU-Mix colonies were identified.

3′). F2 and R7 were used to discriminate between the Evi1^{fl3} (375 bp) and wild type (269 bp) alleles. F1 and R7 were used to detect the Evi1^{δex3} allele (125 bp) (Fig. S1A,B in File S1). Vav-iCre was genotyped using Cre-F (5′-GCCTGCATTACCGGTC-GATGCAACGA-3′) and Cre-R (5′-GTGGCAGATGGCGCG-GCAACACCATT-3′) primers (700 bp amplicon). Blood was obtained by retro-orbital bleeding for adult mice, and by decapitation for embryos. Blood counts were performed with a Hemavet 950 device.

Quantitative real time RT-PCR (qRT-PCR)

RNA was isolated from mouse tissues using Trizol and an RNeasy Mini Kit (Qiagen), and 0.5–2 µg were used for cDNA synthesis (*SuperScript III* First-Strand Synthesis; Invitrogen) with oligodT. qPCR was performed with the ABI-Prism 7500 (Applied Biosystems), SYBR green Master Mix, and primers designed with Primer Express Software v2.0 (Applied Biosystems). A primer list is provided in File S1. We used the $2^{-\delta\delta Ct}$ method [30] to calculate the fold change of expression. Relative expression was normalized to *Tubg1* mRNA levels.

Protein extraction and immunoblotting

Snap frozen tissues were processed for protein extraction as previously described [31]. Immunoblotting was performed using a

protocol previously described [16]. Evi1 antibody was produced in rabbits [19] and γ-tubulin antibody was from Sigma.

HSC characterization

Hematopoietic cells were extracted from the fetal liver or bone marrow. Flow cytometric analyses and cell sorting were performed using a LSR II, a fluorescence activated cell sorter (FACS) Vantage, or a FACSAria as previously described [32]. Antibodies were purchased from BD Biosciences: PE-conjugated anti-Gr1 (RB6-8C5), Mac-1 (M1/70), Ter119 (TER-119), CD4 (RM4-5), CD3 (145-2C11), CD8 (53–6.7), B220 (RA3-6B2), IL7Ra (SB/199), PE-Cy7-conjugated anti-c-Kit (2B8), APC-conjugated anti-Sca-1 (E13-161.7) and FITC-conjugated CD34 (RAM34). Colony forming unit-culture (CFU-C) assays, using fetal liver cells or bone marrow cells, were performed as previously described [32]. Briefly, fetal liver or bone marrow cells were cultured in 35-mm dishes in triplicate in Methocult M3231 methylcellulose medium (StemCell Tec., Vancouver, BC, Canada) supplemented with 20 ng/mL recombinant mouse IL-3, 100 ng/mL mouse SCF, 200 ng/mL mouse G-CSF and 10 ng/mL mouse EPO. Colonies were counted on day 10.

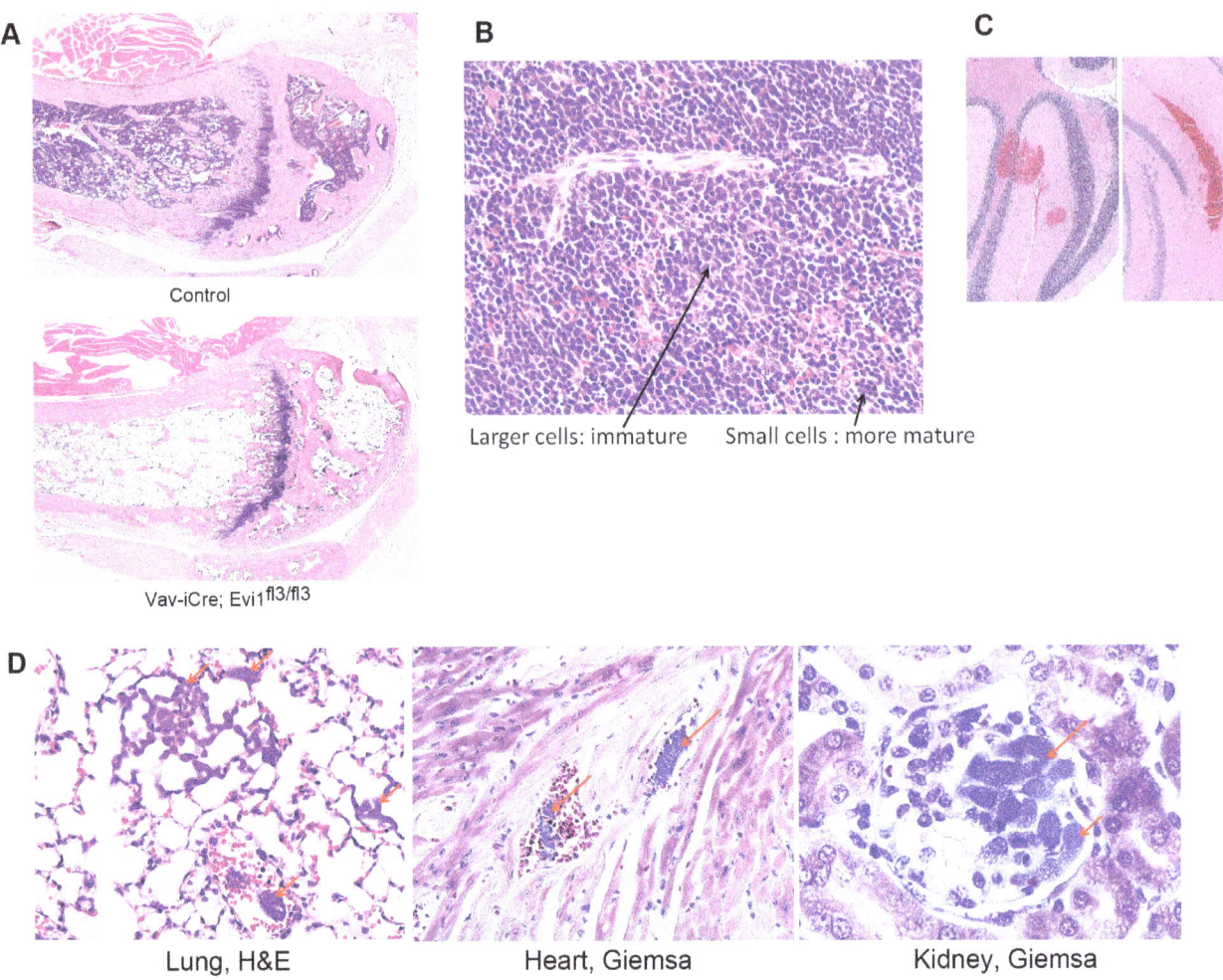

Figure 4. Spontaneous lethal bone marrow depletion in mice harboring an Evi1 exon3 deletion in the hematopoietic system. (A) Histology was performed on sick Vav-iCre; Evi1$^{fl3/fl3}$ and littermate control mice. Bone marrow depletion was observed in the mutant mice. Adipose tissue replaced the hematopoietic cells in the bone marrow. (B) Increased erythropoiesis in the spleen of Vav-iCre; Evi1$^{fl3/fl3}$ mice. No visible border was found between the red pulp and white pulp. Erythroid cells are shown by the arrows. Excess erythropoiesis in spleen likely happens to compensate for bone marrow loss. (C) H&E stained sections of the brain of a dying Vav-iCre; Evi1$^{fl3/fl3}$ mouse. Hemorrhages (red areas) were visible at several locations (also see Fig. S3E in File S1). (D) Histological sections of tissues from dying Vav-iCre; Evi1$^{fl3/fl3}$ animals showing bacteremia. Red arrows indicate the presence of bacteria in alveolar capillaries. Giemsa stains reveal the presence of cocci or small rods within glomerular capillaries. No sign of immune system defense (inflammatory cells) was observed despite the infection.

Histology

Mice received a complete necropsy after which their tissues were fixed in 10% neutral buffered formalin overnight and embedded in paraffin. Embryos were fixed and embedded whole before sectioning. Sections of 5 μm were stained with Hematoxylin and Eosin or Giemsa.

Magnetic Resonance Imaging and 3D reconstruction

Embryos were harvested at E15.5, euthanized and fixed in 4% paraformaldehyde (PFA) with 2 mM Gd-DTPA (gadolinium-diethylenetriaminepentacetate) as a contrast agent. Multi-embryo imaging was conducted as previously described [33]. The raw MR data were reconstructed as described previously [34]. The files were analyzed using Amira 5.3.3 software.

In situ hybridization in embryos

Evi1 mRNA in situ hybridization was carried out using a full length Evi1 cDNA probe [35] using standard protocols. Probes were labeled using a DIG RNA Labeling Kit (Roche Applied Science, Tokyo, Japan). Detection was via an anti-DIG antibody coupled to alkaline phosphatase (Roche, Tokyo, Japan) followed by staining with BCIP-NBT (Bromo-4-chloro-3-indolyl Phosphate/Nitro Blue Tetrazolium) (Nacalai, Tokyo, Japan) as previously described [36].

Results

Deletion of Evi1 exon 3 results in postnatal lethality

Mice homozygous for an Evi1 exon 3 deletion (designed Evi1$^{\delta ex3/\delta ex3}$) have recently been generated and used to access the function of Mecom in hematopoiesis ex vivo [18]. Deletion of exon3 is predicted to prematurely abrogate the expression of Mds1-Evi1 due to the presence of an out-of-frame stop codon in exon 4 (Fig. 1A). Exon 3 also encodes the ATG translation start site for Evi1 and Evi1δ324 (Fig. 1A). Evi1$^{\delta ex3}$ is thus predicted to be a Mecom null allele (Fig. S1A in File S1). We therefore expected that similar to other Evi1 knockout mice [12,13,29], deletion of

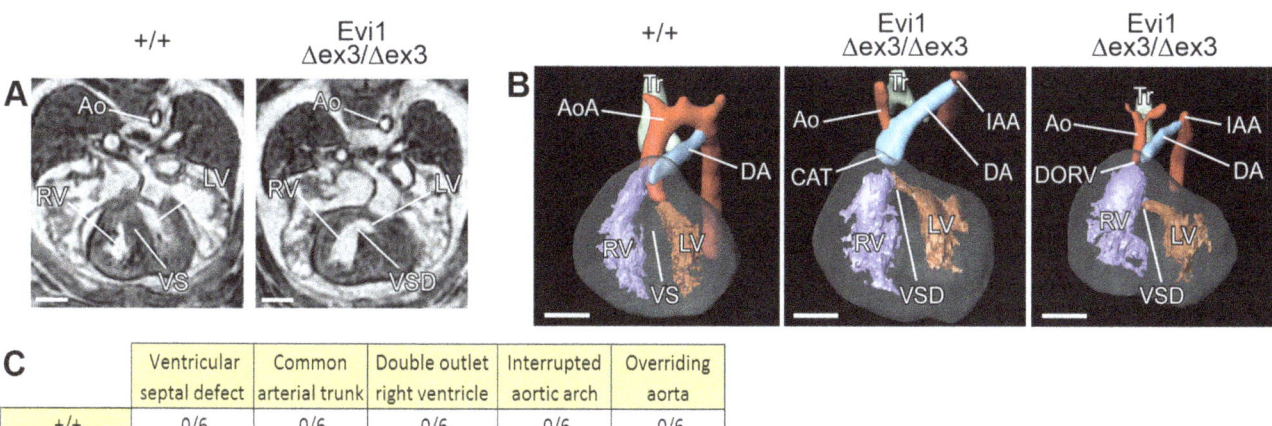

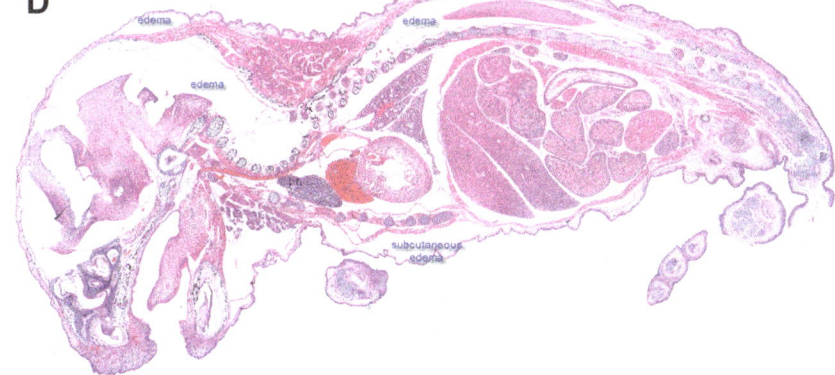

Figure 5. Cardiac malformations and failure in Evi1$^{\delta ex3/\delta ex3}$ mice. (A) Transverse sections and (B) 3D reconstruction (left-ventral oblique view) of hearts from Evi1$^{\delta ex3/\delta ex3}$ or wild type littermate (+/+) E15.5 embryos analyzed by magnetic resonance imaging (MRI). The aorta (Ao), right ventricle (RV), left ventricle (LV), ventricular septum (VS), trachea (Tr), aortic arch (AoA) and ductus arteriosus (DA) are indicated. Ventricular septal defect (VSD), interrupted aortic arch (IAA) and common arterial trunk (CAT) were observed in Evi1$^{\delta ex3/\delta ex3}$ hearts. (C) List of the congenital heart defects identified in fifteen E15.5 embryos of various different genotypes by MRI and 3D reconstruction. (D) Hematoxylin and eosin staining of 5 μm sections of a sick Evi1$^{\delta ex3/\delta ex3}$ pup. Subcutaneous and other tissue edema (white spaces) was present, consistent with heart failure.

exon 3 would lead to embryonic lethality between E10.5 and E16 due to defects in HSC self-renewal and subsequent hematopoietic failure. Surprisingly, this was not the case. Homozygous Evi1$^{\delta ex3/\delta ex3}$ knockout mice (Fig. S1B,C in File S1) were born with a normal Mendelian ratio (Fig. 1B). They were indistinguishable from their control littermates, there were no gross morphological defects and they were normal in size (Fig. S1D in File S1). The presence of grossly visible milk-filled stomachs a few hours after birth also attested to their ability to feed, which was confirmed by histology (Fig. S1E in File S1). However, several hours to a few days after birth, Evi1$^{\delta ex3/\delta ex3}$ mice became weak, lost weight and eventually died, with no Evi1$\delta^{ex3/\delta ex3}$ animals surviving longer than three days (Fig. 1C,D). These results suggest that Evi1^{fl3} might encode a hypomorphic allele rather than a null allele.

Evi1^{fl3} encodes a hypomorphic allele

To determine whether Evi1^{fl3} encodes a hypomorphic allele we used 5′ RACE to confirm that exon3 was deleted from all Mecom transcripts expressed in Evi1$^{\delta ex3/\delta ex3}$ embryos. We also performed RT-qPCR to quantify the level of the Mecom transcripts expressed in Evi1$^{\delta ex3/\delta ex3}$ embryos using primers located in exons 2 and 3, 3 and 4 or 13 and 14. No significant amplification was

detected in Evi1$^{\delta ex3/\delta ex3}$ embryos using the two first sets of primers (Fig. 1E), confirming that exon3 was deleted from all Mecom transcripts in Evi1$\delta^{ex3/\delta ex3}$ animals. Transcripts encoding Evi1 exons 13 and 14 were, however, produced at normal levels, confirming that stable Evi1 transcripts are expressed in Evi1$^{\delta ex3/\delta ex3}$ embryos. Western blot analyses showed that proteins with a similar size to Evi1, Evi1δ105, and Evi1δ324 were also expressed in Evi1$^{\delta ex3/\delta ex3}$ embryos (Fig. 1F). Evi1δ105 is a splice variant present in mouse but not in human tissues [37]. Deletion of exon3 thus did not appear to affect Evi1 protein translation as would have been expected by removal of exon 3. We therefore decided to look for alternative ATG translation start sites that might be located downstream of exon 3. We found a potential ATG start site in exon 4, which contains a Kozak sequence [38] and is in frame with the rest of the protein. This start site is well conserved in higher vertebrates and provides a better Kozak sequence than the start site in exon 3 (Fig. 1G, S2). The use of this alternative start site would remove 42 amino acids from the N-terminus of Evi1 including the first zinc finger motif of the proximal Evi1 zinc finger domain (Fig. S2 in File S1). Evi1δ105, an isoform specifically present in mice [37] and Evi1δ324 would be similarly affected since they share the same transcription start site as Evi1.

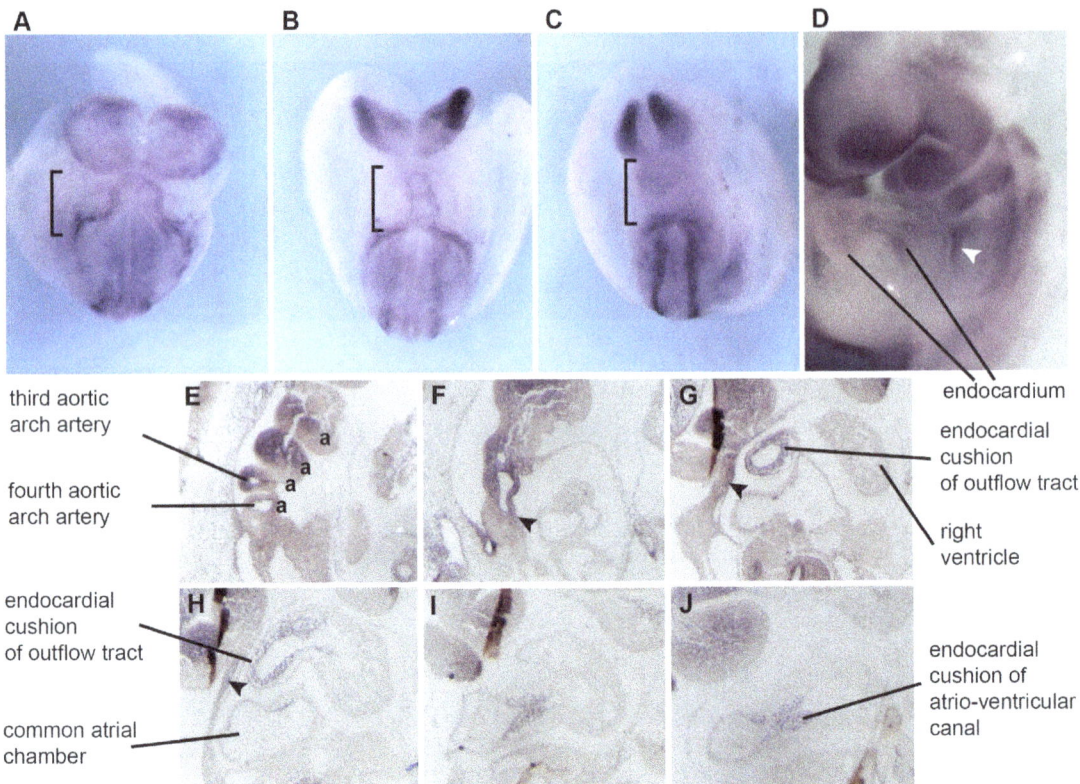

third aortic
arch artery

fourth aortic
arch artery

endocardial
cushion
of outflow tract

common atrial
chamber

endocardium

endocardial
cushion
of outflow tract

right
ventricle

endocardial
cushion of
atrio-ventricular
canal

Figure 6. Expression of Mecom mRNA in cardiac structures of wild type embryos. (A–D) Whole mount mRNA *in situ* hybridization to show Mecom expression. A–C) Expression during subsequent stages of heart tube formation E8.5 (black brackets). D) At E9.5 Evi1 is expressed in the endothelial cells and in the endocardium of the heart and in the mesenchyme of the aortic arches. Expression also includes a population of migrating neural crest cells (white arrowhead). E–J) E10.5 Sagittal sections (from right to left) showing Evi1 in the aortic arches (a), mesenchyme of the secondary heart field (black arrowheads), outflow and atrio-ventricular canal endocardium including the cushions.

These results support the notion that Evi1^{fl3} encodes a hypomorphic allele that results from the expression of an N-terminally truncated Evi1 protein initiated in exon 4.

Evi1$^{\delta ex3/\delta ex3}$ newborn pups have a milder hematopoietic phenotype than that observed in Evi1$^{\delta ex4/\delta ex4}$ embryos

The embryonic lethality in Evi1 exon 4 knockout mice has been ascribed to defective HSC self-renewal and subsequent hematopoietic failure. [12]. To determine whether *Evi1*$^{\delta ex3/\delta ex3}$ embryos have similar defects, we counted the number of two immunophenotypically defined HSC populations, c-Kit+, Sca-1+, lineage- (KSL) and c-Kit+, lineage-, CD34+ (KL-CD34+) cells from E14.5 wild-type, Evi1$^{\delta ex3/+}$ and Evi1$^{\delta ex3/\delta ex3}$ fetal livers (Fig. 2A). The number of KSL HSCs and KL-CD34+ progenitor cells was significantly reduced in Evi1$^{\delta ex3/\delta ex3}$ fetal livers as compared to wild type livers, while Evi1$^{\delta ex3/+}$ fetal livers presented an intermediate phenotype (Fig. 2A). In addition, there was a slight reduction in the number of B220+ B-lymphocytes (Fig. 2B) and colony-forming cells (Fig. 2C) in E14.4 Evi1$^{\delta ex3/+}$ and Evi1$^{\delta ex3/\delta ex3}$ fetal livers. These results show that deletion of Evi1 exon 3 leads to a reduction in the number of HSC and progenitor cells, but this deletion does not affect the differentiation of progenitors once they are formed. This hematopoietic phenotype is milder than that described for *Evi1*$^{\delta ex4/\delta ex4}$ mice [12] as the HSC counts were reduced by only 76% versus 93% for *Evi1*$^{\delta ex4/\delta ex4}$ mice. Blood counts from Evi1$^{+/+}$, Evi1$^{\delta ex3/+}$ and Evi1$^{\delta ex3/\delta ex3}$ newborn animals (Fig. 2D) also showed that erythropoiesis was normal in *Evi1*$^{\delta ex3/\delta ex3}$ newborn animals. Mild leucopenia was however

detected, which equally affected all hematopoietic compartments. Hypoproliferative thrombocytopenia was the most prominent phenotype linked to the Evi1 exon 3 deletion. Histological analyses showed that 31% of the Evi1$^{\delta ex3/\delta ex3}$ pups had grossly visible focal hemorrhages in various tissues at birth (4 out of 13 pups) (Fig. 2E), while no control animals were seen with hemorrhagic lesions (0 out of 8 controls). These hemorrhages were unlikely to be the cause of embryonic lethality, however, because other genetically engineered mouse models with much lower platelet counts have been shown to survive to adulthood [39].

Spontaneous lethal bone marrow failure in the hematopoietic compartment of Evi1$^{\delta ex3/\delta ex3}$ animals

To further characterize the hematopoietic phenotype linked to the Evi1 exon3 deletion, we crossed Evi1$^{fl3/fl3}$ animals with Vav-iCre transgenic mice [40]. Vav-iCre is expressed in all hematopoietic, but few other cell types, and as expected Vav-iCre/+, Evi1$^{fl3/fl3}$ animals displayed a selective loss of Evi1 exon3 in the hematopoietic compartment (Fig. S3A in File S1). These mice did not die during prenatal development but instead died between 2.8 and 24.8 weeks of age (N = 37), with a median survival of 6.3 weeks (Fig. 3A). Heterozygous deletion of exon 3 did not affect the mortality rate compared to control mice (Fig. 3A). Most mice became weak and lost weight before dying (Fig. S3B in File S1). Hemograms were subsequently performed on Vav-iCre/+, Evi1$^{fl3/fl3}$ weak animals and corresponding littermate controls +/+, Evi1$^{fl3/fl3}$. The hematopoietic phenotype was dramatic, with severe thrombocytopenia, anemia and leucopenia in this condi-

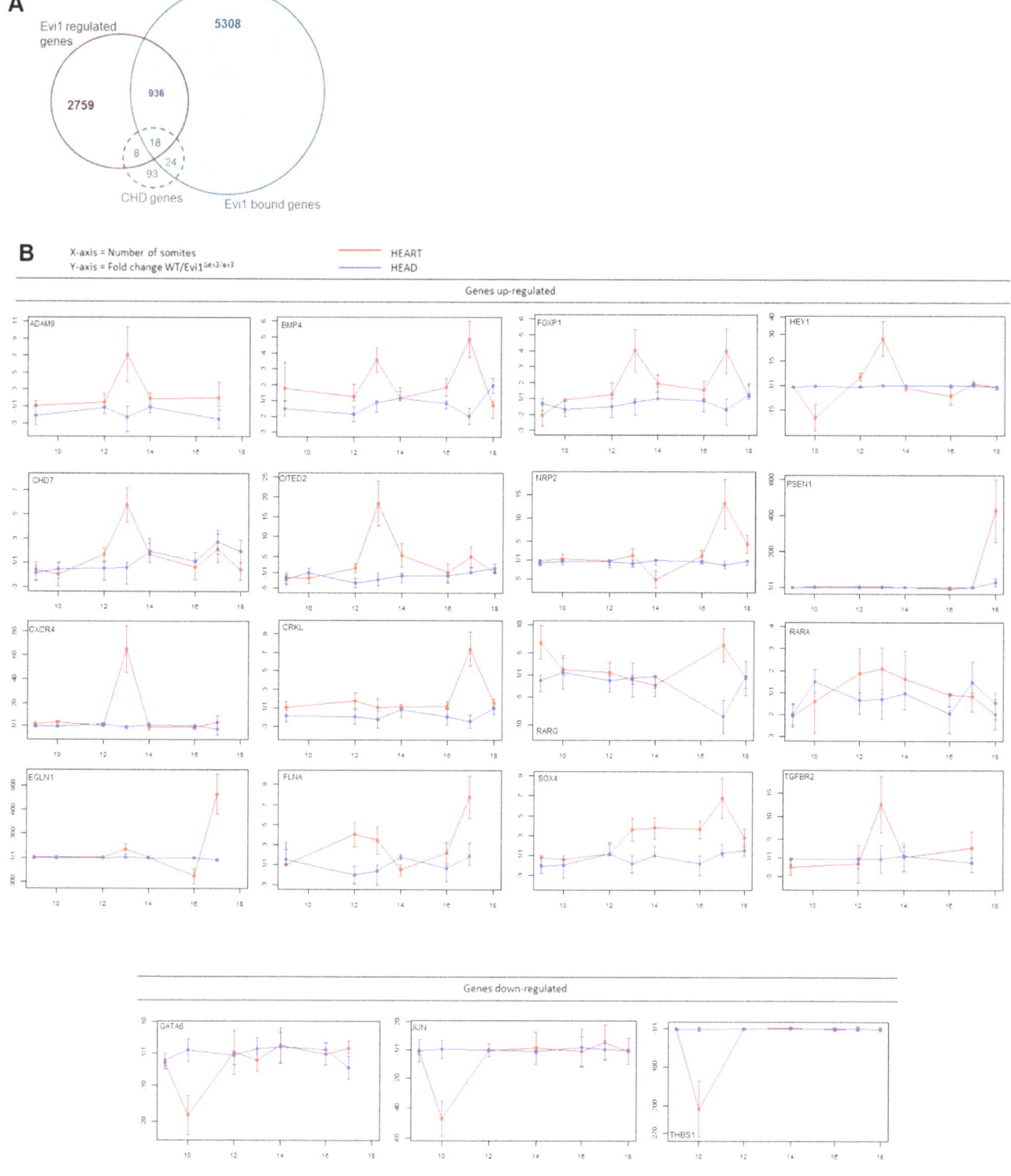

Figure 7. Evi1 regulates the expression of other CHD genes during embryonic heart development. (A) The number of CHD genes represented in Evi1 ChIP-Seq data (Evi1 bound genes) or in the list of genes regulated by Mecom. An enriched number of CHD genes were found bound or regulated by Mecom (50 out of 143 genes), p = 0.0453 and p = 0.0276, respectively. These genes represent potential Mecom target genes in heart development. (B) Mecom regulates the expression of 23 CHD genes, which contain Evi1-binding sites specifically in heart. Heart and head (neural crest) tissues were harvested from WT and Evi1$^{\delta ex3/\delta ex3}$ embryos of somite number 9 to 18. RT-qPCR assays were performed. Genes considered to be mis-regulated in Evi1$^{\delta ex3/\delta ex3}$ hearts were increased or decreased in expression by at least three fold in average for all samples of the same time-point. These graphs are representative of two to five independent experiments.

Table 1. List of 23 congenital heart defect (CHD) genes whose expression is disrupted in Evi1$^{\delta ex3/\delta ex3}$ developing hearts.

mouse gene symbol	human gene symbol	common arterial trunk (MP:0002633)	Ventricular septal defect (MP:0010402)	double outlet right ventricle (MP:0000284)	overriding aorta (MP:0000273)	interrupted aortic arch (MP:0004157)	EVI1 target gene by ChIP-Seq	Regulated by EVI1 (microarray in SKOV3 cells)	Evi1$^{\delta ex3/\delta ex3}$ affects gene expression in embryos hearts
Adam9	ADAM9		yes	yes			yes	up-regulated	up-regulated
Bmp4	BMP4	yes	yes	yes		yes	yes		up-regulated
Bmpr2	BMPR2					yes	yes	down-regulated	up-regulated
Cav1	CAV1						yes	down-regulated	up-regulated
Chd7	CHD7		yes			yes	yes		up-regulated
Cited2	CITED2	yes	yes	yes	yes	yes	yes		up-regulated
Crkl	CRKL		yes	yes	yes	yes	yes		up-regulated
Cxcr4	CXCR4		yes				yes	down-regulated	up-regulated
Egln1	EGLN1	yes	yes			yes	yes	down-regulated	up-regulated
Flna	FLNA	yes	yes	yes		yes	yes		up-regulated
Foxp1	FOXP1	yes	yes	yes			yes		up-regulated
Gata6	GATA6	yes	yes	yes		yes	yes		down-regulated
Hey1	HEY1	yes	yes				yes	up-regulated	up-regulated
Jag1	JAG1						yes	up-regulated	up-regulated
Jun	JUN	yes			yes		yes	down-regulated	down-regulated
Nf1	NF1	yes		yes			yes		up-regulated
Nrp2	NRP2	yes					yes	up-regulated	up-regulated
Psen1	PSEN1			yes			yes	down-regulated	up-regulated
Rarg	RARG	yes		yes			yes	up-regulated	up-regulated
Rxra	RXRA	yes		yes			yes		up-regulated
Sox4	SOX4	yes				yes	yes	up-regulated	up-regulated
Tgfbr2	TGFBR2					yes	yes	up-regulated	up-regulated
Thbs1	THBS1	yes	yes				yes	down-regulated	down-regulated

These genes were previously found targeted by Evi1 in ChIP-Seq and microarray experiments [16], indicating they may be directly regulated by Evi1.

Table 2. Overview of Major Reported Expression Domains.

Gene	Reported Expression Domains	References
Mecom	**AA, CC/HT, End+Csn, NC, SHF**	
Adam9	End+Csn, Myo	[56,57]
Bmp4	AA, Myo, NC, OFT, SHF	[58,59,60]
Bmpr2	AA, End, Myo, NC	[58,59,60]
Cav1	End	[61]
Chd7	AA	[62]
Cited2	AA, CC/HT, End+Csn, Myo, OFT	[63,64]
Crkl	AA, NC	[65]
Cxcr4	AA, Myo	[66]
Flna	AA, End+Csn, NC, OFT	[67]
Foxp1	End+Csn, Myo, OFT	[68]
Gata6	End+Csn, Myo, OFT, NC	[69,70]
Hey1	AA, End, OFT	[71,72,73]
Jag1	AA, End, OFT	[71,74]
Jun	AA, End+Csn, OFT, SHF	[75]
Nf1	AA, End+Csn, Myo, NC	[76]
Nrp2	NC	[77,78]
Psen1	AA, End+Csn, Myo, NC, OFT	[79,80]
Rarg	AA	[81]
Rxra	AA, End+Csn, Myo, NC, OFT	[82]
Sox4	End+Csn, Myo	[68,83]
Tgfbr2	AA, CC/HT, End+Csn, Myo, NC	[84,85,86]
Thbs1	End, Myo	[87]

Key
AA – Aortic Arch and Aortic Arch Arteries.
CC/HT - Cardiac Crescent/Heart Tube.
End – Endocardium (+Csn – including Cushions).
Myo – Myocardium.
NC –Neural Crest (Cardiac).
OFT – Outflow Tract.
SHF – Secondary Heart Field.

tional exon 3 deletion (Fig. 3B). Moreover, the number of KSL HSCs and KL progenitor cells in the bone marrow was close to zero (Fig. 3C). In addition, no colonies could be formed from Vav-iCre/+, Evi1$^{fl3/fl3}$ bone marrow cells ex vivo (Fig. 3D). These results demonstrated a profound depletion of HSC and progenitor cells as well as downstream hematopoietic cells. Histological analysis of the bones of sick animals confirmed the spontaneous bone marrow hypoplasia (Fig. 4A), as hematopoietic cells were few or undetectable in the bone marrow cavity. This phenotype was accompanied by compensatory erythropoiesis in the spleen (Fig. 4B). Erythrophagocytosis with rosettes (Fig. S3C in File S1) was also identified in two animals, demonstrating immune perturbations. Bone marrow depletion can lead to hemorrhages due to lack of megakaryocytes and platelets. Indeed, bleeding in vital organs like the brain was observed in Vav-iCre/+, Evi1$^{fl3/fl3}$ mice and was likely to be one major cause of lethality in these animals (Fig. 4C, S3D in File S1). Another major etiology was severe bacterial infections due to loss of immune defense. Gram-positive bacteria were found in the blood of the lungs, kidneys, and hearts of Vav-iCre/+, Evi1$^{fl3/fl3}$ mice, indicating bacteremia (Fig. 4D). Collectively, these results describe a spontaneous lethal bone marrow failure upon deletion of Evi1 exon3 in the hematopoietic system. This hypomorphic phenotype is consistent with the profound HSC depletion seen in Evi1 exon 4 conditional knockout at E10.5–16.5 [12], but it occurs at a much later stage, in Evi1 exon 3 deleted adult mice.

Congenital heart defects in Evi1$^{\delta ex3/\delta ex3}$ newborn mice

Since it was unlikely that the perinatal lethality observed in Evi1$^{\delta ex3/\delta ex3}$ mice was caused by the hematopoietic defects we looked for other possible causes. We used magnetic resonance imaging (MRI) to visualize organ formation in six Evi1$^{\delta ex3/\delta ex3}$, three Evi1$^{\delta ex3/+}$ and six E15.5 control littermates, as previously described [41]. Structural abnormalities were observed in the hearts of all six Evi1$^{\delta ex3/\delta ex3}$ embryos (Fig. 5A,B), while small benign bilateral cysts were observed in the jugular lymphatic sacks of two Evi1$^{\delta ex3/\delta ex3}$ embryos (Fig. S4 in File S1). No defects were observed in wild type or heterozygous mutant animals. Evi1$^{\delta ex3/\delta ex3}$ embryos displayed several congenital heart defects (Fig. 5C).

All six Evi1$^{\delta ex3/\delta ex3}$ embryos had ventricular septal defects (VSD) - failure to form the septum between the ventricles of the heart (Fig. 5B,C).

Common arterial trunk (CAT), where two great arteries fail to separate and leave the heart as one common vessel, was also observed in 3 out of 6 Evi1$^{\delta ex3/\delta ex3}$ embryos. Double outlet right ventricle (DORV), where both the aorta and pulmonary trunk leave one ventricle, was also observed in half of the Evi1$^{\delta ex3/\delta ex3}$ embryos (Fig. 5B,C). In addition, overriding aorta (aorta originating just above the VSD) was seen in one Evi1$^{\delta ex3/\delta ex3}$ embryo. Finally, aortic arch formation impairments were found in 4 out of 6 Evi1$^{\delta ex3/\delta ex3}$ embryos (Fig. 5B,C). These impairments were manifested as an interrupted aortic arch (IAA), with a complete discontinuation between the ascending and descending parts of the aorta. These type of congenital heart defects are known to be viable *in utero* but lethal during the neonatal phase of life for other mouse knockouts [42], and thus likely represent the major cause of the perinatal lethality seen in Evi1$^{\delta ex3/\delta ex3}$ pups. Consistent with this, heart failure was sometimes accompanied by oedema and congested lungs in Evi1$^{\delta ex3/\delta ex3}$ pups (Fig. 5D).

Mecom expression in the developing heart

We next examined *Mecom* expression by mRNA *in situ* hybridization. At E8.5 *Mecom* was expressed in the forming heart tube (Fig 6A-C). By E9.5-E10.5 *Mecom* expression could clearly be localized to the endothelial cells and in the endocardium (Fig. 6D–J), and its expression was strong in the cushions of the atrio-ventricular canal (AVC). In the outflow tract, *Mecom* was not clearly expressed in the myocardium outer layer, but rather in the mesenchyme cells that are composed of cardiac neural crest. There was also clear expression in the neural crest cells which generates the majority of mesenchyme of aortic arches 1 and 2 (Fig 6E). We also saw *Mecom* in the stream of neural crest cells situated behind the heart (Fig 6D, arrowhead). Finally, there was additional *Mecom* signal in the mesenchyme cells of the secondary heart field (Fig 6E,F).Overall, we found that *Mecom* expression overlaps with the key cell populations in which defects could lead to the heart malformations we have described, especially the endocardium, the endocardial cushions, and the neural crest cells [42,43]

Evi1 controls the expression of genes that regulate heart development

How might Evi1 act to control heart development? Because Evi1 is a transcription factor that can both activate or repress its target genes [16] we hypothesized that it might be part of the transcriptional program that controls heart development. To determine this, we searched the Mouse Genome Informatics (MGI) database [44] and found 143 Congenital Heart Defect (CHD) genes whose mutant heart phenotypes were similar to those observed in Evi1$^{\delta ex3/\delta ex3}$ mice (Table S1). These genes were linked to the MGI Mammalian Phenotype identifications MP:0010402 (VSD), MP:0002633 (persistent truncus arteriosis, another name for CAT), MP:0000284 (DORV), MP:0004157 (IAA), and MP:0000273 (overriding aorta) [45]. We cross-compared these 143 genes with available EVI1 ChIP-Seq and differential microarray data [16]. Forty-two of these 143 genes contain known EVI1-binding sites, which constituted a significant enrichment (p = 0.0453, Chi-square with Yates correction), suggesting them as possible Evi1-target genes in heart (Fig. 7A). Similarly, the expression of 26 genes is known to be affected by Evi1 siRNA knock-down in SKOV3 cells (significant enrichment, p = 0.0276, Chi-square with Yates correction) [16], while 18 genes contain known Evi1-binding sites and are also effected by Evi1 siRNA knockdown (Fig. 7A, Table 1). This represents a very significant enrichment of CHD genes in Evi1 direct target genes (p<0.0001, Chi-square with Yates correction), strongly suggesting a functional involvement of these EVI1 target genes in heart development.

These computational comparative analyses have provided a list of 50 genes that are likely to be enriched for genes that are regulated by Evi1 during heart development (Table S1, Figure 7A). To provide additional evidence for this, we dissected hearts, and heads as a control, from a range of Evi1$^{\delta ex3/\delta ex3}$ embryos between E8 and E10, in order to determine if these candidates are deregulated due to the disruption of *Mecom* activity.

We extracted mRNA from mutant and wild-type embryonic hearts and heads, and performed reverse transcription (RT) and qPCR to quantitate the level of expression of 31 of the Evi1 candidate target genes (Fig. 7B, S5). Due to limited amount of RNA from embryonic heart, we chose to assess the 18 CHD genes previously found occupied and regulated by Evi1, plus 14 CHD genes bound by Evi1. We then used the $2^{-\Delta\Delta Ct}$ method [30] to calculate the fold change in expression between wild type and mutant embryos. We found that the Evi1 exon3 deletion had no effect on the expression of eight genes (Fig. S5 in File S1), while three were downregulated and 20 were upregulated in expression in *Mecom* mutant hearts (Table1, Fig. 7B). This was consistent with MECOM being a known dynamic modulator of transcription that can either activate or repress genes, depending on the recruitment of coactivators or corepressors [46].Of the 13 genes regulated by Evi1 both in cardiac development and in SKOV3 ovarian carcinoma cells, 9 genes showed Evi1-mediated changes in expression level in a similar manner (Jun, Thbs1, Adam9, Hey1, Jag1, Nrp2, Rarg, Sox4, and Tgfbr2). Some of these regulatory relationships were also consistent with previous reports. For instance, in cell line models, Jun expression was found up-regulated by Evi1 through its direct binding to Jun promoter [16,47–50]. The Sox4 transcription factor and Evi1 cooperate to induce myeloid leukemia [51]; and Evi1 was shown to bind to Sox4 promoter and regulate its gene expression [16], providing evidence of transactivation of Sox4 by Evi1. Collectively, these results demonstrate that Evi1 modulates, in embryonic heart, the expression of genes that are important for controlling heart development.

We also performed a literature search to compare the gene expression patterns of these Mecom-deregulated factors to the *Mecom* embryonic heart expression pattern we describe (Fig.6). This analysis (Table 2) confirmed common expression in the endocardium and endocardial cushions, as well as in the aortic arches and outflow tract - especially in the neural crest cells.

Discussion

Our results demonstrate that deletion of Evi1 exon 3 produces a hypomorphic allele compared to previous studies involving Evi1 exons 4 and 7, where their removal produced complete null alleles [12,29]. Deletion of exon 3 indeed does not affect Evi1, Evi1δ105 [37] and Evi1δ324 protein production but does block the generation of Mds1-Evi1 protein production. All Evi1 isoform proteins expressed in these mice are expected to carry a 42 amino acid truncation at the N-terminus that constitutes nearly 4% of the protein. Such truncated proteins would be predicted to lack one zinc finger motif out of the seven present in the proximal DNA-binding site. It is not completely clear if and how this truncation affects Evi1 transcriptional activity or function. Several findings suggest that translation from Evi1 exon4 ATG start site produces a functional protein. First, the exon4 contains the best Kozak sequence with highest cross-species conservation. Thus, it is possible that the exon4 translation start site may be naturally produced in vivo. Secondly, a previous study has suggested that Evi1 protein initiated from exon 4 is oncogenic and able to give rise to leukemic clones in mice [52]. Retroviral insertional mutagenesis screens in mice have identified Evi1 isoform as a targeted mutant gene in myeloid leukemia [53,54]. Sequencing of the retroviral insertion sites from these tumors has shown that the majority of insertions are located upstream of Evi1 coding sequence, where they serve to upregulate the expression of oncogenic Evi1 but block the expression of Mds1-Evi1. The genomic region located between exons 3 and 4 is only 4 kb compared to the rest of the Evi1 upstream region which is 90 kb in size, thus providing 23 times less chance to contain a retrovirus insertion by random chance. However, retroviral insertions located between exon 3 and 4 have been described in tumors, which would serve to activate Evi1 translation from the alternative translation start site located in exon 4 [52].

The profound embryonic lethal disruption of HSC renewal seen in other studies [12,13] was not present in our Evi1$^{\delta ex3/\delta ex3}$ mutant embryos and newborn pups. However, we did identify a dramatic perturbation of hematopoietic repopulation activity in Vav-iCre/+, Evi1$^{fl3/fl3}$ young adult mice. To our knowledge, there is no current genetically-modified mouse model that mimics spontaneous bone marrow failure as seen in the Vav-iCre/+, Evi1$^{fl3/fl3}$ mice. They therefore constitute the first model of spontaneous lethal bone marrow failure in the adult. Surprisingly, the hypomorphic deletion of Evi1 could delay the phenotype of hematopoietic failure and the appearance of bone marrow depletion. This in is line with a previous study [21] that specifically implicated Mds1-Evi1 in the regulation of long term HSC repopulating activity [55] and Evi1 in short term HSC renewal activity [12,29].

The delay in acquisition of the hematological phenotype in Evi1$^{\delta ex3/\delta ex3}$ knockout mice allowed the embryos to survive to the perinatal period and the congenital heart defects found in these mice to be observed. Our results are also consistent with those reported for Evi1 exon 7 knockout mice published in 1997, which reported that E10.5 Evi1$^{-/-}$ mutant embryos displayed heart failure. Although their data based on only one histology section are not clear, Evi1$^{\delta ex7/\delta ex7}$ knockout embryos were reported to display arrested heart development with a looping defect of the posterior part of the heart and a poorly developed constriction between atria and ventricle [29], which is different from our findings. At the time of this previous study, the technologies to study embryonic cardiac development were based only on histological methods, which could not allow precise interpretations of the pathology. In our studies we used MRI and 3D modeling to clearly define the pathology and heart developmental defects in Evi1 exon 3 knockout embryos.

We provide evidence that Mecom belongs to a transcriptional regulatory network that controls heart development. Mecom expression overlaps with the expression of multiple other factors required to form the heart (Table 2). These factors can be Mecom targets, and their expression is deregulated expression in the Evi1$^{\delta ex3/\delta ex3}$ mutant heart. Of particular interest may be factors in the Notch and TGFβ pathways as that Mecom or its homologues interact with these pathways [22]. In the endocardium for example, there is clear overlap of Mecom with the Notch ligand Jag1 and the TGFβ receptor Tgfbr2.

The endocardium is major site of Mecom expression in the heart, and it is possible that Mecom regulates gene expression directly in this tissue. The cushions cells of the AVC originate from endocardium via an epithelial–mesenchymal transition, and they form the partition between the ventricles and the atria (atrioventricular canal and later valves). This partition provides the matrix for the growing ventricular and atrial septa [42,43]. Another possible site of Mecom action is in the neural crest cells. The spectrum of phenotypes seen in the Evi1$^{\delta ex3/\delta ex3}$ knockout heart could also be attributed to defects in these cells causing disrupted remodelling of the aortic arches, and to a failure to septate the outflow tract [43]. Further studies (perhaps using a floxed-Evi1 null allele [12] and specific Cre lines) can be used address if Mecom is required in a particular heart cell population, or in multiple populations to drive heart development.

Supporting Information

File S1 Figure S1, Targeting and knockout of Evi1 exon3. Figure S2, An alternative protein translation site located in Evi1 exon 4 and structure of the translated protein. **Figure S3, Deletion of Evi1 exon 3 in the hematopoietic compartment. Figure S4, Small bilateral cysts in jugular lymphatic sacks of Evi1$^{\delta ex3/\delta ex3}$ embryos. Figure S5, CHD gene expression in Evi1$^{\delta ex3/\delta ex3}$ embryos.**

Table S1 List of 143 congenital heart defect genes with similar heart phenotypes as thosed observed in Evi1$^{\delta ex3/\delta ex3}$ mice. All 143 genes linked to the Mammalian Phenotype identifications MP:0010402 (VSD), MP:0002633 (persistent truncus arteriosis, other name for CAT), MP:0000284 (DORV), MP:0004157 (IAA), MP:0000273 (overriding aorta) in the MGI database [88]. The genes found in previous Evi1 ChIP-Seq and microarray experiments [89] provide potential Mecom target genes in heart development.

Acknowledgments

The authors acknowledge Keith Rogers, Susan Rogers and the IMCB core histopathology laboratory for their necropsy and histotechnology assistance. We also thank Pearlyn Cheok, Nicole Lim and Dorothy Chen for their technical help with mouse breeding and monitoring.

Author Contributions

Conceived and designed the experiments: EAB-C AP NAJ NGC. Performed the experiments: EAB-C DS BJ BQC GCC YZ EK FU SDV. Analyzed the data: EAB-C DS JMW AWM SB MO SA. Contributed reagents/materials/analysis tools: EAB-C DS SDV AWM SB MO AP. Wrote the paper: EAB-C SDV AWM NAJ NGC.

References

1. Koonin EV, Wolf YI (2010) Constraints and plasticity in genome and molecular-phenome evolution. Nat Rev Genet 11: 487–498.
2. Nerlov C (2010) Transcriptional and translational control of C/EBPs: the case for "deep" genetics to understand physiological function. Bioessays 32: 680–686.
3. Lugthart S, van Drunen E, van Norden Y, van Hoven A, Erpelinck CA, et al. (2008) High EVI1 levels predict adverse outcome in acute myeloid leukemia: prevalence of EVI1 overexpression and chromosome 3q26 abnormalities underestimated. Blood 111: 4329–4337.
4. Ogawa S, Kurokawa M, Tanaka T, Mitani K, Inazawa J, et al. (1996) Structurally altered Evi-1 protein generated in the 3q21q26 syndrome. Oncogene 13: 183–191.
5. Goyama S, Kurokawa M (2009) Pathogenetic significance of ecotropic viral integration site-1 in hematological malignancies. Cancer Sci 100: 990–995.
6. Bei JX, Li Y, Jia WH, Feng BJ, Zhou G, et al. (2010) A genome-wide association study of nasopharyngeal carcinoma identifies three new susceptibility loci. Nat Genet 42: 599–603.
7. Brooks DJ, Woodward S, Thompson FH, Dos Santos B, Russell M, et al. (1996) Expression of the zinc finger gene EVI-1 in ovarian and other cancers. Br J Cancer 74: 1518–1525.
8. Choi YW, Choi JS, Zheng LT, Lim YJ, Yoon HK, et al. (2007) Comparative genomic hybridization array analysis and real time PCR reveals genomic alterations in squamous cell carcinomas of the lung. Lung Cancer 55: 43–51.
9. Koos B, Bender S, Witt H, Mertsch S, Felsberg J, et al. (2011) The transcription factor Evi-1 is overexpressed, promotes proliferation and is prognostically unfavorable in infratentorial ependymomas. Clin Cancer Res.
10. Starr TK, Allaei R, Silverstein KA, Staggs RA, Sarver AL, et al. (2009) A transposon-based genetic screen in mice identifies genes altered in colorectal cancer. Science 323: 1747–1750.
11. Yokoi S, Yasui K, Iizasa T, Imoto I, Fujisawa T, et al. (2003) TERC identified as a probable target within the 3q26 amplicon that is detected frequently in non-small cell lung cancers. Clin Cancer Res 9: 4705–4713.
12. Goyama S, Yamamoto G, Shimabe M, Sato T, Ichikawa M, et al. (2008) Evi-1 is a critical regulator for hematopoietic stem cells and transformed leukemic cells. Cell Stem Cell 3: 207–220.
13. Yuasa H, Oike Y, Iwama A, Nishikata I, Sugiyama D, et al. (2005) Oncogenic transcription factor Evi1 regulates hematopoietic stem cell proliferation through GATA-2 expression. EMBO J 24: 1976–1987.
14. Nucifora G, Laricchia-Robbio L, Senyuk V (2006) EVI1 and hematopoietic disorders: history and perspectives. Gene 368: 1–11.
15. Goyama S, Kurokawa M (2010) Evi-1 as a critical regulator of leukemic cells. Int J Hematol 91: 753–757.
16. Bard-Chapeau EA, Jeyakani J, Kok CH, Muller J, Chua BQ, et al. (2012) Ecotopic viral integration site 1 (EVI1) regulates multiple cellular processes important for cancer and is a synergistic partner for FOS protein in invasive tumors. Proc Natl Acad Sci U S A 109: 2168–2173.
17. Delwel R, Funabiki T, Kreider BL, Morishita K, Ihle JN (1993) Four of the seven zinc fingers of the Evi-1 myeloid-transforming gene are required for sequence-specific binding to GA(C/T)AAGA(T/C)AAGATAA. Mol Cell Biol 13: 4291–4300.
18. Perkins AS, Fishel R, Jenkins NA, Copeland NG (1991) Evi-1, a murine zinc finger proto-oncogene, encodes a sequence-specific DNA-binding protein. Mol Cell Biol 11: 2665–2674.
19. Yatsula B, Lin S, Read AJ, Poholek A, Yates K, et al. (2005) Identification of binding sites of EVI1 in mammalian cells. J Biol Chem 280: 30712–30722.
20. Funabiki T, Kreider BL, Ihle JN (1994) The carboxyl domain of zinc fingers of the Evi-1 myeloid transforming gene binds a consensus sequence of GAAGATGAG. Oncogene 9: 1575–1581.
21. Zhang Y, Stehling-Sun S, Lezon-Geyda K, Juneja SC, Coillard L, et al. (2011) PR-domain-containing Mds1-Evi1 is critical for long-term hematopoietic stem cell function. Blood 118: 3853–3861.
22. Hohenauer T, Moore AW (2012) The Prdm family: expanding roles in stem cells and development. Development 139: 2267–2282.
23. Barjesteh van Waalwijk van Doorn-Khosrovani S, Erpelinck C, van Putten WL, Valk PJ, van der Poel-van de Luytgaarde S, et al. (2003) High EVI1 expression predicts poor survival in acute myeloid leukemia: a study of 319 de novo AML patients. Blood 101: 837–845.
24. Nanjundan M, Nakayama Y, Cheng KW, Lahad J, Liu J, et al. (2007) Amplification of MDS1/EVI1 and EVI1, located in the 3q26.2 amplicon, is associated with favorable patient prognosis in ovarian cancer. Cancer Res 67: 3074–3084.
25. Sood R, Talwar-Trikha A, Chakrabarti SR, Nucifora G (1999) MDS1/EVI1 enhances TGF-beta1 signaling and strengthens its growth-inhibitory effect but the leukemia-associated fusion protein AML1/MDS1/EVI1, product of the t(3;21), abrogates growth-inhibition in response to TGF-beta1. Leukemia 13: 348–357.
26. Bartholomew C, Clark AM (1994) Induction of two alternatively spliced evi-1 proto-oncogene transcripts by cAMP in kidney cells. Oncogene 9: 939–942.

27. Bordereaux D, Fichelson S, Tambourin P, Gisselbrecht S (1990) Alternative splicing of the Evi-1 zinc finger gene generates mRNAs which differ by the number of zinc finger motifs. Oncogene 5: 925–927.

28. Morishita K, Parganas E, Parham DM, Matsugi T, Ihle JN (1990) The Evi-1 zinc finger myeloid transforming gene is normally expressed in the kidney and in developing oocytes. Oncogene 5: 1419–1423.

29. Hoyt PR, Bartholomew C, Davis AJ, Yutzey K, Gamer LW, et al. (1997) The Evi1 proto-oncogene is required at midgestation for neural, heart, and paraxial mesenchyme development. Mech Dev 65: 55–70.

30. Schmittgen TD, Livak KJ (2008) Analyzing real-time PCR data by the comparative C(T) method. Nat Protoc 3: 1101–1108.

31. Bard-Chapeau EA, Hevener AL, Long S, Zhang EE, Olefsky JM, et al. (2005) Deletion of Gab1 in the liver leads to enhanced glucose tolerance and improved hepatic insulin action. Nat Med 11: 567–571.

32. Yamashita N, Osato M, Huang L, Yanagida M, Kogan SC, et al. (2005) Haploinsufficiency of Runx1/AML1 promotes myeloid features and leukaemogenesis in BXH2 mice. Br J Haematol 131: 495–507.

33. Schneider JE, Bose J, Bamforth SD, Gruber AD, Broadbent C, et al. (2004) Identification of cardiac malformations in mice lacking Ptdsr using a novel high-throughput magnetic resonance imaging technique. BMC Dev Biol 4: 16.

34. Szumska D, Pieles G, Essalmani R, Bilski M, Mesnard D, et al. (2008) VACTERL/caudal regression/Currarino syndrome-like malformations in mice with mutation in the proprotein convertase Pcsk5. Genes Dev 22: 1465–1477.

35. Palmer S, Brouillet JP, Kilbey A, Fulton R, Walker M, et al. (2001) Evi-1 transforming and repressor activities are mediated by CtBP co-repressor proteins. J Biol Chem 276: 25834–25840.

36. Kinameri E, Inoue T, Aruga J, Imayoshi I, Kageyama R, et al. (2008) Prdm proto-oncogene transcription factor family expression and interaction with the Notch-Hes pathway in mouse neurogenesis. PLoS One 3: e3859.

37. Alzuherri H, McGilvray R, Kilbey A, Bartholomew C (2006) Conservation and expression of a novel alternatively spliced Evi1 exon. Gene 384: 154–162.

38. Harhay GP, Sonstegard TS, Keele JW, Heaton MP, Clawson ML, et al. (2005) Characterization of 954 bovine full-CDS cDNA sequences. BMC Genomics 6: 166.

39. Ware J, Russell S, Ruggeri ZM (2000) Generation and rescue of a murine model of platelet dysfunction: the Bernard-Soulier syndrome. Proc Natl Acad Sci U S A 97: 2803–2808.

40. Ogilvy S, Elefanty AG, Visvader J, Bath ML, Harris AW, et al. (1998) Transcriptional regulation of vav, a gene expressed throughout the hematopoietic compartment. Blood 91: 419–430.

41. MacDonald ST, Bamforth SD, Chen CM, Farthing CR, Franklyn A, et al. (2008) Epiblastic Cited2 deficiency results in cardiac phenotypic heterogeneity and provides a mechanism for haploinsufficiency. Cardiovasc Res 79: 448–457.

42. Conway SJ, Kruzynska-Frejtag A, Kneer PL, Machnicki M, Koushik SV (2003) What cardiovascular defect does my prenatal mouse mutant have, and why? Genesis 35: 1–21.

43. Vincent SD, Buckingham ME (2010) How to make a heart: the origin and regulation of cardiac progenitor cells. Curr Top Dev Biol 90: 1–41.

44. Blake JA, Bult CJ, Kadin JA, Richardson JE, Eppig JT (2011) The Mouse Genome Database (MGD): premier model organism resource for mammalian genomics and genetics. Nucleic Acids Res 39: D842–848.

45. Bentham J, Bhattacharya S (2008) Genetic mechanisms controlling cardiovascular development. Ann N Y Acad Sci 1123: 10–19.

46. Bard-Chapeau EA, Gunaratne J, Kumar P, Chua BQ, Muller J, et al. (2013) EVI1 oncoprotein interacts with a large and complex network of proteins and integrates signals through protein phosphorylation. Proc Natl Acad Sci U S A 110: E2885–2894.

47. Kurokawa M, Ogawa S, Tanaka T, Mitani K, Yazaki Y, et al. (1995) The AML1/Evi-1 fusion protein in the t(3;21) translocation exhibits transforming activity on Rat1 fibroblasts with dependence on the Evi-1 sequence. Oncogene 11: 833–840.

48. Mitani K (2004) Molecular mechanisms of leukemogenesis by AML1/EVI-1. Oncogene 23: 4263–4269.

49. Ogawa S, Kurokawa M, Tanaka T, Tanaka K, Hangaishi A, et al. (1996) Increased Evi-1 expression is frequently observed in blastic crisis of chronic myelocytic leukemia. Leukemia 10: 788–794.

50. Tanaka T, Nishida J, Mitani K, Ogawa S, Yazaki Y, et al. (1994) Evi-1 raises AP-1 activity and stimulates c-fos promoter transactivation with dependence on the second zinc finger domain. J Biol Chem 269: 24020–24026.

51. Boyd KE, Xiao YY, Fan K, Poholek A, Copeland NG, et al. (2006) Sox4 cooperates with Evi1 in AKXD-23 myeloid tumors via transactivation of proviral LTR. Blood 107: 733–741.

52. Modlich U, Schambach A, Brugman MH, Wicke DC, Knoess S, et al. (2008) Leukemia induction after a single retroviral vector insertion in Evi1 or Prdm16. Leukemia 22: 1519–1528.

53. Metais JY, Dunbar CE (2008) The MDS1-EVI1 gene complex as a retrovirus integration site: impact on behavior of hematopoietic cells and implications for gene therapy. Mol Ther 16: 439–449.

54. Wieser R (2007) The oncogene and developmental regulator EVI1: expression, biochemical properties, and biological functions. Gene 396: 346–357.

55. Morrison SJ, Uchida N, Weissman IL (1995) The biology of hematopoietic stem cells. Annu Rev Cell Dev Biol 11: 35–71.

56. Weskamp G, Cai H, Brodie TA, Higashyama S, Manova K, et al. (2002) Mice lacking the metalloprotease-disintegrin MDC9 (ADAM9) have no evident major abnormalities during development or adult life. Mol Cell Biol 22: 1537–1544.

57. Horiuchi K, Zhou HM, Kelly K, Manova K, Blobel CP (2005) Evaluation of the contributions of ADAMs 9, 12, 15, 17, and 19 to heart development and ectodomain shedding of neuregulins beta1 and beta2. Dev Biol 283: 459–471.

58. Liu W, Selever J, Wang D, Lu MF, Moses KA, et al. (2004) Bmp4 signaling is required for outflow-tract septation and branchial-arch artery remodeling. Proc Natl Acad Sci U S A 101: 4489–4494.

59. Beppu H, Malhotra R, Beppu Y, Lepore JJ, Parmacek MS, et al. (2009) BMP type II receptor regulates positioning of outflow tract and remodeling of atrioventricular cushion during cardiogenesis. Dev Biol 331: 167–175.

60. Danesh SM, Villasenor A, Chong D, Soukup C, Cleaver O (2009) BMP and BMP receptor expression during murine organogenesis. Gene Expr Patterns 9: 255–265.

61. Cohen AW, Park DS, Woodman SE, Williams TM, Chandra M, et al. (2003) Caveolin-1 null mice develop cardiac hypertrophy with hyperactivation of p42/44 MAP kinase in cardiac fibroblasts. Am J Physiol Cell Physiol 284: C457–474.

62. Sanlaville D, Etchevers HC, Gonzales M, Martinovic J, Clement-Ziza M, et al. (2006) Phenotypic spectrum of CHARGE syndrome in fetuses with CHD7 truncating mutations correlates with expression during human development. J Med Genet 43: 211–217.

63. Weninger WJ, Lopes Floro K, Bennett MB, Withington SL, Preis JI, et al. (2005) Cited2 is required both for heart morphogenesis and establishment of the left-right axis in mouse development. Development 132: 1337–1348.

64. Lopes Floro K, Artap ST, Preis JI, Fatkin D, Chapman G, et al. (2011) Loss of Cited2 causes congenital heart disease by perturbing left-right patterning of the body axis. Hum Mol Genet 20: 1097–1110.

65. Guris DL, Fantes J, Tara D, Druker BJ, Imamoto A (2001) Mice lacking the homologue of the human 22q11.2 gene CRKL phenocopy neurocristopathies of DiGeorge syndrome. Nat Genet 27: 293–298.

66. Tissir F, Wang CE, Goffinet AM (2004) Expression of the chemokine receptor Cxcr4 mRNA during mouse brain development. Brain Res Dev Brain Res 149: 63–71.

67. Norris RA, Moreno-Rodriguez R, Wessels A, Merot J, Bruneval P, et al. (2010) Expression of the familial cardiac valvular dystrophy gene, filamin-A, during heart morphogenesis. Dev Dyn 239: 2118–2127.

68. Wang B, Weidenfeld J, Lu MM, Maika S, Kuziel WA, et al. (2004) Foxp1 regulates cardiac outflow tract, endocardial cushion morphogenesis and myocyte proliferation and maturation. Development 131: 4477–4487.

69. Brewer AC, Alexandrovich A, Mjaatvedt CH, Shah AM, Patient RK, et al. (2005) GATA factors lie upstream of Nkx 2.5 in the transcriptional regulatory cascade that effects cardiogenesis. Stem Cells Dev 14: 425–439.

70. Lepore JJ, Mericko PA, Cheng L, Lu MM, Morrisey EE, et al. (2006) GATA-6 regulates semaphorin 3C and is required in cardiac neural crest for cardiovascular morphogenesis. J Clin Invest 116: 929–939.

71. Fischer A, Steidl C, Wagner TU, Lang E, Jakob PM, et al. (2007) Combined loss of Hey1 and HeyL causes congenital heart defects because of impaired epithelial to mesenchymal transition. Circ Res 100: 856–863.

72. Nakagawa O, Nakagawa M, Richardson JA, Olson EN, Srivastava D (1999) HRT1, HRT2, and HRT3: a new subclass of bHLH transcription factors marking specific cardiac, somitic, and pharyngeal arch segments. Dev Biol 216: 72–84.

73. Leimeister C, Externbrink A, Klamt B, Gessler M (1999) Hey genes: a novel subfamily of hairy- and Enhancer of split related genes specifically expressed during mouse embryogenesis. Mech Dev 85: 173–177.

74. Loomes KM, Underkoffler LA, Morabito J, Gottlieb S, Piccoli DA, et al. (1999) The expression of Jagged1 in the developing mammalian heart correlates with cardiovascular disease in Alagille syndrome. Hum Mol Genet 8: 2443–2449.

75. Zhang T, Liu J, Zhang J, Thekkethottiyil EB, Macatee TL, et al. (2013) Jun is required in Isl1-expressing progenitor cells for cardiovascular development. PLoS One 8: e57032.

76. Baek ST, Tallquist MD (2012) Nf1 limits epicardial derivative expansion by regulating epithelial to mesenchymal transition and proliferation. Development 139: 2040–2049.

77. Gammill LS, Gonzalez C, Bronner-Fraser M (2007) Neuropilin 2/semaphorin 3F signaling is essential for cranial neural crest migration and trigeminal ganglion condensation. Dev Neurobiol 67: 47–56.

78. Gammill LS, Gonzalez C, Gu C, Bronner-Fraser M (2006) Guidance of trunk neural crest migration requires neuropilin 2/semaphorin 3F signaling. Development 133: 99–106.

79. Lee MK, Slunt HH, Martin LJ, Thinakaran G, Kim G, et al. (1996) Expression of presenilin 1 and 2 (PS1 and PS2) in human and murine tissues. J Neurosci 16: 7513–7525.

80. Nakajima M, Moriizumi E, Koseki H, Shirasawa T (2004) Presenilin 1 is essential for cardiac morphogenesis. Dev Dyn 230: 795–799.

81. Mollard R, Viville S, Ward SJ, Decimo D, Chambon P, et al. (2000) Tissue-specific expression of retinoic acid receptor isoform transcripts in the mouse embryo. Mech Dev 94: 223–232.

82. Dolle P, Fraulob V, Kastner P, Chambon P (1994) Developmental expression of murine retinoid X receptor (RXR) genes. Mech Dev 45: 91–104.

83. Ya J, Schilham MW, de Boer PA, Moorman AF, Clevers H, et al. (1998) Sox4-deficiency syndrome in mice is an animal model for common trunk. Circ Res 83: 986–994.

84. Roelen BA, Lin HY, Knezevic V, Freund E, Mummery CL (1994) Expression of TGF-beta s and their receptors during implantation and organogenesis of the mouse embryo. Dev Biol 166: 716–728.

85. Wang YQ, Sizeland A, Wang XF, Sassoon D (1995) Restricted expression of type-II TGF beta receptor in murine embryonic development suggests a central role in tissue modeling and CNS patterning. Mech Dev 52: 275–289.

86. Mariano JM, Montuenga LM, Prentice MA, Cuttitta F, Jakowlew SB (1998) Concurrent and distinct transcription and translation of transforming growth factor-beta type I and type II receptors in rodent embryogenesis. Int J Dev Biol 42: 1125–1136.

87. Iruela-Arispe ML, Liska DJ, Sage EH, Bornstein P (1993) Differential expression of thrombospondin 1, 2, and 3 during murine development. Dev Dyn 197: 40–56.

88. Bentham J, Bhattacharya S (2008) Genetic mechanisms controlling cardiovascular development. Ann N Y Acad Sci 1123: 10–19.

89. Bard-Chapeau EA, Jeyakani J, Kok CH, Muller J, Chua BQ, et al. (2012) Ecotopic viral integration site 1 (EVI1) regulates multiple cellular processes important for cancer and is a synergistic partner for FOS protein in invasive tumors. Proc Natl Acad Sci U S A 109: 2168–2173.

18

Replication of the 4p16 Susceptibility Locus in Congenital Heart Disease in Han Chinese Populations

Bijun Zhao[1,9], **Yuan Lin**[2,3,9], **Jing Xu**[4], **Bixian Ni**[3], **Min Da**[5], **Chenyue Ding**[6], **Yuanli Hu**[5], **Kai Zhang**[2,3], **Shiwei Yang**[7], **Xiaowei Wang**[4], **Shiqiang Yu**[1], **Yijiang Chen**[4], **Xuming Mo**[5], **Jiayin Liu**[2,6], **Hongbing Shen**[2,3], **Jiahao Sha**[2,8], **Hongxia Ma**[3]*

1 Department of Cardiovascular Surgery, Xijing Hospital, The Fourth Military Medical University, Xi'an, China, **2** State Key Laboratory of Reproductive Medicine, Nanjing Medical University, Nanjing, China, **3** Department of Epidemiology and Biostatistics and Key Laboratory of Modern Toxicology of Ministry of Education, School of Public Health, Nanjing Medical University, Nanjing, China, **4** Department of Thoracic and Cardiovascular Surgery, The First Affiliated Hospital of Nanjing Medical University, Nanjing, China, **5** Department of Cardiothoracic Surgery, Nanjing Children's Hospital, Nanjing Medical University, Nanjing, China, **6** Center of Clinical Reproductive Medicine, First Affiliated Hospital, Nanjing Medical University, Nanjing, China, **7** Department of Cardiology, Nanjing Children's Hospital, Nanjing Medical University, Nanjing, China, **8** Department of Histology and Embryology, Nanjing Medical University, Nanjing, China

Abstract

Congenital heart disease (CHD) is the most common form of congenital human birth anomalies and a leading cause of perinatal and infant mortality. Some studies including our published genome-wide association study (GWAS) of CHD have indicated that genetic variants may contribute to the risk of CHD. Recently, Cordell *et al.* published a GWAS of multiple CHD phenotypes in European Caucasians and identified 3 susceptibility loci (rs870142, rs16835979 and rs6824295) for ostium secundum atrial septal defect (ASD) at chromosome 4p16. However, whether these loci at 4p16 confer the predisposition to CHD in Chinese population is unclear. In the current study, we first analyzed the associations between these 3 single nucleotide polymorphisms (SNPs) at 4p16 and CHD risk by using our existing genome-wide scan data and found all of the 3 SNPs showed significant associations with ASD in the same direction as that observed in Cordell's study, but not with other subtypes- ventricular septal defect (VSD) and ASD combined VSD. As these 3 SNPs were in high linkage disequilibrium (LD) in Chinese population, we selected one SNP with the lowest P value in our GWAS scan (rs16835979) to perform a replication study with additional 1,709 CHD cases with multiple phenotypes and 1,962 controls. The significant association was also observed only within the ASD subgroup, which was heterogeneous from other disease groups. In combined GWAS and replication samples, the minor allele of rs16835979 remained significant association with the risk of ASD (OR = 1.22, 95% CI = 1.08–1.38, P = 0.001). Our findings suggest that susceptibility loci of ASD identified from Cordell's European GWAS are generalizable to Chinese population, and such investigation may provide new insights into the roles of genetic variants in the etiology of different CHD phenotypes.

Editor: Kelvin Yuen Kwong Chan, Hospital Authority, China

Funding: This work was supported by the following sources: National Key Basic Research Program Grant (2011CB944300, 2013CB911400 and 2012CB944902), the National Science Foundation for Distinguished Young Scholars of China (81225020), the New Century Excellent Talents in University (NCET-10-0178), the Organization Department of the CPC Central Committee, the Jiangsu Outstanding Youth Science Foundation (BK2012042), Jiangsu Province Clinical Science and Technology Projects (BL2012008), the Priority Academic Program for the Development of Jiangsu Higher Education Institutions (Public Health and Preventive Medicine) and Collaborative Innovation Center For Cancer Personalized Medicine in Jiangsu Province. The funders had no role in study design, data collection and analysis, decision to publish, or preparation of the manuscript.

Competing Interests: The authors have declared that no competing interests exist.

* Email: hongxiama@njmu.edu.cn

⑨ These authors contributed equally to this work.

Introduction

Congenital heart disease (CHD) usually refers to abnormalities in the heart's structure or function that arise before birth [1]. As the most frequent birth defect, CHD affects about 0.8% of live births [2,3], and it is also a leading cause of perinatal and infant mortality, causing more than 220,000 deaths globally every year [4]. In China, epidemiological studies suggest an obvious increasing trend of CHD mortality with the overall mortality rate increasing from 141 in 2003 to 229 in 2010 per 10,000,000 person-years [5]. CHD can be classified into three broad categories: cyanotic heart disease, left-sided obstruction defects and septation defects [1]. Among them, septation defects are most common and can affect septation of the atria (atrial septal defect, ASD), septation of the ventricle (ventricular septal defect, VSD) or formation of structures in the central part of the heart (atrioventricular septal defect, AVSD) [1]. CHD may occur as part of recognized chromosomal and Mendelian syndromes [6,7]; however, it manifests as a non-syndromic, non-Mendelian condition in 80% of cases and may result from a multifactorial inheritance model that involves environmental factors and genetic predisposition [8]. In the past years, several genes linked to CHD have been identified, including T-box transcription factors (*TBX1*, *TBX5* and *TBX20*), homobox transcription factors (*NKX2.5* and *NKX2.6*), basic helix-loop-helix transcription factors (*HAND1* and *HAND2*), and GATA binding protein 4 (*GATA4*) [9].

More recently, genome-wide association studies (GWAS) have emerged as a powerful tool to identify novel susceptibility loci or genes of disease [10]. In May 2013, our research group conducted a GWA scan with 945 patients of ASD, VSD and ASD combined VSD cases and 1,246 non-CHD controls, followed by a two-stage validation with 2,160 ASD, VSD and ASD combined VSD cases and 3,866 controls [11]. We identified 2 loci at 1p12 (rs2474937 near $TBX15$ gene, odds ratio (OR) = 1.40, $P = 8.44 \times 10^{-10}$) and 4q31.1 (rs1531070 in $MAML3$ gene, OR = 1.40, $P = 4.99 \times 10^{-12}$) associated with CHD significantly ($P < 5.0 \times 10^{-8}$). However, these variants may represent only a very small proportion of SNPs contributing to CHD risk because of the strict criteria of the GWAS significance level ($P = 10^{-7}$ or $P = 10^{-8}$). Simultaneously, a GWAS of multiple CHD phenotypes in European Caucasians was conducted by Cordell et al. In that GWAS, when all CHD phenotypes were considered together, no region achieved genome-wide significant association. However, 3 SNPs were identified to be associated with ASD risk significantly after the stratification analysis was performed in different diagnostic groups (rs870142, $P_{combined} = 2.61 \times 10^{-10}$, odds ratio (OR) = 1.456; rs16835979, $P_{combined} = 2.94 \times 10^{-10}$, OR = 1.452 and rs6824295, $P_{combined} = 9.73 \times 10^{-10}$, OR = 1.437) [12]. However, it is uncertain whether these associations could be applicable to diverse populations. Therefore, we first investigated the association between the 3 SNPs (rs870142, rs16835979 and rs6824295) and CHD risk by using our existing genome-wide scan data and then performed a replication study with additional 1,709 CHD cases with multiple phenotypes and 1,962 controls.

Materials and Methods

Ethics Statement

This study was approved by the institutional review board of Nanjing Medical University. The design and performance of current study involving human subjects were clearly described in a research protocol. All participants over the age of 18 would complete the informed consent in writing before taking part in this research. For the participants under the age of 18, parental written consent was obtained.

Study populations

Study population of GWAS scan has been described previously [11]. For the replication stage, 1,709 CHD cases and 1,962 controls were recruited from the First Affiliated Hospital of Nanjing Medical University and the Affiliated Nanjing Children's Hospital of Nanjing Medical University, Nanjing, China, between March 2009 and May 2013. CHD were diagnosed based on echocardiography, some of which were further confirmed by cardiac catheterization and/or surgery. Cases that had clinical features of developmental syndromes, multiple major developmental anomalies or known chromosomal abnormalities were excluded. Exclusion criteria also included a positive family history of CHD in a first-degree relative (parents, siblings and children), maternal diabetes mellitus, phenylketonuria, maternal teratogen exposures (e.g., pesticides and organic solvents), and maternal therapeutic drugs exposures during the intrauterine period. Controls were non-CHD outpatients from the same geographic areas. They were recruited from the hospitals listed above during the same time period. Controls with congenital anomalies or cardiac disease were excluded. For each participant, approximately 2-ml whole blood was obtained to extract genomic DNA for genotyping analysis.

Quality control for GWAS scan and genotyping of replication study

The GWA scan was conducted using Illumina Omni zhonghua chips followed by a systematic quality control before association analysis [11]. In brief, we removed samples with low call rates, ambiguous gender, familial relationships, and extreme heterozygosity rate. We also detected population outliers and stratification using a PCA-based method. Our PCA analysis showed that the cases and controls were genetically matched, and the genomic control inflation factor (λ) was 1.065 [11]. SNPs were excluded if they are not mapped on autosomal chromosomes, or have a call rate <95%, minor allele frequency (MAF)<0.05 or $P < 1.00 \times 10^{-5}$ for Hardy-Weinberg equilibrium. After quality control procedures, a total of 708,275 SNPs in 945 CHD cases and 1,246 controls were included in the final GWA analysis [11]. The genotyping analyses in the replication study were performed by using the TaqMan allelic discrimination Assay (Applied Biosystems, Inc, USA). The information of the primers and probes were provided in **Table 1**. A series of methods were used to control the quality of genotyping: (i) case and control samples were mixed on each plate; (ii) genotyping was performed without knowing the case or control status; (iii) two water controls were used in each plate as blank control; (iv) five percent of the samples were randomly selected for repeat genotyping. The accurate concordance rate of genotyping for the SNP rs16835979 was 100.00% in the replication stage.

Statistical analysis

Population structure was evaluated by PCA as implemented in the software package EIGENSTRAT 3.1. The significant ($P < 0.05$) top eigenvector was included in the logistic regression model as a covariate for genetic association analysis [11]. Hardy-Weinberg equilibrium was evaluated using the $\chi 2$ test in all of the controls. The genome-wide association analysis was performed using an additive model in a logistic regression analysis in PLINK 1.07 (http://pngu.mgh.harvard.edu/~purcell/plink/). The statistical significance was declared at $\alpha = 0.05$. P values were two-sided, and ORs were estimated with an additive model by logistic regression analyses. The linkage disequilibrium (LD) analysis of the 3 SNPs (rs870142, rs16835979 and rs6824295) was performed in the controls of GWAS by using PLINK 1.07. Other analyses were performed using Stata version 9.2 (StataCorp LP, TX). The Chi-squared based Cochran's Q statistic was calculated to test for heterogeneity between groups in stratified analysis. We used inverse-variance-weighted model for meta-analysis when performing combined analysis. Random-effects model was used when heterogeneity between studies exists, that is, P value for heterogeneity test was less than 0.05; otherwise, fixed-effect model was used.

Results

The characteristics of the 945 CHD cases and the 1,246 non-CHD controls in GWA scan have been described previously [11]. Moreover, selected characteristics of the 1,709 cases and 1,962 non-CHD controls in the replication study were shown in **Table 2** and there were similar distributions of age and sex between cases and controls ($P = 0.221$ and 0.870, respectively).

The genotype distributions of these 3 SNPs in cases and controls of GWA scan were shown in **Table 3**. The observed genotype frequencies were all in Hardy-Weinberg equilibrium in controls ($P = 0.337$ for rs870142, $P = 0.370$ for rs16835979 and $P = 0.385$ for rs6824295). Logistic regression analyses showed that no obvious associations were found between the 3 SNPs and overall

Table 1. Primers and probes of rs16835979.

rs16835979	
F-primer	TGTGGACTCTAGAATGGACTTCCA
R-primer	TGTCAGATTAGGACCATCTCCATCT
FAM-probe	FAM-AGTGACTTTACTGTCCTC-MGB
HEX-probe	HEX-AAGTGACTTTAATGTCC-MGB

risk of CHD in an additive model (**Table 3**). Then, we performed stratification analysis by different diagnostic groups (ASD, VSD and ASD combined VSD) and found that all 3 SNPs showed significant associations with ASD risk (N = 334 cases) in the same direction as that observed in Cordell's study (rs870142: OR = 1.24, 95% CI = 1.04–1.49, $P = 0.016$; rs16835979: OR = 1.25, 95% CI = 1.05–1.50, $P = 0.014$; rs6824295: OR = 1.24, 95% CI = 1.04–1.48, $P = 0.019$). However, no significant association was observed in the other two disease groups (**Table 3**).

As these 3 SNPs were in high LD ($r^2 = 0.86$–0.99) in Chinese population, we selected one SNP with the lowest P value in our GWAS scan (rs16835979) to perform a replication study with additional 1,709 CHD cases of multiple phenotypes (ASD: N = 367; VSD: N = 432, Tetralogy of Fallot (TOF): N = 211, other CHDs: N = 699) and 1,962 controls. Similarly, no significant association was observed when all phenotypes were combined together. In the stratification analysis by disease groups, rs16835979 only showed significant association with the risk of ASD (OR = 1.20, 95% CI = 1.02–1.42, $P = 0.030$), which was heterogeneous from the other subgroups significantly (P for heterogeneity = 0.046) (**Table 4**). In combined GWAS and replication samples, the minor allele of rs16835979 remained significantly associated with ASD risk (OR = 1.22, 95%CI = 1.08–1.38, $P = 0.001$) (**Table 5**).

Discussion

In this study, we attempted to replicate the 4p16 ASD susceptibility loci in Han Chinese population and found that our results were consistent with the results presented by Cordell *et al* to a certain extent. These findings suggest that the susceptibility loci

of diseases may have some similarities among different races and ethnicities.

In Cordell's study, 3 SNPs (rs870142, rs16835979 and rs6824295) were identified to be significantly associated with ASD risk [12]. We performed a LD analysis among the 3 SNPs by the online software of SNAP (http://www.broadinstitute.org/mpg/snap/ldsearchpw.php) and found strong LD between them ($r^2 = 0.89$ to 0.96) in CEU (CEPH- Utah residents with European ancestry). After evaluating the LD between the 3 SNPs in the controls of our GWAS samples, we found that they were also in high LD in Chinese populations ($r^2 = 0.86$–0.99). There were 28 other SNPs in the LD plot of the region containing the 3 mentioned SNPs (chr4:4665181-4698948) and we found that most SNPs were in high LD with the 3 SNPs in European population, while only about half of them were in high LD with the 3 SNPs in Chinese population. Although we included 701 ASD cases and 3,208 controls in this study (334 cases and 1,246 controls in our GWA scan and 367 ASD cases and 1,962 controls in the replication study), the sample size, especially the case sample size was relatively smaller compared to the original Cordell's GWAS. After performing multiple testing corrections with the Bonferroni single-step method (corrected α: 0.05/3 = 0.017), we found the SNPs rs870142 and rs16835979 remained association with ASD risk; however, the SNP rs6824295 lost its association with ASD. Given the high LD of the 3 SNPs, Bonferroni correction might be too strict. Additionally, owing to the genetic heterogeneity, the allele frequency of the SNP rs16835979 in both populations was different (Chinese population: MAF = 0.380 in cases, MAF = 0.334 in controls; European population: MAF = 0.314 in cases, MAF = 0.235 in controls) and the effect size in the current study was weaker than that in European population (OR = 1.22 in

Table 2. Characteristics of CHD cases in validation stage.

Variables	Case (N = 1,709)	Control (N = 1,962)	P
Age (mean ± SD)	3.21 ± 8.70	3.45 ± 7.93	0.221
Sex			
Male	738 (43.2%)	842 (42.9%)	0.870
Female	971 (56.8%)	1,120 (57.1%)	
Phenotype			
ASD	367		
VSD	432		
TOF	211		
Other CHDs	699		

ASD: ostium secundum atrial septal defect; VSD: ventricular septal defect; TOF: tetralogy of fallot; Other CHDs included patent ductus arteriosus, ebstein anomaly, double-chambered right ventricle, bicuspid aortic valve, aortic insufficiency, aortic stenosis, mitral insufficiency, rupture of valsalva sinus aneurysm, etc.
P-values were derived from the χ2 test for the categorical variable (sex) and t-test for the continuous variable (age).

Table 3. Associations of the 3 SNPs with CHD in our GWA scan.

Chr. (cytoband)	Position (bp)	SNP	Study	Cases[b]	Controls[b]	MAF[c] (Cases)	MAF[c] (Controls)	OR (95% CI)[d]	P[d]
4p16.2	4698948	rs870142 G/A[a]	Combined All (945 cases, 1,246 controls)	116/428/399	145/534/558	0.35	0.33	1.08 (0.95–1.22)	0.259
			ASD (334 cases, 1,246 controls)	45/164/123	145/534/558	0.38	0.33	**1.24 (1.04–1.49)**	**0.016**
			VSD (534 cases, 1,246 controls)	63/230/241	145/534/558	0.33	0.33	1.00 (0.86–1.17)	0.969
			ASD/VSD (77 cases, 1,246 controls)	8/34/35	145/534/558	0.32	0.33	0.97 (0.69–1.38)	0.876
4p16.2	4686177	rs16835979 C/A[a]	Combined All (945 cases, 1,246 controls)	116/426/396	144/536/560	0.35	0.33	1.08 (0.95–1.23)	0.212
			ASD (334 cases, 1,246 controls)	44/164/121	144/536/560	0.38	0.33	**1.25 (1.05–1.50)**	**0.014**
			VSD (534 cases, 1,246 controls)	64/228/241	144/536/560	0.33	0.33	1.01 (0.87–1.18)	0.896
			ASD/VSD (77 cases, 1,246 controls)	8/34/34	144/536/560	0.33	0.33	1.00 0.70–1.41	0.986
4p16.2	4665181	rs6824295 G/A[a]	Combined All (945 cases, 1,246 controls)	127/445/372	163/554/525	0.37	0.35	1.07 (0.94–1.21)	0.298
			ASD (334 cases, 1,246 controls)	46/177/111	163/554/525	0.40	0.35	**1.24 (1.04–1.48)**	**0.019**
			VSD (534 cases, 1,246 controls)	71/232/230	163/554/525	0.35	0.35	0.99 (0.85–1.15)	0.878
			ASD/VSD (77 cases, 1,246 controls)	10/36/31	163/554/525	0.36	0.35	1.05 (0.75–1.48)	0.765

[a] major/minor alleles.
[b] variant homozygote/heterozygote/wild type homozygote.
[c] minor allele frequency (MAF).
[d] OR and P were derived from logistic regression analysis in additive model adjusting for the first principal component in GWAS.

Table 4. Associations of rs16835979 with CHD in replication study.

Chr. (cytoband)	Position (bp)	SNP	Study	Cases[b]	Controls[b]	MAF[c] (Cases)	MAF[c] (Controls)	OR (95% CI)[d]	p[d]	p[f]
4p16.2	4686177	rs16835979 C/A[a]	ASD (367 cases, 1,962 controls)	52/165/139	215/888/859	0.38	0.34	**1.20 (1.02–1.42)**	**0.030**	0.046
			VSD (432 cases, 1,962 controls)	56/178/187	215/888/859	0.34	0.34	1.04 (0.89–1.22)	0.635	
			TOF (211 cases, 1,962 controls)	23/76/110	215/888/859	0.29	0.34	0.81 (0.65–1.02)	0.070	
			Other CHDs (699 cases, 1,962 controls)	91/312/287	215/888/859	0.36	0.34	1.10 (0.97–1.26)	0.136	
			Combined subjects[e] (1,709 cases, 1,962 controls)	222/731/723	215/888/859	0.35	0.34	1.05 (0.91–1.20)	0.521	

[a] major/minor alleles.
[b] variant homozygote/Heterozygote/Wild type homozygote.
[c] minor allele frequency (MAF).
[d] estimated in additive model.
[e] combined via random-effects meta-analysis.
[f] P values for heterogeneity test between groups.

Table 5. Associations of rs16835979 with ASD.

Chr. (cytoband)	Position (bp)	SNP	Study	Cases[b]	Controls[b]	MAF[c] (Cases)	MAF[c] (Controls)	OR (95% CI)[d]	p[d]	p[f]
4p16.2	4686177	rs16835979 C/A[a]	**GWAS** (334 ASD cases, 1,246 controls)	44/164/121	144/536/560	0.38	0.33	**1.25 (1.05–1.50)**	**0.014**	0.742
			Replication (367 ASD cases, 1,962 controls)	52/165/139	215/888/859	0.38	0.34	**1.20 (1.02–1.42)**	**0.030**	
			Combined analysis (combined via fixed-effects meta-analysis)	96/329/260	359/1424/1419	0.38	0.33	**1.22 (1.08–1.38)**	**0.001**	

[a] major/minor alleles.
[b] variant homozygote/heterozygote/wild type homozygote.
[c] minor allele frequency (MAF).
[d] estimated in additive model.
[e] P values for heterogeneity test between group.

Chinese population vs. OR = 1.46 in European population). Using Levin's formula [13], we also found that the population-attributable risk of ASD for the SNP rs16835979 was relatively lower in Chinese (7%) than that in Caucasian (9%).

All 3 SNPs locate within an intron of the noncoding RNA gene *LOC100507266* with unknown function. Meanwhile, they also lie in the 320-kb interval between *STX18* (syntaxin 18) and *MSX1* (msh homeobox 1) and locate upstream of both genes. The long non-coding RNA gene *LOC100507266* is known as *STX18* antisense RNA 1 (STX18-AS1). *STX18* is principally located in the endoplasmic reticulum, and it plays roles in transport between the endoplasmic reticulum and Golgi [14]; however, no data are available for its function in heart development. *MSX1* has been showed to be expressed in mesenchymal structures, including the limb buds, pharyngeal arches, neural crest, and endocardial cushions of the heart [15,16]. In Cordell's study, *MSX1* was showed to be expressed in the atrial septum during development, both in mouse and chick [12]. *MSX1* and *MSX2*, which belong to the highly conserved *Nk* family of homeobox genes, display overlapping expression patterns and redundant functions in multiple tissues and organs during vertebrate development [15,16]. The functions of *Msx1* and *Msx2* in endocardial activation prior to EMT via upregulation of *NFATc1* expression have been documented [15]. In addition, *Msx1* has a well-documented role as both a downstream effector and an upstream regulator of Bmp signaling. It has been implicated in regulating epithelial-mesenchymal transition (EMT) during cardiac valve and septa formation [15,17]. *Hand1* and *Hand2* are also candidate target genes regulated by *Msx1* and *Msx2* [18]. Since myocardi-um-specific *Hand1* deficiency leads to thickened atrioventricula (AV) valves, which is associated with impaired valve remodeling [19–21], decreasing *Hand1* expression in the *Msx1/2* double mutant AV myocardium may be associated with defects in remodeling of the AV cushions into mature valve leaflets [15]. In the mouse, loss both of Msx1 and Msx2 leads to a severe endocardial cushion and conotruncal defects [15,18]. In humans, mutations in *MSX1* cause orofacial clefting and tooth agenesis [22,23]. It is speculated that these 3 SNPs may affect the regulation of above genes and thus have associations with the

development of ASD; however, the specific mechanisms of the 3 SNPs affecting the risk of ASD still need to be further investigated.

Like Cordell's study, we did not observe genome-wide significant associations of 4p16 loci with overall CHD risk in our GWAS as well as replication study. The findings suggested that genetic etiology of CHD could have a considerable degree of phenotypic specificity, which was also identified by some recent studies [24,25]. For the various phenotypes of CHD originated from different part of heart, we believe different genetic factors are involved in their pathogenic process.

Interestingly, our previous GWAS has identified 2 susceptibility loci (rs2474937 at 1p12 and rs1531070 at 4q31.1) for CHD in Han Chinese. However, these variants may contribute to the risk of CHD through different pathways. As described previously, the SNP rs2474937 may affect the expression of *TBX15*, a member of T-box transcription factors that have key roles in the development of the embryonic mesoderm, including of the heart and skeleton. Another SNP rs1531070 is in a LD region overlapping the *MAML3* (mastermind-like 3) gene and mastermind (Mam) is one of the essential components of Notch signaling pathway. In the current study, we confirmed the ASD-specific association of SNP rs16835979 in Chinese. This SNP may influence *MSX1* (msh homeobox 1), which belongs to the highly conserved *Nk* family of homeobox genes. *MSX1* has functions in endocardial activation prior to epithelial-mesenchymal transition (EMT) as well as Bmp signaling. Thus, the findings in the current study supplemented the existing results of our GWAS.

In conclusion, we present evidence for association between the common SNP rs16835979 at 4p16 and the ASD-specific risk in Han Chinese, which extends Cordell's results in different populations and suggests that the susceptibility loci of disease indeed have some similarities among different races and ethnicities.

Author Contributions

Conceived and designed the experiments: HM JS HS JL. Performed the experiments: YL BN MD CD YH KZ. Analyzed the data: BZ YL. Contributed reagents/materials/analysis tools: JX YC XM S. Yang XW. Wrote the paper: BZ YL. Oversaw the study design: S. Yu JS HS JL. Contributed to interpretation of results: S. Yu JS HS JL.

References

1. Bruneau BG (2008) The developmental genetics of congenital heart disease. Nature 451: 943–948.

2. van der Linde D, Konings EE, Slager MA, Witsenburg M, Helbing WA, et al. (2011) Birth prevalence of congenital heart disease worldwide: a systematic review and meta-analysis. J Am Coll Cardiol 58: 2241–2247.

3. Reller MD, Strickland MJ, Riehle-Colarusso T, Mahle WT, Correa A (2008) Prevalence of congenital heart defects in metropolitan Atlanta, 1998–2005. J Pediatr 153: 807–813.

4. Lozano R, Naghavi M, Foreman K, Lim S, Shibuya K, et al. (2013) Global and regional mortality from 235 causes of death for 20 age groups in 1990 and 2010: a systematic analysis for the Global Burden of Disease Study 2010. Lancet 380: 2095–2128.

5. Hu Z, Yuan X, Rao K, Zheng Z, Hu S (2014) National trend in congenital heart disease mortality in China during 2003 to 2010: A population-based study. J Thorac Cardiovasc Surg 148: 596–602 e591.

6. Pierpont ME, Basson CT, Benson DW Jr, Gelb BD, Giglia TM, et al. (2007) Genetic basis for congenital heart defects: current knowledge: a scientific statement from the American Heart Association Congenital Cardiac Defects Committee, Council on Cardiovascular Disease in the Young: endorsed by the American Academy of Pediatrics. Circulation 115: 3015–3038.

7. Weismann CG, Gelb BD (2007) The genetics of congenital heart disease: a review of recent developments. Curr Opin Cardiol 22: 200–206.

8. Ware SM, Jefferies JL (2012) New Genetic Insights into Congenital Heart Disease. J Clin Exp Cardiolog S8.

9. Wessels MW, Willems PJ (2010) Genetic factors in non-syndromic congenital heart malformations. Clin Genet 78: 103–123.

10. Shen H, Jin G (2013) Human genome epidemiology, progress and future. J Biomed Res 27: 167–169.

11. Hu Z, Shi Y, Mo X, Xu J, Zhao B, et al. (2013) A genome-wide association study identifies two risk loci for congenital heart malformations in Han Chinese populations. Nat Genet 45: 818–821.

12. Cordell HJ, Bentham J, Topf A, Zelenika D, Heath S, et al. (2013) Genome-wide association study of multiple congenital heart disease phenotypes identifies a susceptibility locus for atrial septal defect at chromosome 4p16. Nat Genet 15: 822–824.

13. Rückinger S, von Kries R, Toschke AM (2009) An illustration of and programs estimating attributable fractions in large scale surveys considering multiple risk factors. BMC Med Res Methodol 9: 7.

14. Hatsuzawa K, Hirose H, Tani K, Yamamoto A, Scheller RH, et al. (2000) Syntaxin 18, a SNAP receptor that functions in the endoplasmic reticulum, intermediate compartment, and cis-Golgi vesicle trafficking. J Biol Chem 275: 13713–13720.

15. Chen YH, Ishii M, Sucov HM, Maxson RE Jr (2008) Msx1 and Msx2 are required for endothelial-mesenchymal transformation of the atrioventricular cushions and patterning of the atrioventricular myocardium. BMC Dev Biol 8: 75.

16. Davidson D (1995) The function and evolution of Msx genes: pointers and paradoxes. Trends Genet 11: 405–411.

17. Bei M, Maas R (1998) FGFs and BMP4 induce both Msx1-independent and Msx1-dependent signaling pathways in early tooth development. Development 125: 4325–4333.

18. Chen YH, Ishii M, Sun J, Sucov HM, Maxson RE Jr (2007) Msx1 and Msx2 regulate survival of secondary heart field precursors and post-migratory proliferation of cardiac neural crest in the outflow tract. Dev Biol 308: 421–437.

19. Iwamoto R, Mekada E (2006) ErbB and HB-EGF signaling in heart development and function. Cell Struct Funct 31: 1–14.

20. Jackson LF, Qiu TH, Sunnarborg SW, Chang A, Zhang C, et al. (2003) Defective valvulogenesis in HB-EGF and TACE-null mice is associated with aberrant BMP signaling. EMBO J 22: 2704–2716.

21. Schroeder JA, Jackson LF, Lee DC, Camenisch TD (2003) Form and function of developing heart valves: coordination by extracellular matrix and growth factor signaling. J Mol Med (Berl) 81: 392–403.

22. Blanco R, Chakraborty R, Barton SA, Carreno H, Paredes M, et al. (2001) Evidence of a sex-dependent association between the MSX1 locus and nonsyndromic cleft lip with or without cleft palate in the Chilean population. Hum Biol 73: 81–89.

23. Vastardis H, Karimbux N, Guthua SW, Seidman JG, Seidman CE (1996) A human MSX1 homeodomain missense mutation causes selective tooth agenesis. Nat Genet 13: 417–421.

24. Soemedi R, Topf A, Wilson IJ, Darlay R, Rahman T, et al. (2012) Phenotype-specific effect of chromosome 1q21.1 rearrangements and GJA5 duplications in 2436 congenital heart disease patients and 6760 controls. Hum Mol Genet 21: 1513–1520.

25. Ching YH, Ghosh TK, Cross SJ, Packham EA, Honeyman L, et al. (2005) Mutation in myosin heavy chain 6 causes atrial septal defect. Nat Genet 37: 423–428.

19

Impact of Sinogram Affirmed Iterative Reconstruction (SAFIRE) Algorithm on Image Quality with 70 kVp-Tube-Voltage Dual-Source CT Angiography in Children with Congenital Heart Disease

Pei Nie[1][9], Haiou Li[1][9], Yanhua Duan[1], Ximing Wang[1]*, Xiaopeng Ji[1], Zhaoping Cheng[1], Anbiao Wang[2], Jiuhong Chen[3]

1 Shandong Provincial Key Laboratory of Diagnosis and Treatment of Cardio-Cerebral Vascular Diseases, Shandong Medical Imaging Research Institute, Shandong University, Jinan, Shandong, China, 2 Department of Cardiovascular Surgery, Shandong Provincial Hospital, Jinan, Shandong, China, 3 CT Research Collaboration, Siemens Ltd. China, Beijing, China

Abstract

Purpose: To compare the image quality and diagnostic accuracy between sinogram affirmed iterative reconstruction (SAFIRE) algorithm and filtered back projection (FBP) reconstruction algorithm at 70 kVp-tube-voltage DSCT angiography in children with congenital heart disease (CHD).

Materials and Methods: Twenty-eight patients (mean age: 13 months; range: 2–48 months; male: 16; female: 12; mean weight: 8 kg) with CHD underwent 70 kVp DSCT angiography. Imaging data were reconstructed with both FBP and SAFIRE algorithms. Subjective image quality was evaluated on a five-point scale. The parameters of image noise, signal-to-noise ratio (SNR) and contrast-to-noise ratio (CNR) on the objective image quality were compared for the two reconstruction algorithms. Surgery was performed in 20 patients, whereas conventional cardiac angiography (CCA) was performed in 8 patients. The diagnostic accuracy was evaluated on the surgical and/or CCA findings. The effective radiation doses were calculated.

Results: Compared to FBP algorithm, SAFIRE algorithm had significantly higher scores for subjective image quality (P<0.05), and lower image noise (P<0.05) as well as higher SNR &CNR values (P<0.05). There was no significant difference in the diagnostic accuracy between the FBP and SAFIRE algorithm ($\chi^2 = 1.793$, P>0.05). The mean effective dose for 70 kVp DSCT angiography was 0.30±0.13 mSv.

Conclusions: The SAFIRE algorithm can significantly reduce image noise and improve the image quality at 70 kVp DSCT angiography for the assessment of CHD in children.

Editor: Carmen San Martin, Centro Nacional de Biotecnologia (CNB-CSIC), Spain

Funding: The authors have no support or funding to report.

Competing Interests: Jiuhong Chen is employed by CT Research Collaboration, Siemens Ltd. China. There are no patents, products in development or marketed products to declare.

* E-mail: Wangximing369@hotmail.com

[9] These authors contributed equally to this work.

Introduction

The recent innovations in multi-detector CT technology with improved spatial and temporal resolution have extended the application of cardiovascular imaging in the assessment of congenital heart disease (CHD) in children [1–6]. Radiation exposure delivered by CT is now of particular concern, especially in paediatric population. In contrast to adults, infants and children are more radiosensitive and have a longer life span to potentially develop radiation-induced carcinogenesis. The "ALARA" (as low as reasonable achievable) principle has to be considered thoroughly before each examination for children. Several dose reduction strategies, such as reduced tube voltage, automated tube current modulation, weight-adjusted tube current, minimization of z-axis coverage as well as use of the prospective ECG-triggering sequential mode and high-pitch mode, have been successfully implemented into paediatric cardiac CT angiography and have been shown to effectively lower the radiation dose [1–3,4–8].

Recently, the second generation DSCT system (Definition Flash, Siemens Healthcare, Forchheim, Germany) provides a new x-ray tube with a tube voltage of 70 kVp. Lowering the tube voltage can reduce the radiation dose and effectively increase the contrast enhancement [9–11]. Using iodine as contrast agent, it is shown that the fraction of photons in the energy range around the k-edge of iodine is the highest for a tube voltage of about 63 kVp. Therefore, a tube voltage between 60 kVp and 70 kVp is the best choice for CT angiography [12]. Although the 80 kVp setting is now routinely used for infants and small children CT examinations [3,4], using 70 kVp instead of 80 kVp should shift the mean photon energy of the x-ray beam closer to the k-edge of iodine and therefore improve the contrast between vessels and the surroundings. The downside of the low-tube-voltage technique is an increase in the image noise, which can be compensated by increasing the tube current and using the iterative reconstruction (IR) algorithm [13]. Gnant R et al. [14] demonstrated that neck CT at 70 kVp was feasible with 34% dose reduction compared to the standard protocol at 120 kVp.

Iterative reconstruction (IR) algorithms have been introduced to help reduce the quantum noise associated with the traditional filtered back projection (FBP) reconstruction algorithm. Recent studies have shown that IR algorithms, such as iterative reconstruction in image space (IRIS; Siemens), iDose (Philips), adaptive statistical iterative reconstruction (ASIR; GE Healthcare) and model-based iterative reconstruction (MBIR; GE Healthcare) etc. can improve the image quality and reduce image noise as well as radiation dose in comparison with FBP reconstruction algorithm [15–21]. Recently, a new IR algorithm- sinogram affirmed iterative reconstruction (SAFIRE; Siemens) has been introduced into clinical use. SAFIRE is a raw-data-based IR algorithm which compares reconstructed and measured data in the raw data domain and iteratively corrects the images [22–27]. Several studies have shown the benefit of SAFIRE algorithm for various clinical applications, including chest [22] and abdominal CT [23], as well as cardiac [24–26] and body CT angiography [27] with the improved image quality and image noise reduction which contributes to the radiation dose saving.

To the best of our knowledge, this is the first study to address the 70 kVp-tube-voltage combined with SAFIRE algorithm for paediatric cardiac DSCT angiography. The purpose of this study was to compare the image quality and diagnostic accuracy of 70 kVp-tube-voltage DSCT angiography in children with CHD by two different reconstruction techniques of sinogram affirmed iterative reconstruction (SAFIRE) algorithm and filtered back projection (FBP) reconstruction algorithm.

Materials and Methods

Patients

Our study received the approval from Shandong Medical Imaging Research Institute Ethics Board and written informed consent was obtained from the parents of all patients. In our institution, DSCT angiography is part of the cardiovascular assessment in patients with CHD besides transthoracic echocardiography.

Between January and October 2013, 34 consecutive patients with CHD referred for DSCT examinations were enrolled in this study. Exclusion criteria were nephropathy (n = 2) and hypersensitivity to iodinated contrast (n = 4). A total of 28 patients have been included in this study. All anomalies were confirmed by the surgical and/or the conventional cardiac angiography (CCA) findings. Surgery was performed in 20 patients, and CCA was performed in 8 patients.

DSCT protocol

All examinations were performed on a second generation DSCT scanner (Somatom Definition Flash, Siemens Healthcare, Forchheim, Germany). Short-term sedation was achieved with oral administration of chloral hydrate. All patients were free-breathing. The scan range was from the bottom of the heart to the thoracic inlet in a caudocranial direction.

Scanning parameters were as follows: 0.28 s gantry rotation time, $2\times64\times0.6$ mm detector collimation, a slice collimation $2\times128\times0.6$ mm by z-flying focal spot technique, 70 kV tube voltage and weight adapted setting for tube current (70–80 mAs/rotation for patients <5 kg body weight, 80–100 mAs/rotation for patients 5–10 kg body weight, 100–130 mAs/rotation for patients >10 kg body weight). In patients with a relatively regular heart rate, prospective ECG-triggered high-pitch spiral scan mode was used with a pitch of 3.4. Data was acquired at 10% of R-R interval in order to obtain a systolic acquisition window for the proximal segments of coronary arteries. In patients with an irregular heart rate, prospective ECG-triggering sequential scan mode was chosen. The acquisition window was set at 40%–40% of R-R interval.

Iodinated contrast medium (Schering Ultravist, Iopromide, 350 mg I/ml, Berlin, Germany) was injected via peripheral veins using a double-head power injector (Stellant; Medrad, Indianola, PA, USA) with a volume of 1.5 ml/kg body weight followed by a saline chaser of 1.0 ml/kg body weight. The interval from injection to data acquisition was set at 25 seconds. Injection rate was calculated with the total injected volume divided by 25 s. For example, a 6-kg baby would be injected with 9 ml of contrast medium and 6 ml saline at flow rate of 0.6 ml/s.

Image reconstruction

All datasets were reconstructed with both FBP and SAFIRE algorithms with a slice thickness of 0.75 mm and an increment of 0.5 mm. In SAFIRE algorithm, 5 presets (strength 1–5) can be adjusted for the level of noise reduction, 1 being the weakest and 5 being the strongest [22]. As recommended by the manufacturer, a medium strength of 3 was applied in all patients in this study. The medium smooth-tissue convolution kernel B26f and I26f were used in FBP and SAFIRE algorithms, respectively.

Image quality analysis

All images were assessed on the subjective and objective image quality with a MMWP (Multiple Modality Workplace, Siemen Healthcare, Forchheim, Germany). Images reconstructed with SAFIRE and FBP algorithms respectively were reviewed in random order. Two radiologists specified on cardiac imaging with more than 5 years' experience independently interpreted the image quality on axial, multiplanar reformation (MPR), maximum intensity projection (MIP) and volume rendering (VR) images.

Subjective image quality analysis regarding to graininess, sharpness and overall image quality was assessed using a 5-grade scoring system (5, excellent; 4, good; 3, adequate; 2, limited diagnostic value; 1, uninterpretable) [28]. For any disagreement between the two observers, consensus agreement was achieved.

The image noise, signal-to-noise ratio (SNR) and contrast-to-noise ratio (CNR) were evaluated as objective image quality parameters. The measurement was done on the 0.75 mm-thick axial images by one observer who was not involved in the subjective image quality evaluation. Regions of interest (ROIs) were drawn in the ascending aorta and the pulmonary trunk as large as the diameter of the lumen, carefully avoiding the vessel wall. The image noise was defined as the standard deviation of the attenuation value and the SNR and CNR were calculated according to the following equations: $SNR = mean\_vessel/SD\_fat$ and $CNR = (mean\_vessel- mean\_fat)/SD\_fat$, respectively, where mean_vessel is the mean CT value of the vessel, mean_fat is the mean CT value of the perivascular fat and SD is the standard deviation of ROI.

Diagnostic performance analysis

Blinded to the results of surgical and/or CCA findings, two radiologists who were not involved in image quality assessment evaluated all images in consensus. Both FBP and SAFIRE series were presented in random order. Using surgical and/or CCA findings as the reference standard, the diagnostic accuracy was calculated compared between FBP and SAFIRE algorithms.

Radiation dose estimations

The volume CT dose index (CTDIvol) and dose-length product (DLP) were obtained from the CT system after each examination. The effective radiation dose (mSv) was calculated from the DLP (mGy·cm) multiplied by 2 to adapt it to the 16-cm phantom (the DLP for the body surface area was given for a 32-cm phantom on the scan protocol). The corrected DLP value was then multiplied by the infant-specific conversion coefficients given for a 16-cm phantom: 0.039 mSv/[mGy·cm] for children up to 4 months, 0.026 mSv/[mGy·cm] between 4 months and 1 year of age, and 0.018 mSv/[mGy·cm] between 1 year and 6 years of age[29].

Statistics

Statistical analysis was performed with SPSS 17.0 software (SPSS, Chicago, IL, USA). Quantitative variables were described as means $\pm$ standard deviations, and categorical variables were given in frequencies or percentages. The subjective image quality scores were compared by using the Mann-Whitney U test. Interobserver agreement on grades of subjective image quality analysis was assessed by kappa statistics ($\kappa > 0.81$, excellent agreement; $\kappa = 0.61$–0.80, good agreement). The independent t test was performed to analyze the differences between the two groups regarding image noise, SNR and CNR. Comparative analysis of the diagnostic performance between FBP and SAFIRE algorithm was obtained by non-parametric chi–square test. $P < 0.05$ was considered statistically significant.

Results

All 28 patients underwent successful low-dose DSCT angiography. The patient demographics are given in Table 1. Prospective ECG-triggered high-pitch spiral scan mode was used in 14 patients; whereas prospective ECG-triggering sequential scan mode was applied in the other 14 patients.

Subjective image quality

The mean scores were significantly higher with SAFIRE algorithm than with FBP algorithm regarding to graininess,

sharpness and overall image quality (Table 2). Diagnostic images (images graded 3 or more) obtained with the SAFIRE algorithm (28/28) were more than those with the FBP algorithm (23/28). Interobserver agreement was good and excellent for FBP ($\kappa = 0.74$) and SAFIRE ($\kappa = 0.83$) series, respectively. Representative cases are shown in Figure 1 and Figure 2.

Objective image quality

The mean image noise in the ascending aorta and pulmonary trunk was significantly lower ($t = 7.1$ and 7.7 respectively, $P < 0.05$) with SAFIRE algorithm than with FBP algorithm. The mean SNR ($t = 4.7$ and 5.1 respectively, $P < 0.05$) and the mean CNR ($t = 4.5$ and 5.0 respectively, $P < 0.05$) in the ascending aorta and pulmonary trunk were significantly higher with SAFIRE algorithm than with FBP algorithm. The details of objective image quality evaluation are shown in Table 3 and Figure 3.

Diagnostic accuracy

A total of 78 separate cardiovascular anomalies were confirmed by surgical and/or CCA findings. The details on separate cardiovascular abnormalities are shown in Table 4. There was no significant difference in the diagnostic accuracy between the FBP and SAFIRE algorithm (98.68% and 99.62%, respectively; $\chi^2 = 1.793$, $P > 0.05$). Both FBP and SAFIRE series misdiagnosed one small atrial septal defect as normal. The FBP series failed to identify 3 cases of atrial septal defect, one ventricular septal defect, one pulmonary artery stenosis and one patent ductus arteriosus, while one small atrial septal defect was missed in SAFIRE series.

Radiation dose

Radiation dose of 70 kVp DSCT angiography is given in Table 1. The mean CTDIvol was 0.47 ± 0.27 mGy. The mean DLP was 6.11 ± 2.70 mGy·cm, corresponding to a mean estimated effective dose of 0.30 ± 0.13 mSv.

The CTDIvol ($t = 6.918$, $P < 0.05$), DLP ($t = 3.625$, $P < 0.05$) and the effective radiation dose ($t = 2.147$, $P < 0.05$) of the high-pitch group were lower than those of the sequential scanning group. The mean CTDIvol of the high-pitch group and the sequential scanning group was 0.26 ± 0.05 mGy and 0.69 ± 0.23 mGy. The mean DLP of the two groups was 4.57 ± 1.22 mGy·cm and 7.64 ± 2.92 mGy·cm, resulting in a mean estimated effective dose of 0.25 ± 0.07 mSv and 0.35 ± 0.16 mSv.

Discussion

The results from our study indicate the feasibility of 70 kVp-tube-voltage DSCT angiography in children with CHD. By applying SAFIRE algorithm with 70 kVp-tube-voltage CT examination, the image quality and diagnostic confidence were

Table 1. Patient demographics, CT acquisition parameters and radiation dose estimates.

Male sex, no. of patients (of total)	16(28)
Age (months), mean±SD	13.25±13.05 (range: 2–48)
Weight (kg), mean±SD	8.14±3.16 (range: 4–16)
Heart rate during scan (bmp), mean±SD	119.86±16.21 (range: 89–149)
Tube voltage (kVp)	70
Tube current (mAs), mean±SD	95.71±16.87 (range: 70–130)
CTDIvol (mGy), mean±SD	0.47±0.27 (range: 0.20–1.14)
DLP (mGy·cm), mean±SD	6.11±2.70 (range: 3–16)
Effective radiation dose (mSv), mean±SD	0.30±0.13 (range: 0.16–0.78)

Table 2. Subjective image quality assessment of filtered back projection (FBP) and sinogram affirmed iterative reconstruction algorithm (SAFIRE) series at 70 kVp dual-source CT (DSCT) angiography.

Subjective measure of image quality	Grade, mean±SD		P
	FBP	SAFIRE	
Graininess	2.82±0.77	3.89±0.74	<0.05
Sharpness	3.14±0.76	4.18±0.72	<0.05
Overall image quality	3.07±0.66	4.07±0.66	<0.05

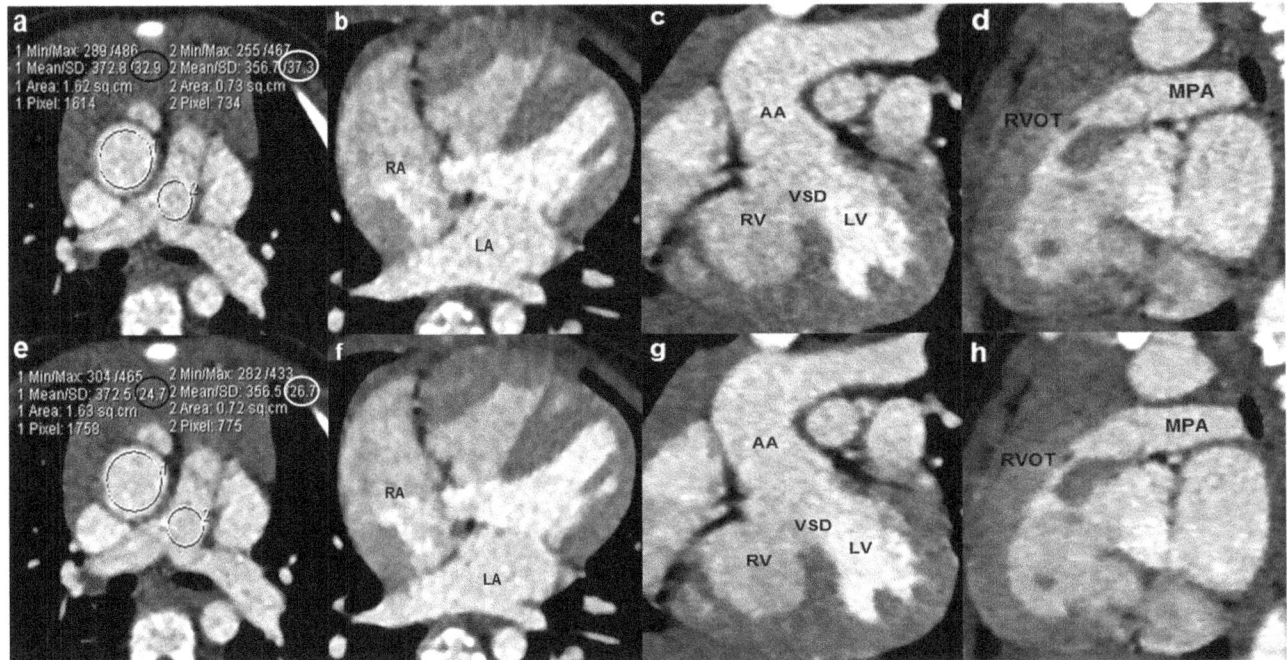

Figure 1. An 18-month boy with the diagnosis of Tetralogy of Fallot and atrial septal defect. The sequential DSCT angiography was performed with 70 kV and 100 mAs/rotation (effective radiation dose, 0.32 mSv). Axial images (a,e), multiplanar reformatted (MPR) images (b–d, f–h) using filtered back projection (FBP) algorithm (a–d) and sinogram affirmed iterative reconstruction (SAFIRE) algorithm (e–h) are shown. Image noise of the ascending aorta and pulmonary trunk which is expressed as the standard deviation (SD) of the attenuation (HU) in the regions of interest is significantly reduced in images reconstructed by SAFIRE (black and white circles in f) in contrast to FBP black and white circles in a). MPR images reconstructed with SAFIRE algorithm exhibit substantially reduced image noise and the improved image quality compared with images obtained with FBP. LA = left atrium, RA = right atrium, RV = right ventricle, LV = left ventricle, VSD = ventricular septal defect, AA = ascending aorta, RVOT = right ventricular outflow tract, MPA = main pulmonary artery.

maintained with significantly image noise reduction and low radiation dose of 0.30±0.13 mSv.

70 kVp-tube-voltage technique

Lowering the tube voltage has the advantage of higher vascular enhancement with a reduced radiation dose. Iodine attenuation increases as the tube voltage decreases because the mean photon energy moves closer to the k-absorption edge of iodine. With the introduction of a new x-ray tube, voltage as low as 70 kVp can now be applied. As the radiation dose is proportional to the square of the tube voltage, the 70 kVp-tube-voltage technique has the potential to further reduce the radiation dose.

Besides 70 kVp-tube-voltage technique, several dose-saving strategies were applied in our study including the adapted tube current to body weight, the prospective ECG-triggering sequential mode and high-pitch mode. Our previous studies [8] demonstrated that the high-pitch mode, in comparison with the sequential mode, further lowers the radiation dose. In this study, the effective

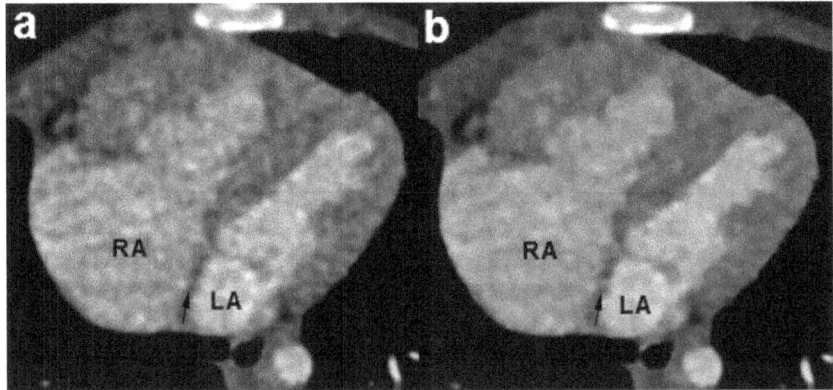

Figure 2. A 7-month girl with a small atrial septal defect. The sequential DSCT angiography was performed with 70 kV and 90 mAs/rotation (effective radiation dose, 0.21 mSv). Multiplanar reformatted (MPR) image reconstructed with sinogram affirmed iterative reconstruction (SAFIRE) algorithm (b) shows the small atrial septal defect (arrow) clearly. However, the lesion was missed on the MPR image using filtered back projection (FBP) algorithm (a). LA = left atrium, RA = right atrium.

Table 3. Image noise, signal-to-noise ratio (SNR) and contrast-to-noise ratio (CNR) in filtered back projection (FBP) and sinogram affirmed iterative reconstruction algorithm (SAFIRE) series at 70 kVp dual-source CT (DSCT) angiography.

Region of interest	Image noise (HU), mean±SD			SNR, mean±SD			CNR, mean±SD		
	FBP	SAFIRE	P	FBP	SAFIRE	P	FBP	SAFIRE	P
Ascending aorta	34.06±6.99	22.07±5.57	<0.05	17.16±7.11	28.33±10.28	<0.05	17.01±7.37	28.11±10.65	<0.05
Pulmonary trunk	32.85±5.78	21.55±5.23	<0.05	15.28±5.51	26.02±9.72	<0.05	15.14±5.65	25.80±9.78	<0.05

dose of high-pitch group and sequential scanning group was 0.25±0.07 mSv and 0.35±0.16 mSv, respectively. However, the high-pitch mode is not the only choice. Because when the indication of DSCT angiography is to evaluate the coronary artery abnormalities, the sequential mode would be recommended as the relatively poorer performance of the high-pitch mode on demonstrating coronary arteries in patients with irregular heart rate.

The downside of the 70 kVp-tube-voltage CT scanning is the increased image noise which may impair diagnostic confidence. To counterbalance the increased image noise, a higher tube current time product compared with our previous study [7,8] was used with the combination application of an iterative reconstruction algorithm.

Sinogram affirmed iterative reconstruction algorithm (SAFIRE)

Conventional CT image reconstruction such as FBP comprises a trade-off between sharpness and noise. Sharpness can only be increased at the expense of higher image noise, or vice versa, noise can only be reduced by decreasing sharpness. This trade-off limits the minimum radiation dose required for a specific diagnostic task since the lower radiation dose is associated with the increased image noise [22,25,27].

SAFIRE, as one recently introduced IR algorithm, represents an iterative optimization process that overcomes the constraint of FBP by using a noise modeling technique supported by the raw data with the aim of decoupling the relationship between sharpness and image noise [22-27]. There are two different correction loops in SAFIRE algorithm. The first loop occurs in the raw data space. After an initial reconstruction used FBP, the detected deviations are corrected by the repeated reconstruction with FBP to generate an updated image. A dynamic raw data-based noise modeling technique is used allowing for noise reduction without noticeable loss of sharpness. The second loop occurs in image space, where the noise is estimated and subtracted from the current dataset. The corrected image is compared with the original data leading to an update image, and added to the previous dataset before the next iteration is performed. This process is repeated a number of times, until the desired image is achieved. [23–25,27]

The benefits of SAFIRE algorithm for various clinical applications have been shown in previous studies [22–27]. In our study, the graininess, sharpness and overall image quality were significantly improved with SAFIRE, in the meanwhile, SAFIRE algorithm yielded a lower image noise and higher SNR and CNR than FBP algorithm. The diagnostic accuracy between FBP and SAFIRE algorithm was not significantly different by Han BK et al. [24], however, there was an incremental improvement in the detection of small atrial septal defect, ventricular septal defect, pulmonary artery stenosis and patent ductus arteriosus with SAFIRE algorithm compared to FBP from our results.

Our study has some limitations. First, a relatively small group of patients were enrolled, a large cohort of population are needed in the future study. Second, the 5 levels of iteration presets of SAFIRE (strength 1–5) associated with its ability of noise reduction were not compared. Third, the potential dose reduction of SAFIRE with 70 kVp tube voltage was not assessed. Last, the amount of contrast material was not considered in this study. Because tube voltage reduction increases the attenuation of iodinated contrast material, it may be possible to reduce the amount of contrast material administered with 70 kVp DSCT angiography.

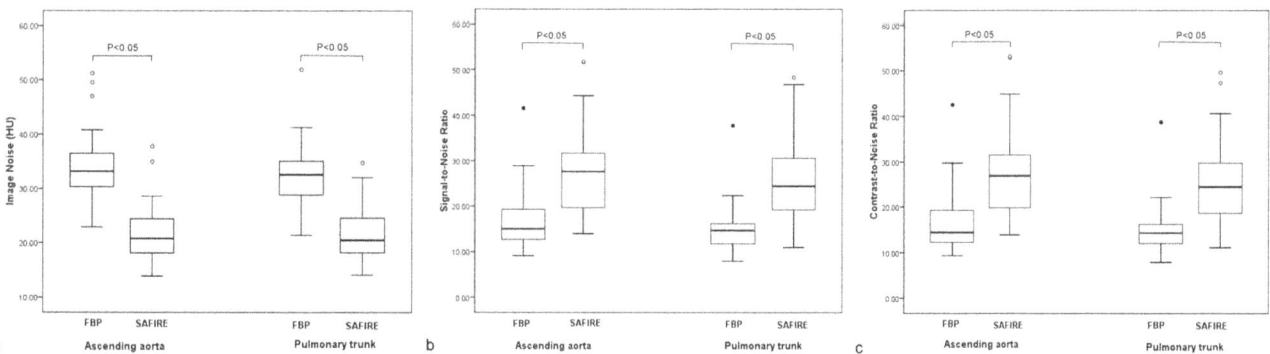

Figure 3. Box-and-whisker plots of objective analysis of image quality acquired with FBP and SAFIRE algorithms. Image noises of ascending aorta and pulmonary trunk were significantly lower with SAFIRE algorithm than with FBP algorithm (a). Signal-to-noise ratios and contrast-to-noise ratios of ascending aorta and pulmonary trunk were significantly higher with SAFIRE algorithm than with FBP algorithm (b,c). Center horizontal lines show median values and whiskers represent upper and lower quartiles. ○/● = outliners.

Table 4. Findings by filtered back projection (FBP) and sinogram affirmed iterative reconstruction algorithm (SAFIRE) series at 70 kVp dual-source CT (DSCT) angiography.

Cardiovascular deformities	FBP				SAFIRE				Surgical/CCA results
	TP	TN	FP	FN	TP	TN	FP	FN	
Atrial septal defect	5	19	1	3	7	19	1	1	8
Ventricular septal defect	12	15	0	1	13	15	0	0	13
Right ventricular outflow tract stenosis	3	25	0	0	3	25	0	0	3
Double outlet right ventricle	2	26	0	0	2	26	0	0	2
Pulmonary artery atresia	3	24	0	1	4	24	0	0	4
Pulmonary artery stenosis	3	25	0	0	3	25	0	0	3
Dilated pulmonary artery	3	25	0	0	3	25	0	0	3
Anomalous origin of pulmonary artery	1	27	0	0	1	27	0	0	1
Anomalous pulmonary venous return	2	26	0	0	2	26	0	0	2
Patent ductus arteriosus	8	19	0	1	9	19	0	0	9
Overriding aorta	5	23	0	0	5	23	0	0	5
Coarctation of the aorta	7	21	0	0	7	21	0	0	7
Interrupted aortic arch	1	27	0	0	1	27	0	0	1
Right aortic arch	4	24	0	0	4	24	0	0	4
Aortopulmonary window	1	27	0	0	1	27	0	0	1
Transposition of the great arteries	3	25	0	0	3	25	0	0	3
Major aortopulmonary collateral artery	3	25	0	0	3	25	0	0	3
Double superior vena cava	2	26	0	0	2	26	0	0	2
Coronary artery anomaly	4	24	0	0	4	24	0	0	4
Total	72	453	1	6	77	453	1	1	78

TP, true positive detection; TN, true negative detection; FP, false positive detection; FN, false negative detection.

In conclusion, the application of SAFIRE algorithm with 70 kVp DSCT angiography significantly reduces the image noise and improves the image quality in comparison with FBP algorithm. The combination of low-tube-voltage DSCT angiography with the SAFIRE algorithm in children with CHD is recommended.

Author Contributions

Conceived and designed the experiments: PN XW. Performed the experiments: PN HL YD XJ. Analyzed the data: HL AW. Contributed reagents/materials/analysis tools: ZC. Wrote the paper: PN. Provided technical support and polished the manuscript: JC.

References

1. Mahesh M. (2011) Advances in CT technology and application to pediatric imaging. Pediatr Radiol. 41 Suppl 2:493–497.
2. Siripornpitak S, Pornkul R, Khowsathit P, Layangool T, Promphan W, et al. (2011) Cardiac CT angiography in children with congenital heart disease. Eur J Radiol. doi.org/10.1016/j.ejrad.2011.11.042.
3. Paul JF, Rohnean A, Sigal-Cinqualbre A. (2010) Multidetector CT for congenital heart patients:what a paediatric radiologist should know. Pediatr Radiol. 40:869–875.
4. Young C, Taylor AM, Owens CM. (2011) Paediatric cardiac computed tomography: a review of imaging techniques and radiation dose consideration. Eur Radiol. 21:518–529.
5. Goo HW. (2010) State-of-the-art CT imaging techniques for congenital heart disease. Korean J Radiol. 11:4–18.
6. Goo HW. (2011) Cardiac MDCT in children: CT technology overview and interpretation. Radiol Clin North Am. 49:997–1010.
7. Cheng Z, Wang X, Duan Y, Wu L, Wu D, et al. (2010) Low-dose prospective ECG-triggering dual-source CT angiography in infants and children with complex congenital heart disease: first experience. Eur Radiol. 20:2503–2011.
8. Nie P, Wang X, Cheng Z, Ji X, Duan Y, et al. (2012) Accuracy, image quality and radiation dose comparison of high-pitch spiral and sequential acquisition on 128-slice dual-source CT angiography in children with congenital heart disease. Eur Radiol. 22:2057–2066.
9. Alkadhi H, Leschka S. (2011) Radiation dose of cardiac computed tomography - what has been achieved and what needs to be done. Eur Radiol. 21:505–509.
10. Alkadhi H, Schindera ST. (2011) State of the art low-dose CT angiography of the body. Eur J Radiol. 80:36–40.
11. Leschka S, Stolzmann P, Schmid FT, Scheffel H, Stinn B, et al. (2008) Low kilovoltage cardiac dual-source CT: attenuation, noise, and radiation dose. Eur Radiol. 18:1809–1817.
12. Bahner ML, Bengel A, Brix G, Zuna I, Kauczor HU, et al. (2005) Improved vascular opacification in cerebral computed tomography angiography with 80 kVp. Invest Radiol. 40:229–234.
13. Park EA, Lee W, Kim KW, Kim KG, Thomas A, et al. (2012) Iterative reconstruction of dual-source coronary CT angiography: assessment of image quality and radiation dose. Int J Cardiovasc Imaging. 28:1775–1786.
14. Gnannt R, Winklehner A, Goetti R, Schmidt B, Kollias S, et al. (2012) Low Kilovoltage CT of the Neck with 70 kVp: Comparison with a Standard Protocol. AJNR Am J Neuroradiol. 33:1014–1019.
15. Bittencourt MS, Schmidt B, Seltmann M, Muschiol G, Ropers D, et al. (2011) Iterative reconstruction in image space (IRIS) in cardiac computed tomography: initial experience. Int J Cardiovasc Imaging. 27:1081–1087.
16. Singh S, Kalra MK, Shenoy-Bhangle AS, Saini A, Gervais DA, et al. (2012) Radiation dose reduction with hybrid iterative reconstruction for pediatric CT. Radiology. 263:537–546.
17. Utsunomiya D, Weigold WG, Weissman G, Taylor AJ. (2012) Effect of hybrid iterative reconstruction technique on quantitative and qualitative image analysis at 256-slice prospective gating cardiac CT. Eur Radiol. 22:1287–1294.
18. Korn A, Fenchel M, Bender B, Danz S, Hauser TK, et al. (2012) Iterative reconstruction in head CT: image quality of routine and low-dose protocols in comparison with standard filtered back-projection. AJNR Am J Neuroradiol. 33:218–224.
19. Katsura M, Matsuda I, Akahane M, Sato J, Akai H, et al. (2012) Model-based iterative reconstruction technique for radiation dose reduction in chest CT:

comparison with the adaptive statistical iterative reconstruction technique. Eur Radiol. 22:1613–1623.

20. Marin D, Nelson RC, Schindera ST, Richard S, Youngblood RS, et al. (2010) Low-tube-voltage, high-tube-current multidetector abdominal CT: improved image quality and decreased radiation dose with adaptive statistical iterative reconstruction algorithm–initial clinical experience. Radiology. 254:145–153.

21. Ren Q, Dewan SK, Li M, Li J, Mao D, et al. (2012) Comparison of adaptive statistical iterative and filtered back projection reconstruction techniques in brain CT. Eur J Radiol. 81:2597–2601.

22. Baumueller S, Winklehner A, Karlo C, Goetti R, Flohr T, et al. (2012) Low-dose CT of the lung: potential value of iterative reconstructions. Eur Radiol. 22:2597–2606.

23. Kalra MK, Woisetschläger M, Dahlström N, Singh S, Lindblom M, et al. (2012) Radiation dose reduction with Sinogram Affirmed Iterative Reconstruction technique for abdominal computed tomography. J Comput Assist Tomogr. 36:339–346.

24. Han BK, Grant KL, Garberich R, Sedlmair M, Lindberg J, et al. (2012) Assessment of an iterative reconstruction algorithm (SAFIRE) on image quality in pediatric cardiac CT datasets. J Cardiovasc Comput Tomogr. 6:200–204.

25. Moscariello A, Takx RA, Schoepf UJ, Renker M, Zwerner PL, et al. (2011) Coronary CT angiography: image quality, diagnostic accuracy, and potential for radiation dose reduction using a novel iterative image reconstruction technique-comparison with traditional filtered back projection. Eur Radiol. 21:2130–2138.

26. Ebersberger U, Tricarico F, Schoepf UJ, Blanke P, Spears JR, et al. (2012) CT evaluation of coronary artery stents with iterative image reconstruction: improvements in image quality and potential for radiation dose reduction. Eur Radiol. doi 10.1007/s00330-012-2580-5.

27. Winklehner A, Karlo C, Puippe G, Schmidt B, Flohr T, et al. (2011) Raw data-based iterative reconstruction in body CTA: evaluation of radiation dose saving potential. Eur Radiol. 21:2521–2526.

28. Oda S, Utsunomiya D, Funama Y, Yonenaga K, Namimoto T, et al. (2012) A hybrid iterative reconstruction algorithm that improves the image quality of low-tube-voltage coronary CT angiography. AJR Am J Roentgenol. 198:1126–1131.

29. Pache G, Grohmann J, Bulla S, Arnold R, Stiller B, et al. (2011) Prospective electrocardiography-triggered CT angiography of the great thoracic vessels in infants and toddlers with congenital heart disease: Feasibility and image quality. Eur J Radiol. doi: 10.1016/j.ejrad.2011.01.032.

20

Characterization of Nodal/TGF-Lefty Signaling Pathway Gene Variants for Possible Roles in Congenital Heart Diseases

Xia Deng[1,9], Jing Zhou[2,9], Fei-Feng Li[1]*, Peng Yan[3], Er-Ying Zhao[1], Ling Hao[4], Kai-Jiang Yu[2]*, Shu-Lin Liu[1,5]*

1 Genomics Research Center (one of the State-Province Key Laboratory of Biopharmaceutical Engineering, China), Harbin Medical University, Harbin, China, **2** Intensive Care Unit, the Second Affiliated Hospital of Harbin Medical University, Harbin, China, **3** Department of Colorectal Surgery, the Second Affiliated Hospital of Harbin Medical University, Harbin, China, **4** Department of Oncology, the Fourth Affiliated Hospital of Harbin Medical University, Harbin, China, **5** Department of Microbiology and Infectious Diseases, University of Calgary, Calgary, Canada

Abstract

Background: Nodal/TGF-Lefty signaling pathway has important effects at early stages of differentiation of human embryonic stem cells in directing them to differentiate into different embryonic lineages. LEFTY, one of transforming growth factors in the Nodal/TGF-Lefty signaling pathway, plays an important role in the development of heart. The aim of this work was to find evidence on whether *Lefty* variations are associated with congenital heart diseases (CHD).

Methods: We sequenced the *Lefty* gene for 230 Chinese Han CHD patients and evaluated SNPs rs2295418, rs360057 and g.G169A, which are located within the translated regions of the genes. The statistical analyses were conducted using Chi-Square Tests as implemented in SPSS (version 13.0). The Hardy-Weinberg equilibrium test of the population was carried out using online software OEGE, and multiple-sequence alignments of LEFTY proteins were carried out using the Vector NTI software.

Results: Two heterozygous variants in *Lefty1* gene, g.G169A and g.A1035C, and one heterozygous variant in *Lefty2* gene, g.C925A, were identified. Statistical analyses showed that the rs2295418 (g.C925A) variant in *Lefty2* gene was obviously associated with the risk of CHD (P value = 0.016 < 0.05). The genotype frequency of rs360057 (g.A1035C) variant in *Lefty1* gene was associated with the risk of CHD (P value = 0.007 < 0.05), but the allele frequency was not (P value = 0.317 > 0.05).

Conclusions: The SNP rs2295418 in the *Lefty2* gene is associated with CHD in Chinese Han populations.

Editor: Reiner Albert Veitia, Institut Jacques Monod, France

Funding: This work was supported by a grant from Heilongjiang Innovation Research Foundation for Graduate Studies (YJSCX2012-199HLJ) to XD; a grant from Heilongjiang Province (ZD200917) to KJY; a grant from Pharmacy College of Harbin Medical University to FFL for training undergraduate students; and grants of National Natural Science Foundation of China (NSFC81271786, 81110378, 30970119, 81030029) to SLL. The funders had no role in study design, data collection and analysis, decision to publish, or preparation of the manuscript.

Competing Interests: The authors have declared that no competing interests exist.

* Email: drkaijiang@163.com (K-JY); lff-1981@163.com (F-FL); slliu@ucalgary.ca (S-LL)

9 These authors contributed equally to this work.

Introduction

Congenital heart diseases (CHD) are a group of common and complex illnesses with high morbidity and mortality. Despite the enormous advances in surgical treatments over the past decades, the genetic etiology is still largely unknown [1]. The incidence of moderate and severe forms of CHD is about 6/1,000 of live births. If tiny muscular ventricular septal defects and other trivial lesions are included, the total incidence is about 75/1,000 of live births [2]. For the CHD patients, about one percent would require intervention [3] and about thirteen percent show recognizable chromosomal variants [4]. Most adult CHD patients are predisposed to cardiac complications, such as coronary heart diseases, arrhythmias or heart failure [5]. Although extensive genetic studies and high-resolution technologies have revealed the genetic defects in many familiar and sporadic CHD cases [6,7], the genetic abnormalities in the majority of CHD patients remain largely unknown.

In the embryonic development, heart is the first formed organ, strictly controlled by gene regulatory networks, involving transcription factors, signaling pathways, epigenetic factors, and miRNAs [8,9]. During the last few decades, a variety of CHD-causing gene mutations have been identified, such as those in *CITED2* [10], *CFC1* [11], *GATA4* [12] and *TBX1* [13]. These genes play critical roles in cardiac development; mutations in these genes lead to cardiovascular malformations and contribute to

CHD [14]. Human embryonic stem (HES) cells may differentiate to various cell types and develop to different embryonic lineages, including those of ectoderm (neurons and epidermal cells), endoderm (hepatocytes and pancreatic cells), and mesoderm (muscle cells and cardiomyocytes cells) under the control of certain factors[15]. LEFTY negatively regulates the Nodal/TGF-Lefty signaling pathway [16] and inhibits cellular proliferation and differentiation [17,18]. It has been shown that when the Nodal/TGF-Lefty pathway goes wrong, serious malignant transformation may occur. In malignant melanoma cells, for example, LEFTY inhibits the malignant properties of melanoma cells [19] [20,21]. During the early differentiation of HES cells, LEFTY is expressed in a subset of cells, playing an important role in mesodermal cell differentiation [22]. The Nodal/TGF-Lefty signaling pathway also has an important effect in early stages of HES cell differentiation, directing specific cells into different embryonic lineages. LEFTY, as one of the important transforming growth factors in the Nodal/TGF-Lefty signaling pathway, inhibits the signaling of NODAL, which may play an important role in the development of heart.

To elucidate possible associations of *Lefty* genes with CHD, we analyzed the transcribed region and splicing sites of the *Lefty1* and *Lefty2* genes and compared the *Lefty* gene sequences between 230 Chinese Han CHD patients and 263 controls. We found that the rs2295418 (g.C925A) variant in the *Lefty2* gene was closely associated with the risk of CHD.

Materials and Methods

The study population

For this study, a total of 230 CHD patients and 263 control subjects with no reported cardiac phenotypes were recruited from Linyi People's Hospital and the Second Affiliated Hospital of Harbin Medical University, Harbin, China (Table 1). The 263 control subjects were enrolled at the Medical Examination Center of the Second Affiliated Hospital of Harbin Medical University. All these subjects had physical and electrocardiogram examinations and ultrasonic echocardiogram examination, and none of them showed any defects in the heart or other parts of the body. A written informed consent was obtained from each participant, and this work had been approved by the Ethics Committee of Harbin Medical University, consistent with the 1975 Declaration of Helsinki. Detailed records on their medical history, physical examination and chest X-ray examination, electrocardiogram, and ultrasonic echocardiogram were obtained. We deposited our data in the NIH Short Read Archive dataset, with the accession number SRP043439.

DNA analysis

Genomic DNA was extracted from peripheral blood leukocytes using standard protocols. The human *Lefty1* and *Lefty2* genes are located on 1q42.1 and are encoded by four exons. The four exons and the splicing sites of the two genes were amplified by polymerase chain reaction (PCR) with the primers shown in Table 2. PCR products were sequenced using the BigDye Terminator Cycle Sequencing kit (Applied Biosystems, Foster City, CA, USA) and the ABI 3130XL (Applied Biosystems) sequencer for mutational analysis.

Rs2295418, Rs360057 and g.G169A *Lefty* SNP genotyping analysis and Statistical methods

Genotypes of the rs2295418 and rs360057, g.G169A SNPs, within the *Lefty2* or *Lefty1* genes (Figure 1), were determined using two stage methods. We amplified rs2295418, rs360057 and g.G169A (Table 2, Lefty2exon4; Lefty1exon4 and exon1) and sequenced the PCR products to determine the genotype. The statistical analyses were conducted using Chi-Square Tests to calculate odds ratios and P value as implemented in SPSS (version 13.0). We also used online software OEGE to conduct the Hardy-Weinberg equilibrium test of the CHD and control population.

Multiple sequence alignments

From the NCBI website (http://www.ncbi.nlm.nih.gov/), the LEFTY protein sequences of various species were obtained, and using the Vector NTI software, multiple-sequence alignments of LEFTY proteins were carried out.

Results

Patients

Clinical diagnosis of the recruited patients was confirmed in Linyi People's Hospital and The Second Affiliated Hospital of Harbin Medical University. There was no history of other systemic abnormalities in these CHD patients, and their mothers did not have a history of taking medicines or attracting infections during pregnancy. The 230 CHD patients contained 12 pulmonary stenosis, 14 tetralogy of Fallot, 14 patent ductus arteriosus, 22 mitral valve insufficiency, 41 atrial septal defect, 95 ventricular septal defect and 32 other complex congenital heart diseases.

Lefty gene analysis

We sequenced *Lefty* to test the hypothesis that germline common genetic variants in *Lefty* may confer susceptibility to CHD. We first compared the transcribed region and splicing sites of *Lefty* and found two variations in the *Lefty1* gene [g.G169A (p.Arg33Gln) and g.A1035C-rs360057 (p.Asp322Ala)] and one variation in the *Lefty2* gene [g.C925A-rs2295418 (p.Pro286Leu)] in the CHD cases (Figure 1). These variations were located within the translated region of the genes, and the g.A1035C-rs360057 and g.C925A-rs2295418 variations were located within the transforming growth factor-β-like domain of LEFTY protein (Figure 2).

Rs2295418, Rs360057 and g.G169A Lefty SNP genotyping and Statistical analysis

To further test any possible associations between *Lefty* and CHD, we conducted SNP analyses and found that the rs2295418 (g.C925A) variant in *Lefty2* gene was obviously associated with the risk of CHD; the genotype frequency of the rs360057 (g.A1035C) variant in *Lefty1* gene was associated with the risk of CHD, but there was no statistical significance in the allele frequency. The g.G169A variant in *Lefty1* gene was not associated with the risk of CHD in the Chinese Han population (Tables 3, 4). We also conducted the Hardy-Weinberg equilibrium test for the CHD patients and controls and our results were in line with the Hardy-Weinberg equilibrium.

Table 1. Clinical characteristics of study population.

Parameter	CHD	Control
Sample (n)	230	263
Male/Female (n)	142/88	171/92
Age (years)	16.18±10.22	8.36±9.98

Data are shown as mean±SD.

Table 2. PCR primers used for Lefty sequence analysis.

Gene	Exon	Forward primer	Reverse primer	Size	Tm
LEFTY1	1	TGCCTGAGACCCTCCTGC	CCCTCACTCAGCCTCCCA	436	59.9
	2	TTTGCCCCAGAAATAGAACAGG	GACCCAGCGCCGCTTGAG	499	62.1
	3	CAACCGCACCTCCCTCAT	CATTCATTCCCACAGCACTC	513	59.2
	4	TAAATCTCCATCCCAGACGC	ACCCTCGAACACTTCAGAAACA	499	57.9
LEFTY2	1	CTCCCTCTTCCCTTCACCC	ACAGCCTCCCACAGAGTCCC	511	60.5
	2	GCCTGGCTGCCAGCTCAG	GACCCAGCGCCGCTTGAG	462	62.7
	3	CAACCGCACCTCCCTCATC	GCAATCGCTGGCATCCTG	570	61.7
	4	CCTCCCAGGTGCCCACTA	GGGATGGAGTAACTTGCTAA	549	56.5

Conservation of the protein in evolution

Comparison of the LEFTY1 and LEFTY2 protein sequences from species including birds, fishes and mammals by multiple-sequence alignment analysis showed that the 286Pro residue in LEFTY2 was highly conserved among the mammals but the 33Arg and 322Asp residues in LEFTY1 were just conserved in Chimpanzee and Humans (Figure 3).

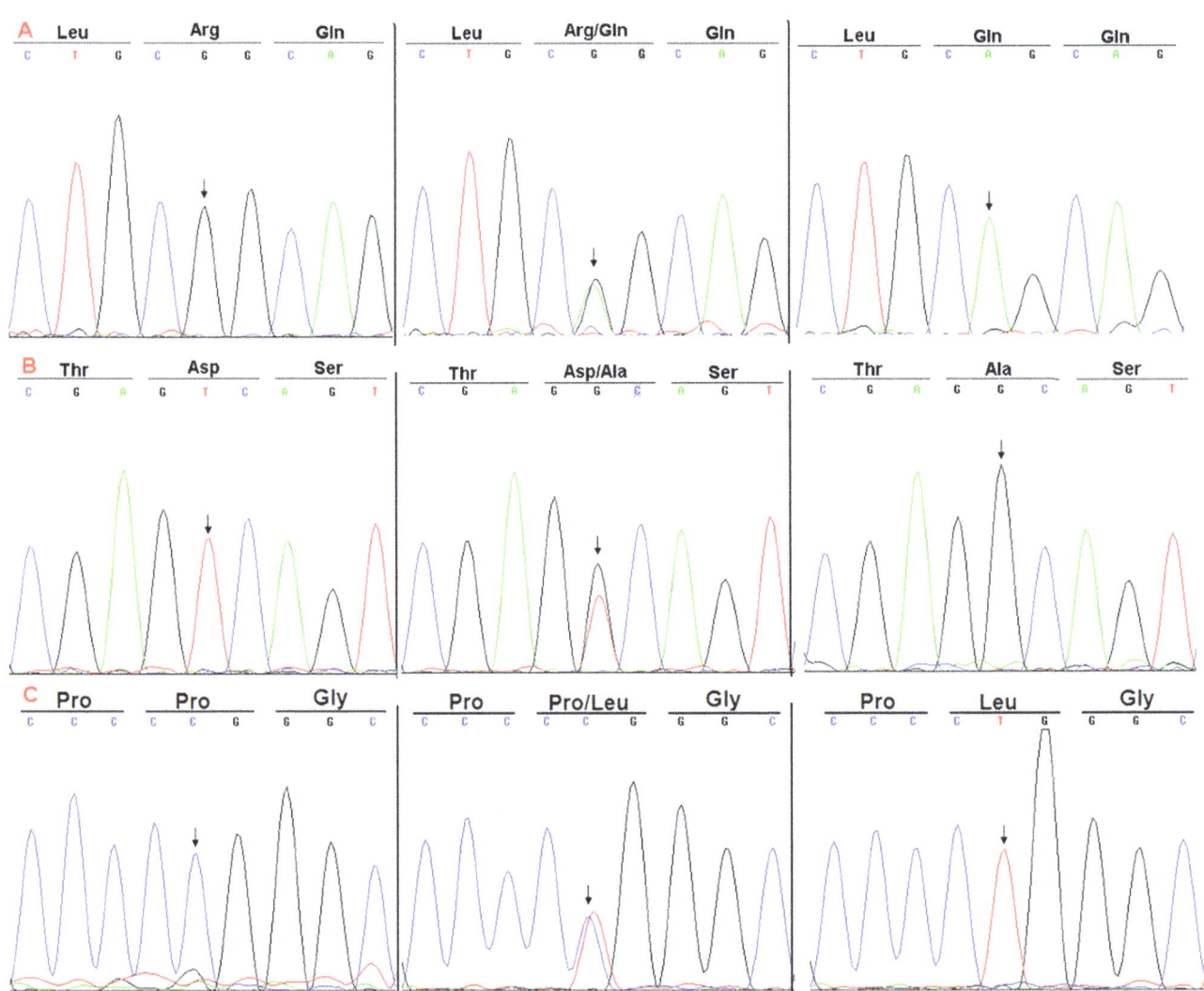

Figure 1. DNA sequence chromatograms of the *Lefty-1* and *Lefty -2* genes. A: g.G169A (p.Arg33Gln); B: g.A1035C-rs360057 (p.Asp322Ala); C: g.C925A-rs2295418 (p.Pro286Leu).

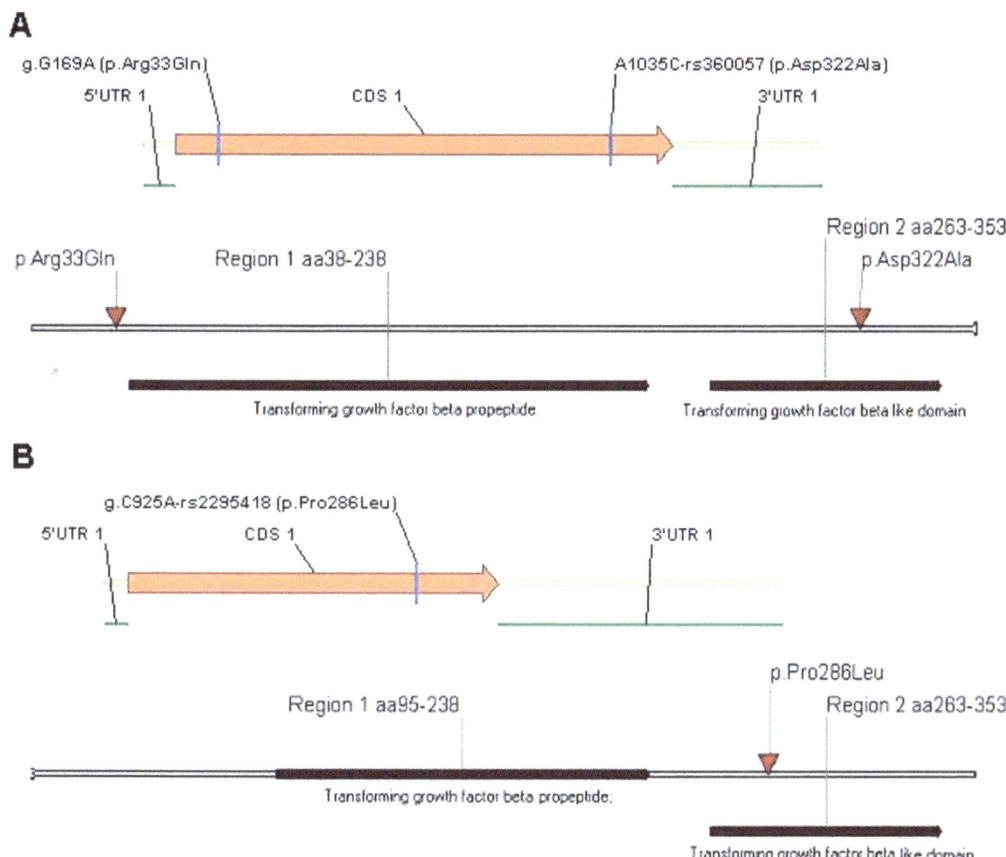

Figure 2. Schematic diagrams of rs2295418 and rs360057 locations within the translated region of *Lefty-2* and *Lefty -1* genes and transforming growth factor-β-like domain of the proteins. A: Lefty-1; B: Lefty-2.

Discussion

In this study, we analyzed the transcribed regions and splicing sites of the *Lefty* genes in large cohorts of CHD patients and controls and found that two variants, rs2295418 (g.C925A) and rs360057 (g.A1035C), were associated with the risk of CHD in the Chinese Han population, demonstrating the involvement of the *Lefty* genes in the CHD etiology.

The formation of the human heart starts on day 18 or 19 in the mesoderm after fertilization and involves strict temporal, spatial, and sequential gene expressions. Nodal/TGF-Lefty signaling pathway acts upon gastrulation, which develops to progenitor cells of the mesoderm and endoderm [22]. In mice, the formation of mesendoderm was affected by the expression level of Nodal/TGF-Lefty signaling pathway [23], and mutations in the Nodal gene can affect the formation of primitive streak, which is formed by mesendoderm progenitor cells. The vascular systems of the mouse arise from extraembryonic mesoderm that migrate through the primitive streak to the presumptive yolk sac [24]. At later stages of embryonic development, Nodal expression initiates a series of signal transduction and induces its own and *Lefty* gene expression, and the LEFTY negatively regulates the Nodal/TGF-Lefty signaling pathway [16,22].

We analyzed genes of the Nodal/TGF-Lefty signaling pathway, which has been demonstrated to play vital roles in mouse mesoderm differentiation and heart formation; such genes are also temporally expressed in the differentiation of the HES cells [22]. We here demonstrated that the rs2295418 (g.C925A) and the

rs360057 (g.A1035C) variants in *Lefty2* and *Lefty1* genes were associated with the risk of CHD in the Chinese Han population. These nucleotides were conserved only between Chimpanzee and man among the species compared. SNP-rs1904589 within the Nodal gene, which we also analyzed in the study, was not found to be significantly associated with the risk of CHD in the population (data not show).

Of great interest, although the translated regions of the two genes are 97.18% similar in nucleotide sequence, *Lefty2* plays a more central role in the mesoderm differentiation [25], which may at least partly explain why the rs2295418 variants in *Lefty2* gene were so closely associated with the risk of CHD. In contrast to *Lefty2*, *Lefty1* seems to be less involved: although the genotype frequency of the rs360057 variant in *Lefty1* gene was apparently associated with the risk of CHD, its allele frequency was not. Further work will be needed on the Nodal/TGF-Lefty signaling pathway for their involvement in the pathogenesis of CHD at the molecular level.

Acknowledgments

The authors thank the patients and family members for their cooperation and participation in this study.

Patient consent. Obtained.

Ethics approval. Ethics Committee of Harbin Medical University.

Table 3. The genotype and allele frequency of SNP rs2295418, rs360057 and g.G169A in 230 Chinese Han CHD patients and 263 non-CHD controls.

SNP	Group		Genotype frequency (%)			Allele frequency (%)	
rs2295418	Genotype		G/G	G/A	A/A	G	A
	CHD	230	173(75.2)	45(19.6)	12(5.2)	391(85.0)	69(15.0)
	Controls	263	223(84.8)	35(13.3)	5(1.9)	481(91.4)	45(8.6)
rs360057	Genotype		T/T	T/G	G/G	T	G
	CHD	230	148(64.3)	62(27.0)	20(8.7)	358(77.8)	102(22.2)
	Controls	263	167(63.5)	89(33.8)	7(2.7)	423(80.4)	103(19.6)
g.G169A	Genotype		G/G	G/A	A/A	G	A
	CHD	230	179(77.8)	47(20.4)	4(1.7)	405(88.0)	55(12.0)
	Controls	263	203(77.2)	56(21.3)	4(1.5)	462(87.8)	64(12.2)

Table 4. SNP rs2295418, rs360057 within Lefty-2 and Lefty-1 associated with the risk of congenital heart diseases in Chinese populations.

Genotyped SNP	Associated gene		Pearson Chi-square				Pearson's R			
			Value	Min count[a]	df	Asymp. Sig. (2-sided)	Value	Asymp. Std. error[b]	Approx. T[c]	Approx. Sig
rs2295418	LEFTY2	Genotype	8.274	7.93	2	0.016	−0.129	0.044	−2.893	0.004[d]
		Allele	9.968	53.18	1	0.002	−0.101	0.032	−3.170	0.002[d]
rs360057	LEFTY1	Genotype	10.069	12.60	2	0.007	−0.044	0.045	−0.966	0.334[d]
		Allele	1.001	95.64	1	0.317	−0.032	0.032	−1.000	0.318[d]
g.G169A	LEFTY1	Genotype	0.086	3.73	2	0.958	0.005	0.045	0.100	0.920[d]
		Allele	0.010	55.52	1	0.919	0.003	0.032	0.101	0.919[d]

a: The minimum expected count;
b: Not assuming the null hypothesis;
c: Using the asymptotic standard error assuming the null hypothesis;
d: Based on normal approximation.

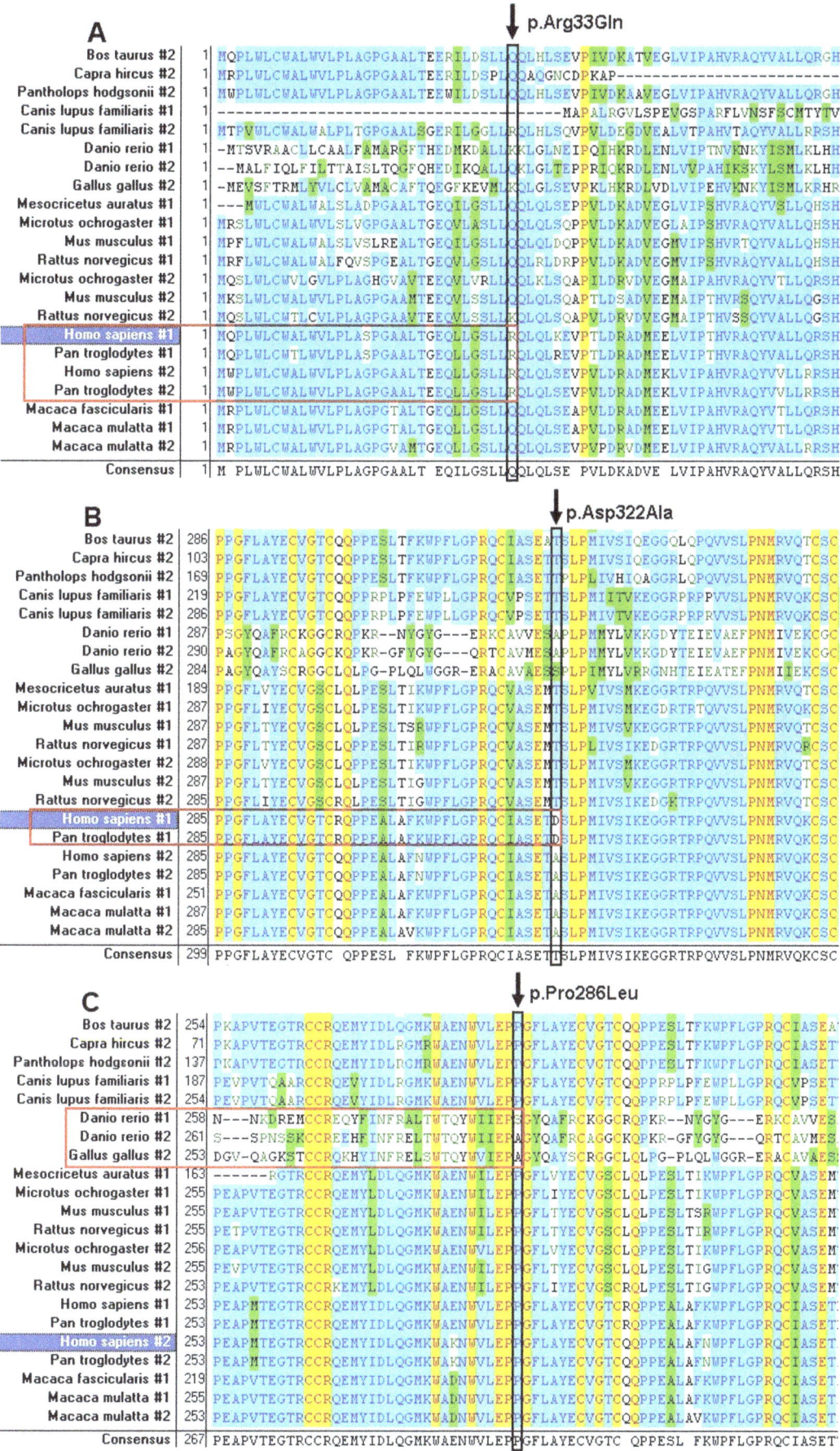

Figure 3. Multiple-sequence alignment of Lefty-1(#1) and -2(#2) from birds, fishes and mammals (including *Homo sapiens, Pan troglodytes, Macaca mulatta* **etc.).** A: p.Arg33Gln; B: p.Asp322Ala; C: p.Pro286Leu.

Author Contributions

Conceived and designed the experiments: FFL SLL. Performed the experiments: JZ XD PY EYZ. Analyzed the data: FFL KJY SLL. Contributed reagents/materials/analysis tools: JZ LH. Contributed to the writing of the manuscript: FFL SLL. Funding: KJY SLL.

References

1. Verheugt CL, Uiterwaal CS, van der Velde ET, Meijboom FJ, Pieper PG, et al. (2010) Mortality in adult congenital heart disease. Eur Heart J 31: 1220–1229.
2. Hoffman JI, Kaplan S (2002) The incidence of congenital heart disease. J Am Coll Cardiol 39: 1890–1900.
3. Hoffman JI, Kaplan S, Liberthson RR (2004) Prevalence of congenital heart disease. Am Heart J 147: 425–439.
4. Pierpont ME, Basson CT, Benson DW, Jr., Gelb BD, Giglia TM, et al. (2007) Genetic basis for congenital heart defects: current knowledge: a scientific statement from the American Heart Association Congenital Cardiac Defects Committee, Council on Cardiovascular Disease in the Young: endorsed by the American Academy of Pediatrics. Circulation 115: 3015–3038.
5. van der Bom T, Zomer AC, Zwinderman AH, Meijboom FJ, Bouma BJ, et al. (2011) The changing epidemiology of congenital heart disease. Nat Rev Cardiol 8: 50–60.
6. Bruneau BG (2008) The developmental genetics of congenital heart disease. Nature 451: 943–948.
7. Richards AA, Garg V (2010) Genetics of congenital heart disease. Curr Cardiol Rev 6: 91–97.
8. Buckingham M, Meilhac S, Zaffran S (2005) Building the mammalian heart from two sources of myocardial cells. Nat Rev Genet 6: 826–835.
9. van Weerd JH, Koshiba-Takeuchi K, Kwon C, Takeuchi JK (2011) Epigenetic factors and cardiac development. Cardiovasc Res 91: 203–211.
10. Sperling S, Grimm CH, Dunkel I, Mebus S, Sperling HP, et al. (2005) Identification and functional analysis of CITED2 mutations in patients with congenital heart defects. Hum Mutat 26: 575–582.
11. Wang B, Wang J, Liu S, Han X, Xie X, et al. (2009) CFC1 mutations in Chinese children with congenital heart disease. Int J Cardiol.
12. Butler TL, Esposito G, Blue GM, Cole AD, Costa MW, et al. (2010) GATA4 Mutations in 357 Unrelated Patients with Congenital Heart Malformation. Genet Test Mol Biomarkers.
13. Wang H, Chen D, Ma L, Meng H, Liu Y, et al. (2012) Genetic analysis of the TBX1 gene promoter in ventricular septal defects. Mol Cell Biochem 370: 53–58.
14. Gong W, Gottlieb S, Collins J, Blescia A, Dietz H, et al. (2001) Mutation analysis of TBX1 in non-deleted patients with features of DGS/VCFS or isolated cardiovascular defects. J Med Genet 38: E45.
15. Schuldiner M, Benvenisty N (2003) Factors controlling human embryonic stem cell differentiation. Methods Enzymol 365: 446–461.
16. Tabibzadeh S, Hemmati-Brivanlou A (2006) Lefty at the crossroads of "stemness" and differentiative events. Stem Cells 24: 1998–2006.
17. Ikushima H, Miyazono K (2010) TGFbeta signalling: a complex web in cancer progression. Nat Rev Cancer 10: 415–424.
18. Heldin CH, Landstrom M, Moustakas A (2009) Mechanism of TGF-beta signaling to growth arrest, apoptosis, and epithelial-mesenchymal transition. Curr Opin Cell Biol 21: 166–176.
19. Postovit LM, Margaryan NV, Seftor EA, Kirschmann DA, Lipavsky A, et al. (2008) Human embryonic stem cell microenvironment suppresses the tumorigenic phenotype of aggressive cancer cells. Proc Natl Acad Sci U S A 105: 4329–4334.
20. Costa FF, Seftor EA, Bischof JM, Kirschmann DA, Strizzi L, et al. (2009) Epigenetically reprogramming metastatic tumor cells with an embryonic microenvironment. Epigenomics 1: 387–398.
21. Malchenko S, Galat V, Seftor EA, Vanin EF, Costa FF, et al. (2010) Cancer hallmarks in induced pluripotent cells: new insights. J Cell Physiol 225: 390–393.
22. Dvash T, Sharon N, Yanuka O, Benvenisty N (2007) Molecular analysis of LEFTY-expressing cells in early human embryoid bodies. Stem Cells 25: 465–472.
23. Schier AF (2003) Nodal signaling in vertebrate development. Annu Rev Cell Dev Biol 19: 589–621.
24. Barroso-delJesus A, Lucena-Aguilar G, Sanchez L, Ligero G, Gutierrez-Aranda I, et al. (2011) The Nodal inhibitor Lefty is negatively modulated by the microRNA miR-302 in human embryonic stem cells. FASEB J 25: 1497–1508.
25. Meno C, Gritsman K, Ohishi S, Ohfuji Y, Heckscher E, et al. (1999) Mouse Lefty2 and zebrafish antivin are feedback inhibitors of nodal signaling during vertebrate gastrulation. Mol Cell 4: 287–298.

21

Modelling Survival and Mortality Risk to 15 Years of Age for a National Cohort of Children with Serious Congenital Heart Defects Diagnosed in Infancy

Rachel L. Knowles[1]*, Catherine Bull[2], Christopher Wren[3], Angela Wade[1], Harvey Goldstein[1], Carol Dezateux[1], on behalf of the UKCSCHD (UK Collaborative Study of Congenital Heart Defects) collaborators[¶]

1 Population Policy and Practice Programme, Institute of Child Health, University College London, London, United Kingdom, 2 Cardiac Unit, Great Ormond Street Hospital for Children NHS Trust, London, United Kingdom, 3 Department of Paediatric Cardiology, Freeman Hospital, Newcastle-upon-Tyne, United Kingdom

Abstract

Background: Congenital heart defects (CHDs) are a significant cause of death in infancy. Although contemporary management ensures that 80% of affected children reach adulthood, post-infant mortality and factors associated with death during childhood are not well-characterised. Using data from a UK-wide multicentre birth cohort of children with serious CHDs, we observed survival and investigated independent predictors of mortality up to age 15 years.

Methods: Data were extracted retrospectively from hospital records and death certificates of 3,897 children (57% boys) in a prospectively identified cohort, born 1992–1995 with CHDs requiring intervention or resulting in death before age one year. A discrete-time survival model accounted for time-varying predictors; hazards ratios were estimated for mortality. Incomplete data were addressed through multilevel multiple imputation.

Findings: By age 15 years, 932 children had died; 144 died without any procedure. Survival to one year was 79.8% (95% confidence intervals [CI] 78.5, 81.1%) and to 15 years was 71.7% (63.9, 73.4%), with variation by cardiac diagnosis. Importantly, 20% of cohort deaths occurred after age one year. Models using imputed data (including all children from birth) demonstrated higher mortality risk as independently associated with cardiac diagnosis, female sex, preterm birth, having additional cardiac defects or non-cardiac malformations. In models excluding children who had no procedure, additional predictors of higher mortality were younger age at first procedure, lower weight or height, longer cardiopulmonary bypass or circulatory arrest duration, and peri-procedural complications; non-cardiac malformations were no longer significant.

Interpretation: We confirm the high mortality risk associated with CHDs in the first year of life and demonstrate an important persisting risk of death throughout childhood. Late mortality may be underestimated by procedure-based audit focusing on shorter-term surgical outcomes. National monitoring systems should emphasise the importance of routinely capturing longer-term survival and exploring the mechanisms of mortality risk in children with serious CHDs.

Editor: Zaccaria Ricci, Piazza S, Italy

Funding: This work was supported by a British Heart Foundation project grant (reference PG/02/065/13934). RLK was awarded an MRC Special Training Fellowship in Health of the Public and Health Services Research (reference G106/1083). HG and the Centre for Paediatric Epidemiology and Biostatistics benefited from Medical Research Council funding support to the MRC Centre of Epidemiology for Child Health (reference G04005546). Great Ormond St Hospital for Children NHS Trust and the UCL Institute of Child Health receives a proportion of funding from the Department of Health's NIHR Biomedical Research Centres scheme. The funders had no role in the study design, data analysis and interpretation, writing or publication of this paper.

Competing Interests: The authors have declared that no competing interests exist.

* Email: rachel.knowles@ucl.ac.uk

¶ Membership of the UKCSCHD (UK Collaborative Study of Congenital Heart Defects) is provided in the Acknowledgments.

Introduction

Serious congenital heart defects (CHDs), requiring surgery in the first year of life, affect around 1% of births each year in the UK [1–3] and include a broad spectrum of complexity and severity. Without intervention in early life, serious CHDs are often incompatible with long-term survival. Continuous improvement in medical, intensive care and surgical technologies have significantly reduced infant mortality and around 80% of affected babies now survive the first year of life [4–7]. Despite the rising number of paediatric cardiac procedures being undertaken [8], surgical mortality is decreasing and the number of UK adults with CHDs is steadily growing [9]. Nevertheless, long-term survival for individuals within most CHD subgroups remains below that of the unaffected population [10].

Recognising the growing population of adolescents and adults with CHDs, recent research has focused on the epidemiology and health experience of adult survivors. It is generally assumed that

Table 1. Inclusion and exclusion criteria for the UKCSCHD cohort.

Inclusion criteria (for the UKCSCHD and original register). Live born infants:
1) born between 1st January 1992 and 31st December 1995
2) resident in the United Kingdom (UK) at birth
3) with a serious congenital heart defect, defined as a structural malformation of the heart or great vessels, requiring an intervention or resulting in death during the first year of life.
Exclusion criteria (for the UKCSCHD and original register). Live born infants with:
1) isolated cardiovascular defects such as persistent ductus arteriosus, vascular ring or anomalous coronary arteries
2) myocardial dysfunction, arrhythmia or tumours in a structurally normal heart
3) a congenital heart defect that did not require an intervention or result in death during the first year of life.
Excluded from the UKCSCHD but included in the original register:
Babies with a fetal diagnosis of serious congenital heart defect made at prenatal ultrasound but not subsequently live born.

additional mortality between infancy and 15 years of age is extremely low and likely to be related to further surgery, yet observational studies with prospective long-term follow-up of the transition of children with CHDs from infancy through school, adolescence and into adulthood are lacking. While short-term surgical outcome studies provide extensive detail about post-operative survival and mortality, particularly within specific CHD subgroups, the factors associated with mortality risk that are common to all diagnostic subgroups and their significance at different ages are poorly defined [11]. Developing a life course approach [12] to children and adults surviving with CHDs is a vital step in recognising that they experience complex interactions between intrinsic early life factors, cardiac diagnosis and the pressures of the external environment, which have a significant impact on their growth, development and late outcomes. There remains a crucial lack in our understanding of the relevance of different risk factors and exposures at each stage of the lifecourse and how these may modify long-term outcomes, not only when they occur in relation to critical periods but also when experienced as repeated exposures such as multiple surgical interventions. Such information is key to future interventions to improve survival and health outcomes and ensure a smooth transition to adult life for affected children.

The UK Collaborative Study of Congenital Heart Defects (UKCSCHD) was established as a UK-wide multi-centre cohort involving almost 4000 children, diagnosed with serious CHDs during their first year of life, to determine prospectively survival, health, educational and quality of life outcomes. In this paper we examine survival from birth to 15 years of age, characterise the timing and causes of death during childhood and investigate the relative importance of patient-specific and early life factors to mortality risk during childhood for this national cohort that is largely representative of contemporary surgical and medical management.

Materials and Methods

Ethics statement

Ethics approval was granted by Trent Multicentre Research Ethics Committee (MREC 04/4/017). Case notes review was undertaken within collaborating centres under the supervision of the local responsible cardiologist; the names and addresses of the children were not provided to the central study team who carried out analyses on de-identified data.

Methods

The UKCSCHD includes children with serious CHDs born between 1992 and 1995 and prospectively notified to a UK-wide study evaluating fetal diagnosis by paediatric cardiologists (British Congenital Cardiac Association [BCCA] members) in all 17 UK paediatric cardiac surgical centres [13]. Serious CHDs were defined as structural heart malformations requiring intervention or resulting in death during the first year of life [13].

A retrospective hospital records review of 3897 children was co-ordinated by the central research team; 268 children from the original register were excluded as there were insufficient details in the case notes to confirm that all inclusion criteria (Table 1) for the UKCSCHD were met. Local clinicians extracted data and completed a standardised proforma for 3698 (95%) of 3897 children. Record retrieval varied by centre, reflecting local record-keeping, and retrieval was less successful for children who were reported by local clinicians to have died (difference 6% [95% CI 4%, 8%]).

Deaths were traced within hospital systems then validated through the Office for National Statistics (England and Wales) and General Register Office (Scotland). A primary cardiac diagnosis (Table 2) was assigned to every child using a hierarchical classification prioritising the most severe structural defect adapted from Wren et al. [14]; three clinical raters (CB, CW, RK) independently assigned diagnoses (generalised kappa (κ) for rater agreement = 0.83) and the final diagnosis was agreed by consensus. Two cardiologists (CB, CW) designated one procedure for each child as 'definitive', defined as the procedure which would approximate normal anatomy and restore biventricular function or provide long-term palliation without expectation of further surgery during childhood, thus the final stage of a multi-stage repair was considered definitive. The definitive procedure may have taken place at any time during follow-up. Children were assigned to a cardiac prognostic severity (CPS) group, adapted from Lane [15], based on primary diagnosis and whether their definitive procedure was presumed curative, corrective or palliative (Table 2).

Statistical analysis

Descriptive statistics are presented as numbers and percentages, or median and interquartile ranges (IQR), and 95% confidence intervals (CI) were estimated for the difference between two proportions. Table 3 provides information about the numbers of children who died or were censored alive (last seen) during each

Table 2. Cardiac diagnosis and severity for all children in the cohort.

PRIMARY CHD DIAGNOSIS*		Number of children	Cardiac Prognostic Severity Group** (% of children within diagnostic group)				
			Curative	Corrective	Palliative	No intervention	Insufficient information
HLH/MA	Hypoplastic left heart/mitral atresia	199	0	0	65%	32%	4%
TA	Tricuspid atresia	67	0	0	97%	3%	0
DIV	Double inlet ventricle	85	0	0	96%	4%	0
PA+IVS	Pulmonary atresia with intact ventricular septum	33	0	0	99%	1%	0
PA+VSD	Pulmonary atresia with ventricular septal defect	151	0	34%	62%	3%	1%
CAT	Common arterial trunk (Truncus arteriosus)	99	0	89%	6%	5%	0
CAVSD	Complete atrioventricular septal defect	460	0	74%	21%	5%	0
TGA	Transposition of the great arteries	597	0	83%	17%	0%	0
TOF	Tetralogy of Fallot	361	0	81%	17%	1%	1%
TAPVC	Total anomalous pulmonary venous connection	150	93%	4%	1%	1%	0
VSD	Ventricular septal defect	760	63%	25%	11%	2%	0
AS	Aortic stenosis	107	0	92%	7%	2%	0
PS	Pulmonary stenosis	194	95%	2%	2%	1%	0
COA	Coarctation of the aorta	395	0	97%	1%	1%	0
Misc	Miscellaneous	189	21%	25%	46%	8%	1%
	Total	**3,897**					

Notes:

*adapted from Wren [14];

**adapted from Lane [15].

Assignment of primary CHD diagnosis: The methodology for assigning primary diagnoses to 1,768 children with multiple defects was validated independently by three raters (RK, CB, CW). Based on cardiac diagnoses in medical records, children assigned a primary diagnosis were 1,738 (98%), 1,610 (91%) and 1,146 (65%) for each rater; this increased to 1,761 (99.7%), 1,689 (95.5%) and 1,658 (93.8%) respectively using records of surgical procedures (Interrater agreement: k = 0.83). A 'miscellaneous' category included defects found in fewer than 40 children: congenitally corrected transposition of the great arteries (n = 24), partial atrioventricular septal defect (n = 20), aortopulmonary window (n = 26), atrial septal defect (n = 36) and rarer diagnoses (n = 83).

CPS groups were: no intervention-children who received ro surgical intervention prior to death during first year of life; curative-children who had successful repair of atrial or ventricular septal defect, pulmonary stenosis or total anomalous pulmonary veins and had no additional cardiac defects; corrective-children who had a procedure which approximated normal anatomy and restored biventricular function, with no expectation of future surgery during childhood; palliative-children whose surgery did not restore biventricular function, including children for whom all stages of multi-stage repair were not achieved, who had a valve replacement which would require later revision, or for whom only a single functional ventricle circulation was possible.

Table 3. Number of children dying or last seen (censored) during each year of follow-up.

Year of follow-up	Number at risk	Deaths	Censored (last seen)
(from birth = 0)	n	n	n
0–1 year	3897	727	681
1–2 years	2489	78	103
2–3 years	2308	35	55
3–4 years	2218	28	46
4–5 years	2144	16	58
5–6 years	2070	11	53
6–7 years	2006	8	48
7–8 years	1950	8	64
8–9 years	1878	3	106
9–10 years	1769	5	168
10–11 years	1596	4	405
11–12 years	1187	4	520
12–13 years*	663	4	424
13–14 years*	235	1	214
14–15 years*	20	0	20

*All children in the cohort were aged 12 years or older at the time of ascertainment of deaths in 2007, thus losses from follow-up at younger ages were due to death or censoring alive on the date last seen (as recorded in hospital case notes). Between 12 and 15 years there are fewer children under follow-up ('at risk') in the older age groups as many children had not reached these ages and this reduced the precision of survival estimates after 12 years.

year of follow-up. The Kaplan-Meier survival function was estimated up to 15 years of age; five children, whose date of death was not known, were censored alive on the date of the last hospital visit.

A multilevel discrete time event history model was developed to investigate the factors influencing survival; this was a binomial logit model with the response variable, death or censoring, coded as a binary variable. The discrete time hazard function represented the conditional probability of an event in each interval given that the event had not occurred in a previous interval: $h(t) = \Pr(T = t \mid T \geq t)$. The period of observation was divided into 24 discrete intervals; 12 intervals of one month duration for the first year of life when the majority of events occurred, then 11 intervals of one year from one to 12 years of age and a final interval of three years duration representing the interval 12 to 15 years of age, in which events were rare. In the final model including multiple predictors, three 'smoothed' categories (representing the first year of life, one to 12 years, and 12 to 15 years of age) were developed by estimating the log-transformed midpoint of each variable and dividing by the number of months within each category. Although the 24 category model had marginally better fit than the 'smoothed' category model (DIC 8887.9 and 8946.8 respectively), the smoothed category model improved model convergence and was therefore used.

Within each interval, it was assumed that the hazards were constant and the binary response variable indicated whether death occurred during the final interval. Covariates specific to the child, such as sex or preterm birth, remained constant whilst factors recorded at each procedure, such as cardiopulmonary bypass duration, were permitted to vary between intervals. Weight and height were converted to age- and sex-standardised z-scores (British 1990 growth reference) [16]. Each predictor was explored in univariable analyses then multivariable models were constructed to determine joint associations.

Missing data were imputed using a hierarchical imputation model developed with MLwiN 2.18–2.20 [17] and Realcom-

Impute [18]. The imputation procedure used Markov-chain Monte Carlo (MCMC) procedure to generate 20 imputed datasets during 2500 iterations. Imputation was conditioned on centre availability of records, as this significantly influenced missingness. Imputation excluded 28 children whose date of death or censoring was unknown, and variables with more than 50% missing data; the included variable with the most missing data was clinical status on admission (46%; Table 4). Distributions of continuous variables before and after imputation were compared using density plots (data not shown).

Hierarchical models of mortality risk were developed to take account of the grouping of individual children within cardiac centres and the correlation of procedure-related data within the individual child. For each imputed dataset multilevel discrete-time event models [19,20] were constructed to predict mortality risk from birth to follow-up in 2007, when all surviving children were aged 12 to 15 years. The final results reported are those averaged over these datasets according to 'Rubin's rules'. The results from these analyses using imputed datasets were compared with those using the 'complete case' datasets (including only those children with complete data).

Analyses were undertaken using Stata SE 11 (Timberlake Consulting) and MLwiN 2.18–2.20 [17].

Results

Almost one-quarter of the cohort died (n = 932 deaths) and, of these, 727 (78%) deaths occurred within the first year and 323 (35%) within the first month of life. Although the risk of death was lower after the first year of life, 20% of all cohort deaths occurred after one year of age. Death occurred before intervention, or parents chose palliative care, for 144 (4%) children who died without any procedure; most (n = 63; 44%) of these children had hypoplastic left heart and/or mitral atresia (HLH/MA). The median age at death for children who died without undergoing an

Table 4. Patient-specific characteristics by diagnostic group (n = 3897).

Primary CHD Diagnosis	Boys	Preterm	DS: Down's syndrome	Non-DS non-cardiac malformation	Add. cardiac defects	Unstable clinical status	Age at first intervention* Median (IQR) days	Death without intervention n
	as % of all non-missing values†							
HLH/MA	67%	7%	0	4%	26%	75%	5 (2,14)	63
TA	52%	6%	0	6%	88%	57%	23 (5,83)	2
DIV	71%	4%	0	7%	92%	64%	14 (5,46)	3
PA+IVS	64%	8%	0	5%	29%	82%	3 (2,6)	1
PA+VSD	45%	10%	0	18%	52%	61%	8 (3,81)	5
CAT	52%	10%	0	17%	40%	61%	29 (12,65)	5
CAVSD	47%	8%	43%	5%	43%	42%	103 (55,169)	22
TGA	68%	5%	0	2%	51%	65%	3 (1,14)	1
TOF	59%	10%	3%	12%	29%	33%	133 (42,249)	4
TAPVC	64%	7%	0	6%	19%	76%	16 (3,62)	2
VSD	51%	9%	9%	10%	54%	57%	97 (34,180)	13
AS	70%	2%	2%	5%	44%	60%	15 (3,61)	2
PS	45%	6%	1%	8%	27%	23%	72 (8,71)	2
COA	63%	8%	0	8%	45%	55%	17 (8,71)	4
Misc	52%	9%	7%	7%	63%	65%	81 (14,174)	15
Total	57%	8%	8%	7%	46%	55%	38 (6,121)	144

Notes:

*excludes 144 children who did not have an intervention;

†**Number (%) of children with missing data:** Sex n = 129(3%); Unstable clinical status n = 1784(46%); non-cardiac malformations/Additional cardiac defects: no missing data.

Key: IQR interquartile range; **preterm** <37 completed weeks gestation at birth; **Add. cardiac defects** - in addition to primary CHD diagnosis; **unstable clinical status** on first admission was defined as unstable if one or more of the following symptoms/signs were present: unwell = significant pallor, breathlessness or sweating, intubated, mechanically ventilated, hypotension = systolic blood pressure [SBP] <50 mmHg, hypertensive = SBP >100 mmHg, cardiac or respiratory arrest, metabolic acidosis, requiring adrenaline or high dose inotropic support; **HLH/MA** hypoplastic left heart and/or mitral atresia; **TA** tricuspid atresia; **DIV** double inlet ventricle; **PA+IVS** pulmonary atresia with intact ventricular septum; **PA+VSD** pulmonary atresia with ventricular septal defect; **CAT** common arterial trunk; **CAVSD** complete atrioventricular septal defect; **TGA** transposition of the great arteries; **TOF** tetralogy of Fallot; **TAPVC** total anomalous pulmonary venous connection; **VSD** ventricular septal defect; **AS** aortic stenosis; **PS** pulmonary stenosis; **COA** coarctation of the aorta; **Misc** miscellaneous cardiac defects (not included within other categories).

Table 5. Characteristics of individuals in the cohort (n = 3897).

Patient-specific factors	N (% of 3897)	Missing N (% of 3897)
Sex		129 (3%)
Boys	2147 (55%)	
Girls	1621 (42%)	
Preterm birth		0
Gestation <37 weeks	296 (8%)	
Gestation ≥37 weeks	3601 (92%)	
Non-cardiac malformations		0
Down's syndrome (DS)	293 (8%)	
Non-DS non-cardiac malformations	290 (7%)	
No non-cardiac malformations	3314 (85%)	
Additional cardiac defects		0
Isolated CHD	1826 (47%)	
Additional cardiac defects	1488 (53%)	
Antenatal diagnosis of CHD		0
Antenatal diagnosis	177 (5%)	
Postnatal diagnosis	3720 (95%)	
Factors related to management		
Clinical status on first admission		1784 (46%)
Stable	953 (24%)	
Unstable	1160 (30%)	
Age at first procedure (*median [IQR]*)	38 (6, 121) days	
Weight z-score at first procedure (*median [IQR]*)	−1.7 (IQR −2.83, −0.58)	
Height z-score at first procedure (*median [IQR]*)	−0.8 (IQR −2.03, 0.42)	
Number of procedures (*median [IQR]*)	1 (1, 2)	

Notes:
IQR interquartile range;
Preterm birth - before 37 completed weeks of gestation;
Additional cardiac defects - children who had at least one structural cardiac defect in addition to their primary cardiac diagnosis;
Non-Down's syndrome non-cardiac malformations - a further 290 children had non-cardiac congenital malformations that were not Down's syndrome, including recognised syndromes such as Di George's (n = 61).
Clinical status on first admission was defined as unstable if one or more of the following symptoms/signs were present: unwell = significant pallor, breathlessness or sweating, intubated, mechanically ventilated, hypotension = systolic blood pressure [SBP] <50 mmHg, hypertensive = SBP >100 mmHg, cardiac or respiratory arrest, metabolic acidosis, requiring adrenaline or high dose inotropic support.

intervention was 8.5 days (IQR 3, 75.5 days) and only one-third survived beyond the first month of life. Of 723 children who survived to one year without having undergone a definitive corrective or palliative procedure, 578 (80%) died between age one and 15 years. There was no significant difference in the proportion of girls and boys who died without a procedure. Characteristics of the cohort children and procedure-related factors are presented in Table 5 and Table 6 respectively.

Overall 80% (95% CI 78%–81%) of children were alive at one year and 72% [70%, 73%] at 15 years of age. Survival varied by primary cardiac diagnosis (Figure 1; Table 7). For 2,489 children remaining under follow-up after one year of age, survival between one and 15 years was 90% (95% CI 88%, 91%) overall, however for children within six diagnostic subgroups (HLH/MA, tricuspid atresia [TA], double inlet ventricle [DIV], pulmonary atresia with intact ventricular septum [PA+IVS], PA+VSD and CAVSD), survival post-infancy was lower than 90%.

In univariable models involving *all* children followed from birth, preterm birth (hazard ratio [HR] 1.43 [95% CI: 1.16, 1.77]), non-Down's syndrome non-cardiac malformations (HR 1.56 [1.27,

1.93]), cardiac defects additional to the primary diagnosis (HR 1.24 [1.09, 1.41]) and unstable clinical status on first admission (HR 1.43 [1.07, 1.90]) were statistically significant predictors of higher mortality. Relative to the largest subgroup (ventricular septal defect [VSD]), all primary diagnostic subgroups except pulmonary stenosis (PS) and aortic coarctation (COA) were associated with increased mortality.

In the multivariable model including all children and adjusted for centre effects, higher mortality up to age 15 years was associated with female sex (HR 1.25 [1.06, 1.47]), preterm birth (HR 1.44 [1.15, 1.79]), non-Down's syndrome non-cardiac malformations (HR 1.49 [1.20, 1.86]), additional cardiac defects (HR 1.23 [1.07, 1.42]) and, relative to VSD, all primary diagnoses except for PS and COA (data not shown). When procedure-related risk factors were included in the multivariable model, thus excluding children who died without a procedure, independent predictors of higher mortality risk were female sex, preterm birth, additional cardiac defects, pre-procedure sepsis or hypertension, post-procedure seizures, cardiac arrest, renal failure, stroke, sepsis or disseminated intravascular coagulopathy (DIC), lower weight or

Table 6. Characteristics of procedure-related factors (6351 procedures in 3753 individuals).

Procedure-related factors	Details of procedures	
	N (% of 6351 procedures)	
Pre-procedure variables:		
Any pre-procedure complications/support	786 (12%)*	
Intubated	590	
Inotropic support	252	
Acidosis	159	
Hypotensive (systolic BP <50 mmHg)	111	
Sepsis	93	
Hypertensive (systolic BP >100 mmHg)	51	
Seizures	46	
Intra-procedure variables:		
Procedures not requiring bypass‡	2486 (39%)	
Cardiopulmonary bypass (CPB) time†	2346	median = 87(IQR 60,129) minutes
Circulatory arrest (CA) time†	1059	median = 30 (IQR 14,49) minutes
Aortic cross-clamp (XC) time†	1980	median = 52 (IQR 32,75) minutes
Post-procedure variables:		
Any post-procedure complications	816 (13%)*	
Sepsis	356	
Re-intubated (after 24 hrs extubation)	224	
Renal failure	202	
Cardiac arrest	169	
Seizures	113	
ECMO (extracorporeal membrane oxygenation)	47	
DIC (disseminated intravascular coagulopathy)	31	
Stroke	22	

Notes:

IQR interquartile range; BP blood pressure; hrs hours.

*Procedures at which there was more than one pre-procedure (or post-procedure) complication are only counted once in the totals so the sum of individual complications is greater.

‡Procedures for which cardiopulmonary bypass would not be required, e.g. catheter intervention.

†Excludes procedures in which duration is recorded as 0 minutes.

height z-score, younger age at first procedure, or longer duration of cardiopulmonary bypass or cardiac arrest (Table 8). Non-Down's syndrome non-cardiac malformation and postoperative ECMO were not significant predictors of higher mortality. Mortality risk for children with TGA and COA was similar to VSD, and significantly higher than VSD for all other CHD subgroups.

In sensitivity analyses results from the imputed models were compared with those using complete cases; the imputed data analyses provided greater precision with no significant difference in the magnitude and direction of effect. During stepwise development of the model, the variable representing definitive surgery did not significantly improve the model and was excluded. However in a sensitivity analysis involving only 606 children who had complete data and were alive at age one year, mortality risk was significantly lower for those who had experienced definitive surgery by age one year than for those who did not (HR 0.19, 95%CI 0.05, 0.73; p = 0.015).

Discussion

In this UK-wide cohort involving 3897 children with serious CHDs, mortality was 20% in the first year of life. An additional 8% of the cohort died between one and 15 years of age, thus 20% of all deaths within the cohort occurred after the first year of life. There were 144 children in the cohort who died without any intervention during the first year of life. Overall survival was 79.8% at one year and 71.7% at 15 years of age with variation by primary cardiac diagnosis, thus for children who survived the first year survival into adulthood was generally good. Children with functional single ventricles (HLH/MA, TA and DIV) experienced the highest mortality overall but for children surviving to one year of age, those with PA+VSD and CAVSD had the worst post-infant survival rates.

Primary cardiac diagnosis was an important independent predictor of mortality risk up to 15 years; children with TGA, COA and VSD had the lowest mortality risk. Higher mortality risk regardless of intervention was independently associated with female sex, preterm birth and having a cardiac defect in addition to the primary cardiac diagnosis. For children who had at least one procedure, higher mortality risk was associated with earlier age at

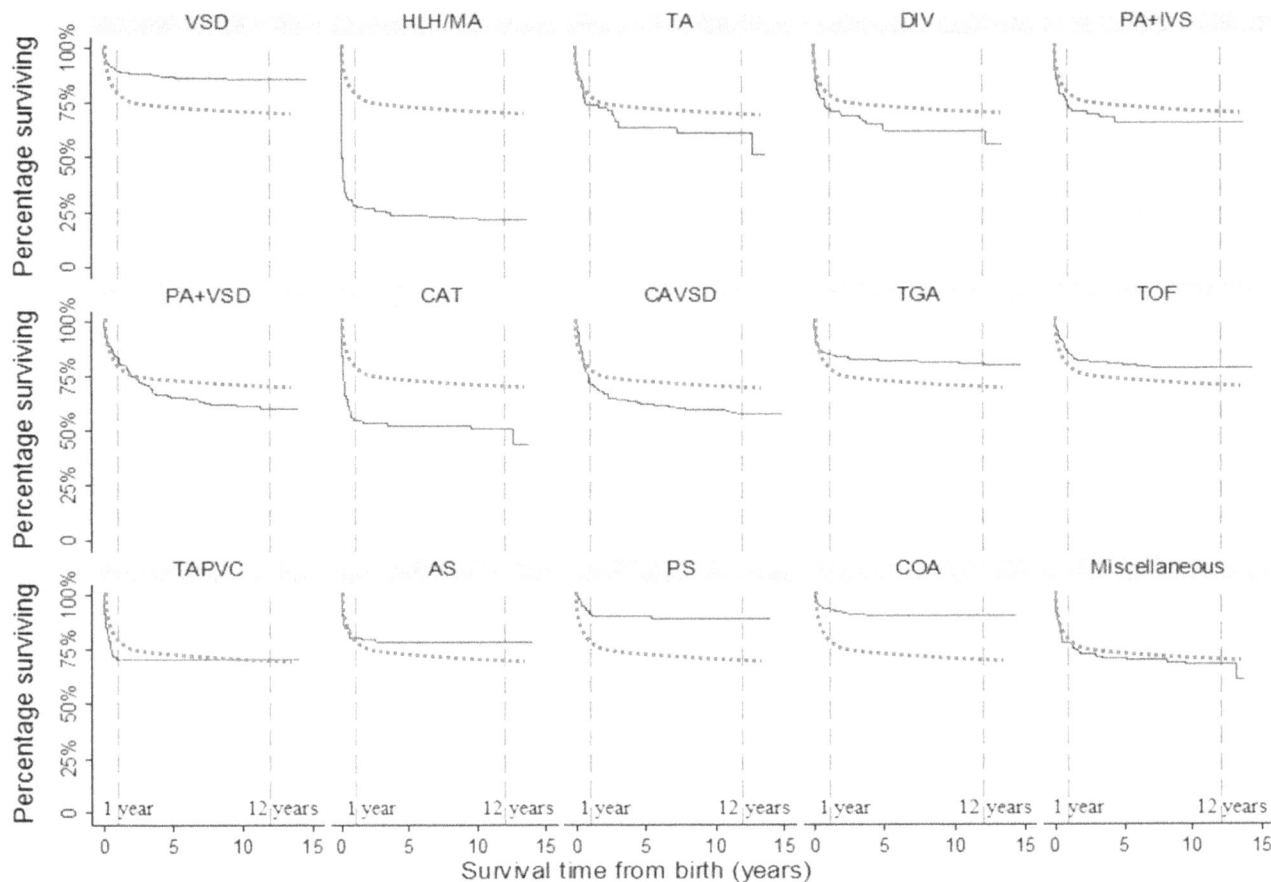

Notes: Interrupted vertical lines represent survival at 1 and 12 years.
The survival curve for all children within the cohort is represented by a **dotted** line.
The survival curve for children with each specific cardiac diagnosis is represented by a **solid** line.

Abbreviations: HLH/MA hypoplastic left heart and/or mitral atresia; **TA** tricuspid atresia; **DIV** double inlet ventricle; **PA+IVS** pulmonary atresia with intact ventricular septum; **PA+VSD** pulmonary atresia with ventricular septal defect; **CAT** common arterial trunk; **CAVSD** complete atrioventricular septal defect; **TGA** transposition of the great arteries; **TOF** tetralogy of Fallot; **TAPVC** total anomalous pulmonary venous connection; **VSD** ventricular septal defect; **AS** aortic stenosis; **PS** pulmonary stenosis; **COA** coarctation of the aorta; **Misc** miscellaneous cardiac defects.

Figure 1. Survival from birth to 15 years by primary diagnosis (for individual diagnoses). Notes: Interrupted vertical lines represent survival at 1 and 12 years. The survival curve for all children within the cohort is represented by a **dotted** line. The survival curve for children with each specific cardiac diagnosis is represented by a **solid** line. **Abbreviations: HLH/MA** hypoplastic left heart and/or mitral atresia; **TA** tricuspid atresia; **DIV** double inlet ventricle; **PA+IVS** pulmonary atresia with intact ventricular septum; **PA+VSD** pulmonary atresia with ventricular septal defect; **CAT** common arterial trunk; **CAVSD** complete atrioventricular septal defect; **TGA** transposition of the great arteries; **TOF** tetralogy of Fallot; **TAPVC** total anomalous pulmonary venous connection; **VSD** ventricular septal defect; **AS** aortic stenosis; **PS** pulmonary stenosis; **COA** coarctation of the aorta; **Misc** miscellaneous cardiac defects.

first procedure, pre-procedural sepsis and hypertension (systolic BP>100 mHg), post-procedural complications (including cardiac arrest, stroke, renal failure, seizures and sepsis) and increased duration of cardiopulmonary bypass or cardiac arrest.

Longitudinal cohort studies present important methodological challenges for survival analysis, including the need to model hierarchical data structures, repeated procedures, and to address missing data. An important strength of our study is the development of multilevel models that allowed us to link procedure-related factors across the child's lifecourse and to explicitly order these in time. Children in the cohort underwent varying numbers of procedures, which did not occur at fixed ages, and earlier postoperative experience could influence later management. Despite recognition of the complexity of survival analysis in children with CHDs, for whom both predictors and mortality are time-dependent [11], examples of survival models including

time-varying covariates are rare and few previous studies have explicitly stated the temporal ordering of childhood factors and their inter-relationships, directly or through mediating factors, with mortality. We addressed the methodological challenges of repeat observations, and also adjusted for the effects of clustering by cardiac centre, through the development of discrete-time hierarchical survival models [19,20] and multilevel multiple imputation [44,45] of missing values. The use of imputed datasets, by allowing us to include all cohort children and procedures in the analyses, reduced the likelihood of bias that can result from restricting analyses to the small proportion of children with complete data [21]. Our sensitivity analyses evaluating the effect of multiple imputation in comparison with complete-case datasets, demonstrated that imputed data contributed to greater precision in mortality estimates and ensured that the impact of less

Table 7. Data Table for Figure 1.

PRIMARY CARDIAC DIAGNOSIS	Number at birth	Survivor function	
		(95% confidence intervals)	
	n	At 1 year	At 12 years
Hypoplastic left heart/mitral atresia	199	**28%**(22%,35%)	**21%**(15%,27%)
Tricuspid atresia	67	**74%**(62%,83%)	**61%**(48%,72%)
Double inlet ventricle	85	**72%**(61%,80%)	**62%**(50%,71%)
Pulmonary atresia with intact ventricular septum	83	**73%**(62%,82%)	**65%**(53%,74%)
Pulmonary atresia with ventricular septal defect	151	**84%**(77%,89%)	**60%**(51%,68%)
Common arterial trunk (truncus arteriosus)	99	**55%**(44%,64%)	**51%**(40%,61%)
Complete atrioventricular septal defect	460	**71%**(67%,76%)	**57%**(52%,62%)
Transposition of the great arteries	597	**85%**(82%,88%)	**81%**(77%,84%)
Tetralogy of Fallot	361	**85%**(81%,88%)	**79%**(74%,83%)
Total anomalous pulmonary venous connection	150	**71%**(62%,78%)	**71%**(62%,78%)
Ventricular septal defect	760	**90%**(87%,92%)	**86%**(83%,88%)
Aortic stenosis	107	**81%**(72%,87%)	**78%**(69%,85%)
Pulmonary stenosis	194	**91%**(85%,94%)	**89%**(83%,93%)
Coarctation of the aorta	395	**94%**(90%,96%)	**90%**(86%,93%)
Miscellaneous	189	**77%**(70%,83%)	**68%**(60%,75%)

commonly reported factors, such as pre- and post-procedural complications, was quantifiable.

Although we were prevented by our governance permissions [22] from accessing routine mortality data to check for deaths amongst children who clinicians presumed to be surviving, all reported deaths were confirmed against public death registrations. As children with serious CHDs remain under review throughout life, we believe that our ascertainment of deaths through cardiologists, hospital records and GPs was complete.

The heterogeneity of CHDs also presents a significant problem for population-based analyses [23,24] and variability in classification systems often limits comparisons between studies. Our simple hierarchical classification adapted from Wren [14] and validated on data available from medical case notes, ensured that each child was assigned to only one CHD subgroup and avoided double-counting of children with multiple cardiac defects. As similar classifications have been successfully applied in other UK studies [9,25] [26], this provides a sound basis for cross-study comparisons.

Patients do not pay for care within the UK healthcare system, thus there were no financial barrier to accessing surgery and deaths in children who were offered only palliative medical care were related to the inoperability of the defect. As with all long-term follow-up, early management of cohort members who were born in 1992–1995 was determined by clinical era. Although our cohort has its inception after the introduction of neonatal cardiac surgery and key procedures, such as the arterial switch operation, paediatric cardiac surgical and intensive care technologies have continued to advance, notably for children with HLH for whom Norwood-type surgery is now widely available, or with TOF for whom neonatal surgery is now common. Nonetheless, surgical management has not altered markedly for many CHD subgroups. Advances in fetal screening s well as surgery may also alter the proportion of children who would be offered palliative medical care in current practice compared our cohort. Whereas fetal screening detected around 23% of severe CHDs in 1993–94 [13],

this has now increased to detection of around one-third of cases [27], which may mean that more children born today would commence specialist care at birth than in our cohort. The findings from our cohort should therefore be interpreted with caution within specific diagnostic subgroups where surgical techniques or screening detection have altered significantly as there may be improved survival for children born today. Nevertheless we believe our results are still likely to remain relevant overall to children born and operated with CHDs today, particularly for diagnostic subgroups in which significant improvements in early postoperative survival have not been seen.

There are relatively few population-based observational cohort studies that describe mortality and survival up to age 12–15 years for children affected by CHDs (Table 9). Although we also present some findings from our model including children who remained unoperated at the time of death, the majority of these children died in the first month after birth, many had HLH and palliative care was chosen by some parents; management of such severe and complex cases has continued to advance in the last decade. Thus our main model excludes these unoperated cases and focuses on survival from birth for the majority of children in the cohort, who did undergo an intervention.

Reviewing all child CHD deaths in Bohemia between 1952 and 1979, Samanek reported that 'natural' survival before the widespread introduction of paediatric cardiac surgery was 67% at 15 years [28]. Three further studies investigated survival in large surgical cohorts [10,29,30], including a Finnish population-based study between 1953 and 1989 in which survival was reported as 78% at 45 years after surgery, significantly lower than for the unaffected population. Only three studies have reported survival after diagnosis in early life, including children who remained unoperated as well as those undergoing surgery, of which two present directly observed survival from diagnosis [31] [32]. These two studies, representing contemporary management, documented better overall survival (Table 10) than we observed but up to 40% of children survived without any interventions suggesting

Table 8. Multivariable survival analysis using multiple imputation (n = 3725*).

Variable	Reference Category	Category	Hazard Ratio	95% CI		P-value
				lower	upper	
Sex	Boys					
		Girls	1.51	1.24	1.84	<0.0001
Birth gestation	Term (≥37 weeks)					
		Preterm (<37 weeks gestation)	1.31	1.01	1.69	0.042
Non-cardiac malformations	None					
		Downs Syndrome	0.87	0.62	1.21	0.403
		Non- Downs Syndrome	1.26	0.97	1.64	0.085
Additional cardiac defects	Isolated CHDs					
		Additional defects	1.34	1.13	1.57	0.001
Clinical status on admission	Stable					
		Unstable	1.17	0.82	1.66	0.383
Primary diagnoses	VSD					
		Hypoplastic left heart/mitral atresia	7.58	5.20	11.04	<0.0001
		Tricuspid atresia	4.05	2.45	6.69	<0.0001
		Double inlet ventricle	3.31	2.07	5.29	<0.0001
		Pulmonary atresia with intact ventricular septum	2.98	1.75	5.08	<0.0001
		Pulmonary atresia with ventricular septal defect	2.98	2.01	4.42	<0.0001
		Common arterial trunk (truncus arteriosus)	2.53	1.65	3.89	<0.0001
		Complete atrioventricular septal defect	3.96	2.88	5.42	<0.0001
		Transposition of the great arteries	1.36	0.97	1.90	0.074
		Tetralogy of Fallot	2.55	1.78	3.66	<0.0001
		Total anomalous pulmonary venous connection	2.11	1.35	3.32	0.001
		Aortic stenosis	1.85	1.10	3.13	0.021
		Pulmonary stenosis	1.85	1.06	3.22	0.030
		Coarctation of the aorta	1.11	0.71	1.75	0.645
		Miscellaneous	2.52	1.67	3.80	<0.0001
Procedure- related variables: constant						
Age at first procedure		per month increase	0.90	0.86	0.93	<0.0001
Procedure- related variables: time-varying						
Pre-procedure complications	None					
		Inotropic support	1.57	0.83	2.97	0.162

Table 8. Cont.

Variable	Reference Category	Category	Hazard Ratio	95% CI		P-value
				lower	upper	
		Intubation	0.83	0.48	1.42	0.497
		Seizures	1.38	0.48	4.01	0.551
		Sepsis	2.69	1.27	5.71	0.010
		Metabolic acidosis	0.93	0.43	2.04	0.859
		Hypertension	3.78	1.23	11.60	0.020
		Hypotension	1.84	0.99	3.43	0.053
Post-procedure complications	None					
		Seizures	1.54	1.05	2.26	0.027
		Cardiac arrest	4.98	3.78	6.55	<0.0001
		Renal failure	1.78	1.27	2.48	0.001
		Stroke	2.03	1.05	3.90	0.034
		Sepsis	1.46	1.09	1.95	0.010
		Disseminated intravascular coagulopathy (DIC)	6.44	3.78	10.95	<0.0001
		Extra-corporeal membrane oxygenation (ECMO)	1.42	0.83	2.45	0.200
		Re-intubation (after 24 hours extubation)	0.97	0.73	1.30	0.851
Weight and height						
z-score weight		per one z-score unit increase	0.92	0.85	1.00	0.048
z-score height		per one z-score unit increase	0.87	0.81	0.93	<0.0001
Intra-procedure						
Cardiopulmonary bypass duration		per 10 min increase	1.03	1.01	1.05	0.001
Cardiac arrest duration		per 10 min increase	1.10	1.08	1.12	<0.0001
Aortic cross-clamping duration		per 10 min increase	0.98	0.95	1.01	0.243

*Adjusted for specialist cardiac centre; excludes children who did not have an intervention or who died on same day as birth.

Table 9. Population-based cohort studies reporting mid- and long-term survival for children with congenital heart defects.

Lead author, publication year	Region/State, Country	Period	Study population (n)	Method/Design; Outcome measure	Period of follow-up	Survival/mortality
Morris, 1991 [29]	Oregon, US	Operated 1958–1989	Children aged <18 years (n = 2,701)	Retrospective review of paediatric cardiac procedures (for 8 CHD types); Death after surgery	Up to 25 years after surgery	Varying by CHD: 64% survival at 15 years after surgery (transposition) to 98% survival (atrial septal defect)
Samanek, 1992 [28]	Bohemia, Czech Republic	Diagnosed 1952–1979	Deaths aged ≤15 years (n = 946)	Retrospective review of death registrations; Death ≤15 years old	Up to 16 years of age	71% survival at 1 year of age; 67% survival at 15 years of age
Meberg, 2000 [31]	Vestfold County, Norway	Diagnosed 1982–1996	Children diagnosed clinically or at post-mortem (n = 360)	Prospective follow-up after diagnosis; Death ≤18 years old	Mean 9.5 years (range 3–18 years)	Overall 12% mortality at end of follow-up
Nieminen, 2001 [10]	Finland	Operated 1953–1989	Children aged <15 years old at surgery (n = 6,461)	Retrospective review of paediatric cardiac procedures (all CHDs); Death after surgery	Mean 22 years after surgery (range 9–45 years)	Overall 7% surgical mortality; 78% survival at 45 years after surgery
Wren, 2001 [9]	Northern Region, UK	Born 1985–1994	Children diagnosed clinically or at post-mortem (n = 1,942)	Prospective follow-up from birth/diagnosis; Death ≤15 years old	Up to 16 years of age	82% survival at 1 year of age; *Predicted 78% survival to 16 years of age*
Moons, 2009 [32]	Belgium	Born 2002	Children diagnosed clinically (n = 921)	Prospective follow-up from birth/diagnosis; Death ≤5 years old	Up to 5 years of age	96% survival at 5 years of age
Larsen, 2011 [30]	Western Region, Denmark	Operated 1996–2002	Children operated for CHD (n = 801)	Prospective follow-up after cardiac surgery; Death after surgery	Median 8.2 years after surgery (range 6–12 years)	86% survival at 8.2 years after surgery

Table 10. Childhood survival by primary cardiac diagnosis reported within population-based cohort studies published since 1990.

PRIMARY CARDIAC DIAGNOSIS	UKCSCHD	Samanek, 1992 [28]	Meberg, 2000 [31]	Wren, 2001 [9]
	At age 12 years ('observed')	At age 15 years ('natural')*	At age 9.5 years ('observed')	At age 15 years ('predicted')§
Hypoplastic left heart	21%	11%	22%	0
Pulmonary atresia	60–65%	30%	75%	40%
Common arterial trunk (truncus arteriosus)	51%	11%	50%	31%
Complete atrioventricular septal defect	57%	49%	55%	55%
Transposition of the great arteries	81%	38%	85%	67%
Tetralogy of Fallot	79%	86%	82%	84%
Total anomalous pulmonary venous connection	71%	0	-	70%
Ventricular septal defect	86%	76%	97%	91%
Aortic stenosis	78%	84%	92%	66%
Pulmonary stenosis	89%	94%	93%	92%
Coarctation of the aorta	90%	68%	84%	85%

Notes:
This table compares defect-specific survival reported in childhood within four population-based cohorts that include all children diagnosed in infancy even if no intervention was performed. Most studies present 'observed' cohort survival from diagnosis or first surgery during infancy, with the exception of:
*Samanek presents 'natural' survival in an era prior to widespread surgical correction.
§Wren presents 'predicted' survival up to age 15 years based on observed survival to age 1 year and survival from 1 to 15 years estimated from a review of the published literature.

that, in comparison with the UKCSCHD, they included a higher proportion of mild CHDs that were compatible with survival without intervention.

Surgical case series have highlighted important associations between increased postoperative mortality risk and factors such as low birth weight [33,34], preterm birth [35], sudden clinical deterioration in the neonatal period [36,37], and procedure-associated complications, including sepsis and renal failure [38]. Several studies have demonstrated the detrimental impact of longer intra-procedure duration of cardiopulmonary bypass and cardiac arrest [39–42], also observed in our cohort, although most previous authors estimated the effect at a single procedure only rather than repeated exposure over multiple procedures. Moreover Kang has cautioned that longer duration of cardiopulmonary bypass may only reflect technically more difficult surgery [41].

Although our findings indicate that girls with CHDs are at significantly higher risk of death, published evidence for sex differences in mortality for individuals with CHDs remains inconclusive. Morris [29] demonstrated that girls with COA and TGA had higher mortality prior to intervention, whereas Fyler [43] reported a higher death rate for boys during the first year of life. Other authors have highlighted that girls experience higher perioperative mortality related to paediatric cardiac surgery [44–47]. As the ratio of boys to girls affected varies by specific cardiac defect, these sex differences may be confounded by the severity of cardiac diagnosis. Nevertheless children's cardiac size and function, lung development and immune responses have been shown to vary by sex [47–51], therefore biological differences also provide a plausible explanation for sex differences in mortality risk and would merit further research.

In accordance with previous reports [52,53], we found no independent influence on mortality associated with Down's syndrome. Eskedal [52] has highlighted that children with CHDs who have non-cardiac malformations other than Down's syndrome experience higher mortality than those with isolated cardiac defects. In our cohort, non-Down's non-cardiac malfor-

mations were significant predictors of mortality when children who died without intervention were included in the analysis, suggesting that these malformations do contribute to mortality in this subgroup.

It is now over a decade since the Bristol Inquiry addressed concerns about the care of children receiving cardiac surgery at the Bristol Royal Infirmary [54]. Expert evidence presented to the Inquiry emphasised the lack of data on long-term outcomes relevant to children and their families [55]. The Central Cardiac Audit Database (CCAD) now routinely collects national outcome data for cardiac procedures, including survival up to one year after paediatric cardiac intervention; these data are published through the National Institute for Cardiac Outcomes Research (NICOR) Congenital Heart Disease Portal [56].

While routine audit remains essential to monitoring outcomes for children receiving interventions for CHDs in the UK [57], a procedure-based system excludes children who never receive an intervention and often fails to capture late mortality and broader health outcomes, such as educational achievement or quality of life. Improved record linkage between multiple routinely collected data sources, supplemented by focused observational or clinical studies, could enrich current routine data collection and provide more efficient use of existing resources for extended follow-up.

Conclusions

The UKCSCHD has provided a unique opportunity to observe survival and wider health outcomes throughout childhood in a prospectively ascertained UK-wide cohort that is largely representative of contemporary management. We found that infant mortality under age one year for children with serious CHDs was over 30 times greater than for the general population, estimated at six per 1,000 live births [58]. It is also clear from our data that whilst children with CHDs were still most likely to die in infancy in this cohort, over 20% of CHD-related deaths in childhood took place after the first year of life. Surgical management of serious

CHDs carries an initial perioperative risk of death or neurological injury in childhood, but the altered physiology of the operated heart may also result in reduced ability to cope with ageing or cardiac stressors arising in adult life. Long-term survival and health outcomes are influenced by health events across the lifecourse thus optimising the health experience of preschool and school-age children with CHDs is as relevant to future improvements in survival and quality of life of adults with CHDs as successful early surgical repair. Crucially cardiac diagnosis remained an important predictor of outcome particularly as this influenced the type of definitive procedure, whether this was palliative or corrective, and the age at which it was performed. However, we also identified procedure-related predictors of mortality that may be amenable to modification in order to effect further advances in survival or improve health outcomes after surgery. Investigation into the biological mechanisms contributing to higher mortality for girls is warranted to explore the potential for improving future outcomes and reducing health inequalities.

Acknowledgments

We are very grateful to the local cardiologists and members of the British Congenital Cardiac Association (BCCA) within the UKCSCHD collaborating centres without whom this study would not have been possible: We are very grateful to the local cardiologists and members of the British Congenital Cardiac Association (BCCA) in each UKCSCHD collaborating centre, without whom this study would not have been possible: Dr S Adwani, Dr F Bu'Lock, Dr B Craig, Dr P Daubeney, Dr G Derrick, Dr M Elliott, Dr R Franklin, Dr J Gibbs, Dr B Knight, Dr J Lim, Dr A Magee, Dr R Martin, Dr P Miller, Dr S Qureshi, Dr E Rosenthal, Dr A Salmon, Dr I Sullivan, Dr P Thakker, Dr J Thomson, Dr D Wilson, Dr A Wong. UKCSCHD collaborating centres included: Belfast, Birmingham, Bristol, Cardiff, Edinburgh, Glasgow, Leeds, Leicester, Liverpool, London, Manchester, Newcastle, Nottingham, Oxford and Southampton. We would also like to thank Dr Huiqi Pan for her advice and support for the programming of the MLwiN models and the UKCSCHD research assistants (Ms Ugochi Nwulu, Dr Carly Rich and others) for their valuable contribution and hard work. In addition, we appreciate very much the support that we received from Heartline (parent support group).

Author Contributions

Conceived and designed the experiments: RLK CD CB CW. Performed the experiments: RLK CD CB CW. Analyzed the data: RLK AW HG. Contributed reagents/materials/analysis tools: HG. Wrote the paper: RLK. Reviewed and developed the analyses: RLK CD CB CW AW HG. Reviewed and agreed the manuscript: RLK CD CB CW AW HG.

References

1. Dadvand P, Rankin J, Shirley MD, Rushton S, Pless-Mulloli T (2009) Descriptive epidemiology of congenital heart disease in Northern England. Paediatr Perinat Epidemiol 23: 58–65.

2. Lee K, Khoshnood B, Chen L, Wall SN, Cromie WJ, et al. (2001) Infant mortality from congenital malformations in the United States, 1970–1997. Obstet Gynecol 98: 620–627.

3. Khoshnood B, De Vigan C, Vodovar V, Goujard J, Lhomme A, et al. (2005) Trends in prenatal diagnosis, pregnancy termination, and perinatal mortality of newborns with congenital heart disease in France, 1983–2000: a population-based evaluation. Pediatrics 115: 95–101.

4. Samanek M, Voriskova M (1999) Congenital heart disease among 815,569 children born between 1980 and 1990 and their 15-year survival: a prospective Bohemia survival study. Pediatr Cardiol 20: 411–417.

5. Macmahon B, McKeown T, Record RG (1953) The incidence and life expectation of children with congenital heart disease. Br Heart J 15: 121–129.

6. Dastgiri S, Gilmour WH, Stone DH (2003) Survival of children born with congenital anomalies. Arch Dis Child 88: 391–394.

7. Freedom RM, Lock J, Bricker JT (2000) Pediatric cardiology and cardiovascular surgery: 1950–2000. Circulation 102(20 Suppl 4): IV58–68.

8. NHS Information Centre (2009) National Audit of Congenital Heart Disease: Executive Summary 2009. Leeds, UK: NHS Information Centre. Available: http://www.hscic.gov.uk/catalogue/PUB02661/nati-cong-hear-dise-exec-summ-audi-2009-rep.pdf Accessed: 17 July 2014.

9. Wren C, O'Sullivan JJ (2001) Survival with congenital heart disease and need for follow up in adult life. Heart 85: 438–443.

10. Nieminen HP, Jokinen EV, Sairanen HI (2001) Late results of pediatric cardiac surgery in Finland: a population-based study with 96% follow-up. Circulation 104: 570–575.

11. McCrindle BW (2001) Considerations in the appraisal of mortality associated with congenital cardiac lesions. Semin Thorac Cardiovasc Surg Pediatr Card Surg Annu 4: 244–255.

12. Ben-Shlomo Y, Kuh D (2002) A life course approach to chronic disease epidemiology: conceptual models, empirical challenges and interdisciplinary perspectives. Int J Epidemiol 31: 285–293.

13. Bull C (1999) Current and potential impact of fetal diagnosis on prevalence and spectrum of serious congenital heart disease at term in the UK. British Paediatric Cardiac Association. Lancet 354: 1242–1247.

14. Wren C, Richmond S, Donaldson L (2000) Temporal variability in birth prevalence of cardiovascular malformations. Heart 83: 414–419.

15. Lane DA, Lip GY, Millane TA (2002) Quality of life in adults with congenital heart disease. Heart 88: 71–75.

16. Cole TJ, Freeman JV, Preece MA (1998) British 1990 growth reference centiles for weight, height, body mass index and head circumference fitted by maximum penalized likelihood. Stat Med 17: 407–429.

17. Rasbash J, Charlton C, Browne WJ, Healy M, Cameron B (2009) MLwiN version 2.1. University of Bristol, UK: Centre for Multilevel Modelling.

18. Goldstein H (2009) REALCOM-Impute: Multiple Imputation using MLwiN, User Guide. University of Bristol: Centre for Multilevel Modelling.

19. Goldstein H, Browne W, Rasbash J (2002) Multilevel modelling of medical data. Stat Med 21: 3291–3315.

20. Goldstein H (2011) Multilevel Statistical Models. Chichester, UK: John Wiley and Sons.

21. Kenward MG, Carpenter J (2007) Multiple imputation: current perspectives. Stat Methods Med Res 16: 199–218.

22. Knowles RL, Bull C, Wren C, Dezateux C (2011) Ethics, governance and consent in the UK: implications for research into the longer-term outcomes of congenital heart defects. Arch Dis Child 96: 14–20.

23. Brown KL, Crowe S, Pagel C, Bull C, Muthialu N, et al. (2013) Use of diagnostic information submitted to the United Kingdom Central Cardiac Audit Database: development of categorisation and allocation algorithms. Cardiol Young 23: 491–498.

24. Riehle-Colarusso T, Strickland MJ, Reller MD, Mahle WT, Botto LD, et al. (2007) Improving the quality of surveillance data on congenital heart defects in the metropolitan Atlanta congenital defects program. Birth Defects Res A Clin Mol Teratol 79: 743–753.

25. Billett J, Majeed A, Gatzoulis M, Cowie M (2008) Trends in hospital admissions, in-hospital case fatality and population mortality from congenital heart disease in England, 1994 to 2004. Heart 94: 342–348.

26. Crowe S, Brown KL, Pagel C, Muthialu N, Cunningham D, et al. (2013) Development of a diagnosis- and procedure-based risk model for 30-day outcome after pediatric cardiac surgery. J Thorac Cardiovasc Surg 145: 1270–1278.

27. Wren C, Reinhardt Z, Khawaja K (2008) Twenty-year trends in diagnosis of life-threatening neonatal cardiovascular malformations. Arch Dis Child Fetal Neonatal Ed 93: F33–35.

28. Samanek M (1992) Children with congenital heart disease: probability of natural survival. Pediatr Cardiol 13: 152–158.

29. Morris CD, Menashe VD (1991) 25-year mortality after surgical repair of congenital heart defect in childhood. A population-based cohort study. JAMA 266: 3447–3452.

30. Larsen SH, Emmertsen K, Johnsen SP, Pedersen J, Hjortholm K, et al. (2011) Survival and morbidity following congenital heart surgery in a population-based cohort of children–up to 12 years of follow-up. Congenit Heart Dis 6: 322–329.

31. Meberg A, Otterstad JE, Froland G, Lindberg H, Sorland SJ (2000) Outcome of congenital heart defects–a population-based study. Acta Paediatr 89: 1344–1351.

32. Moons P, Sluysmans T, De WD, Massin M, Suys B, et al. (2009) Congenital heart disease in 111 225 births in Belgium: birth prevalence, treatment and survival in the 21st century. Acta Paediatr 98: 472–477.

33. Oppido G, Napoleone CP, Formigari R, Gabbieri D, Pacini D, et al. (2004) Outcome of cardiac surgery in low birth weight and premature infants. Eur J Cardiothorac Surg 26: 44–53.

34. Padley JR, Cole AD, Pye VE, Chard RB, Nicholson IA, et al. (2011) Five-year analysis of operative mortality and neonatal outcomes in congenital heart disease. Heart Lung Circ 20: 460–467.

35. Tanner K, Sabrine N, Wren C (2005) Cardiovascular malformations among preterm infants. Pediatrics 116: e833–e838.

36. Brown KL, Ridout DA, Hoskote A, Verhulst L, Ricci M, et al. (2006) Delayed diagnosis of congenital heart disease worsens pre-operative condition and outcome of surgery in neonates. Heart 92: 1298–1302.

37. Bonnet D, Coltri A, Butera G, Fermont L, Le Bidois J, et al. (1999) Detection of transposition of the great arteries in fetuses reduces neonatal morbidity and mortality. Circulation 99: 916–918.

38. Brown KL, Ridout DA, Goldman AP, Hoskote A, Penny DJ (2003) Risk factors for long intensive care unit stay after cardiopulmonary bypass in children. Crit Care Med 31: 28–33.

39. Vogt PR, Carrel T, Pasic M, Arbenz U, von Segesser LK, et al. (1994) Early and late results after correction for double-outlet right ventricle: uni- and multivariate analysis of risk factors. Eur J Cardiothorac Surg 8: 301–307.

40. Nollert G, Fischlein T, Bouterwek S, Bohmer C, Klinner W, et al. (1997) Long-term survival in patients with repair of tetralogy of Fallot: 36- year follow-up of 490 survivors of the first year after surgical repair. J Am Coll Cardiol 30: 1374–1383.

41. Kang N, Cole T, Tsang V, Elliott M, de Leval M (2004) Risk stratification in paediatric open-heart surgery. Eur J Cardiothorac Surg 26: 3–11.

42. Greeley WJ, Kern FH, Ungerleider RM, Boyd JL, 3rd, Quill T, et al. (1991) The effect of hypothermic cardiopulmonary bypass and total circulatory arrest on cerebral metabolism in neonates, infants, and children. J Thorac Cardiovasc Surg 101: 783–794.

43. Fyler DC (1980) Report of the New England Regional Infant Cardiac Program. Pediatrics 65: 375–461.

44. Chang RK, Chen AY, Klitzner TS (2002) Female sex as a risk factor for in-hospital mortality among children undergoing cardiac surgery. Circulation 106: 1514–1522.

45. Klitzner TS, Lee M, Rodriguez S, Chang RK (2006) Sex-related disparity in surgical mortality among pediatric patients. Congenit Heart Dis 1: 77–88.

46. Seifert HA, Howard DL, Silber JH, Jobes DR (2007) Female gender increases the risk of death during hospitalization for pediatric cardiac surgery. J Thorac Cardiovasc Surg 133: 668–675.

47. Kochilas LK, Vinocur JM, Menk JS (2014) Age-Dependent Sex Effects on Outcomes After Pediatric Cardiac Surgery. J Am Heart Assoc 3: e000608.

48. Sarikouch S, Boethig D, Beerbaum P (2013) Gender-specific algorithms recommended for patients with congenital heart defects: review of the literature. Thorac Cardiovasc Surg 61: 79–84.

49. Dezateux C, Stocks J (1997) Lung development and early origins of childhood respiratory illness. Br Med Bull 53: 40–57.

50. Postma DS (2007) Gender differences in asthma development and progression. Gend Med 4 Suppl B: S133–146.

51. Falagas ME, Mourtzoukou EG, Vardakas KZ (2007) Sex differences in the incidence and severity of respiratory tract infections. Respir Med 101: 1845–1863.

52. Eskedal L, Hagemo P, Eskild A, Aamodt G, Seiler KS, et al. (2004) A population-based study of extra-cardiac anomalies in children with congenital cardiac malformations. Cardiol Young 14: 600–607.

53. Frid C, Bjorkhem G, Jonzon A, Sunnegardh J, Anneren G, et al. (2004) Long-term survival in children with atrioventricular septal defect and common atrioventricular valvar orifice in Sweden. Cardiol Young 14: 24–31.

54. Bristol Royal Infirmary Inquiry (2001) Learning from Bristol: the report of the public inquiry into children's heart surgery at the Bristol Royal Infirmary 1984 - 1995. Norwich, UK: The Stationery Office Ltd.

55. Bull C (2001) Key Issues in Retrospective Evaluation of Morbidity Outcomes Following Paediatric Cardiac Surgery. Final Report of the Bristol Royal Infirmary Inquiry (CM 5207). Norwich, UK: The Stationery Office Ltd.

56. NICOR (2012) National Institute for Cardiovascular Outcomes Research: Congenital Heart Disease Website. London, UK: University College London. Available: https://nicor4.nicor.org.uk/CHD/an_paeds.nsf/vwContent/home?Opendocument Accessed: 17 July 2014.

57. Gibbs JL, Monro JL, Cunningham D, Rickards A (2004) Survival after surgery or therapeutic catheterisation for congenital heart disease in children in the United Kingdom: analysis of the central cardiac audit database for 2000-1. BMJ 328: 611.

58. Office for National Statistics (2010) Infant and perinatal mortality by health areas in England and Wales, 2009. Office for National Statistics Statistical Bulletin. Newport, UK: Office for National Statistics.

22

Uncovering the Rare Variants of *DLC1* Isoform 1 and their Functional Effects in a Chinese Sporadic Congenital Heart Disease Cohort

Bin Lin[1,9], **Yufeng Wang**[1,9], **Zhen Wang**[2], **Huilian Tan**[2], **Xianghua Kong**[3], **Yang Shu**[1], **Yuchao Zhang**[1], **Yun Huang**[1], **Yufei Zhu**[1], **Heng Xu**[1], **Zhiqiang Wang**[1], **Ping Wang**[1], **Guang Ning**[4], **Xiangyin Kong**[1,4]*, **Guohong Hu**[1]*, **Landian Hu**[1,4]*

1 The Key Laboratory of Stem Cell Biology, Institute of Health Sciences, Shanghai Jiao Tong University School of Medicine (SJTUSM) and Shanghai Institutes for Biological Sciences (SIBS), Chinese Academy of Sciences (CAS), Shanghai, People's Republic of China, **2** Diagnosis and Treatment Center of Congenital Heart Disease, the First Hospital of Hebei Medical University, Shijiazhuang, Hebei, People's Republic of China, **3** Clinical Laboratory, Affiliated Hospital of Binzhou Medical College, Binzhou, Shandong, People's Republic of China, **4** State Key Laboratory of Medical Genomics, Ruijin Hospital Affiliated to Shanghai Jiao Tong University School of Medicine, Shanghai, People's Republic of China

Abstract

Congenital heart disease (CHD) is the most common birth defect affecting the structure and function of fetal hearts. Despite decades of extensive studies, the genetic mechanism of sporadic CHD remains obscure. Deleted in liver cancer 1 (*DLC1*) gene, encoding a GTPase-activating protein, is highly expressed in heart and essential for heart development according to the knowledge of *Dlc1*-deficient mice. To determine whether *DLC1* is a susceptibility gene for sporadic CHD, we sequenced the coding region of *DLC1* isoform 1 in 151 sporadic CHD patients and identified 13 non-synonymous rare variants (including 6 private variants) in the case cohort. Importantly, these rare variants (8/13) were enriched in the N-terminal region of the DLC1 isoform 1 protein. Seven of eight amino acids at the N-terminal variant positions were conserved among the primates. Among the 9 rare variants that were predicted as "damaging", five were located at the N-terminal region. Ensuing *in vitro* functional assays showed that three private variants (Met360Lys, Glu418Lys and Asp554Val) impaired the ability of DLC1 to inhibit cell migration or altered the subcellular location of the protein compared to wild-type DLC1 isoform 1. These data suggest that *DLC1* might act as a CHD-associated gene in addition to its role as a tumor suppressor in cancer.

Editor: Yong-Gang Yao, Kunming Institute of Zoology, Chinese Academy of Sciences, China

Funding: This work is supported by the National Basic Research Program of China (No. 2007CB512103, 2011CB510100) (http://www.973.gov.cn/English/Index.aspx), the National Natural Science Foundation of China (No. 81030015) (http://www.nsfc.gov.cn/Portal0/default166.htm), and the E-Institutes of Shanghai Municipal Education Commission. The funders had no role in study design, data collection and analysis, decision to publish, or preparation of the manuscript.

Competing Interests: The authors have declared that no competing interests exist.

* E-mail: xykong@sibs.ac.cn (XK); ghhu@sibs.ac.cn (GH); ldhu@sibs.ac.cn (LH)

9 These authors contributed equally to this work.

Introduction

Congenital heart disease (CHD) presents a variety of structural malformations of the heart or great vessels at birth, constituting a major cause of birth defect-related deaths [1]. Although decades of research have revealed that both environmental and genetic factors contribute to the etiology of CHD, increasing evidence supports an important role of a genetic predisposition to the disease [1–4]. Indeed, many disease-causing genes, which follow Mendelian patterns of inheritance (e.g., *TBX5*, *JAG1*, *NKX2-5*, *GATA4*, *NOTCH1*), have been identified by pedigree analysis [5–10]; however, the genetic mechanism of most sporadic CHD cases remains elusive [11].

In our previous mutational screen in a Chinese sporadic CHD cohort, a low-coverage (100×) exome sequencing of 18 pooled samples identified a splice-site mutation (chr8:13072284, C>G, reference assembly: hg19) of the deleted in liver cancer 1 (*DLC1*) gene in a patient who has atrial septal defect (ASD). This variant is not recorded in The 1000 Genomes Project database and the dbSNP 137 database; after validation assays, it is absent in 800 control samples, suggesting that this splicing site mutation is unique in the CHD cohort (unpublished data).

DLC1, which encodes a GTPase-activating protein, is considered to be a tumor suppressor gene in several types of tumors (e.g., primary hepatocellular carcinoma, breast cancer, prostate cancer, non-small cell lung cancer and meningioma tumors) [12–18]. The migration and proliferation of some tumor cells are reported to be inhibited by DLC1 [19–22]. DLC1 can interact with tensin family proteins [23,24] and is localized to focal adhesions [25], which together indicate that DLC1 is essential for the cytoskeletal organization and morphology of cells. Interestingly, *Dlc1*$^{-/-}$ mice are embryonic lethal, and histologically, the heart is incompletely developed with a distorted architecture of the chambers [26]. Another study reported that *Dlc1* homozygous gene-trapped mice demonstrated abnormalities in the embryonic heart and blood vasculature of the yolk sac [27]. These results, which were derived from observations of knockout mice, unequivocally prove that *DLC1* is of paramount importance to the developmental events occurring in the embryonic heart.

The human *DLC1* gene encodes four transcript variants: isoforms 1–4 encode protein products of 1528 aa, 1091 aa, 463 aa and 1017 aa, respectively. Although there have been numerous investigations focused on characterizing the multi-faceted function of *DLC1* isoform 2, the properties of the other isoforms remain unclear. In particular, *DLC1* isoform 1, the longest isoform of the *DLC1* gene (NCBI Reference Sequence: NM_182643.2), is abundantly expressed in human heart tissues [28].

The evidence described above logically leads to the hypothesis that, in addition to its role as a tumor suppressor in cancer, DLC1 might play another role in the pathogenesis of CHD. Therefore, to verify the rare variant frequency of *DLC1* isoform 1 in a CHD cohort, we sequenced the coding regions and intron boundaries of *DLC1* isoform 1 in 151 CHD patients (not including the initial screening CHD cohort of our previous work). Functional experiments were then performed to determine the consequences of the identified mutations.

Materials and Methods

Ethics statement

The written informed consent for the genetic analysis was obtained from all the subjects who participated in this study, and the research was approved by the ethics committee at Institute of Health Sciences, Shanghai Institutes for Biological Sciences, Chinese Academy of Sciences.

Sample preparation

A total of 151 patients with congenital heart disease were enrolled in the study at the First Hospital of Hebei Medical University. All the subjects were examined by experienced cardiologists, and the cardiac phenotypes were determined using standard transthoracic echocardiography and other tests according to the ICD-10 diagnostic criteria (Table S1 in File S1). The patients' basic medical situation and family history were recorded. The karyotypes of all patients were examined; with the exception of three individuals with trisomy 21, all others were normal. Most of the patients did not have extra-cardiac manifestations except the three individuals with Down syndrome. Most of the patients had undergone cardiac catheterization or surgery. After recruitment in Hebei and Shanghai of normal individuals without CHD, control blood samples ($n = 500$) were collected. Genomic DNA was extracted from peripheral blood using QIAamp DNA Blood Mini Kits.

Mutational analysis

The exons and portions of 5′UTR and 3′UTR regions of *DLC1* isoform 1 were amplified using the primers shown in Table S2 in File S1. The PCR products were then purified using ExoSAP-IT reagent (USB) and sequenced with an ABI 3730 Genetic Analyzer. The results were analyzed using the ABI software suite and the identified variants were re-sequenced and validated.

Mutation simulation

The method of O'Roak *et al.* [29] was used to calculate the mutation weight of each base of the *DLC1* isoform 1 coding sequence. Because the simulation only focused on the *DLC1* gene, the locus-specific substitution rate was not considered. Thus the mutation weight for each base and each substitution can be calculated as follows:

$$W_m = W_n * W_s$$

where W_n is the weight measuring the nucleotide-specific substitution rates and has two values according to the base composition [30]:

$$W_{n=AT} = 0.884$$

$$W_{n=CG} = 0.942$$

For the weight W_s, which represents the relative transition or transversion substitution rates [31]:

$$W_{missense,ti} = 2.31,\ W_{missense,ti} = 2.31,\ W_{missense,tv} = W_{nonsense,tv} = 1$$

We mutated each base to the other three bases and predicted the class of mutation (i.e., synonymous, missense or nonsense) that would be introduced. For the sake of convenience, only the missense and nonsense classes were considered. We then obtained the mutation weight of each base for missense and nonsense classes using:

$$W_m = W_n * (W_{s,missense} + W_{s,nonsense})$$

To address whether the cluster of mutations we observed was identical to that expected by chance, after the common SNP sites were eliminated from the coding sequence, 13 non-synonymous rare mutations were randomly introduced into the gene based on the mutation weights in one simulation. We then recorded how often the number of mutations residing within the identical range of our cluster was larger than or equal to 8. The range of the cluster was defined as 639 bp (the length from substitution Ala220Val to Thr433Asn in the coding sequence). The significance was estimated as $P = (n+1)/(m+1)$, where n is the number of instances where the randomized number was greater than the observed number and m was the number of randomizations (we employed $m = 1,000,000$). Thus, we could estimate the probability of the identical cluster occurring by chance.

Plasmids construction

The wild-type *DLC1* isoform 1 expression plasmid was purchased from OpenBiosystems. Seven missense mutants of *DLC1* isoform 1 (threonine substitution of alanine-350, lysine substitution of methionine-360, methionine substitution of leucine-413, lysine substitution of glutamic acid-418, valine substitution of aspartic acid-554, valine substitution of leucine-952 and leucine substitution of valine-1371) were generated by site-directed mutagenesis. The wild type *DLC1* isoform 1 and these mutants were cloned into the pEGFP(N1) plasmid, and the DLC1-GFP fusion constructs were transferred into the retroviral plasmid pBabe-puro.

Cell culture

The human umbilical vein endothelial cell line (HUVEC, acquired from Lonza) was maintained in basal medium 199 (Invitrogen) with 20% fetal bovine serum (FBS), heparin (25 µg/ mL, Sigma) and endothelial cell growth supplement (ECGS)

(50 μg/mL, Sigma). The human bone marrow endothelial cell line (HBMEC-60) [32] was maintained in basal medium 200 (Invitrogen) with 20% FBS and a low-serum growth supplement (Invitrogen). The amphotropic Phenix packaging cell line, H29 was maintained in Dulbecco's modified Eagle's medium (DMEM, Invitrogen) with 10% FBS (HyClone), 100 units/mL penicillin, 100 μg/mL streptomycin (Invitrogen) and 1 μg/mL tetracycline (Sigma) in 5% CO_2 at 37°C.

Transwell migration assay

To test the effects of the DLC1 wild-type and mutant proteins on cell migration, pBabe-puro overexpression plasmids were transfected into the amphotropic Phenix packaging cell line, and the viruses were collected as previously described [32]. When the cells (HUVEC or HBMEC-60) grew to 30~40% confluency, the culture medium was replaced with a 1:1 mixture of fresh medium and the above virus-containing medium in the presence of 5 μg/mL polybrene for infection and this operation was repeated every 24 h until the infection rate of the target cells reached ~80%, as judged by GFP-positive cells. After infection, 10^5 infected endothelial cells were resuspended in fresh media containing 0.5% serum, and the cells were seeded in inserts (Costar) containing 8 μm pores. These inserts were placed in Transwell cartridges that contained 300 μL of medium with 10% FBS in the bottom wells. At 24 h after seeding, the medium was aspirated, and 350 μL of trypsin was added into the wells to trypsinize the cells that had passed through the pores. After serum neutralization of the trypsin, the trypsinized cells were centrifuged for 4 min at 1000 rpm, resuspended in 100 μL phosphate-buffered saline (PBS) and counted using a hemocytometer.

Proliferation assay

When the virus infection rate reached ~80%, 5×10^4 infected cells were seeded. After 2 days, the resulting cells were trypsinized and counted using a hemocytometer. Then, 5×10^4 of these cells were reseeded for another round of counting. The process was repeated for at least three cycles.

Active rho assay

Cells at 80% confluence were gently rinsed once with ice-cold Tris-buffered saline (TBS) and lysed. The lysate was centrifuged at $16,000\times g$ at 4°C for 15 min, and the supernatant was subjected to active Rho purification and detection with the Active Rho Kit (Pierce, Cat No. 16116) according to the manufacturer's protocol.

Stress fiber staining and DLC1 subcellular localization

When the cells reached 40% confluence, they were transfected with pEGFP(N1) plasmids harboring DLC1 wild-type or mutant cDNA. After 24 h, the cells were fixed with 10% formalin for 15 min, permeated with 0.1% Triton X-100 for 10 min and stained with 5 units/mL rhodamine phalloidin (Invitrogen) for 20 min. The stained cells were imaged with using a laser confocal microscope. A total of 100 randomly selected transfected cells in each sample were assessed for subcellular localization of the DLC1-GFP fusion protein. The selected cells were also assessed for the percentage of cells with visible stress fibers as previously described [33].

Angiogenesis (tube-formation) assay

A total of 5×10^4 cells infected with DLC1-expressing viruses were suspended in 300 μL of DMEM supplemented with 10% FBS and 10 ng/mL FGF (Invitrogen). The cell suspension was seeded on 300 μL of pregelled Matrigel (10.8 mg/mL, Becton,

Dickinson and Company). After 24 h, 10 microscopic fields were randomly selected for each well. Angiogenesis in each well was determined by counting the branch points of the formed tubes, as previously described [34].

Apoptosis assay

Cell apoptosis analysis was performed using an Apoptosis Assay Kit (Keygen Biotech) according to the manufacturer's instructions. Briefly, 1×10^6 cells infected with virus expressing wild-type or mutant DLC1 were trypsinized and resuspended in 500 μL of $1\times$ binding buffer. Then, fluorochrome-conjugated Annexin V was added to the cell suspension and was incubated for 10 min at room temperature, followed by incubation with 5 μL of 7-AAD viability staining solution for 10 min at room temperature. The cells were then subjected to flow cytometry using a FACSAria (BD Biosciences).

Results

Identification of rare variants in the DLC1 gene of CHD patients

DLC1 isoform 1 contains 18 exons and spans 431,558 base pairs (bp). Each exon of DLC1 isoform 1 was amplified from the genomic DNA of 151 CHD patients and the PCR products were then sequenced by Sanger sequencing. After eliminating the common single-nucleotide polymorphisms (SNPs) (SNPs with minor allele frequency $\geq 1\%$) found in the dbSNP database, 13 rare non-synonymous variants were identified. One of these variants was found in 2 patients and each of the rest 12 variant was found in 1 patient. We then assessed the frequency of these rare variants in the control cohort by sequencing the corresponding sites in 500 normal samples using Sanger sequencing method. These data were combined with an additional exome sequencing dataset of 400 individuals (average depth $60\times$) (G.N., unpublished data) to widen the control cohort to 900 individuals. Consequently, only 3 rare variants identified in the CHD cohort were also found in the controls. In addition, 6 of the 13 variants were SNPs with very low frequency recorded in dbSNP build 137 (Table 1). Altogether, we identified 6 private variants that were absent in 900 controls and the dbSNP database (Table 1, Fig. 1A). The clinical information of 14 patients who carried these rare variants of DLC1 were reviewed, and ten of the fourteen patients had septal defects. We also reviewed the health status information of the parents of these patients, and all of them had no cardiac defects. However, it's a great pity that we could not obtained the blood samples of these parents because they came to the hospital years ago and we lost touch with these families.

DLC1 rare variants cluster in the N-terminus of the protein

Compared to DLC1 isoform 2, which is the most studied isoform, the coding product of isoform 1 has an N-terminal end of 447 amino acids prior to the SAM domain (including an extended region of 437 amino acids and 10 amino acids which are different from the corresponding parts of DLC1 isoform 2) (Fig. 1B). Although several domains have been identified in the DLC1 protein, the function of the N-terminus is still undefined. Interestingly, 8 (61.5%) of the amino acid-altering variants identified in sporadic CHD were located in this region (Fig. 1A). To evaluate the rare variant frequency of this region in other populations, the rare variant information of DLC1 in the 1000 Genomes Project [35] and the Exome Sequencing Project [31] were collected and analyzed ($samplesize=7592$). As described before, we defined amino acids 1-447 as the N-terminal region and

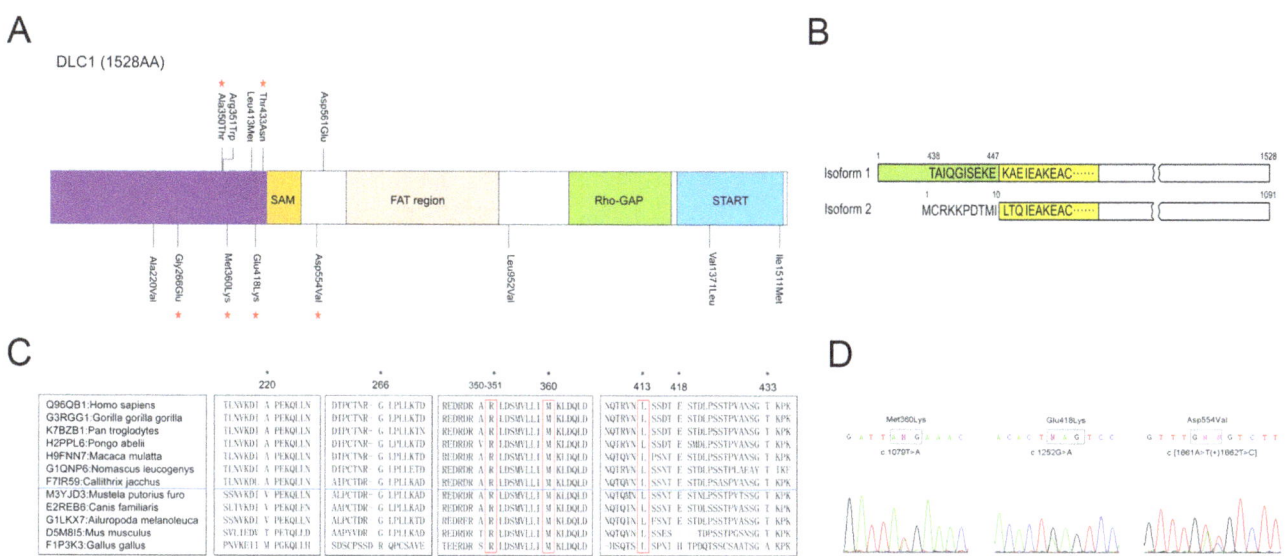

Figure 1. Rare variants identified in *DLC1* isoform 1. (A) The locations of the rare variants are indicated by black lines on the DLC1 isoform 1 protein. FAT (focal adhesion targeting) region, SAM (sterile alpha motif), Rho-Gap (Rho-GTPase-activating protein) and START (steroidogenic acute regulatory protein related lipid transfer) domains are indicated by different colors. Stars denote the private variants identified in the CHD cohort. (B) DLC1 isoform 1 possesses an extended N-terminal region compared to isoform 2. The first 437 residues of isoform 1 are missing in isoform 2, and the sequence 'TAIQGISEKEKAE' is replaced by 'MCRKKPDTMILTQ' in isoform 2. The yellow box indicates the SAM domain in DLC1, and the green box shows the N-terminal region. (C) The conservation of residues in the N-terminal region was analyzed in different species. The primates and non-primates are separated by the blue lines in the boxes. Asterisks indicate the residues that are conserved among the primates. The residues that are conserved in the primates and non-primates locate in the red boxes. The UniProt accession ID is followed by a colon and the corresponding species name. (D) The private variants that altered the regulation of cell migration function of DLC1 are shown.

found that 60 (29.6%) of the 203 rare protein-altering variants were localized in this region (Table S3 in File S1). Consequently, Fisher's exact test (two-tail) showed that, compared to variants found in the 1000 Genomes Project and the Exome Sequencing Project mentioned above, the rare variants identified in our CHD cohort significantly clustered at the N-terminus ($P = 0.027$), revealing that this might be a disease-associated mutation hot spot. We then used the methods from O'Roak *et al.* [29] to measure the mutation weight of each base of the *DLC1* isoform 1 coding sequence. Subsequently 13 missense or nonsense mutations were randomly introduced into the gene in a simulation according to the mutation weights. After one million simulations, we found that the probability of mutation enrichment similar to the observed cases (at least 8 mutations in a range of 639 bp) was very low ($P = 0.004$), which illustrated that the existence of this mutation cluster in the case cohort was not a spontaneous phenomenon.

Most rare variants are predicted to be deleterious

We then BLAST-searched the N-terminal sequence in the UniProt database and aligned the homologous sequences [36]. The alignment showed that, seven of eight amino acids at the N-terminal variant positions were conserved among the primates, and it's worth noting that Arg351, Met360 and Leu413 were conserved in the primates and non-primates (Fig. 1C). The SIFT scores were also calculated to predict the effects of the rare variants on protein function [37] (Table 1, Table S3 in File S1). Among the 9 rare variants that were predicted as "damaging" in the case cohort (*SIFT score* < 0.05), 5 were located at the N-terminal region. As for other five rare variants beyond the N-terminal end, there were three amino acid substitutions in the region between the sterile alpha motif (SAM) and Rho-GTPase-activating protein (GAP) domains, but none in the focal adhesion targeting region

[38,39]. The other two amino acid substitutions (Val1371Leu and Ile1511Met) were located in the steroidogenic acute regulatory protein related lipid transfer (START) domain. All of these substitutions were predicted to be deleterious except the c.1683C>A transition (Table 1). We also evaluated the effects of these 13 rare variants found in the case cohort by multiple prediction methods (PolyPhen-2, LRT, Mutation Taster, etc.), and the prediction results from PolyPhen-2 were similar to the SIFT results (Table S4 in File S1).

Three mutations affect the role of DLC1 in cell migration

To study whether the rare variants identified in the CHD cohort affect the protein function of DLC1, we cloned 7 of the variants, including 4 private variants and 3 other rare variants, by introducing the point mutations into the wild-type *DLC1* isoform 1. These variants are as the following: Mutant 1, Ala350Thr; Mutant 2, Met360Lys; Mutant 3, Leu413Met; Mutant 4, Glu418Lys; Mutant 5, Asp554Val; Mutant 6, Leu952Val; and Mutant 7, Val1371Leu. These seven variants were selected because they were absent in 900 control samples (altogether 10 rare variants were absent in 900 control samples, but mutant vectors of Gly266Glu, Thr433Asn and Ile1511Met were failed to construct for technical reasons). Cell migration inhibition is one of the most studied functions of DLC1. However, most studies focused on the isoform 2 of DLC1 (1091 aa) and the effect of isoform 1 and its mutants on cell migration has not been reported. Therefore, we assessed the functions of DLC1 isoform 1 and its mutants on migration in human umbilical vein endothelial cells (HUVEC) and human bone marrow endothelial cells 60 (HBMEC-60), the two cell lines widely used in cardiovascular disease studies. The wild-type isoform 1, mutants 1–7, and the control vector were transfected into HUVEC and HBMEC-60 cells (Fig. 2A), following by transwell migration assays to analyze

Table 1. The rare variants identified in *DLC1* isoform 1.

Variant type	Patient ID	Gender	Age of diagnosis	Diagnosis	Exon	Nucleotide alteration[a]	Amino acid alteration	SIFT score	SIFT prediction (cutoff = 0.05)	Number of mutations in patients	Number of mutations in controls	In dbSNP[b]	ALT allele frequency in dbSNP[c]
Private variants	67	M	5	VSD&PFO	2	c.797G>A	p.Gly266Glu	0.406	Tolerated	1/151	0/900	Na	Na
	153	F	8	VSD	3	c.1048G>A*	p.Ala350Thr	0.368	Tolerated	1/151	0/900	Na	Na
	168	F	5	ASD	3	c.1079T>A*	p.Met360Lys	0.001	Damaging	1/151	0/900	Na	Na
	169	F	22	PS	4	c.1252G>A*	p.Glu418Lys	0.027	Damaging	1/151	0/900	Na	Na
	89	F	2	PDA	4	c.1298C>A	p.Thr433Asn	0.02	Damaging	1/151	0/900	Na	Na
	131	F	8	PDA	9	c.[1661A>T(+)1662T>C]*	p.Asp554Val	0.014	Damaging	1/151	0/900	Na	Na
	190	F	7	VSD	9	c.[1661A>T(+)1662T>C]*	p.Asp554Val	0.014	Damaging	1/151	0/900	Na	Na
Other rare variants	49	F	9	TOF	2	c.659C>T	p.Ala220Val	1	Tolerated	1/151	1/900	Na	Na
	61	F	6	TOF	3	c.1051C>T	p.Arg351Trp	0	Damaging	1/151	2/900	rs144283917	2.324/5869
	42	F	17	VSD	4	c.1237T>A*	p.Leu413Met	0.005	Damaging	1/151	0/900	rs143447199	1/4545
	55	F	26	PDA	9	c.1683C>A	p.Asp561Glu	0.171	Tolerated	1/151	2/900	rs201661577	5/2174
	124	F	4	VSD	9	c.2854C>G*	p.Leu952Val	0.003	Damaging	1/151	0/900	rs184157214	1/2000
	28	M	1	VSD	16	c.4111G>C*	p.Val1371Leu	0.016	Damaging	1/151	0/900	rs142865083	1/2000
	8	M	12	VSD	18	c.4533C>G	p.Ile1511Met	0.001	Damaging	1/151	0/900	rs78322853	Na

Note. Na, no available data; M, male; F, female; VSD, ventricular septal defect; PFO, patent foramen ovale; ASD, atrial septal defect; PS, pulmonary stenosis; PDA, patent ductus arteriosus; TOF, tetralogy of Fallot. a, Nucleotide numbering is according to the RefSeq database NM_182643.2. b, The version of dbSNP used in the table is dbSNP build 137. c, The alternative allele frequency from the dbSNP database is calculated by the alternative allele count/ two times the number of individuals assayed. *The mutant vectors were constructed according to these variants.

the migratory abilities of the cells. As shown in Figure 2, DLC1 isoform 1 suppressed the migration abilities of HUVEC and HBMEC-60 *in vitro*. Mutants 2, 4 and 5 (Fig. 1D), which either changed the polarity (Met360 and Asp554) or altered the electric charge (Glu418) of the amino acids, rescued the migration suppression by the wild-type DLC1 protein, as the migration of the cells transfected by these mutants was similar to the control cells. The other mutants appeared to have no significant differences from the wild type to suppress cell migration (Fig. 2B, 2C). In addition, the migration rescue effect of Mutants 2, 4 and 5 could not be accounted for by their effect on cell proliferation, because the mutants and the wild-type protein similarly suppressed the growth of endothelial cells (Fig. S1 in File S1).

The Glu418Lys mutant changes subcellular localization of DLC1

DLC1 is an inhibitor protein of small GTPases including RhoA/B/C and CDC42. Such an inhibitory effect was thought to be mainly mediated by the GAP domain of DLC1. Interestingly, none of the variants identified in CHD lay within the GAP domain. Since a recent study reported that the protein sequences outside of GAP domain may also affect the Rho-inhibiting activity of DLC1 [40], we studied whether the CHD variants affect the GAP activity of DLC1. It was found all the mutants and the wild-type protein efficiently suppressed the activation of RhoA (Fig. 2A). Then we considered whether the small GTPases in the endothelial cells were regulated by DLC1 *in situ* by analyzing the formation of stress fibers in the cells, a process that is regulated by Rho activities. The *DLC1* constructs were tagged with GFP, and the stress fiber formation was analyzed by the high-affinity F-actin probe Rhodamine phalloidin. The data showed that when the wild-type and mutant DLC1 were expressed in the endothelial cells, the formation of stress fibers were prevented to similar levels (Fig. 3A, Fig. S3 in File S1).

Although the variants in DLC1 did not lead to any difference in the regulation of endothelial cytoskeleton, we observed Mutant 4 (Glu418Lys) markedly altered the localization of the protein in the cells. Fluorescent confocal microscopy revealed that DLC1 isoform 1 was primarily located in the cytoplasm, as were Mutants 1–3 and 5–7. Mutant 4 was found in both the cytoplasm and nucleus. Compared to the wild type and the other 6 mutant proteins which were excluded from the nucleus of 73% – 84% endothelial cells, the Mutant 4 protein was not seen in only 11% of the nucleus, suggesting the protein nuclear translocation (PNT) caused by the Glu418Lys substitution (Fig. 3). It was previously reported that PNT occurred in 10% of tumor cells after transfection with *DLC1* isoform 2 and was accompanied by morphological changes, and then these cells progressed to apoptosis stage [41]. Although no difference was observed between the cells transfected by Mutant 4 and those by other *DLC1* constructs in our apoptosis analysis, all the wild type and mutant DLC1 led to markedly enhanced percentages of apoptotic cells (Fig. S2 in File S1).

Discussion

Congenital heart disease is complex. Although key mutations have been identified by pedigree research, the great heterogeneity of CHD makes it very difficult to identify the responsible genes,

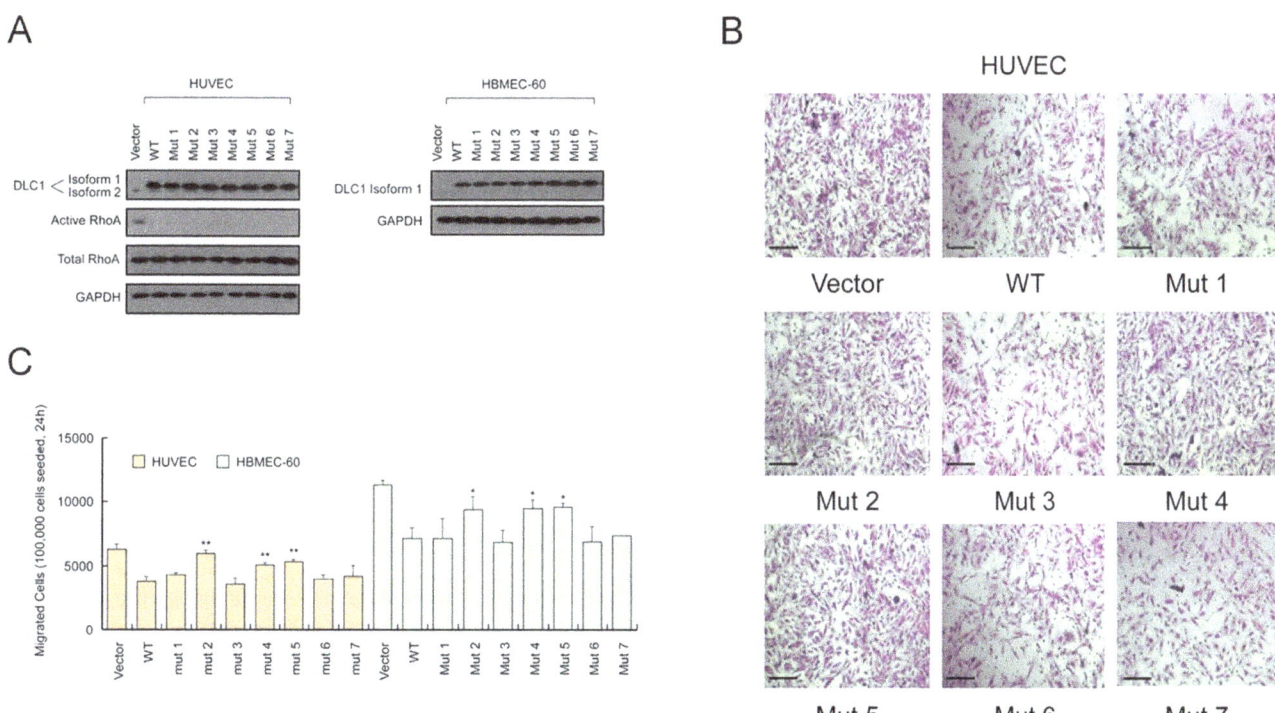

Figure 2. *DLC1* isoform 1 mutants had different effects on cell migration compared with the wild type protein. (A) Western blot analyses of *DLC1* isoform 1 mutant overexpression in two endothelial cell lines, HUVEC and HBMEC-60. In HUVECs, the effect of *DLC1* isoform 1 mutation on the GAP activity of the protein was detected by western blotting. (B) Representative images of the Transwell migration assay using HUVECs cells are shown. (C) The quantification of HUVEC and HBMEC-60 migration showed significant differences between wild-type DLC1 and Mutants 2, 4 and 5, whereas the other mutants showed no significant difference from wild-type DLC1. Wild-type DLC1 also showed an inhibitory effect on cell migration compared to the control vector. *Student's t-test $P < 0.05$; ** $P < 0.01$. Scale bars, 100 μm. Ns, not significant.

A

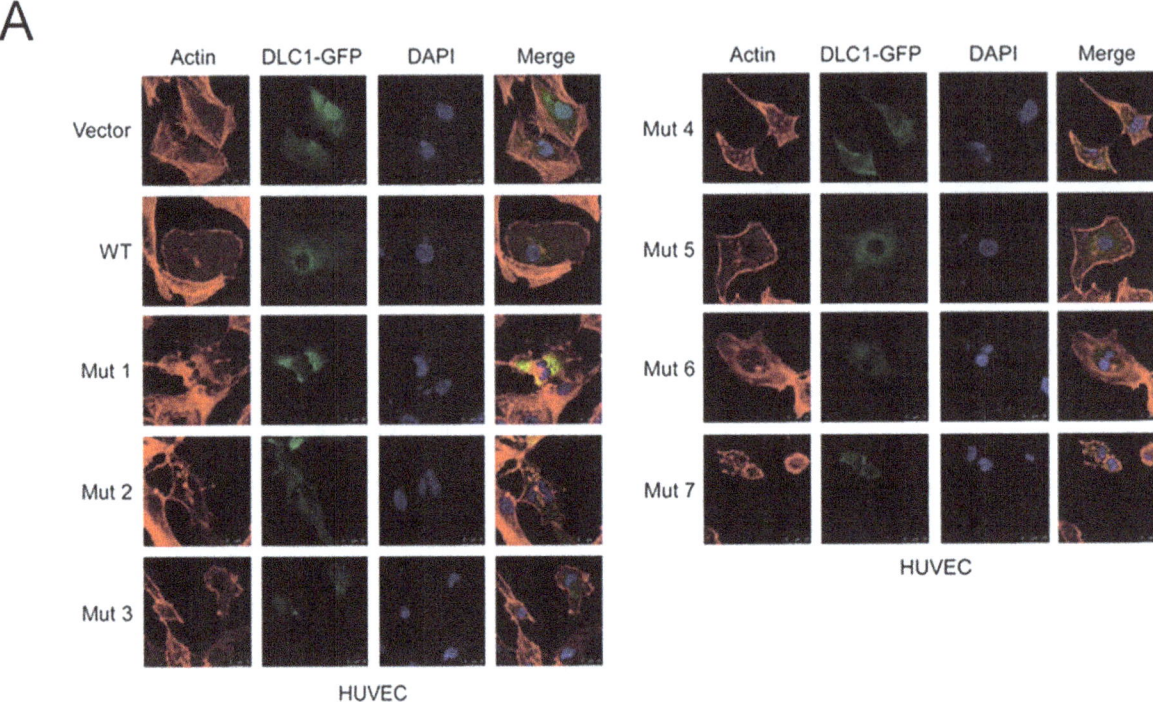

B

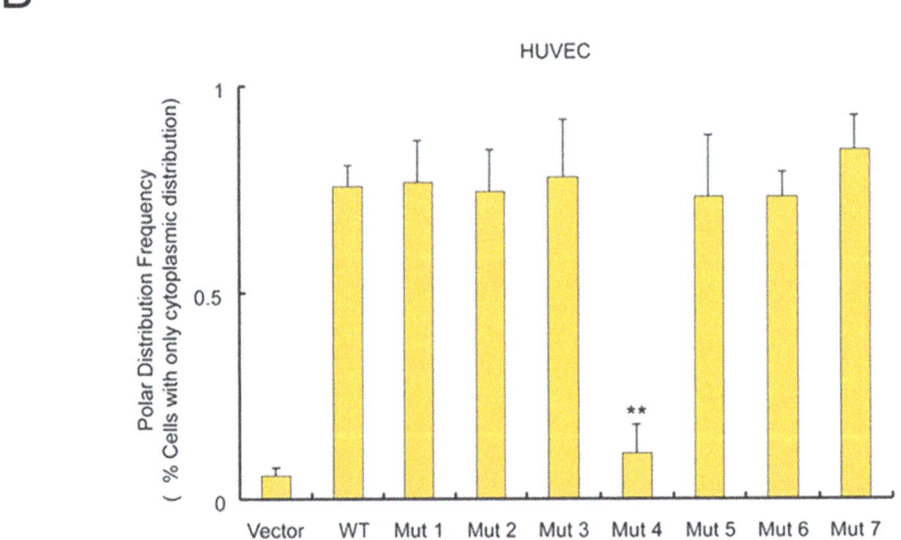

Figure 3. The subcellular localization of wild-type DLC1 and mutants in HUVECs. (A) Images of wild-type and mutant DLC1 distribution in HUVECs using laser scanning confocal microscopy. (B) The percentage of cells with wild-type and mutant DLC1 proteins with exclusive cytoplasmic-localization. Mutant 4 showed a significant difference from the wild type, as opposed to the control vector. *Student's t-test $P<0.05$; ** $P<0.01$. Scale bar, 25 μm. Ns, not significant.

particularly among sporadic CHD cohorts. However, disease or deleterious alleles could be rare [42], and rare variants that have obvious functional consequences will show the largest effect size for the disease [43]. Therefore, we focused on the identification of rare variants in a case cohort. We successfully identified 13 rare variants in a sporadic CHD cohort and provide clear evidence that 8 rare variants are clustered in the N-terminal region of the protein. However, we should note that, the reference variant data

from the 1000 Genomes Project and the Exome Sequencing Project were produced by different platforms, most of which were next generation sequencing platforms. The sequencing depth, coverage and data analysis pipelines might affect the variant detection rate. It is the consideration that the variant number from different platforms might not be compared directly. So we focused on the locations of the rare variants on the protein, and the analysis strategy is feasible in our study. More importantly, in our *in vitro* assays, three private variants (corresponding to Mutants 2, 4 and 5) were shown to alter the ability of DLC1 to inhibit cell migration or the subcellular localization of the protein, which supported the notion that private variants might also play major roles in the pathological process of complex diseases [43]. In addition, the extended N-terminal region of DLC1 isoform 1 harbors 83% (5/6) of the private variants identified in the CHD cohort in a non-random manner. The relatively high transcriptional level of *DLC1* isoform 1 in human heart tissues [28] implies that the unique N-terminal region may possess a tissue-specific function in the cardiovascular system. However, future studies are necessary to elucidate the details.

Cell migration is an evolutionarily conserved mechanism that includes four steps: polarization, protrusion, adhesion and retraction [44]. Actin is primarily involved in the last three steps. Studies have confirmed that DLC1 can function in the regulation of actin cytoskeletal organization and cell migration [45], suggesting that DLC1 acts as an important regulator of migration. It is essential for endothelial cells in the outflow tract (OT) and atrioventricular (AV) regions to migrate into the cardiac jelly during embryonic heart development [46]. Similarly, the migration of cardiac neural crest cells is also a crucial event during heart development, and the inappropriate timing or path of cardiac neural crest cell migration will cause cardiac congenital anomalies [47]. Thus, if the migration regulatory ability of DLC1 is impaired in the early stage of fetal cardiac development, it is reasonable to speculate that inaccurate developmental consequences, such as defects or malformations, will occur. Although DLC1 is generally considered to affect cell motility and focal adhesion via the Rho-Gap domain and focal adhesion targeting region, respectively [38,39,45], the SAM domain has also been reported to regulate cell migration [48]. We demonstrated that three private variants near the SAM domain could reduce the inhibitory effect of wild-type DLC1, suggesting that these mutations might be implicated in regulating the function of the SAM domain.

Although *DLC1* isoform 2 has been well studied during the past ten years, the functions of *DLC1* isoform 1 still need to be characterized. A series of assays were performed to verify whether DLC1 isoform 1 had a function similar to isoform 2. As shown above, all the mutant and wild-type protein had suppression effects on Rho (Fig. 2A), and similarly regulated the cytoskeleton rearrangement and prevented the formation of stress fiber in the endothelial cells (Fig. 3A, Fig. S3 in File S1). Considering that endocardium formation in the primitive heart tube is affected by vasculogenesis [49], we conducted an angiogenesis assay *in vitro*, and DLC1 isoform 1 and the mutants had similar prohibitive effects on angiogenesis (Fig. S4 in File S1). Although the mutants showed no difference from the wild-type protein, these negative results only indicate that the variations did not affect these specific features in certain cells. Indeed, the variants might impair the function of DLC1 in other ways or in other cardiac cells. Furthermore, to the best of our knowledge, this is the first report using in vitro assays to demonstrate that DLC1 isoform 1 manifests a function analogous to isoform 2. In conclusion, our mutational analysis of *DLC1* isoform 1 presents a spectrum of rare variants in a CHD cohort and shows a mutation cluster in the N-terminus of the DLC1 protein. Our functional assays prove that the ability to inhibit cell migration or the subcellular localization of the protein are altered by three private variants. These findings provide novel insight that *DLC1* may be a high-priority candidate gene associated with CHD.

Supporting Information

File S1   Tables S1–S4 and Figures S1–S4. Table S1. The statistics of phenotype information of 148 non-trisomy CHD patients; Table S2. The primers for PCR to amplify the exons and portions of 5′UTR and 3′UTR regions of *DLC1* isoform 1; Table S3. Rare variants of *DLC1* isoform 1 identified in The 1000 Genomes project and Exome sequencing project; Table S4. The effects of 13 rare variants identified in the CHD cohort were predicted using multiple prediction algorithms; Figure S1. Effect of wild-type DLC1 isoform 1 and mutants on HUVEC proliferation; Figure S2. The apoptosis analysis of wild-type DLC1 isoform 1 and mutants in HUVECs; Figure S3. Percentage of cells overexpressing wild-type DLC1 isoform 1 and mutants that exhibited stress fibers; Figure S4. Wild-type DLC1 isoform 1 and mutants had similar effects on angiogenesis.

Acknowledgments

We are grateful to all of the patients and their families and the control individuals described herein for their contributions to this study. We thank Dr. Lei Bu for critical reading and helpful discussions of this manuscript.

Author Contributions

Conceived and designed the experiments: XK LH GH. Performed the experiments: BL YW YS YH HX Zhiqiang Wang. Analyzed the data: XK LH GH BL YW Y. Zhang PW GN. Contributed reagents/materials/analysis tools: Zhen Wang HT XK Y. Zhu BL. Wrote the paper: BL YW GH LH XK.

References

1. Pierpont ME, Basson CT, Benson DW, Jr., Gelb BD, Giglia TM, et al. (2007) Genetic basis for congenital heart defects: current knowledge: a scientific statement from the American Heart Association Congenital Cardiac Defects Committee, Council on Cardiovascular Disease in the Young: endorsed by the American Academy of Pediatrics. Circulation 115: 3015–3038.

2. Payne RM, Johnson MC, Grant JW and Strauss AW (1995) Toward a molecular understanding of congenital heart disease. Circulation 91: 494–504.

3. Garg V (2006) Insights into the genetic basis of congenital heart disease. Cell Mol Life Sci 63: 1141–1148.

4. Richards AA and Garg V (2010) Genetics of congenital heart disease. Curr Cardiol Rev 6: 91–97.

5. Basson CT, Bachinsky DR, Lin RC, Levi T, Elkins JA, et al. (1997) Mutations in human TBX5 [corrected] cause limb and cardiac malformation in Holt-Oram syndrome. Nat Genet 15: 30–35.

6. Li L, Krantz ID, Deng Y, Genin A, Banta AB, et al. (1997) Alagille syndrome is caused by mutations in human Jagged1, which encodes a ligand for Notch1. Nat Genet 16: 243–251.

7. Oda T, Elkahloun AG, Pike BL, Okajima K, Krantz ID, et al. (1997) Mutations in the human Jagged1 gene are responsible for Alagille syndrome. Nat Genet 16: 235–242.

8. Schott JJ, Benson DW, Basson CT, Pease W, Silberbach GM, et al. (1998) Congenital heart disease caused by mutations in the transcription factor NKX2-5. Science 281: 108–111.

9. Garg V, Kathiriya IS, Barnes R, Schluterman MK, King IN, et al. (2003) GATA4 mutations cause human congenital heart defects and reveal an interaction with TBX5. Nature 424: 443–447.

10. Garg V, Muth AN, Ransom JF, Schluterman MK, Barnes R, et al. (2005) Mutations in NOTCH1 cause aortic valve disease. Nature 437: 270–274.

11. Wessels MW, Willems PJ (2010) Genetic factors in non-syndromic congenital heart malformations. Clin Genet 78: 103–123.

12. Liao YC, Lo SH (2008) Deleted in liver cancer-1 (DLC-1): a tumor suppressor not just for liver. Int J Biochem Cell Biol 40: 843–847.

13. Wong CM, Yam JW, Ching YP, Yau TO, Leung TH, et al. (2005) Rho GTPase-activating protein deleted in liver cancer suppresses cell proliferation and invasion in hepatocellular carcinoma. Cancer Res 65: 8861–8868.

14. Ng IO, Liang ZD, Cao L and Lee TK (2000) DLC-1 is deleted in primary hepatocellular carcinoma and exerts inhibitory effects on the proliferation of hepatoma cell lines with deleted DLC-1. Cancer Res 60: 6581–6584.

15. Yuan BZ, Zhou X, Durkin ME, Zimonjic DB, Gumundsdottir K, et al. (2003) DLC-1 gene inhibits human breast cancer cell growth and in vivo tumorigenicity. Oncogene 22: 445–450.

16. Guan M, Tripathi V, Zhou X and Popescu NC (2008) Adenovirus-mediated restoration of expression of the tumor suppressor gene DLC1 inhibits the proliferation and tumorigenicity of aggressive, androgen-independent human prostate cancer cell lines: prospects for gene therapy. Cancer Gene Ther 15: 371–381.

17. Yuan BZ, Jefferson AM, Baldwin KT, Thorgeirsson SS, Popescu NC, et al. (2004) DLC-1 operates as a tumor suppressor gene in human non-small cell lung carcinomas. Oncogene 23: 1405–1411.

18. Hankins GR, Sasaki T, Lieu AS, Saulle D, Karimi K, et al. (2008) Identification of the deleted in liver cancer 1 gene, DLC1, as a candidate meningioma tumor suppressor. Neurosurgery 63: 771–780; discussion 780–771.

19. Goodison S, Yuan J, Sloan D, Kim R, Li C, et al. (2005) The RhoGAP protein DLC-1 functions as a metastasis suppressor in breast cancer cells. Cancer Res 65: 6042–6053.

20. Wu PP, Jin YL, Shang YF, Jin Z, Wu P, et al. (2009) Restoration of DLC1 gene inhibits proliferation and migration of human colon cancer HT29 cells. Ann Clin Lab Sci 39: 263–269.

21. Zhang T, Zheng J, Jiang N, Wang G, Shi Q, et al. (2009) Overexpression of DLC-1 induces cell apoptosis and proliferation inhibition in the renal cell carcinoma. Cancer Lett 283: 59–67.

22. Feng M, Huang B, Du Z, Xu X, Chen Z (2011) DLC-1 as a modulator of proliferation, apoptosis and migration in Burkitt's lymphoma cells. Mol Biol Rep 38: 1915–1920.

23. Yam JW, Ko FC, Chan CY, Jin DY and Ng IO (2006) Interaction of deleted in liver cancer 1 with tensin2 in caveolae and implications in tumor suppression. Cancer Res 66: 8367–8372.

24. Qian X, Li G, Asmussen HK, Asnaghi L, Vass WC, et al. (2007) Oncogenic inhibition by a deleted in liver cancer gene requires cooperation between tensin binding and Rho-specific GTPase-activating protein activities. Proc Natl Acad Sci U S A 104: 9012–9017.

25. Liao YC, Si L, deVere White RW, Lo SH (2007) The phosphotyrosine-independent interaction of DLC-1 and the SH2 domain of cten regulates focal adhesion localization and growth suppression activity of DLC-1. J Cell Biol 176: 43–49.

26. Durkin ME, Avner MR, Huh CG, Yuan BZ, Thorgeirsson SS, et al. (2005) DLC-1, a Rho GTPase-activating protein with tumor suppressor function, is essential for embryonic development. FEBS Lett 579: 1191–1196.

27. Sabbir MG, Wigle N, Loewen S, Gu Y, Buse C, et al. (2010) Identification and characterization of Dlc1 isoforms in the mouse and study of the biological function of a single gene trapped isoform. BMC Biol 8: 17.

28. Ko FC, Yeung YS, Wong CM, Chan LK, Poon RT, et al. (2010) Deleted in liver cancer 1 isoforms are distinctly expressed in human tissues, functionally different and under differential transcriptional regulation in hepatocellular carcinoma. Liver Int 30: 139–148.

29. O'Roak BJ, Vives L, Fu W, Egertson JD, Stanaway IB, et al. (2012) Multiplex targeted sequencing identifies recurrently mutated genes in autism spectrum disorders. Science 338: 1619–1622.

30. Lynch M (2010) Rate, molecular spectrum, and consequences of human mutation. Proc Natl Acad Sci U S A 107: 961–968.

31. Tennessen JA, Bigham AW, O'Connor TD, Fu W, Kenny EE, et al. (2012) Evolution and functional impact of rare coding variation from deep sequencing of human exomes. Science 337: 64–69.

32. Hu G, Chong RA, Yang Q, Wei Y, Blanco MA, et al. (2009) MTDH activation by 8q22 genomic gain promotes chemoresistance and metastasis of poor-prognosis breast cancer. Cancer Cell 15: 9–20.

33. Theisen CS, Wahl JK, 3rd, Johnson KR, Wheelock MJ (2007) NHERF links the N-cadherin/catenin complex to the platelet-derived growth factor receptor to modulate the actin cytoskeleton and regulate cell motility. Mol Biol Cell 18: 1220–1232.

34. Leung KW, Cheung LW, Pon YL, Wong RN, Mak NK, et al. (2007) Ginsenoside Rb1 inhibits tube-like structure formation of endothelial cells by regulating pigment epithelium-derived factor through the oestrogen beta receptor. Br J Pharmacol 152: 207–215.

35. Consortium TGP (2010) A map of human genome variation from population-scale sequencing. Nature 467: 1061–1073.

36. Consortium U (2012) Reorganizing the protein space at the Universal Protein Resource (UniProt). Nucleic Acids Research 40: D71–D75.

37. Kumar P, Henikoff S, Ng PC (2009) Predicting the effects of coding non-synonymous variants on protein function using the SIFT algorithm. Nat Protoc 4: 1073–1082.

38. Kawai K, Yamaga M, Iwamae Y, Kiyota M, Kamata H, et al. (2004) A PLCdelta1-binding protein, p122RhoGAP, is localized in focal adhesions. Biochem Soc Trans 32: 1107–1109.

39. Kawai K, Iwamae Y, Yamaga M, Kiyota M, Ishii H, et al. (2009) Focal adhesion-localization of START-GAP1/DLC1 is essential for cell motility and morphology. Genes Cells 14: 227–241.

40. Cao X, Voss C, Zhao B, Kaneko T, Li SS (2012) Differential regulation of the activity of deleted in liver cancer 1 (DLC1) by tensins controls cell migration and transformation. Proc Natl Acad Sci U S A 109: 1455–1460.

41. Yuan BZ, Jefferson AM, Millecchia L, Popescu NC, Reynolds SH (2007) Morphological changes and nuclear translocation of DLC1 tumor suppressor protein precede apoptosis in human non-small cell lung carcinoma cells. Exp Cell Res 313: 3868–3880.

42. Gibson G (2011) Rare and common variants: twenty arguments. Nat Rev Genet 13: 135–145.

43. Cirulli ET, Goldstein DB (2010) Uncovering the roles of rare variants in common disease through whole-genome sequencing. Nat Rev Genet 11: 415–425.

44. Kurosaka S, Kashina A (2008) Cell biology of embryonic migration. Birth Defects Res C Embryo Today 84: 102–122.

45. Kim TY, Vigil D, Der CJ, Juliano RL (2009) Role of DLC-1, a tumor suppressor protein with RhoGAP activity, in regulation of the cytoskeleton and cell motility. Cancer Metastasis Rev 28: 77–83.

46. Sakabe M, Matsui H, Sakata H, Ando K, Yamagishi T, et al. (2005) Understanding heart development and congenital heart defects through developmental biology: a segmental approach. Congenit Anom (Kyoto) 45: 107–118.

47. Keyte A, Hutson MR (2012) The neural crest in cardiac congenital anomalies. Differentiation 84: 25–40.

48. Zhong D, Zhang J, Yang S, Soh UJ, Buschdorf JP, et al. (2009) The SAM domain of the RhoGAP DLC1 binds EF1A1 to regulate cell migration. J Cell Sci 122: 414–424.

49. Coffin JD, Poole TJ (1991) Endothelial cell origin and migration in embryonic heart and cranial blood vessel development. Anat Rec 231: 383–395.

23

Maternal Parity and the Risk of Congenital Heart Defects in Offspring: A Dose-Response Meta-Analysis of Epidemiological

Yu Feng[1,9], Di Yu[1,9], Tao Chen[2], Jin Liu[2], Xing Tong[3], Lei Yang[1], Min Da[1], Shutong Shen[4], Changfeng Fan[1], Song Wang[1], Xuming Mo[1]*

1 Department of Cardiothoracic Surgery, The Affiliated Children's Hospital of Nanjing Medical University, Nanjing, Jiangsu, China, **2** Department of Epidemiology and Biostatistics, School of Public Health, Nanjing Medical University, Nanjing, Jiangsu, China, **3** Atherosclerosis Research Center, Key Laboratory of Cardiovascular Disease and Molecular Intervention, Nanjing Medical University, Nanjing, Jiangsu, China, **4** Department of Cardiology, The First Affiliated Hospital of Nanjing Medical University, Nanjing, Jiangsu, China

Abstract

Background: Epidemiological studies have reported conflicting results regarding maternal parity and the risk of congenital heart defects (CHDs). However, a meta-analysis of the association between maternal parity and CHDs in offspring has not been conducted.

Methods: We searched MEDLINE and EMBASE for articles catalogued between their inception and March 8, 2014; we identified relevant published studies that assessed the association between maternal parity and CHD risk. Two authors independently assessed the eligibility of the retrieved articles and extracted data from them. Study-specific relative risk estimates were pooled by random-effects or fixed-effects models. From the 11272 references, a total of 16 case-control studies and 3 cohort studies were enrolled in this meta-analysis.

Results: The overall relative risk of CHD in parous versus nulliparous women was 1.01 (95% CI, 0.97–1.06; $Q = 32.34$; $P = 0.006$; $I^2 = 53.6\%$). Furthermore, we observed a significant association between the highest versus lowest parity number, with an overall RR = 1.20 (95% CI, 1.10–1.31; ($Q = 74.61$, $P < 0.001$, $I^2 = 82.6\%$). A dose–response analysis also indicated a positive effect of maternal parity on CHD risk, and the overall increase in relative risk per one live birth was 1.06 (95% CI, 1.02–1.09); $Q = 68.09$; $P < 0.001$; $I^2 = 80.9\%$). We conducted stratified and meta-regression analyses to identify the origin of the heterogeneity among studies. A Galbraith plot was created to graphically assess the sources of heterogeneity.

Conclusion: In summary, this meta-analysis provided a robust estimate of the positive association between maternal parity and risk of CHD.

Editor: Zaccaria Ricci, Bambino Gesù Children's Hospital, Italy

Funding: The authors have no support or funding to report.

Competing Interests: The authors have declared that no competing interests exist.

* Email: mohsuming15@sina.com

9 These authors contributed equally to this work.

Introduction

Congenital heart defects (CHD) are the most common human birth defects and the leading cause of perinatal mortality, with an incidence of approximately 4 to 50 per 1000 live birth or even higher [1]. The etiology of CHD is complex and may involve the interaction of environmental exposure and inherited factors [2]. A multitude of studies have identified both chromosomal and gene mutations as the cause of the syndromic version of the heart malfunction [1]. In contrast, the origin of non-syndromic CHD, which accounts for most congenital cardiac abnormalities, remains unknown.

Maternal phenylketonuria, diabetes mellitus, maternal terato-gen exposure, and maternal therapeutic drug exposure during pregnancy may increase the risk of congenital malformations in offspring [3]. Apart from these influences, previous studies have indicated that inherent maternal characteristics, such as parity, may be responsible for certain categories of congenital defects. Some studies have observed a positive association between nulliparity and the risk of various birth defects [4–10]. In contrast, other studies have observed that multiparity is associated with an increased risk of specific birth defects [11–13]. The results for CHD are similar; no consensus has been reached, and some studies show positive associations while others find null results. The association between maternal parity and CHDs might be explained by unmeasured environmental risk factors which are more common among multiparous women than nulliparous women. Both biological and psychosocial interpretations can be proposed, including maternal stress, maternal uterus condition and serum levels of estradiol [14–17].

To date, an increasing number of studies has focused on the association between maternal parity and CHDs; however, the results have been ambiguous, possibly because of inadequate sample sizes. Therefore, we conducted a dose-response meta-analysis to quantitatively assess the effects of maternal parity on CHDs.

Methods

Literature Search

To identify relevant epidemiological studies, two independent researchers (Feng and Yu) conducted a computerized literature search in MEDLINE and EMBASE to retrieve articles that were catalogued between the databases' inception and March 8, 2014.The search terms for the exposure were: 'Parity', 'Pregnancy', 'Live Birth', 'Reproduction', 'Reproductive' and 'Reproductive Factors' and the search terms for the outcome were: 'Congenital Heart Defect', 'Heart Abnormality', 'Malformation Of Heart' and 'CHD'. In addition, we conducted a search for a broad range of environmental teratogens and CHDs and examined the relevant references and review articles; in this way, we could identify information from other related studies. We followed standards of quality for conducting and reporting meta-analyses [18].

Eligibility Criteria

We selected articles that (1) were original epidemiologic studies (i.e., case–control and cohort), (2) examined the association between maternal parity and CHDs overall or any one of the CHD subtypes in infants, (3) were published in the English language, (4) reported RRs (i.e., risk ratios or odds ratios) and associated 95% confidence intervals (CIs) or standard errors or provided the data necessary to recalculate these factors, and (5) defined CHDs or one of the CHD subtypes as an outcome. Articles that reported results from more than one population were considered to be separate studies. When multiple articles from the same study were provided, we used the article with the most applicable information and the largest number of cases. We excluded non-peer-reviewed articles, experimental animal studies, ecological assessments, correlation studies and mechanistic studies.

Data Extraction

Data extraction was carried out separately by two reviewers (Feng and Yu) working independently. When differences of opinion arose, they were resolved by a discussion between the two reviewers or by the involvement of a third reviewer (Chen) for adjudication. Parity was defined as the number of live births before the index delivery [19]. Nulliparous women were defined as those with no previous live births before the index delivery. Primiparous women were those with one live birth, and multiparous women were those with two or more prior live births. The studies that met the inclusion criteria were reviewed to retrieve the information of interest. The characteristics of interest included authors, year of

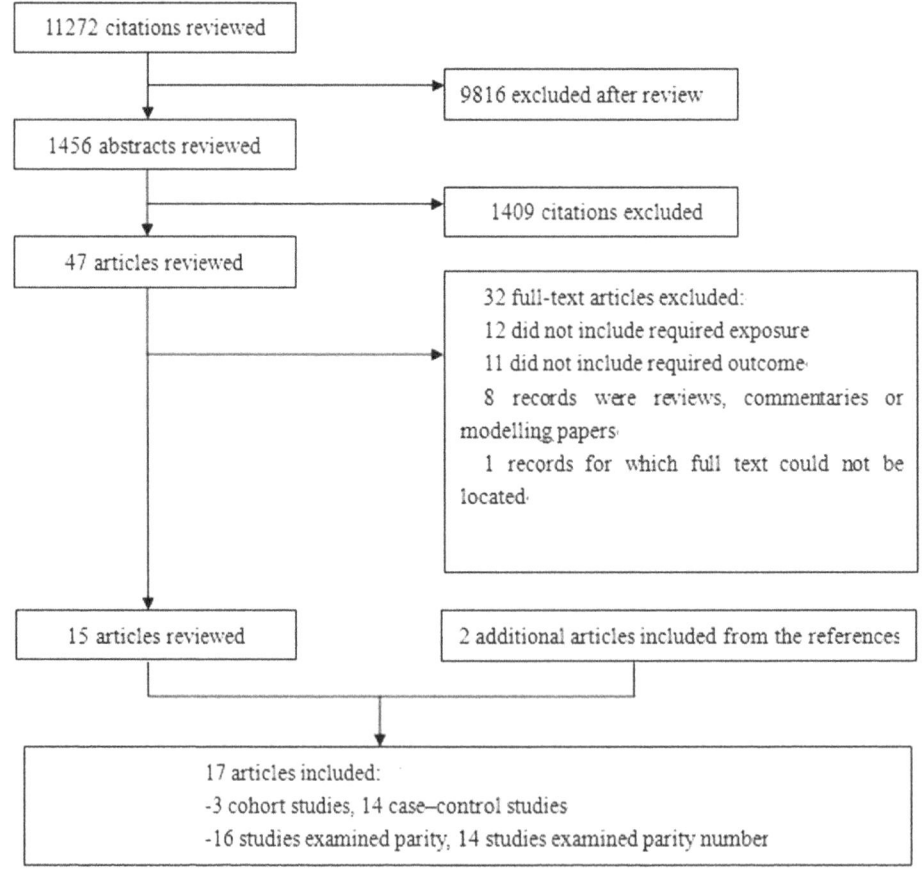

Figure 1. Study selection procedures for a meta-analysis of maternal parity and congenital heart defects (CHDs) in offspring.

publication, geographic region, periods of data collection, study design, sample size, case classification, exposure and outcome assessment (including parity as both a binary and categorical variable), adjusted estimates and their corresponding 95% CIs for parous versus nulliparous women, highest versus lowest number of previous births, and confounding factors that were controlled for by matching cases or adjustments in the data analysis. We back-calculated the point estimate and 95% CI if the original study did not report the risk estimates in this order. When no adjusted estimates were available, we extracted the crude estimate. If no estimate was provided in a given study, we recalculated odds ratios or risk ratios and 95% CIs from the presented raw data using standard equations.

To assess the study quality, we used a 9-star system on the basis of the Newcastle-Ottawa Scale [20]. This system judges a study based on three broad characteristics: the selection of study groups, comparability of study groups and ascertainment of the exposure or outcome of interest for case-control and cohort studies, respectively. The highest score was 9, and we defined a high quality study as one with a quality score greater than or equal to 7.

Statistical Analysis

We used study-specific relative risks as a summary statistic of the association between maternal parity and CHD risk. To simplify the procedure, a RR was used to represent all reported study-specific results from cohort studies and an OR to represent results from case-control studies. If a study did not use the lowest parity number as the reference category, the effective count method proposed by Hamling and colleagues [21] was used to recalculate the RRs.

For the dose–response analysis, which considers parity as a continuous variable, the method proposed by Greenland and colleagues [22] and Orsini and colleagues [23] was used to calculate study-specific slopes (i.e., linear trends) and 95% CIs. For studies which reported duration as a range, the midpoint, determined by calculating the average of the lower and upper bounds, was used. When the highest category was open-ended, the width of the open-ended interval was taken to be the same as that of the category immediately previous to it. When the lowest category did not have a lower bound, we considered the lower bound to be zero. We presented the dose–response results in forest plots on the basis of increments of 1 live birth with regard to parity.

Cochran's Q and I^2 statistics were used to test for heterogeneity among studies [24]. If there was evidence of heterogeneity ($P < 0.05$ or $I^2 \geq 56\%$), a random-effects model was used, which provided a more appropriate summary estimate for heterogeneous study-specific estimates. If the study revealed no evidence of heterogeneity, the fixed-effects analysis was used, an inverse variance weighting was applied to calculate summary RR estimates [25].

We conducted subgroup analyses based on study design (i.e., cohort versus case–control studies), geographical region (i.e., North America, Europe, and Asia), number of cases (i.e., ≤1000 versus >1000), publication period (i.e., before 2010 versus 2010 or after), maternal age (i.e., ≤27 versus >27), primary interest (i.e., whether the title or abstract refers to the reproductive factors as their research interest, yes versus no), and study quality (i.e., low versus high quality). We evaluated heterogeneity between subgroups by meta-regression. A P value less than 0.05 from the meta-regression was considered representative of a significant difference between subgroups. Finally, we conducted sensitivity analyses to explore whether a specific study strongly influenced the results by excluding one study at a time.

Publication bias was assessed via visual inspection of a funnel plot with asymmetry using both Egger's linear regression [26] and Begg's rank correlation [27] methods. Significant statistical publication bias was defined as a P value of <0.05 for the two above-mentioned tests. All statistical analyses were performed with STATA (version 11.0; StataCorp, College Station, Texas, USA).

Results

Study Characteristics

The search strategy generated 11272 citations; from these, 17 were used in the final analysis, representing 43880 incident cases (Figure 1). All of the studies were published between 1989 and 2013. There were 14 case–control studies [28–41] and 3 cohort studies [42–44]. The main characteristics of the included studies are presented in Table S1. As shown, 10 studies [28–30,32,33,35,36,39,43,44] were conducted in the United States or Canada, 6 in Europe [31,37,38,40–42], and 1 in Asia [34]. Among these studies, 16 investigated the association between maternal parity as a binary variable and CHD risk [28–43], and 14 examined the association of maternal parity number with CHD risk [28,30–34,36,38–44]. In the 3 cohort studies, cohort sizes varied from 22,365 [44] to 1,625,945 [43], and the number of CHD cases ranged from 4,123 [44] to 12,101 [43]. In the 16 case–control studies, the number of cases varied from 81 [28] to 7,575 [32], and the number of control subjects ranged from 302 [39] to 38,151 [41]. The highest parity number ranged from 2 [28] to more than 4 [39].

Parous versus Nulliparous

A total of 14 case–control studies and 2 cohort studies examined the association between parity as a binary variable and CHD risk. The overall relative risk of CHD for parous versus nulliparous women was 1.01 (95% CI, 0.97–1.06), with moderate heterogeneity ($Q = 32.34$; $P = 0.006$; $I^2 = 53.6\%$; **Table 1** and **Fig. 2**). There was no indication of publication bias based on the Egger test ($P = 0.295$) or visual inspection of the funnel plot (data not shown). In a sensitivity analysis, we sequentially excluded one study at a time and reanalyzed the data. The 16 study-specific relative risks for the parous versus nulliparous women ranged from a low of 1.01 (95% CI, 0.97–1.05; $Q = 34.59$; $P = 0.007$; $I^2 = 50.9\%$) after omission of the study by Padula and colleagues [36] to a high of 1.02 (95% CI, 0.99–1.06; $Q = 31.44$; $P = 0.018$; $I^2 = 45.9\%$) after omission of the study by Luo and colleagues [34]. As shown in **Table 1**, similar risks were observed between subgroup stratified by maternal age for association between maternal ever parity and CHD in offspring (P for heterogeneity = 0.12).

Highest versus Lowest Parity Number

A total of 11 case–control studies and 3 cohort studies examined the association between high and low parity and CHD risk. The estimate of the relative risk of CHD for the highest versus lowest parity categories was 1.20 (95% CI, 1.10–1.31). Statistically significant heterogeneity was detected ($Q = 74.61$, $P < 0.001$, $I^2 = 82.6\%$; Table 2 and Fig. 3) with no publication bias (Begg's test: $P = 0.443$, Egger's test: $P = 0.883$). The 13 study-specific relative risks when considering the parity number ranged from a low of 1.17 (95% CI, 1.07–1.27; $Q = 61.84$; $P = 0.000$; $I^2 = 80.6\%$) after omission of the study by Vereczkey and colleagues [40] to a high of 1.22 (95% CI, 1.12–1.34; $Q = 59.74$; $P = 0.000$; $I^2 = 79.9\%$) after omission of the study by Batra and colleagues [30].

Table 1. Summary risk estimates of the association between maternal ever parity and CHD risk in offspring.

Subgroup analysis	No. of studies	No. of cases	Summary RR (95% CIs)	P^1	I^2 (%)	P^2
Summary pooled estimate	16	39757	1.01(0.97–1.06)	0.006	53.6	
Geographical region						0.202
North America	9	31090	1.01(0.98–1.05)	0.313	14.5	
Europe	6	7974	1.14(0.98–1.33)	0.014	64.9	
Asia	1	693	0.82(0.71–0.97)	-	-	
Number of cases						0.438
≤1000	9	3691	1.14(0.98–1.32)	0.007	62.3	
>1000	7	36066	1.00(0.98–1.03)	0.165	34.5	
Publication period						0.719
Before 2010	8	26457	1.00(0.96–1.04)	0.119	39.1	
2010 or after	8	13300	1.05(0.95–1.17)	0.004	66.4	
Design						0.744
Case-control	14	20747	1.02(0.96–1.09)	0.027	46.9	
Cohort	2	19010	1.00(0.93–1.08)	0.006	86.6	
Maternal age(year)						0.12
≤27	8	18296	1.05(0.99–1.12)	0.169	32.4	
>27	7	21461	0.98(0.92–1.04)	0.063	49.8	
Primary interest						0.69
Yes	9	23805	1.01(0.94–1.09)	0.020	54.2	
No	7	15952	1.03(1.00–1.06)	0.144	39.2	
Quality assessment						0.362
High quality studies (scores≥7)	11	30300	1.03(0.99–1.07)	0.060	43.6	
Low quality studies (scores<7)	7	9457	0.96(0.92–1.00)	0.161	36.8	

[1]p-value for heterogeneity within each subgroup.
[2]p-value for heterogeneity between subgroups with meta-regression analysis.
Abbreviations: RR: relative risk; CI: confidence interval.

Dose–Response Analysis

A total of 11 case–control studies and 3 cohort studies were included in the dose-response analysis. The estimate of relative risk per live birth was 1.06 (95% CI, 1.02–1.09), and there was statistically significant heterogeneity ($Q = 68.09$; $P < 0.001$; $I^2 = 80.9\%$; Table 2 and Fig. 4). Publication bias was not evident based on the Egger test ($P = 0.973$) or Begg test ($P = 0.101$), and no asymmetry was observed in the funnel plots. The 13 study-specific relative risks of parity ranged from a low of 1.05 (95% CI, 1.02–1.08; $Q = 56.94$; $P = 0.000$; $I^2 = 78.9\%$) after omission of the study by Vereczkey and colleagues [40] to a high of 1.06 (95% CI, 1.03–1.10; $Q = 51.12$; $P = 0.000$; $I^2 = 76.5\%$) after omission of the study by Cedergren and colleagues [42].

Heterogeneity Analysis

We conducted stratified and meta-regression analyses to identify the origin of the heterogeneity among studies. In subgroup analyses of parity as a binary variable and CHD risk, there was no indication of significant heterogeneity between subgroups according to meta-regression analyses (**Table 1**). However, significant heterogeneity existed in the dose-response analyses of the association between parity number and CHD risk. To clarify the sources of heterogeneity, we conducted a sensitivity analysis; however, I^2 did not decrease much by removing each study in turn. Subsequently, a meta-regression was performed with a Knapp-Hartung modification, and we found that differing numbers of cases may contribute to the heterogeneity

($p = 0.060$). We further created a Galbraith plot to graphically assess the sources of heterogeneity (Figures S1, S2). A total of 7 studies [30,32,34,40–42,44] were identified as the primary sources of heterogeneity (i.e., 6 studies [30,32,40–42,44] from the high versus low parity number analysis and 6 studies [30,34,40–42,44] from the dose-response analysis). Once the outlying studies were excluded, the heterogeneity was effectively removed (i.e., for the high versus low parity number analysis, $I^2 = 0.0\%$; for the dose-response analysis, $I^2 = 0.0\%$); however, the corresponding pooled RRs were not materially altered in any comparisons (i.e., for the high versus low parity analysis: RR = 1.23, 95% CI = 1.17–1.29; for the dose-response analysis: RR = 1.05, 95% CI = 1.03–1.07).

Discussion

To the best of our knowledge, this is the first quantitative meta-analysis evaluating the association between maternal parity and the risk of congenital heart defects. Overall, the findings of our meta-analysis suggested that maternal parity (i.e., the highest category compared to the lowest category, RR = 1.20, 95% CI = 1.10–1.31) was significantly associated with CHD risk. Meanwhile, in the dose-response meta-analysis, we found that the risk of CHD increased by 6% per live birth. However, there was no evidence that verified the association between parous versus nulliparous women (RR = 1.01, 95%CI = 0.97–1.06) and the risk of CHDs. Additionally, the results were consistent across most of the subgroup analyses (Table 1 and 2).

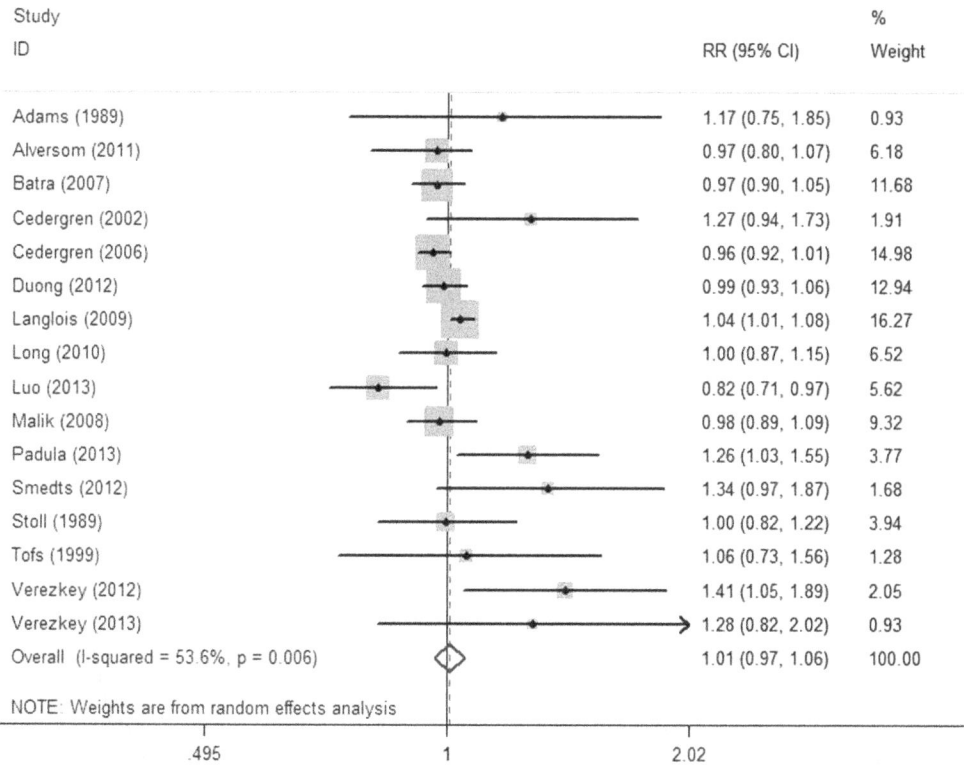

Figure 2. Relative risk (RR) estimates for the association between ever parity and CHD risk. Meta-analysis random-effects estimates were used. The sizes of the squares reflect the weighting of the included studies. Bars represent 95% confidence intervals (CIs). The center of the diamond represents the summary effect; left and right points of the diamond represent the 95% confidence interval.

Although the specific biological mechanism underlying maternal parity and the risk of CHDs remains unclear, some relevant evidence has been published. Nutrient depletion was more likely to occur among mothers who had given birth to live fetuses than those who had never delivered. Folic acid is one of the most important vitamins, and the association between folic acid and birth defects has been widely studied. It has been confirmed that lack of it would cause severe congenital malformation [45], especially CHDs [46] and neural tube defects [47]. Additionally, mothers who gave birth to more fetuses were more likely to have shorter inter-pregnancy intervals, which have been verified to increase the risk of major congenital malformations, including CHDs [48]. Moreover, having young children who carry respiratory viruses in the household would increase the risk of an embryo's in utero exposure to viruses, such as rubella, which was confirmed to contribute to CHD more than half a century ago [49,50]. Moreover, changes in the intrauterine environment that affect embryonic development and eventually lead to birth defects may be explained by multiparity. In addition to biological interpretations, psychosocial explanations should also be explored. Multiparity would cause an increased burden on families and increased mental stress in parents. Moreover, Zhu et al [14] found that mothers who were exposed to stress during pregnancy were at an increased risk of having offspring with CHD.

When stratified by geographic region, a significant increase in CHD risk in North America and Europe was found to be associated with increases in parity number, and similar results

were found in a dose-response meta-analysis. However, the pooled RRs for North America and Europe differed when considering parity as a binary variable. Considering the fact that only one study from Asia was included, the influence of parity in this region needs further research. In the subgroup analysis to assess study quality, we observed statistically significant results in high quality studies that included analyses of both parity number and dose-response, while no significant association was found among low quality studies. For the subgroup analysis of study design, the pooled RR from case-control studies was different from cohort studies in the analysis of dose-response. Selection and information biases might account for the observed difference. Furthermore, compared to the cohort studies, the case-control studies had a lower median quality score (7 versus 8), which may have an influence on the results.

Some limitations of our study must be taken into account. First, a total of 14 case-control studies and 3 cohort studies were recruited into our meta-analysis, and we extracted our raw data primarily from case-control studies, which are susceptible to selection and information biases. Additionally, our meta-analysis was limited to studies published in English; the results may therefore have been affected by the lack of data from studies performed in other languages. Thus, general conclusions must be considered carefully and cannot be regarded as the final word on the matter. Second because we lacked a large data set, we did not conduct a subgroup analysis of CHD subtypes; however, different CHD subtypes have different etiologies. Maternal parity may be

Table 2. Summary risk estimates of the association between maternal parity number and CHD risk in offspring.

Subgroup analysis	Highest versus lowest						Dose-response analysis (per 1 live birth)					
	No. of studies	No. of cases	Summary RR (95% CIs)	P¹	I²(%)	P²	No. of studies	No. of cases	Summary RR (95% CIs)	P¹	I²(%)	P²
Summary pooled estimate	14	38027	1.21(1.11–1.31)	<0.001	83.8		14	38027	1.06(1.02–1.09)	<0.001	80.9	
Geographical region						0.924						0.379
North America	8	29621	1.18(1.07–1.30)	<0.001	84.3		8	29621	1.05(1.02–1.08)	<0.001	75	
Europe	5	7713	1.49(1.06–2.09)	<0.001	83.6		5	7713	1.17(1.02–1.34)	<0.001	83.1	
Asia	1	693	0.95(0.71–1.28)	-	-		1	693	0.92(0.82–1.04)	-	-	
Number of cases						0.140						0.060
≦1000	8	3430	1.41(1.12–1.79)	<0.001	66.1		8	3430	1.14(1.03–1.25)	<0.001	71.6	
>1000	6	34597	1.13(1.03–1.25)	<0.001	90.4		6	34597	1.04(1.00–1.07)	<0.001	88	
Publication period						0.340						0.665
Before 2010	7	23390	1.13(1.02–1.25)	<0.001	65.2		7	23390	1.03(1.02–1.05)	0.110	42	
2010 or after	7	14637	1.30(1.12–1.53)	<0.001	87.4		7	14637	1.09(1.02–1.16)	<0.001	82.7	
Design						0.829						0.626
Case-control	11	15539	1.22(1.07–1.39)	<0.001	70.1		11	15539	1.05(0.97–1.13)	<0.001	96.4	
Cohort	3	22488	1.21(1.09–1.34)	<0.001	88.8		3	22488	1.05(1.01–1.10)	<0.001	93.5	
Maternal age(year)						0.106						0.157
≤27	7	15229	1.37(1.16–1.63)	0.004	68.6		7	15229	1.12(1.04–1.20)	0.001	72.5	
>27	7	22798	1.11(0.97–1.27)	<0.001	88.8		7	22798	1.03(0.99–1.08)	<0.001	86.9	
Primary interest						0.774						0.737
Yes	10	21534	1.23(1.08–1.40)	<0.001	84.7		10	21534	1.06(1.02–1.11)	<0.001	84.1	
No	4	16493	1.18(1.01–1.37)	0.003	78.6		4	16493	1.05(1.00–1.10)	0.049	61.9	
Quality assessment						0.252						0.673
High quality studies (scores≥7)	8	28570	1.27(1.13–143)	0.000	88.6		8	28570	1.08(1.03–1.12)	0.000	83.6	
Low quality studies (scores<7)	6	9457	1.08(0.99–1.16)	0.735	0		6	9457	1.01(1.00–1.04)	0.251	24.4	

¹p-value for heterogeneity within each subgroup.
²p-value for heterogeneity between subgroups with meta-regression analysis.
Abbreviations: RR: relative risk; CI: confidence interval.

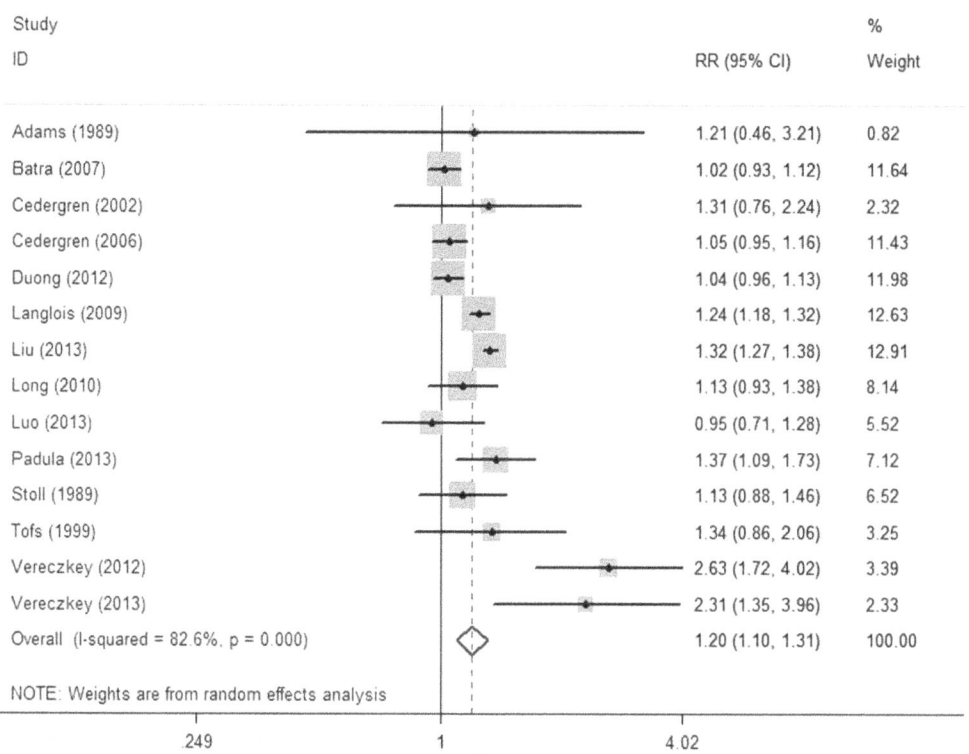

Figure 3. Relative risk (RR) estimates for the association between parity number (highest versus lowest) and CHD risk. Meta-analysis random-effects estimates were used. The sizes of the squares reflect the weighting of the included studies. Bars represent 95% confidence intervals (CIs). The center of the diamond represents the summary effect; left and right points of the diamond represent the 95% confidence interval.

not associated with all subtypes of CHD. Therefore, further research, including more high quality studies, is needed. Thirdly, although no evidence of publication bias was found, heterogeneity exists among the studies included in these analyses of both parity number and dose response; this heterogeneity may affect the interpretation of the overall results. In this study, we conducted sensitivity analyses to explore the sources of heterogeneity by deleting one study at a time from the pooled analysis. However, heterogeneity still could not be fully removed. Moreover, geographical region, sample size, CHD subtypes and other risk factors may result in heterogeneity. Therefore, we performed meta-regression and subgroup analyses to further investigate the sources of heterogeneity. In the dose-response analysis, we found that the heterogeneity stemmed partly from the number of cases. In contrast, no cause was found for the heterogeneity in the parity number meta-analysis. Furthermore, we created a Galbraith plot to assess the heterogeneity and to identify potentially outlying studies. A total of 6 were identified as the primary contributors to heterogeneity in both the analysis of parity number [30,32,40–42,44] and dose-response [30,34,40–42,44]. After excluding the outlying studies, the above-mentioned heterogeneity was effectively removed while the corresponding pooled RRs were not materially altered, indicating that the overall results regarding parity number and dose-response were statistically stable. Meanwhile, in the subgroup analysis to assess quality, heterogeneity was present in the high quality studies but not in the low quality ones. Of the 7 studies that were the main sources of heterogeneity, 5

[31,33,41,42,45] were high quality studies, which could explain the discrepancy. Finally, maternal age may be a major confounder, but in our study, similar risks were observed between subgroup stratified by maternal age for association between maternal parity and CHD in offspring (P for heterogeneity = 0.12 in maternal ever parity; P for heterogeneity = 0.106 and P for heterogeneity = 0.157 in maternal parity number). So we consider that maternal age may have no significant confounding effect on association between maternal parity and CHD in offspring. However, because of the limiting number of included studies, more studies are needed to validate our results.

Additionally, there are several important strengths of our study. First, to our knowledge, this is the first meta-analysis to report an association between maternal parity and CHDs. Moreover, our literature search was conducted on multiple databases, and the references from the retrieved articles were fully scrutinized to obtain any missing data. Therefore, our study included 43880 cases, enough to have sufficient statistical power to investigate the potential association between maternal parity and the risk of CHDs. Another strength of our study is that, although heterogeneity exists in our meta-analysis, we conducted a number of sensitivity, subgroup and Galbraith plot analyses and found that the results were stable.

In summary, this study provides evidence that maternal parity number was positively associated with the risk of CHDs. However, more prospective studies, particularly in developing countries, are needed to further investigate the association between maternal

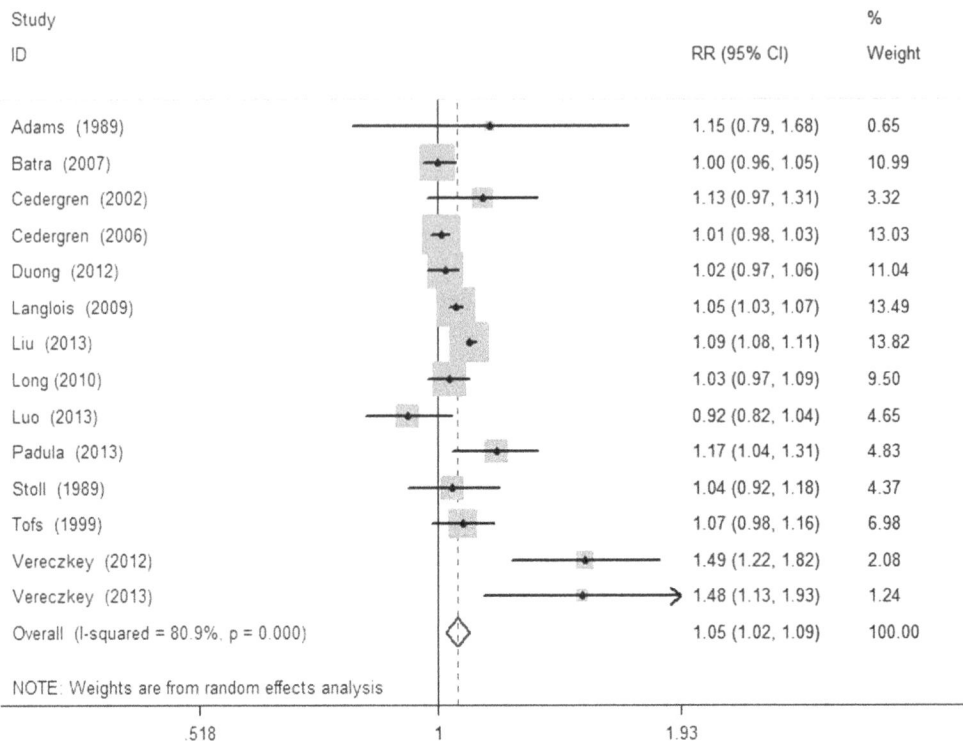

Figure 4. Relative risk (RR) estimates for the association between parity number (per 1 live birth) and CHD risk. Meta-analysis random-effects estimates were used. The sizes of the squares reflect the weighting of the included studies. Bars represent 95% confidence intervals (CIs). The center of the diamond represents the summary effect; left and right points of the diamond represent the 95% confidence interval.

parity and CHDs, especially with regard to the different subtypes of CHDs.

Supporting Information

Figure S1 Galbraith plots for parity number (highest versus lowest) and CHD risk.

Figure S2 Galbraith plots for parity number (per 1 live birth) and CHD risk.

Table S1 Characteristics of studies of maternal parity and CHD risk.

Checklist S1 PRISMA checklist.

Acknowledgments

We sincerely thank Dr. Hongcheng Zhu and Dr. Xi Yang for their help with this manuscript.

Author Contributions

Conceived and designed the experiments: XM. Performed the experiments: YF DY TC JL. Analyzed the data: YF DY XT. Contributed reagents/materials/analysis tools: LY MD SS CF SW. Wrote the paper: YF DY XM.

References

1. Pierpont ME, Basson CT, Benson DW Jr., Gelb BD, Giglia TM, et al. (2007) Genetic basis for congenital heart defects: current knowledge: a scientific statement from the American Heart Association Congenital Cardiac Defects Committee, Council on Cardiovascular Disease in the Young: endorsed by the American Academy of Pediatrics. Circulation 115: 3015–3038.
2. van der Bom T, Zomer AC, Zwinderman AH, Meijboom FJ, Bouma BJ, et al. (2011) The changing epidemiology of congenital heart disease. Nat Rev Cardiol 8: 50–60.
3. Jenkins KJ, Correa A, Feinstein JA, Botto L, Britt AE, et al. (2007) Noninherited risk factors and congenital cardiovascular defects: current knowledge: a scientific statement from the American Heart Association Council on Cardiovascular Disease in the Young: endorsed by the American Academy of Pediatrics. Circulation 115: 2995–3014.
4. Hay S, Barbano H (1972) Independent effects of maternal age and birth order on the incidence of selected congenital malformations. Teratology 6: 271–279.
5. Agopian A, Marengo L, Mitchell LE (2009) Descriptive epidemiology of nonsyndromic omphalocele in Texas, 1999–2004. Am J Med Genet A 149A: 2129–2133.
6. Bianca S, Ettore G (2003) Isolated esophageal atresia and perinatal risk factors. Dis Esophagus 16: 39–40.
7. Benjamin BG, Ethen MK, Van Hook CL, Myers CA, Canfield MA (2010) Gastroschisis prevalence in Texas 1999–2003. Birth Defects Res A Clin Mol Teratol 88: 178–185.
8. Pradat P, Francannet C, Harris JA, Robert E (2003) The epidemiology of cardiovascular defects, part I: a study based on data from three large registries of congenital malformations. Pediatr Cardiol 24: 195–221.

9. Werler MM, Bosco JL, Shapira SK, National Birth Defects Prevention S (2009) Maternal vasoactive exposures, amniotic bands, and terminal transverse limb defects. Birth Defects Res A Clin Mol Teratol 85: 52–57.

10. Carmichael SL, Shaw GM, Laurent C, Olney RS, Lammer EJ, et al. (2007) Maternal reproductive and demographic characteristics as risk factors for hypospadias. Paediatr Perinat Epidemiol 21: 210–218.

11. Vieira AR (2004) Birth order and neural tube defects: a reappraisal. J Neurol Sci 217: 65–72.

12. Hashmi SS, Waller DK, Langlois P, Canfield M, Hecht JT (2005) Prevalence of nonsyndromic oral clefts in Texas: 1995–1999. Am J Med Genet A 134: 368–372.

13. Canfield MA, Marengo L, Ramadhani TA, Suarez L, Brender JD, et al. (2009) The prevalence and predictors of anencephaly and spina bifida in Texas. Paediatr Perinat Epidemiol 23: 41–50.

14. Zhu JL, Olsen J, Sorensen HT, Li J, Nohr EA, et al. (2013) Prenatal maternal bereavement and congenital heart defects in offspring: a registry-based study. Pediatrics 131: e1225–1230.

15. Chubak J, Tworoger SS, Yasui Y, Ulrich CM, Stanczyk FZ, et al. (2004) Associations between reproductive and menstrual factors and postmenopausal sex hormone concentrations. Cancer Epidemiol Biomarkers Prev 13: 1296–1301.

16. Rovas L, Sladkevicius P, Strobel E, Valentin L (2006) Reference data representative of normal findings at three-dimensional power Doppler ultrasound examination of the cervix from 17 to 41 gestational weeks. Ultrasound Obstet Gynecol 28: 761–767.

17. Bernstein L, Depue RH, Ross RK, Judd HL, Pike MC, et al. (1986) Higher maternal levels of free estradiol in first compared to second pregnancy: early gestational differences. J Natl Cancer Inst 76: 1035–1039.

18. Stroup DF, Berlin JA, Morton SC, Olkin I, Williamson GD, et al. (2000) Meta-analysis of observational studies in epidemiology: a proposal for reporting. Meta-analysis Of Observational Studies in Epidemiology (MOOSE) group. JAMA 283: 2008–2012.

19. Baird JT Jr., Quinlivan LG (1972) Parity and hypertension. Vital Health Stat 11: 1–28.

20. Wells GA, Shea B, O'Connell D, Peterson J, Welch V, et al. (2013) The Newcastle-Ottawa Scale (NOS) for assessing the quality of nonrandomized studies in meta-analyses.comparison. Available: http://wwwohrica/programs/clinical_epidemiology/oxfordasp Accessed May 3, 2013.

21. Hamling J, Lee P, Weitkunat R, Ambuhl M (2008) Facilitating meta-analyses by deriving relative effect and precision estimates for alternative comparisons from a set of estimates presented by exposure level or disease category. Stat Med 27: 954–970.

22. Greenland S, Longnecker MP (1992) Methods for trend estimation from summarized dose-response data, with applications to meta-analysis. Am J Epidemiol 135: 1301–1309.

23. Orsini N, Li R, Wolk A, Khudyakov P, Spiegelman D (2012) Meta-analysis for linear and nonlinear dose-response relations: examples, an evaluation of approximations, and software. Am J Epidemiol 175: 66–73.

24. Higgins JP, Thompson SG, Deeks JJ, Altman DG (2003) Measuring inconsistency in meta-analyses. BMJ 327: 557–560.

25. Woolf B (1955) On estimating the relation between blood group and disease. Ann Hum Genet 19: 251–253.

26. Egger M, Davey Smith G, Schneider M, Minder C (1997) Bias in meta-analysis detected by a simple, graphical test. BMJ 315: 629–634.

27. Begg CB, Mazumdar M (1994) Operating characteristics of a rank correlation test for publication bias. Biometrics 50: 1088–1101.

28. Adams MM, Mulinare J, Dooley K (1989) Risk factors for conotruncal cardiac defects in Atlanta. J Am Coll Cardiol 14: 432–442.

29. Alverson CJ, Strickland MJ, Gilboa SM, Correa A (2011) Maternal smoking and congenital heart defects in the Baltimore-Washington Infant Study. Pediatrics 127: e647–653.

30. Batra M, Heike CL, Phillips RC, Weiss NS (2007) Geographic and occupational risk factors for ventricular septal defects: Washington State, 1987–2003. Arch Pediatr Adolesc Med 161: 89–95.

31. Cedergren MI, Selbing AJ, Kallen BA (2002) Risk factors for cardiovascular malformation–a study based on prospectively collected data. Scand J Work Environ Health 28: 12–17.

32. Duong HT, Hoyt AT, Carmichael SL, Gilboa SM, Canfield MA, et al. (2012) Is maternal parity an independent risk factor for birth defects? Birth Defects Res A Clin Mol Teratol 94: 230–236.

33. Long J, Ramadhani T, Mitchell LE (2010) Epidemiology of nonsyndromic conotruncal heart defects in Texas, 1999–2004. Birth Defects Res A Clin Mol Teratol 88: 971–979.

34. Luo YL, Cheng YL, Gao XH, Tan SQ, Li JM, et al. (2013) Maternal age, parity and isolated birth defects: a population-based case-control study in Shenzhen, China. PLoS One 8: e81369.

35. Malik S, Cleves MA, Honein MA, Romitti PA, Botto LD, et al. (2008) Maternal smoking and congenital heart defects. Pediatrics 121: e810–816.

36. Padula AM, Tager IB, Carmichael SL, Hammond SK, Yang W, et al. (2013) Ambient air pollution and traffic exposures and congenital heart defects in the San Joaquin Valley of California. Paediatr Perinat Epidemiol 27: 329–339.

37. Smedts HP, van Uitert EM, Valkenburg O, Laven JS, Eijkemans MJ, et al. (2012) A derangement of the maternal lipid profile is associated with an elevated risk of congenital heart disease in the offspring. Nutr Metab Cardiovasc Dis 22: 477–485.

38. Stoll C, Alembik Y, Roth MP, Dott B, De Geeter B (1989) Risk factors in congenital heart disease. Eur J Epidemiol 5: 382–391.

39. Torfs CP, Christianson RE (1999) Maternal risk factors and major associated defects in infants with Down syndrome. Epidemiology 10: 264–270.

40. Vereczkey A, Kosa Z, Csaky-Szunyogh M, Urban R, Czeizel AE (2012) Birth outcomes of cases with left-sided obstructive defects of the heart in the function of maternal socio-demographic factors: a population-based case-control study. J Matern Fetal Neonatal Med 25: 2536–2541.

41. Vereczkey A, Kosa Z, Csaky-Szunyogh M, Czeizel AE (2013) Isolated atrioventricular canal defects: birth outcomes and risk factors: a population-based Hungarian case-control study, 1980–1996. Birth Defects Res A Clin Mol Teratol 97: 217–224.

42. Cedergren MI, Kallen BA (2006) Obstetric outcome of 6346 pregnancies with infants affected by congenital heart defects. Eur J Obstet Gynecol Reprod Biol 125: 211–216.

43. Langlois PH, Scheuerle A, Horel SA, Carozza SE (2009) Urban versus rural residence and occurrence of septal heart defects in Texas. Birth Defects Res A Clin Mol Teratol 85: 764–772.

44. Liu S, Joseph KS, Lisonkova S, Rouleau J, Van den Hof M, et al. (2013) Association between maternal chronic conditions and congenital heart defects: a population-based cohort study. Circulation 128: 583–589.

45. Brentlinger PE (2001) Folic acid antagonists during pregnancy and risk of birth defects. N Engl J Med 344: 933–934; author reply 934–935.

46. Rosenquist TH, Ratashak SA, Selhub J (1996) Homocysteine induces congenital defects of the heart and neural tube: effect of folic acid. Proc Natl Acad Sci U S A 93: 15227–15232.

47. Czeizel AE, Dudas I, Vereczkey A, Banhidy F (2013) Folate deficiency and folic acid supplementation: the prevention of neural-tube defects and congenital heart defects. Nutrients 5: 4760–4775.

48. Grisaru-Granovsky S, Gordon ES, Haklai Z, Samueloff A, Schimmel MM (2009) Effect of interpregnancy interval on adverse perinatal outcomes–a national study. Contraception 80: 512–518.

49. Gibson S, Lewis KC (1952) Congenital heart disease following maternal rubella during pregnancy. AMA Am J Dis Child 83: 317–319.

50. Stuckey D (1956) Congenital heart defects following maternal rubella during pregnancy. Br Heart J 18: 519–522.

Permissions

All chapters in this book were first published in PLOS ONE, by The Public Library of Science; hereby published with permission under the Creative Commons Attribution License or equivalent. Every chapter published in this book has been scrutinized by our experts. Their significance has been extensively debated. The topics covered herein carry significant findings which will fuel the growth of the discipline. They may even be implemented as practical applications or may be referred to as a beginning point for another development.

The contributors of this book come from diverse backgrounds, making this book a truly international effort. This book will bring forth new frontiers with its revolutionizing research information and detailed analysis of the nascent developments around the world.

We would like to thank all the contributing authors for lending their expertise to make the book truly unique. They have played a crucial role in the development of this book. Without their invaluable contributions this book wouldn't have been possible. They have made vital efforts to compile up to date information on the varied aspects of this subject to make this book a valuable addition to the collection of many professionals and students.

This book was conceptualized with the vision of imparting up-to-date information and advanced data in this field. To ensure the same, a matchless editorial board was set up. Every individual on the board went through rigorous rounds of assessment to prove their worth. After which they invested a large part of their time researching and compiling the most relevant data for our readers.

The editorial board has been involved in producing this book since its inception. They have spent rigorous hours researching and exploring the diverse topics which have resulted in the successful publishing of this book. They have passed on their knowledge of decades through this book. To expedite this challenging task, the publisher supported the team at every step. A small team of assistant editors was also appointed to further simplify the editing procedure and attain best results for the readers.

Apart from the editorial board, the designing team has also invested a significant amount of their time in understanding the subject and creating the most relevant covers. They scrutinized every image to scout for the most suitable representation of the subject and create an appropriate cover for the book.

The publishing team has been an ardent support to the editorial, designing and production team. Their endless efforts to recruit the best for this project, has resulted in the accomplishment of this book. They are a veteran in the field of academics and their pool of knowledge is as vast as their experience in printing. Their expertise and guidance has proved useful at every step. Their uncompromising quality standards have made this book an exceptional effort. Their encouragement from time to time has been an inspiration for everyone.

The publisher and the editorial board hope that this book will prove to be a valuable piece of knowledge for researchers, students, practitioners and scholars across the globe.

List of Contributors

Yan Liu, Qiaolian Wen, Xiaomei Zhu, Xi Wang, Xu Ma and Hong Pan
Graduate School, Peking Union Medical College, Beijing, China
National Research Institute for Family Planning, Beijing, China

Fengyu Wang and Congmin Li
Henan Research Institute of Population and Family Planning, Key Laboratory of Population Defects Intervention Technology of Henan Province, Zhengzhou, China

Yuan Wu
Cardiac Surgery Department, Xiamen Heart Center, Organ Transplantation Institute of Xiamen University, Xiang'an District, Xiamen, China

Sainan Tan
Key Laboratory of Genetics and Birth Health of Hunan Province, Family Planning Institute of Hunan Province, Chang sha, China

Jing Wang
Department of Medical Genetics, School of Basic Medical Sciences, Capital Medical University, Beijing, China

Xu Ma
World Health Organization Collaborating Centre for Research in Human Reproduction, Beijing, China

Rachael Maree Hunter, Kate Brown and Kate Bull
University College London, London, United Kingdom

Mark Isaac, Alessandra Frigiola, Kate Brown and Kate Bull
Great Ormond St Hospital NHS Foundation Trust, London, United Kingdom

David Blundell
Leeds School of Medicine, Leeds, United Kingdom

Fernando A. Poletta, Jorge S. López Camelo, Juan A. Gili and Eduardo E. Castilla
ECLAMC (Estudio Colaborativo Latinoamericano de Malformaciones Congénitas) at Centro de Educación Médica e Investigaciones Clínicas (CEMIC) (CONICET), Buenos Aires, Argentina

Jorge S. López Camelo
ECLAMC at Instituto Multidisciplinario de Biología Celular (IMBICE) (CIC-CONICET), La Plata, Argentina

Emmanuele Leoncini and Pierpaolo Mastroiacovo
Headquarters of the International Clearinghouse for Birth Defects Surveillance and Research, Rome, Italy

Eduardo E. Castilla
ECLAMC at Instituto Oswaldo Cruz, Rio de Janeiro, Brazil

Fernando A. Poletta, Jorge S. López Camelo and Eduardo E. Castilla
INAGEMP (Instituto Nacional de Genética Médica Populacional), Rio de Janeiro, Brazil

Dandan Wu, Yang Chen, Chen Xu and Guomin Wang
Department of Oral & Cranio-maxillofacial Science, Shanghai 9th People's Hospital, College of Stomatology, School of Medicine, Shanghai Jiao Tong University, Shanghai Key Laboratory of Stomatology, Shanghai, P. R. China

Ke Wang
Department of Oral and Maxillofacial Surgery, The Affiliated Hospital, Medical School, Qingdao University, Qingdao, P. R. China

Huijun Wang and Duan Ma
Children's Hospital, Fudan University, Shanghai, P. R. China

Fengyun Zheng and Duan Ma
Key Laboratory of Molecular Medicine, Ministry of Education, Department of Biochemistry and Molecular Biology, Institute of Medical Sciences, Shanghai Medical College, Fudan University, Shanghai, P. R. China

Christoph Gerhardt, Johanna M. Lier, Stefanie Kuschel and Ulrich Rüther
Institute for Animal Developmental and Molecular Biology, Heinrich Heine University, Düsseldorf, Germany

Philip R. Buskohl
Department of Mechanical and Aerospace Engineering, Cornell University, Ithaca, New York, United States of America

Michelle L. Sun and Jonathan T. Butcher
Department of Biomedical Engineering, Cornell University, Ithaca, New York, United States of America

Robert P. Thompson
Department of Cell Biology and Regenerative Medicine, Medical University of South Carolina, Charleston, South Carolina, United States of America

Erli Wang, Shuhua Xu and Li Jin
Chinese Academy of Sciences Key Laboratory of Computational Biology, Chinese Academy of Sciences and Max Planck Society (CAS-MPG) Partner Institute for Computational Biology, Shanghai Institutes for Biological Sciences, Chinese Academy of Sciences, Shanghai, China

Erli Wang, Yufang Zheng, Zhixi Su, Xun Gu, Li Jin and Hongyan Wang
The State Key Laboratory of Genetic Engineering and MOE Key Laboratory of Contemporary Anthropology, School of Life Sciences, Fudan University, Shanghai, China

Shuna Sun, Guoying Huang and Yu An
Children's Hospital of Fudan University, Shanghai, China

Bin Qiao and Wenyuan Duan
Institute of Cardiovascular Disease General Hospital of Jinan Military Region, Jinan, China

Yu An and Hongyan Wang
The Institutes of Biomedical Sciences, Fudan University, Shanghai, China

Tao Zhang, Eldhose B. Thekkethottiyil and Jason Z. Stoller
Division of Neonatology, Department of Pediatrics, Perelman School of Medicine at the University of Pennsylvania, Children's Hospital of Philadelphia, Philadelphia,Pennsylvania, United States of America

Junchen Liu and Fen Wang
Center for Cancer and Stem Cell Biology, Institute of Biosciences and Technology, Texas A & M Health Science Center, Houston, Texas, United States of America

Jue Zhang
Morgridge Institute for Research, Madison, Wisconsin, United States of America

Timothy L. Macatee
Department of Pathology and Laboratory Medicine, Perelman School of Medicine at the University of Pennsylvania, Philadelphia, Pennsylvania, United States of America

Fraz A. Ismat
Division of Cardiology, Department of Pediatrics, Perelman School of Medicine at the University of Pennsylvania, Children's Hospital of Philadelphia, Philadelphia, Pennsylvania, United States of America

Vikas Bansal, Cornelia Dorn, Marcel Grunert and Silke R. Sperling
Department of Cardiovascular Genetics, Experimental and Clinical Research Center, Charité - Universitätsmedizin Berlin and Max Delbrück Center (MDC) for Molecular Medicine, Berlin, Germany

Vikas Bansal
Department of Mathematics and Computer Science, Free University of Berlin, Berlin, Germany

Cornelia Dorn and Silke R. Sperling
Department of Biology, Chemistry, and Pharmacy, Free University of Berlin, Berlin, Germany

Sabine Klaassen
For the National Register for Congenital Heart Defects, Berlin, Germany
Experimental and Clinical Research Center, Charité - Universitätsmedizin Berlin and Max Delbrü ck Center (MDC) for Molecular Medicine, Berlin, Germany

Sabine Klaassen and Felix Berger
Department of Pediatric Cardiology, Charité - Universitätsmedizin Berlin, Berlin, Germanys

Roland Hetzer
Department of Cardiac Surgery, German Heart Institute Berlin, Berlin, Germany

Felix Berger
Department of Pediatric Cardiology, German Heart Institute Berlin, Berlin, Germany

Zahi Abdul-Sater, Amin Yehya, Jean Beresian, Elie Salem, Amina Kamar, Serine Baydoun, Kamel Shibbani, Ayman Soubra and Georges Nemer
Department of Biochemistry and Molecular Genetics, American University of Beirut, Beirut, Lebanon

Fadi Bitar
Department of Pediatrics and Adolescent Medicine, American University of Beirut, Beirut, Lebanon

Penny S. Thomas, Somyoth Sridurongrit and Vesa Kaartinen
Department of Biologic and Materials Sciences, University of Michigan, Ann Arbor, Michigan, United States of America

Pilar Ruiz-Lozano
Department of Pediatrics, Stanford University School of Medicine, Stanford, California, United States of America

Douglas C. Bittel, Nataliya Kibiryeva, James E. O'Brien Jr. and Jennifer Marshall
The Ward Family Heart Center, Children's Mercy Hospitals and Clinics and University of Missouri-Kansas City School of Medicine, Kansas City, Missouri, United States of America

Xin-Gang Zhou and Hong-Yu Liu
Section of Cardiovascular Surgery, The First Affiliated Hospital of Harbin Medical University, Harbin, China

Stephanie Fiedler
Department of Pathology, Children's Mercy Hospitals and Clinics and University of Missouri-Kansas City School of Medicine, Kansas City, Missouri, United States of America

Shihui Yu
Department of Laboratory Medicine and Pathology, Seattle Children's Hospital and Department of Laboratory Medicine, University of Washington School of Medicine, Seattle, Washington, United States of America

Klaartje van Engelen and Barbara J. M. Mulder
Department of Cardiology, Academic Medical Center, Amsterdam, The Netherlands

Klaartje van Engelen and Marieke J. H. Baars
Department of Clinical Genetics, Academic Medical Center, Amsterdam, The Netherlands

Klaartje van Engelen and Barbara J. M. Mulder
Interuniversity Cardiology Institute of The Netherlands (ICIN), Utrecht, The Netherlands

Mathilda T. M. Mommersteeg, Aho Ilgun, Vincent M. Christoffels and Alcx V. Postma
Heart Failure Research Centre, Department of Anatomy and Embryology, Academic Medical Center, Amsterdam, The Netherlands

Jan Lam
Department of Pediatric Cardiology, Academic Medical Center, Amsterdam, The Netherlands,

A. S. Paul van Trotsenburg
Department of Pediatric Endocrinology, Academic Medical Center, Amsterdam, The Netherlands

Anne M. J. B. Smets
Department of Radiology, Academic Medical Center, Amsterdam, The Netherlands

Clara Serra-Juhé, Ivon Cuscó and Luis A. Pérez-Jurado
Unitat de Genètica, Universitat Pompeu Fabra, Barcelona, Spain

Clara Serra-Juhé and Ivon Cuscó
Centro de Investigación Biomédica en Red de Enfermedades Raras (CIBERER), Barcelona, Spain

Benjamín Rodríguez-Santiago
Quantitative Genomic Medicine Laboratories (qGenomics), Barcelona, Spain

Teresa Vendrell
Programa de Medicina Molecular i Genetica, Hospital Barcelona, Spain

Núria Camats and Núria Torán
Servei d'Anatomia Patologica, Hospital Universitari Vall d'Hebron, Barcelona, Spain

Minjuan Zheng, Micheal Schaal, Xiaokui Li, Weihui Shentu, Pengyuan Zhang, Muhammad Ashraf and David J. Sahn
Pediatric Cardiology, Oregon Health and Science University, Portland, Oregon, United States of America

Minjuan Zheng
Department of Ultrasound, Xijing Hospital/Fourth Military Medical University, Xi'an, China

Yan Chen
Department of Oncology, Xijing Hospital/Fourth Military Medical University, Xi'an, China

Shuping Ge
Section of Cardiology, St. Christopher's Hospital for Children/Drexel University College of Medicine, Philadelphia, Pennsylvania, United States of America

Chiann-mun Chen, Jamie Bentham, Catherine Cosgrove, Jose Braganca, Simon D. Bamforth, Jürgen E. Schneider, Hugh Watkins and Shoumo Bhattacharya
Department of Cardiovascular Medicine, Wellcome Trust Centre for Human Genetics, University of Oxford, Oxford, United Kingdom

Chiann-mun Chen, Jamie Bentham, Catherine Cosgrove, Jose Braganca, Simon D. Bamforth, Jürgen E. Schneider, Hugh Watkins, Benjamin Davies and Shoumo Bhattacharya
Wellcome Trust Centre for Human Genetics, University of Oxford, Oxford, United Kingdom

Simon D. Bamforth and Bernard Keavney
Institute of Genetic Medicine, Newcastle University, Newcastle, United Kingdom

Ana Cuenda
Centro Nacional de Biotecnología, CSIC, Madrid, Spain

Emilie A. Bard-Chapeau, Belinda Q. L. Chua, Jerrold M. Ward, Sayadi Ahmed, Nancy A. Jenkins and Neal G. Copeland
Institute of Molecular and Cell Biology, Singapore, Singapore

Dorota Szumska and Shoumo Bhattacharya
Welcome Trust Centre for Human Genetics, Oxford, United Kingdom

Bindya Jacob and Motomi Osato
Cancer Science Institute, Singapore, Singapore

Gouri C. Chatterjee
MYSM School of Medicine, Yale University School of Medicine, New Haven, Connecticut, United States of America

Yi Zhang and Archibald S. Perkins
Department of Pathology and Laboratory Medicine, University of Rochester Medical Center, Rochester, New York, United States of America

Fatma Urun, Emi Kinameri and Adrian W. Moore
RIKEN Brain Science Institute, 2-1 Hirosawa, Wako-shi, Saitama, Japan

Stéphane D. Vincent
Department of Development and Stem Cells, Institut de Génétique et de Biologie Moléculaire et Cellulaire, CNRS UMR 7104, Inserm U964, Universitéde Strasbourg, Illkirch, France

Bijun Zhao and Shiqiang Yu
Department of Cardiovascular Surgery, Xijing Hospital, The Fourth Military Medical University, Xi'an, China

Yuan Lin, Kai Zhang, Jiayin Liu, Hongbing Shen and Jiahao Sha
State Key Laboratory of Reproductive Medicine, Nanjing Medical University, Nanjing, China

Yuan Lin, Bixian Ni, Kai Zhang, Hongbing Shen and Hongxia Ma
Department of Epidemiology and Biostatistics and Key Laboratory of Modern Toxicology of Ministry of Education, School of Public Health, Nanjing Medical University, Nanjing, China

Jing Xu and Xiaowei Wang
Department of Thoracic and Cardiovascular Surgery, The First Affiliated H ospital o f N anjing Medical University, Nanjing, China

Min Da, Yuanli Hu and Xuming Mo
Department of Cardiothoracic Surgery, Nanjing Children's Hospital, Nanjing Medical University, Nanjing, China

Chenyue Ding and Jiayin Liu
Center of Clinical Reproductive Medicine, First Affiliated Hospital, Nanjing Medical University, Nanjing, China

Shiwei Yang
Department of Cardiology, Nanjing Children's Hospital, Nanjing Medical University, Nanjing, China

Jiahao Sha
Department of Histology and Embryology, Nanjing Medical University, Nanjing, China

Pei Nie, Haiou Li, Yanhua Duan, Ximing Wang, Xiaopeng Ji and Zhaoping Cheng
Shandong Provincial Key Laboratory of Diagnosis and Treatment of Cardio-Cerebral Vascular Diseases, Shandong Medical Imaging Research Institute, Shandong University, Jinan, Shandong, China

Anbiao Wang
Department of Cardiovascular Surgery, Shandong Provincial Hospital, Jinan, Shandong, China

Jiuhong Chen
CT Research Collaboration, Siemens Ltd. China, Beijing, China

Xia Deng, Fei-Feng Li, Er-Ying Zhao and Shu-Lin Liu
Genomics Research Center (one of the State-Province Key Laboratory of Biopharmaceutical Engineering, China), Harbin Medical University, Harbin, China

Jing Zhou and Kai-Jiang Yu
Intensive Care Unit, the Second Affiliated Hospital of Harbin Medical University, Harbin, China

Peng Yan
Department of Colorectal Surgery, the Second Affiliated Hospital of Harbin Medical University, Harbin, China

Ling Hao
Department of Oncology, the Fourth Affiliated Hospital of Harbin Medical University, Harbin, China

Shu-Lin Liu
Department of Microbiology and Infectious Diseases, University of Calgary, Calgary, Canada

Rachel L. Knowles, Angela Wade, Harvey Goldstein and Carol Dezateux
Population Policy and Practice Programme, Institute of Child Health, University College London, London, United Kingdom

Catherine Bull
Cardiac Unit, Great Ormond Street Hospital for Children NHS Trust, London, United Kingdom

Christopher Wren
Department of Paediatric Cardiology, Freeman Hospital, Newcastle-upon-Tyne, United Kingdom

Bin Lin, Yufeng Wang, Yang Shu, Yuchao Zhang, Yun Huang, Yufei Zhu, Heng Xu, Zhiqiang Wang, Ping Wang, Xiangyin Kong, Guohong Hu and Landian Hu
The Key Laboratory of Stem Cell Biology, Institute of Health Sciences, Shanghai Jiao Tong University School of Medicine (SJTUSM) and Shanghai Institutes for Biological
Sciences (SIBS), Chinese Academy of Sciences (CAS), Shanghai, People's Republic of China

Zhen Wang and Huilian Tan
Diagnosis and Treatment Center of Congenital Heart Disease, the First Hospital of Hebei Medical University, Shijiazhuang, Hebei, People's Republic of China

Xianghua Kong
Clinical Laboratory, Affiliated Hospital of Binzhou Medical College, Binzhou, Shandong, People's Republic of China

Guang Ning, Xiangyin Kong and Landian Hu
State Key Laboratory of Medical Genomics, Ruijin Hospital Affiliated to Shanghai Jiao Tong University School of Medicine, Shanghai, People's Republic of China

Yu Feng, Di Yu, Lei Yang, Min Da, Changfeng Fan, Song Wang and Xuming Mo
Department of Cardiothoracic Surgery, The Affiliated Children's Hospital of Nanjing Medical University, Nanjing, Jiangsu, China

Tao Chen and Jin Liu
Department of Epidemiology and Biostatistics, School of Public Health, Nanjing Medical University, Nanjing, Jiangsu, China

Xing Tong
Atherosclerosis Research Center, Key Laboratory of Cardiovascular Disease and Molecular Intervention, Nanjing Medical University, Nanjing, Jiangsu, China

Shutong Shen
Department of Cardiology, The First Affiliated Hospital of Nanjing Medical University, Nanjing, Jiangsu, China

Index

www.ingramcontent.com/pod-product-compliance
Lightning Source LLC
Chambersburg PA
CBHW080411190526
45161CB00003B/202